labyrinth, maze: bony labyrinth
lacri-, tears: lacrimal gland
lacun-, pool: lacuna
lamell-, layer: lamella
lanug-, fine hair: lanugo
-lemm, rind or peel: neurolemma
leuko-, white: leukocyte
lingu-, tongue: lingual tonsil
-logy, study of: physiology
lord-, bent back: lordosis
lun-, moon: semilunar valve
lut-, yellow: macula lutea
lys-, to break up: lysosome
macro-, large: macrophage
macula, spot: macula lutea
malle-, hammer: malleus
mamm-, breast: mammary gland
man-, hand: manubrium
mandib-, jaw: mandible
mast-, breast: mastitis
maxill, jawbone: maxillary bone
meat-, passage: auditory meatus
medull-, in the middle: adrenal
  medulla
melan-, black: melanin
mening-, membrane: meninges
ment-, chin: mental foramen
meso-, middle: mesoderm
micr-, small: microfilament
mid-, middle: midbrain
milli-, one-thousandth: millimeter
mit-, thread: mitosis
mono-, one: monozygotic
mons-, an eminence: mons pubis
moto-, moving: motor neuron
multi-, many: multipolar neuron
myo-, muscle: myofibril
nas-, nose: nasal
nat-, to be born: prenatal
neo-, new: neonatal period
nephr-, pertaining to the kidney:
  nephron
neuro-, nerve: neuron
nod-, knot: nodule
nucle-, kernal: nucleus
occipit-, back of head: occipital lobe
oculi-, eye: orbicularis oculi
odont-, tooth: odontoid process

-oid, a thing like: odontoid process
olfact-, to smell: olfactory
oligo-, few: oligodendrocyte
oo-, egg: oogenesis
or-, mouth: oral cavity
orb-, circle: orbital
osseo-, bone: osseous tissue
-ous, having qualities of: cancerous
ov-, egglike: synovial fluid
palpebra-, eyelid: levator palpebrae
  superioris
papill-, nipple: papillary muscle
para-, beside: parathyroid glands
pariet-, wall: parietal membrane
patho-, disease: pathogen
pelv-, basin: pelvic cavity
peri-, around: pericardial membrane
pept-, digestive: peptic ulcer
phleb-, vein: phlebitis
phot-, light: photoreceptor
phren-, diaphragm: phrenic nerve
pia-, delicate: pia mater
pleur-, rib: pleural membrane
plex-, interweaving: choroid plexus
plic-, to fold: plicae circularis
poie-, making: hematopoesis
popl-, knee: popliteal artery
por-, channel: pore
post-, after: postnatal period
pre-, before: prepatellar bursa
prim-, first: primordial follicle
pro-, before: prophase
prox-, nearest: proximal
pseudo-, false: pseudostratified
  epithelium
pter-, wing: pterygoid process
pulm-, lung: pulmonary artery
pylor-, gatekeeper: pyloric sphincter
quadri-, four: quadriceps femoris
ram-, branch: gray ramus
rect-, straight: rectum
ren-, kidney: renal cortex
rete-, net: rete testis
reticul-, net: sarcoplasmic reticulum
rhin-, nose: rhinitis
scler-, hard: sclera
seb-, grease: sebaceous gland
sect-, to cut: section

sella-, saddle: sella turcica
semi-, one-half: semitendinosus
sens-, feeling: sensory neuron
sin-, hollow: sinus
-som, body: ribosome
-sorpt-, to soak up: absorption
squam-, scale: squamous epithelium
stria-, groove: striated muscle
sulc-, furrow: sulcus
super-, above: superior
supra-, above: supraspinatus muscle
sutur-, sewing: suture
syn-, together: synthesis
syndesm-, binding together: syndesmosis
systol-, contraction: systole
tal-, ankle: talus
therm-, heat: thermoreceptor
thalam-, chamber: thalamus
theo-, sheath: theca externa
thyr-, shield: thyroid gland
-tomy, cutting: anatomy
trans-, across: transverse
tri-, three: tricuspid valve
trigon-, triangular shape: trigone
-troph, well fed: hypertrophy
tuber-, swelling: tuberculosis
tympano-, drum: tympanic membrane
umbil-, navel: umbilical cord
uni-, one: unipolar neuron
uter-, womb: uterine tube
vag-, to wander: vagus nerve
vas-, vessel: vasa recta
vesic-, blister: vesicle
vill-, hair: villus
visc-, internal organs: viscera
vitre-, glass: vitreous humor
voluntar-, of one's free will: voluntary
  muscle
xiph-, sword: xiphoid process
zon-, belt: zona pellucida

H U M A N

ANATOMY

A personal library is a lifelong source of enrichment and distinction. Consider this book an investment in your future, and add it to your personal library.

HUMAN
ANATOMY
SECOND EDITION

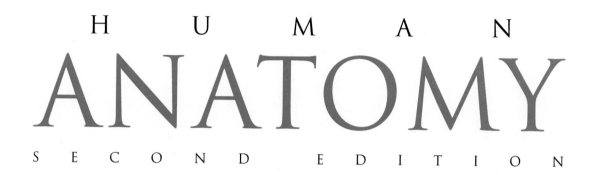

JOHN W. HOLE, JR.

KAREN A. KOOS
Rio Hondo College

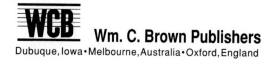

WCB Wm. C. Brown Publishers

Dubuque, Iowa•Melbourne, Australia•Oxford, England

Book Team

Editor *Colin Wheatley*
Developmental Editor *Jane DeShaw*
Production Editor *Kennie Harris*
Designer *Eric Engelby*
Art Editor *Mary E. Powers*
Photo Editor *Diane S. Saeugling*
Permissions Coordinator *Gail I. Wheatley*
Art Processor *Amy L. Ley*
Visuals/Design Developmental Consultant *Donna Slade*

Wm. C. Brown Publishers
A Division of Wm. C. Brown Communications, Inc.

Vice President and General Manager *Beverly Kolz*
Vice President, Publisher *Kevin Kane*
Vice President, Director of Sales and Marketing *Virginia S. Moffat*
Marketing Manager *Christopher T. Johnson*
Advertising Manager *Janelle Keeffer*
Director of Production *Colleen A. Yonda*
Publishing Services Manager *Karen J. Slaght*

Wm. C. Brown Communications, Inc.

President and Chief Executive Officer *G. Franklin Lewis*
Corporate Vice President, President of WCB Manufacturing *Roger Meyer*
Vice President and Chief Financial Officer *Robert Chesterman*

Cover photo © Dave Siegel/Siegel Photographic

Copyedited by Sarah Aldridge

The credits section for this book begins on page 647 and is
considered an extension of the copyright page.

A Times Mirror Company

Library of Congress Catalog Card Number: 92–75379

ISBN 0–697–12252–2

Printed in the United States of America by Wm. C. Brown Communications, Inc.,
2460 Kerper Boulevard, Dubuque, IA 52001

10   9   8   7   6   5   4   3   2   1

*To the memory of Ed Jaffe,
editor and friend, who provided
the inspiration for this book.*

BRIEF
CONTENTS

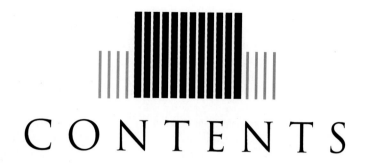

CONTENTS

UNIT 1

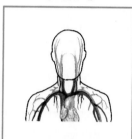

Levels of Organization 1

1
An Introduction to Human Anatomy 2

2
Body Organization and Terminology 27

UNIT 2

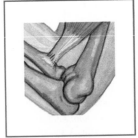

Support and Movement 119

6
The Skeletal System 120

7
Joints of the Skeletal System 188

8
The Muscular System 213

Contents   ix

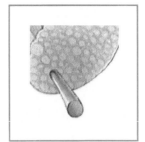

Integration and Coordination 263

UNIT 4

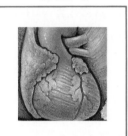

Processing and Transporting 383

12

The Digestive System 384

13

The Respiratory System 419

14

The Cardiovascular System 447

15
The Lymphatic System 498

16
The Urinary System 518

UNIT 5

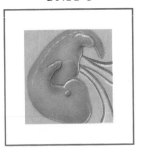

The Human Life Cycle 539

17
The Reproductive Systems 540

18

Human Growth and Development 570

REFERENCE PLATES

PREFACE

Human Anatomy, second edition, was prepared to provide a comprehensive introduction to the study of human body structure in an interesting and easily readable manner. It is especially designed for students pursuing careers in allied health fields, who have minimal backgrounds in the biological sciences and who need to understand the basic principles of human anatomy.

Human Anatomy takes a systematic approach to the study of the human body. Each chapter presents in detail the structure of certain body parts and describes more briefly the relationship between the structure and functions of these parts, clinical implications, and ways in which anatomic features vary normally from individual to individual.

Organization

The textbook is organized into units, each containing several chapters. These chapters are arranged traditionally, beginning with a discussion of basic terminology and proceeding through levels of increasing complexity.

Unit 1 introduces the human body and its major parts. It is also concerned with anatomic terminology and the structure of cells and tissues. It presents membranes as organs and the integumentary system as an organ system. Unit 2 concerns the parts of the skeletal and muscular systems; unit 3 deals with the organization of the nervous and endocrine systems; unit 4 discusses the structures of the digestive, respiratory, circulatory, lymphatic, and urinary systems; unit 5 describes the reproductive systems as well as growth and development of human offspring.

Terminology
The importance of anatomic terminology is emphasized throughout the book. Basic terms appear in boldface or italic type, and the phonetic pronunciation of many anatomic words has been included within the narratives of certain chapters as those terms are introduced.

Illustration Program
In recognition of the visual nature of human anatomy, the chapters are richly illustrated with line drawings, medical illustrations, photographs, X rays, and a variety of scanning and transmission electron micrographs. In addition, sets of reference plates are positioned between selected chapters. These include drawings of the human torso with various layers of organs exposed, photographs of the human skull with special features identified, photographs of human dissection, photographs of models with their surface features labeled, photographs of human brains sectioned in various planes, and drawings of the development of various organs. These illustrations will help the reader visualize anatomic structures macroscopically, as well as on the histological, cytological, and ultrastructural levels of organization.

Readability
Readability is an important asset of this text. The writing style is intentionally informal and easy to read. Technical vocabulary has been minimized, and summary paragraphs and review questions occur frequently within the narrative. Numerous illustrations and summary charts are carefully positioned near the discussions they complement.

Pedagogical Devices
The text includes an unusually large number of pedagogical devices intended to increase readability and to involve students in the learning process, to stimulate their interests in the subject matter, and to help them relate their classroom knowledge to their future clinical experiences. For an annotated listing of these devices, see To the Reader, which follows this preface.

Special Features of the Second Edition

Human Anatomy has been carefully reviewed for this second edition. The chapters have been revised and updated, the illustration program has been improved, and the clinical features have been expanded. The major improvements in this edition include:

1. Many figures have been improved or replaced. Examples of new artwork can be found in chapter 4 (tissues), chapter 6 (skeleton), chapter 8 (muscles), chapter 9 (nervous system), and the reference plates following chapter 18 (development).
2. Discussions of many topics have been revised or expanded. Among these topics are transport of intracellular membranes, neuromuscular junctions, muscles of the neck, back, legs, and hands, association tracts in the brain, pathways of cranial nerves, and valves of the heart.
3. All of the clinical boxed asides have been reviewed, and more than twenty new boxed asides have been added. The topics of these asides include endoscopy, skin cancer, wound healing, osteoporosis, knee ligament tears and repair, ALS (amyotrophic lateral sclerosis), pituitary gland development, and newborn lung function.
4. More than twenty-five new clinical application of knowledge questions have been added. The answers to all of the Clinical Application of Knowledge questions have been included in Appendix B. In addition, the Review Activities portion of certain chapters has been expanded to include a short answer section (Part B).

5. New summary charts dealing with neck, back, and laryngeal muscles have been added. Also, figure references have been added to appropriate charts.

Supplementary Materials
Supplementary materials designed to help the instructor plan class work and presentations and to aid students in their learning activities are also available. They include the following:

Instructor's Resource Manual and Test Item File by John W. Hole, Jr., and Karen A. Koos, which contains chapter overviews, instructional techniques, suggested schedules, discussions of chapter elements, lists of related films, and directories of suppliers of audiovisual and laboratory materials. It also contains test items for each chapter of the text.

WCB TestPak is a computerized testing service offered free upon request to adopters of this textbook. It provides a call-in/mail-in test preparation service. A complete test item file is also available on computer diskette for use with IBM compatible, Apple IIe or IIc, or Macintosh computers.

Transparencies include a set of 150 acetate transparencies designed to complement classroom lectures or to be used for short quizzes.

Color slides include a set of 72 micrographs of tissues, organs, and other body features described in the textbook to complement classroom instruction.

Laboratory Manual to Accompany Human Anatomy by John W. Hole, Jr., and Karen A. Koos is designed specifically to accompany *Human Anatomy*.

Dissection Video demonstrates for students the procurement, maintenance, and utilization of cadavers, as well as prosection of abdominal and thoracic cavities, and arm and leg extremities. The video was prepared by Terry Martin and Hassan Rastegar of Kishwaukee College.

Extended Lecture Outline Software consists of detailed outlines of each chapter on disk. Instructors can add their own lecture notes for convenience in lecture preparation. Available for use with IBM, Apple, or Macintosh.

Also available from WCB . . .
• Study Cards for Human Anatomy and Physiology by Van De Graaff/Rhees/Creek
• *The Coloring Review Guide to Human Anatomy* by McMurtrie/Rikel
• *Atlas of the Skeletal Muscles* by Robert and Judith Stone
• The WCB Anatomy and Physiology Video Series
• *Anatomy and Physiology of the Heart* videodisc
• *Computer Review of Human Anatomy and Physiology* software by Davis/Zimmerman/Van De Graaff
• *Knowledge Map of Human Anatomy Systems* software (Macintosh) by Craig Gundy of Weber State College
• *Slice of Life, Vol. V.* videodisc

TO THE READER

This textbook includes a variety of aids to the reader that should make your study of human anatomy more effective and enjoyable. These aids are included to help you master the basic concepts of human anatomy that are needed before progressing to more difficult material.

Unit Introductions

Each unit opens with a brief description of the general content of the unit and a list of chapters included within the unit (see page 1 for an example). This introduction provides an overview of the chapters that make up a unit and tells how the unit relates to the other aspects of human anatomy.

Chapter Introductions

Each chapter introduction previews the chapter's contents and relates that chapter to the others within the unit (see page 2).

After reading an introduction, browse through the chapter, paying particular attention to topic headings and illustrations so that you get a feeling for the kinds of ideas included within the chapter.

Chapter Outlines

The chapter outline includes all the major topic headings and subheadings within the body of the chapter (see page 3). It provides an overview of the chapter's contents and helps you locate sections dealing with particular topics.

Chapter Objectives

Before you begin to study a chapter, carefully read the chapter objectives (see page 3). These indicate what you should be able to do after mastering the information within the narrative. The review activities at the end of each chapter (see page 18) are phrased like detailed objectives, and it

is helpful to read them before beginning your study. Both sets of objectives are guides that indicate important sections of the narrative.

Aids to Understanding Words

The aids to understanding words section at the beginning of each chapter also helps build your vocabulary. This section includes a list of word roots, stems, prefixes, and suffixes that help you discover word meanings. Each root and an example word using that root are defined (see page 3). Knowing the roots from these lists will help you discover and remember scientific word meanings. A complete list of word roots can be found inside the front and back covers of the book.

Review Questions within the Narrative

Review questions occur at the ends of major sections within each chapter (see page 5). When you reach such questions, try to answer them. If you succeed, then you probably understand the previous discussion and are ready to proceed. If you have difficulty answering the questions, reread that section before proceeding.

Illustrations and Charts

Numerous illustrations and charts occur in each chapter and are placed near their related textual discussion. They are designed to help you visualize structures and processes, clarify complex ideas, and summarize sections of the narrative.

As mentioned earlier, it is a good idea to skim through the chapter before beginning to read it, paying particular attention to these figures. Then, as you read for detail, carefully study each figure to gain a better understanding of the material presented.

Sometimes the figure legends contain questions that will help you apply your knowledge to the object or process the figure illustrates. The ability to apply information to new situations is of prime importance. These questions will provide practice in this skill.

There are also sets of special reference figures that you may want to refer to from time to time. The first set (see pages 19–26) is designed to illustrate the structure and location of the major internal organs of the body. Other sets (see pages 179–187) will help you locate major features of the skull, human muscles, the body surface, the brain, and stages in the development of certain organs.

Boxed Information

Shaded boxes occur throughout each chapter (see page 7). These boxed asides often contain information that will help you apply the ideas presented in the narrative to clinical situations. Some boxes contain information about changes that occur in the body's structure (and its function) as a person passes through the various phases of the human life cycle. These will help you understand how certain body conditions change as a person grows older.

Clinical Applications and Normal Variations

Other, longer asides are entitled "Clinical Applications" and "Normal Variations." These discuss pathological disorders and pertinent information of more general interest.

Clinical Terms

At the ends of certain chapters are lists of related terms and phonetic pronunciations sometimes used in clinical situations (see page 175). Although these lists and the word definitions are often brief, they will be a useful addition to your understanding of medical terminology.

Chapter Summaries

A summary in outline form at the end of each chapter will help you review the major ideas presented in the narrative (see page 17). Scan this section a few days after you have read the chapter. If you find portions that seem unfamiliar, reread the related sections of the narrative.

Clinical Application of Knowledge

End-of-chapter questions dealing with clinical situations (see page 18) will help you gain experience in the critical thinking skills necessary to apply information presented in the text. You may find it useful to discuss your answers with other students or with an instructor. Answers to these questions are located in Appendix B.

Review Activities

The review activities at the end of each chapter (see page 18) will check your understanding of the major ideas presented in the narrative. After studying the chapter, read the review activities; if you can perform the tasks suggested, you have accomplished the goals of the chapter. If not, reread the sections of the narrative that need clarification.

Appendixes, Glossary, and Index

The Appendixes following chapter 18 contain: A, lists of various units of measurement and their equivalents, together with a description of how to convert one unit into another (see page 629); B, answers to Clinical Application of Knowledge questions (see page 630); C, suggestions for additional reading to help you locate library materials that can extend your understanding of topics discussed within the chapters (see page 634). If a particular idea interests you, check the list of readings for items related to it.

The Glossary defines the more important textual terms and provides their phonetic pronunciations. It also contains an explanation of phonetic pronunciation on page 636.

The Index is complete and comprehensive.

ACKNOWLEDGMENTS

We wish to express our gratitude to the reviewers for the second edition. They provided detailed criticisms and ideas for improving the manuscript. They include:

Carol S. Annibale
University of Toronto

Dianne Y. Bell
Avila College

Carolyn Williamson Burroughs
Bossier Parish Community College

Douglas Duff
Indiana University at South Bend

Larry Ganion
Ball State University

Shirley A. Gansen
Northeast Iowa Community College

Mac F. Given
Neumann College

Lyle W. Konigsberg
University of Tennessee–Knoxville

Jean E. Magney
University of Minnesota

Daniel R. Olson
Northern Illinois University

Carlos F. A. Pinkham
Norwich University

Brian R. Shmaefsky
Kingwood College

We also wish to acknowledge the contribution of Anne Lesak, R.N., M.S., M.S.N., Moraine Valley Community College. Professor Lesak helped prepare many of the answers to the Clinical Application of Knowledge questions, which appear in Appendix B.

U N I T 1
Levels of Organization

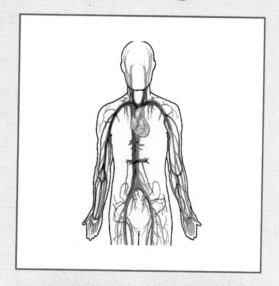

The chapters of unit 1 introduce the study of human anatomy. They are concerned with the basic methods and terminology of this branch of science, and the way the body is constructed of parts with increasing degrees of complexity.

They describe each of the levels of organization within the body—atoms, molecules, cellular organelles, cells, tissues, organs, organ systems, and the human organism—and prepare the reader for the more detailed study of the organ systems presented in units 2–5.

C H A P T E R 1

An Introduction
to Human Anatomy

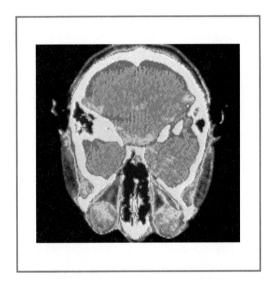

Human anatomy is the study of body structures. It includes the form and arrangement, microscopic structure, functions, and development of body parts.

Anatomists make use of a variety of tools and techniques to aid their investigations of various aspects of body structure. They have also devised a complex set of terms that help them communicate with one another and aid them in organizing information.

Chapter Outline

Introduction

Anatomy and Physiology

Types of Anatomy
    Gross Anatomy
    Microscopic Anatomy
    Developmental Anatomy

Methods of Anatomy
    Microscopy
    Radiography
    Tomography
    Ultrasonography
    Scintigraphy
    Magnetic Resonance Imaging

Language of Anatomy
    Origin of Terms
    Problems of Nomenclature

Chapter Objectives

After you have studied this chapter, you should be able to

1. Distinguish between anatomy and physiology.

2. Explain why the topics of anatomy and physiology are closely related.

3. List three types of anatomy and explain how each type can be further subdivided.

4. List four types of microscopes and describe the qualities of images produced by each.

5. List five noninvasive procedures used to study internal body parts and explain how an image is produced by each.

6. Explain why Latin was used as the basis for anatomic nomenclature.

7. Describe how anatomic structures are named.

8. Define *Nomina Anatomica* and explain its importance.

9. Complete the review activities at the end of this chapter. Note that the items are worded in the form of specific learning objectives. You may want to refer to them before reading the chapter.

Aids to Understanding Words

ana-, apart: *ana*tomy—study of structure that often involves cutting structures apart.

cyt-, cell: *cyt*ology—study of cells.

endo-, within: *endo*scope-device used to observe the interior of an organ or cavity.

-graph, written: radio*graph*y—making of X-ray pictures.

hist-, fabric: *hist*ology—study of tissues, which are composed of groups or layers of cells.

-logy, the study of: physio*logy*—study of body functions.

macro-, large: *macro*scopic—large enough to be seen with the unaided eye.

micro-, small: *micro*scopic—too small to be seen with the unaided eye.

scop-, to look at: macro*scop*ic—large enough to be seen with the unaided eye.

son-, sound: ultra*son*ography—method by which high-frequency sound waves are used to visualize internal body parts.

-tomy, cutting: ana*tomy*—the study of structure that often involves cutting body structures apart.

ultra-, in excess: *ultra* sonography—method by which high-frequency sound waves are used to visualize internal body parts.

Introduction

Human anatomy is the branch of science that deals with the human body structure (morphology) and the relationships of body parts. This study has a long and interesting history, because even in ancient times people were concerned about the well-being of their bodies and their physical capabilities (figure 1.1).

At first those who were interested in examining the human body closely depended upon *dissection*—the separation of parts for the purpose of observing their characteristics and arrangement. In fact, the word anatomy originated from a Greek term that meant "to cut up," and today the words *anatomize* and *dissect* have the same meaning (figure 1.2).

Although early investigators developed a variety of tools to aid dissection, they lacked the means to magnify objects, and thus their observations were limited to relatively large structures—structures that were visible to their unaided eyes. However, following the development of lens grinding techniques and the invention of the light microscope a few hundred years ago, interest in minute body structures grew.

When the use of lenses and microscopes became more common, newly gained information concerning microscopic body parts was incorporated into the growing science of anatomy (figure 1.3). Then, as still better tools and techniques for investigating various aspects of the body were developed, human anatomy came to include facts obtained from a variety of means, some of which are described in subsequent sections of this chapter.

Anatomy and Physiology

Although anatomy began as the study of body structure, it is clear from writings of early investigators that they often speculated about the importance of various parts and wondered about their functions.

As knowledge of body functions expanded and became more and more complex, this portion of the information was separated from anatomy to become a new branch of science called **physiology**—the study of body functions.

Actually, it is difficult to separate the topics of anatomy and physiology because the structures of body parts are so closely associated with their functions. These parts are arranged to form a well-organized unit—the human

FIGURE 1.1

Study of the human body has a long history, as indicated by these illustrations from the second book of *De Humani Corporis Fabrica* by Andreas Vesalius, issued in 1543.

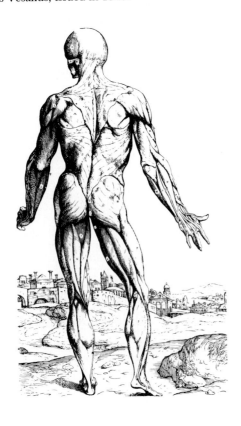
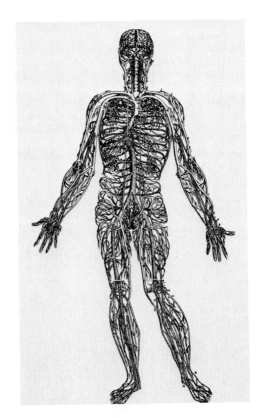

FIGURE 1.2

Early investigators depended upon cadaver dissection to observe human body parts.

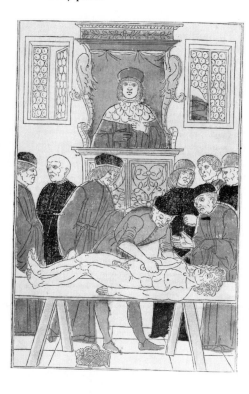

FIGURE 1.3

(a) The earliest microscopes, from the 1600s, allowed investigators to first observe cells; (b) a microscope of the type in use during the late 1800s.

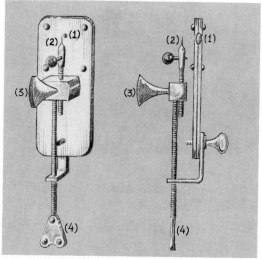

(a)

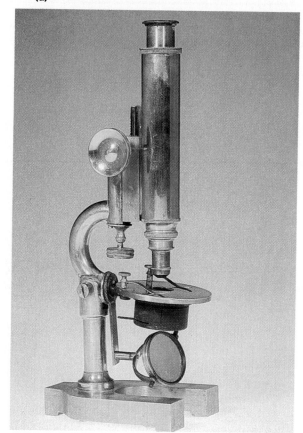

(b)

organism—and each part plays a role in the operation of the unit as a whole. This role, which is the part's function, depends upon the way the part is constructed or the way its subparts are organized. For example, the arrangement of parts in the human hand with its long, jointed fingers is related to the function of grasping objects. Blood vessels of the heart allow transport of blood to and from its hollow chambers; the heart's powerful muscular walls are structured to contract and cause blood to move out of the chambers; and the valves associated with the vessels and chambers ensure that the blood will move in a certain direction. The shape of the mouth is related to the function of receiving food; teeth act to break solids into smaller pieces; and the muscular tongue and cheeks are constructed in ways that help mix food particles with saliva and prepare it for swallowing (figure 1.4).

While reading about the human body, keep the connection between anatomy and physiology in mind. Although the relationship between structure and function is not always obvious, nevertheless it is sure to exist.

---

1. What is meant by anatomy?
2. What were the early methods used to study the human body?
3. Why is it difficult to separate the topics of anatomy and physiology?

FIGURE 1.4

The structures of body parts are closely related to their functions. (*a*) The hand is adapted for grasping; (*b*) the heart for pumping blood; and (*c*) the mouth for receiving food.

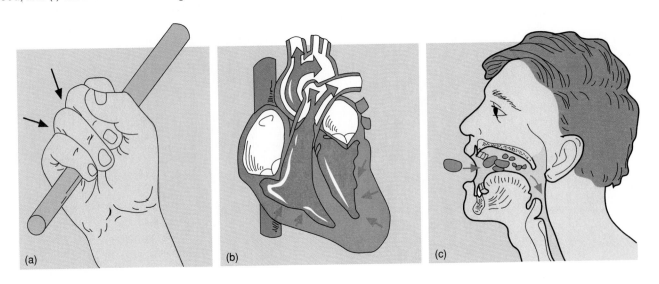

FIGURE 1.5

Some types of gross anatomy: (*a*) systematic anatomy—cardiovascular system; (*b*) regional anatomy—organs of the thorax; and (*c*) surface anatomy—palpating abdominal organs.

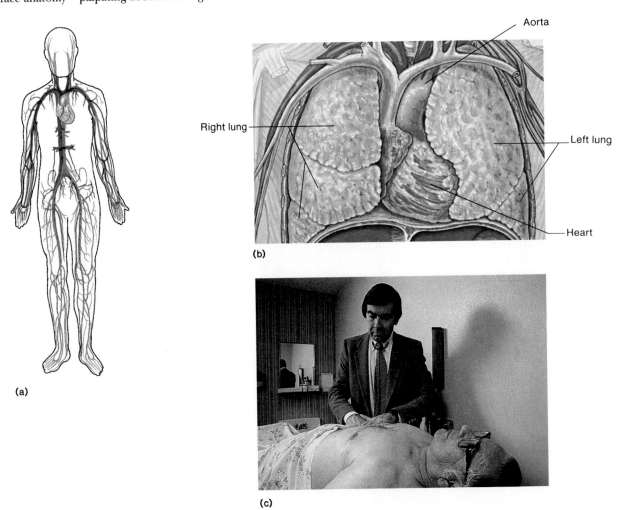

Types of Anatomy

As in the case of other major branches of science, anatomy can be subdivided into special types. These types include gross anatomy, microscopic anatomy, and developmental anatomy.

Gross Anatomy

Gross anatomy is the study of *macroscopic* body structures—those that are visible to the unaided eye or by using a hand lens. This type, of course, is the oldest of the anatomical subdivisions and depends largely upon observations made while dissecting dead human bodies or *cadavers*. Gross anatomy can be subdivided into systematic anatomy, regional anatomy, and surface anatomy (figure 1.5).

Systematic anatomy is usually studied in introductory anatomy courses. In it, body parts are organized according to their functions so that those with common functions are studied together. Systematic anatomy also provides the basis for the organization of this textbook, in which separate chapters are used to describe each of the organ systems—the skeletal system, muscular system, and nervous system, for example.

Regional anatomy is the type most commonly presented in advanced courses and professional schools. In such courses, all of the structures located in a specific body region—such as the head, neck, thorax, abdomen, pelvis, and limb—are studied together. Also, cadavers usually are dissected regionally, and regional anatomy is of special interest to physicians and surgeons who must treat injuries and diseases in particular areas of the body.

Endoscopy is a technique for directly examining the interior of body cavities and hollow organs. It differs from many other surgical techniques because it requires only a very small incision in the body wall.

The endoscope, which is a tubular device and includes a miniature camera, is inserted into the small incision and images of internal body structures appear on a viewing screen (figure 1.6). Small surgical instruments can also be inserted through such an incision and portions of body parts may be removed or repaired. For example, endoscopic surgery can be used to remove a diseased vermiform appendix, a gallbladder, or a damaged piece of cartilage from a knee joint. These devices may also be used to repair the wall of a body cavity (hernia repair).

Surface anatomy concerns the use of body features that can be observed or felt (palpated) on the surface. Such features or markings serve as aids for locating and visualizing the form and arrangement of internal parts. This type of anatomy is of particular interest to physicians who often examine their patients by palpation or feeling the contours of structures beneath the skin.

FIGURE 1.6

(*a*) Endoscopy allows a direct view of internal organs while requiring only a small incision in the body wall. (*b*) A view of the uterine tube and ovarian cyst as seen through the endoscope.

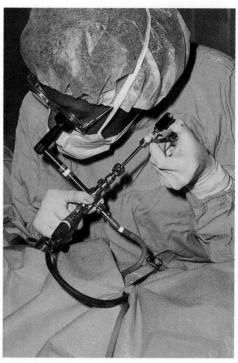

(a)

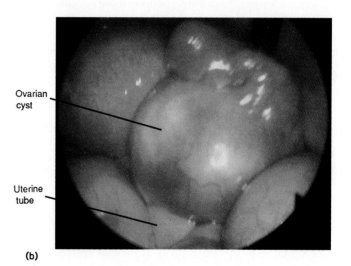

Ovarian cyst

Uterine tube

(b)

FIGURE 1.7
Cytology is the study of cells, and histology is the study of tissues.

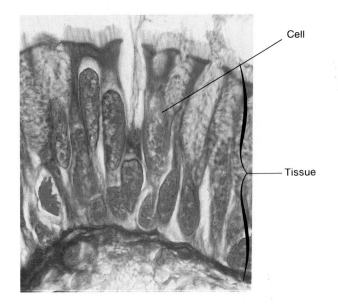

FIGURE 1.8
Developmental anatomy includes the study of growth and development before birth. These figures depict changes that occur between the fourth and seventh weeks of development.

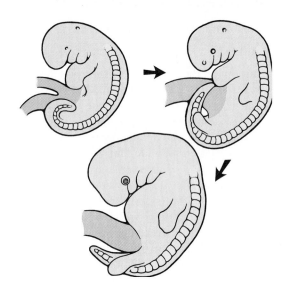

Microscopic Anatomy

Microscopic anatomy is concerned with minute body structures and requires the use of a microscope. This type of anatomy can be subdivided into cytology and histology.

Cytology is the study of cells—the basic units of structure and function of the body—and the parts of these cells (organelles). **Histology** is the study of tissues—groups or layers of similar cells—that, in turn, comprise larger parts called organs (figure 1.7).

By using an electron microscope to study very thin slices (sections) of cells, it is possible to examine the *fine structure* (ultrastructure) of cellular parts magnified many thousands of times.

Developmental Anatomy

Developmental anatomy is the study of changes that occur as the body grows and differentiates from a single cell (fertilized egg) into the adult form. It is concerned with such processes as the replacement of tissues following injuries and diseases; changes in bones and muscles resulting from use and disuse; changing rates of growth accompanying various phases of development; and the maturation of the reproductive organs occurring at puberty. Developmental anatomy also includes *embryology*, which is the study of growth and development that takes place before birth (prenatal development) (figure 1.8).

1. What is meant by gross anatomy?
2. How are systematic and regional anatomy distinguished?
3. What method is used to study the fine structure of cellular parts?
4. What studies are included in developmental anatomy?

Methods of Anatomy

As was mentioned, anatomists often use dissection to examine macroscopic body structures. They also use microscopy to investigate microscopic parts, and they use a variety of noninvasive methods (procedures that do not involve entering the body) to visualize macroscopic internal organs. Such noninvasive procedures include radiography, tomography, ultrasonography, scintigraphy, and magnetic resonance imaging. These techniques produce a variety of visual representations of internal body parts. Physicians often use such techniques in diagnosing disease conditions and in evaluating their progress.

Microscopy

Microscopy involves the use of a **microscope** to magnify small structures. Since the human eye is unable to perceive objects that have a diameter of less than 0.1 mm, a microscope is an essential tool for the study of tissues, cells, and cellular organelles.

FIGURE 1.9

(*a*) Light microscope; (*b*) dissecting microscope. How do the images from these microscopes differ?

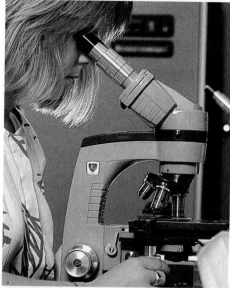

(a)

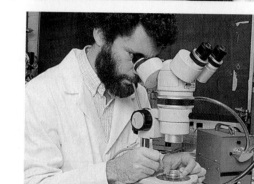

(b)

The instrument most commonly used for microscopy is the *light microscope* (compound microscope). It utilizes ordinary light to produce two-dimensional images of transparent objects that may be magnified from ten to about 1,000 times (10×–1,000×). Typically, these thin slices of objects are stained to increase the visibility of the structures.

The *dissecting microscope* (binocular-stereoscopic microscope) is a type of light microscope that is adapted to magnify surface features and opaque objects. Although a dissecting microscope achieves a relatively low magnification, it has the advantage of producing a three-dimensional image rather than the flat, two-dimensional image characteristic of the compound microscope. Thus, a dissecting microscope may be used to view larger body structures during a dissection (figure 1.9).

FIGURE 1.10

A transmission electron microscope can magnify objects up to 1,000,000 times.

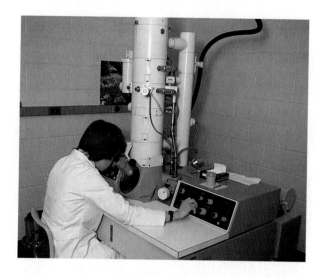

Another type of microscope makes use of an electron beam instead of ordinary light to produce magnified images. In one form of this instrument, the *transmission electron microscope* (TEM), the beam of electrons is passed through an extremely thin section of an object. As a result, an image that can be magnified up to 1,000,000 times is formed on a viewing screen or photographic film (figure 1.10). In a second form of the instrument, the *scanning electron microscope* (SEM), the electron beam scans over an object. Electrons reflecting from the object's surface are detected electronically and used to create an image that may be magnified up to about 50,000 times.

Although images created by a transmission electron microscope typically are two-dimensional, those obtained with a scanning electron microscope have three-dimensional qualities (figure 1.11).

The electron beam generated within the column of an electron microscope must travel in a vacuum. Consequently, specimens to be examined must also be placed in the vacuum. For this reason, the specimens must first be fixed (killed) and dehydrated, and since this treatment may alter their structure, it is sometimes difficult to visualize precisely the lifelike characteristics of the specimens.

The transmission electron microscope is further limited by the fact that an electron beam has little power to penetrate matter. As a result, a specimen to be examined must be extremely thin—usually no more than 50 to 100 nanometers in thickness. (A nanometer is equal to one-billionth of a meter.) Thus, before the structure of a cell can be studied it must be cut into very thin sections, and then the sections are observed individually.

An Introduction to Human Anatomy 9

FIGURE 1.11

A human red blood cell as viewed using (*a*) a stained light microscope (×1,000); (*b*) a transmission electron microscope (×5,000); and (*c*) a falsely colored scanning electron microscope (×3,500). How do these images differ?

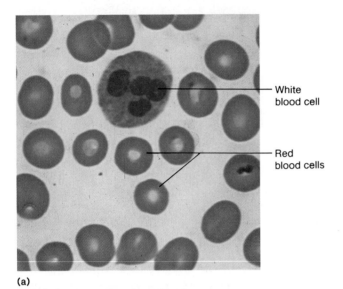

White blood cell

Red blood cells

(a)

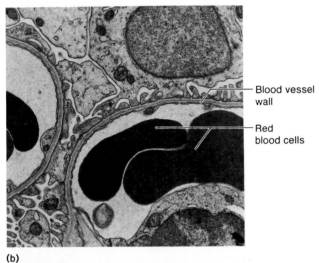

Blood vessel wall

Red blood cells

(b)

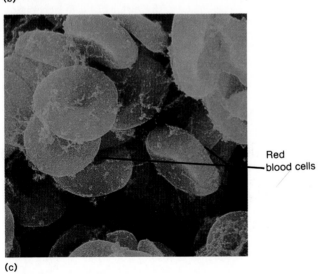

Red blood cells

(c)

FIGURE 1.12

An X-ray machine in use.

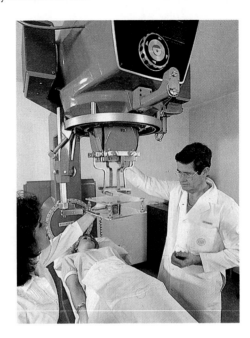

FIGURE 1.13

An X-ray film of the left hand. The arrow indicates a sesamoid bone at the base of the thumb.

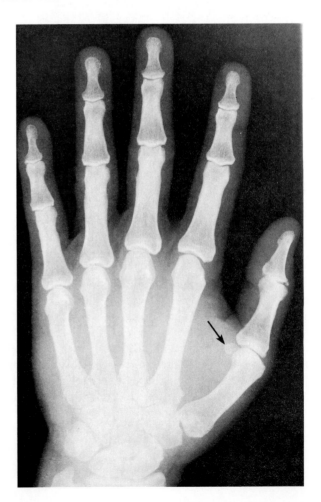

Radiography

Radiography involves the production of images of internal body structures by using X ray. In radiographic procedures, X ray from an X-ray tube is passed through a body part and allowed to expose photographic film on the other side (figure 1.12). The image that appears on the film when it is developed reveals the presence of parts with different densities. Bone, for example, contains very dense tissue and is a good absorber of X ray. Consequently, bone generally appears light on the film. Air-filled spaces, on the other hand, absorb almost no X ray, and they appear as dark areas. Liquids and soft tissues absorb intermediate quantities of X ray, so they usually appear in various shades of gray (figure 1.13).

Sometimes substances that are opaque to X ray (radiopaque substances), such as compounds of barium or iodine, are introduced into body fluids or body cavities before the X-ray film is exposed. When the film is developed, a shadow of the opaque substance may allow the investigator to visualize an otherwise indistinct internal part (figure 1.14).

Angiography is a specialized radiographic technique used to study blood vessels. In this procedure, a substance that is opaque to X ray is introduced into the blood. Then, by passing X ray through a body part and exposing X-ray film or by using a fluoroscope (an instrument with a fluorescent screen that produces light in the presence of X ray), the vessels filled with the radiopaque fluid can be visualized.

Angiography is often used to study the condition of blood vessels supplying the brain (cerebral angiography) or of those supplying the heart (coronary angiography).

1. How do images produced by a compound microscope and a dissecting microscope differ?
2. What is the difference between images obtained from a transmission electron microscope and a scanning electron microscope?
3. How can X ray be used to visualize internal body structures?

Tomography

Tomography is a method by which X ray is used to produce sectional images of the body. In one procedure, called *computed tomography* (CT; also called computerized axial tomography—CAT) an X-ray-emitting part is moved around the body region being examined. As a result, an X-ray beam is passed through the body from hundreds of different angles. At the same time, an X-ray detector is moved in the opposite direction on the other side of the body. Since tissues and organs of varying densities within the body absorb X ray differently, the amount of X ray reaching the detector varies from position to position. The measurements made by the detector are recorded in the memory of a computer, which later combines them mathematically

FIGURE 1.14

An X-ray film of the large intestine, exposed after a radiopaque substance was introduced into the intestine.

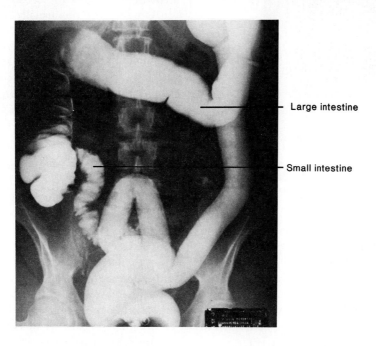

Large intestine

Small intestine

FIGURE 1.15

(*a*) A CT scan produced by equipment such as this shows sectional images of the body. (*b*) False color CT scan of the head and (*c*) false color scan of the abdomen.

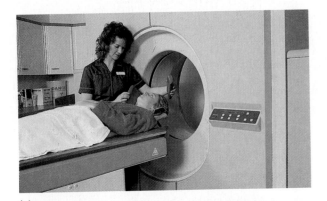

(a)

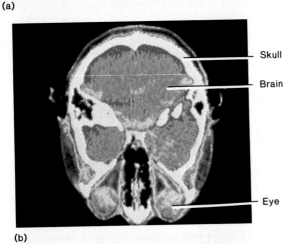

Skull

Brain

Eye

(b)

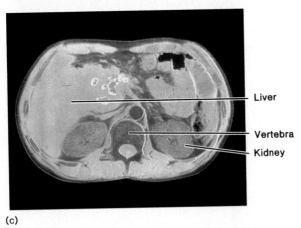

Liver

Vertebra

Kidney

(c)

FIGURE 1.16

A three-dimensional image can be obtained when several CT scans are combined by a computer. This CT scan shows a skull with a fracture of the right maxillary bone.

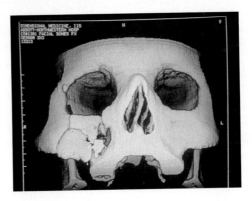

Ultrasonography

Ultrasonography makes use of high-frequency sound waves—those that are beyond the range of human hearing. In this procedure, a *transducer* that emits sound waves is pressed firmly against the skin and moved over the surface of the region being examined.

The sound waves travel into the body, and when they reach a border (interface) between structures of slightly different densities, some of the waves are reflected back to the transducer. Other sound waves continue into deeper tissues, and some of them are reflected back by still other interfaces.

As the reflected sound waves reach the transducer, they are converted into electrical impulses that are amplified and used to create a sectional image of the body's internal structure on a viewing screen.

Ultrasonography usually is not used to examine very compact organs such as bones or those containing air-filled spaces such as lungs, because resulting images are of poor quality. However, useful images of medium-density organs often can be obtained, making it possible to locate a fetus in its mother's uterus, abnormal masses of tissue, accumulations of fluids, or hard, stonelike objects (figure 1.17).

Scintigraphy

Scintigraphy involves the use of radioactive isotopes—substances that give off atomic radiation. To obtain an image of a particular internal organ, a small quantity of a certain isotope—one that is known to become concentrated in the part being examined—is introduced into the body. After a time, a *scintillation counter,* which can detect the presence of atomic radiation, is scanned over the part and the measurements from the counter are used to generate an image. In this way, the location and shape of organs such as bones, the heart, and the thyroid gland can be visualized (figure 1.18). This technique is often used to distinguish normal tissue from cancerous tissue.

and generates an image of a body section on a viewing screen (figure 1.15). CT scanning makes it possible to differentiate clearly between soft tissues of slightly different densities, which cannot be visualized with conventional X-ray film.

While ordinary X-ray techniques usually produce two-dimensional images, several CT scans may be combined to produce a three-dimensional image (figure 1.16).

FIGURE 1.17

(*a*) Ultrasonography creates images from reflected sound waves; (*b*) an ultrasonogram of a fetus within the uterus of its mother.

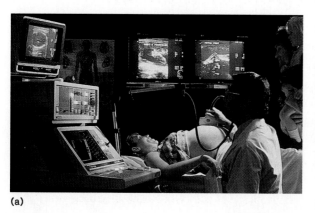

(a)

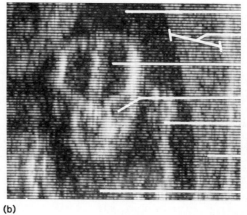

Amniotic fluid

Placenta

Left cerebral hemisphere of brain

Orbit of eye

Left hand

Uterine wall

Thorax

(b)

FIGURE 1.18

(*a*) Scintillation counters such as this are used to detect the presence of radioactive isotopes; (*b*) a scan of the thyroid gland; (*c*) the shape of the thyroid gland.

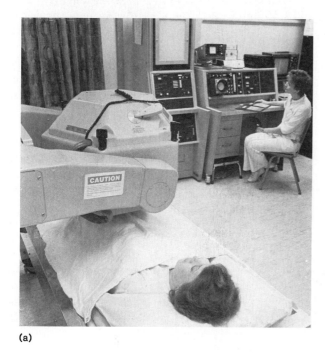

(a)

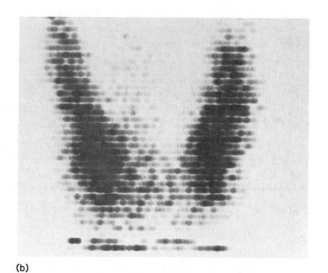

(b)

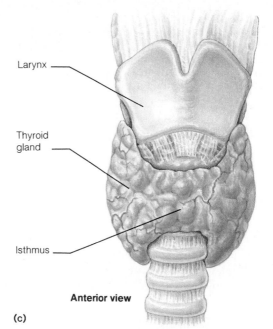

Larynx

Thyroid gland

Isthmus

Anterior view

(c)

FIGURE 1.19

In a PET image of a human brain, areas that are most active are shown in yellow and orange.

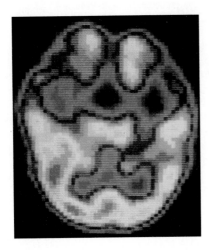

PET, or *positron emission tomography,* is a type of scintigraphy that makes use of a special group of radioactive isotopes. To produce an image of a body part, a person is given a substance to which a radioactive isotope has been chemically bound. Often nutrient molecules, such as a sugar, are used so that body parts that are most active in utilizing the nutrient accumulate the most radioactive isotope. After the substance is taken up by the tissues, radiation detectors are used to record atomic radiation. The data obtained by the detectors are combined by a computer, which, in turn, generates a cross-sectional image with those body regions that are most active shown in particular colors (figure 1.19). This allows physicians to distinguish between normal regions and abnormal or injured regions of certain organs.

Radiography, tomography, and scintigraphy make use of a form of energy called ionizing radiation. Such radiation includes X ray and radioactive isotopes. While there are medical benefits from using these techniques, there are also dangers, because ionizing radiation damages cellular structures and may cause cells to die. For this reason, precautions should be taken to minimize the number of exposures and the amount of ionizing radiation to which a person is exposed.

Magnetic Resonance Imaging

In the procedure called **magnetic resonance imaging,** or **MRI,** the body or part being examined is placed in a chamber surrounded by a powerful magnet and a special radio antenna. When the device is operating, the magnetic field created by the magnet affects alignment and spin of certain types of atoms within the living material. At the same time, a second rotating magnetic field is adjusted to cause particular kinds of atoms (such as hydrogen atoms in body fluids and various chemical compounds) to release

FIGURE 1.20

(*a*) An MRI device produces a sectional image of a body region without exposing the patient to radiation; (*b*) an MRI image of the human knee.

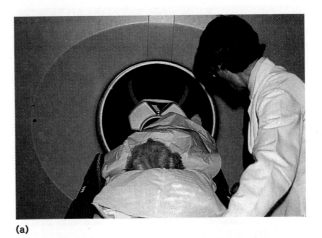

(a)

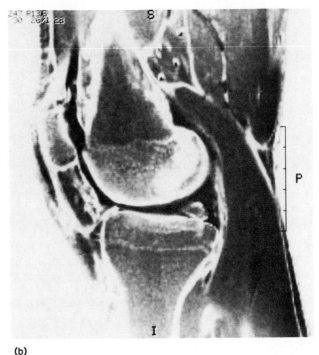

(b)

weak radio waves with characteristic frequencies. The radio waves are received by the antenna and amplified. The amplified signals are then processed by a computer, and the computer generates a cross-sectional image. (See figure 1.20.)

Unlike CT scans and PET images, MR images are obtained without exposing a patient to X ray or radiation. MRI scans are particularly useful for distinguishing normal and cancerous tissues, depicting blood vessels, assessing damage sustained by the heart muscle as a result of a heart attack, evaluating damage to the cartilage of the knee joint, and observing changes in the structure of the brain, spinal cord, and nerves.

Anatomical Characteristics

Anatomical studies reveal that normal body parts differ somewhat from one individual to another. These differences are called **variations** in body structures. Such parts vary in size, shape, location, and number. Most of these variations are produced by an interaction between each person's inheritance and environment.

The most obvious variations are in a person's external characteristics, such as height, weight, and skin and hair color. However, variations also occur in the internal organs (figure 1.21). For example, there is no single "normal" size or shape of the human stomach; instead, there is a range of sizes and shapes. Such variation occurs in all body structures and the term *normal* usu-

ally means what is most common or what is found in healthy individuals. However, variation in body parts also appears as a result of aging, so that the normal range for a characteristic may be different at different times in a person's life.

The concept of variation is important to health care personnel, who work with a variety of patients. Physicians and researchers must be able to distinguish normal variations of body structures from changes caused by injuries and disease processes. Variation is also important in the study of basic anatomy, because specimens of organs and tissues will vary.

FIGURE 1.21
Human stomachs vary in size and in shape.

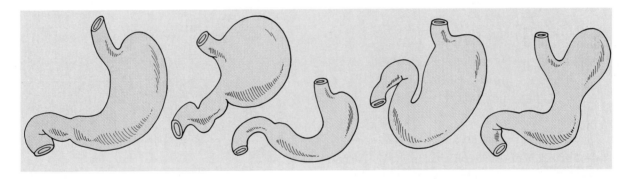

Many of the anatomical methods described in the previous section have been used to produce figures in this textbook. For example, some diagrams of organs have been drawn by observing dissected organs; photographs taken using different kinds of microscopes (micrographs) are included to illustrate microscopic parts; and X-ray films are used to visualize internal organs. As you study the figures, review for yourself the methods employed to produce the images.

1. How can a body section be visualized by using tomography?
2. How is the image obtained by a CT scan different from that produced on an X-ray film?
3. What types of internal parts can be visualized by using ultrasonography?
4. What is meant by scintigraphy?
5. Why is MRI less likely to affect the patient than CT scanning?

Language of Anatomy

As the science of anatomy evolved, anatomists devised new terms to describe body parts. These terms were needed so that the scientists could communicate more effectively with one another, and so that they could more easily organize the growing body of anatomic information.

Origin of Terms

The majority of anatomic terms originated from Greek and Latin words, largely because the Greeks and Romans developed early interests in anatomy. However, since the Latin language remained relatively unchanged and its terms were commonly understood throughout the world, Latin was used as the basis for international anatomic terminology, or *nomenclature*. For this reason, anatomic terms typically are latinized.

As a rule, anatomic terms are descriptive. Thus, a knowledge of Greek and Latin prefixes, word roots, and

FIGURE 1.22

Word roots, prefixes, and suffixes are combined to create descriptive anatomic terms, such as those applied to the anatomy of the heart.

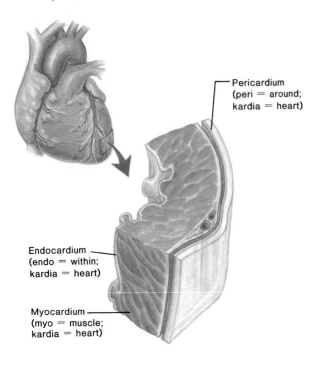

Pericardium
(peri = around;
kardia = heart)

Endocardium
(endo = within;
kardia = heart)

Myocardium
(myo = muscle;
kardia = heart)

FIGURE 1.23

Some body structures such as the middle ear bones were named for objects that they were thought to resemble.

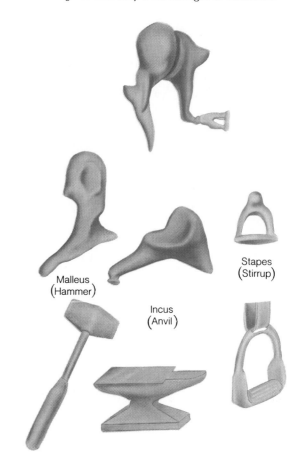

Malleus
(Hammer)

Incus
(Anvil)

Stapes
(Stirrup)

suffixes often makes it possible to visualize the parts represented by the words. For example, the term *endocardium* refers to the delicate inner lining of the heart. It originated from the Greek prefix *endo-* that means within, the Greek word *kardia* that means heart, and the Latin suffix *-ium* that often is used to end scientific terms. Similarly, the term *pericardium*, which refers to the outer covering of the heart, makes use of the Greek prefix *peri-* that means all around. The term *myocardium*, which is used to describe the muscular wall of the heart, contains part of the Greek word for muscle, *mys* (figure 1.22).

In other instances anatomic structures are named for familiar objects that they seem to resemble. Thus, the three small bones in the middle ear are called the *malleus, incus,* and *stapes*—terms that roughly describe their shapes—after the Latin words for hammer (malleus), anvil (incus), and stirrup (stapes). (See figure 1.23.) Other body parts that are named for objects include the *cricoid cartilage* (a ring-shaped structure) from the Greek word for ring, *krikos;* the *ethmoid bone* (a bone with many holes passing through it) after the Greek word for sieve, *ethmos;* the *frenulum* (a thin, membranous fold that attaches the tongue to the floor of the mouth) from the Latin word for bridle (a restraint), *frenum;* and *pelvis* (a hollow ring of bone) from the Latin word for basin, *pelvis.*

At the beginning of each chapter in this textbook there is a section called "Aids to Understanding Words." It contains a list of prefixes, word roots, and suffixes, along with examples to illustrate their uses that may help you discover the meanings of certain words within the chapter.

Still other anatomic structures have been named to honor individuals—usually anatomists or physicians who made important discoveries. Thus, there are Stensen's ducts (parotid ducts), Eustachian tubes (auditory tubes), crypts of Lieberkühn (intestinal glands), and islets of Langerhans (pancreatic islets). Unfortunately for beginning students, such names (eponyms) provide no information about the characteristics or locations of the parts they represent. Most of these terms have been replaced with more descriptive terms.

Problems of Nomenclature

During the history of anatomy, some body parts received more than one name; in fact, many parts were given several names. This, of course, led to disagreements among anatomists and confusion among students. In time, the need for an organized system of nomenclature was realized, and various groups of anatomists prepared standardized lists of anatomic terms.

The list most recently approved by the International Congress of Anatomists is called the *Nomina Anatomica*. It resulted from a thorough review of anatomic terms in use before 1955, and the list has been reevaluated and revised every few years by the International Nomenclature Committee. However, even today some anatomists and physicians, who were trained before the *Nomina Anatomica* was prepared, are likely to use older terms with which they are more familiar. In this textbook, the fifth edition of *Nomina Anatomica* is used as the standard.

---

1. Why was Latin used as the basis for anatomic nomenclature?
2. How are body parts named?
3. Why was the *Nomina Anatomica* prepared?

Chapter Summary

Introduction (page 4)
1. Human anatomy is the study of body structure.
2. Investigators depended upon dissection to observe body parts until the invention of the microscope.

Anatomy and Physiology (page 4)
1. Early anatomists speculated about the functions of body parts.
2. As knowledge of body functions grew, this information was separated from anatomy to become physiology, the study of body functions.
3. The structure of a body part is closely associated with its function.

Types of Anatomy (page 7)
The science of anatomy can be subdivided into three major types.

1. Gross anatomy is the study of macroscopic structure and can be further subdivided into systematic, regional, and surface anatomy.
   a. In systematic anatomy, body parts are organized according to their functions.
   b. In regional anatomy, all structures located in a specific region are studied together.
   c. In surface anatomy, features that can be observed or felt from the surface are used to visualize internal parts.
2. Microscopic anatomy is the study of structures that can be observed only with a microscope.
   a. Cytology is the study of cells.
   b. Histology is the study of tissues.
   c. The fine structure of cells can be examined by using an electron microscope.

3. Developmental anatomy is the study of changes that occur as the body grows and differentiates into the adult form.
   a. This type of anatomy also includes the study of tissue replacement, changes in bone and muscle due to use and disuse, changes in growth rate, and maturation of the reproductive organs.
   b. Embryology is the study of growth and development of the body before birth.

Methods of Anatomy (page 8)
In addition to dissection and microscopy, anatomists use various noninvasive procedures to visualize macroscopic structures.

1. Microscopy involves the use of a microscope to magnify small objects.
   a. The light microscope is most commonly used and can magnify two-dimensional images up to about 1,000 times.
   b. A dissecting microscope, which produces a three-dimensional image of low magnification, is often used to observe surface features.
   c. A transmission electron microscope requires an extremely thin specimen and can magnify images up to 1,000,000 times.
   d. A scanning electron microscope produces a three-dimensional image of surface features that can be magnified up to about 50,000 times.
2. Radiography uses X ray to visualize internal structures.
   a. X-ray images on photographic film reveal the presence of parts with different densities.
   b. Substances that are opaque to X ray are sometimes used to visualize internal parts that otherwise are indistinct.
3. Tomography is a method by which X ray is used to produce sectional images of the body.
   a. In computed tomography, an X-ray beam is passed through the body from many angles while an X-ray detector moves in the opposite direction on the other side.
   b. Measurements of varying tissue density are recorded in a computer memory and are combined to produce a sectional image.
4. Ultrasonography makes use of high-frequency sound waves to visualize internal parts.
   a. Sound waves from the body surface reflect from borders between structures with different densities.
   b. Reflected sound waves are received by a transducer and converted into electrical impulses that are used to produce an image.
   c. This method produces useful images of organs with medium densities.
5. Scintigraphy uses radioactive isotopes to visualize internal organs.
   a. An isotope that is known to be concentrated in the organ being observed is introduced into the body.
   b. After a time, a scintillation counter, which can detect the presence of atomic radiation, is scanned over the organ.

c. Measurements from the scintillation counter are used by a computer to produce an image of the organ.

d. Positron emission tomography is a type of scintigraphy that produces a cross-sectional image.

6. Magnetic resonance imaging makes use of a magnetic field and weak radio waves to generate a sectional image of the body.

a. A powerful magnet creates a magnetic field that affects certain atoms that release weak radio waves.

b. The radio signals are amplified and processed by computer to produce a cross-sectional image.

Language of Anatomy (page 15)

Anatomists have devised many terms to help them communicate with one another and to organize information.

1. Origin of terms

a. The majority of anatomic terms originated from Greek and Latin words.

b. Latin is used as the basis for international anatomic nomenclature.

c. Many anatomic terms are descriptive; some parts are named for objects they resemble; others are named to honor individuals.

2. Problems of nomenclature

a. Some body structures have been given many names.

b. To avoid disagreements and confusion, standardized lists of anatomic terms have been prepared.

c. The *Nomina Anatomica* is the list approved by the International Congress of Anatomists.

Clinical Application of Knowledge

1. Assuming that the same information could be obtained by either method, what would be the advantages of using ultrasonography rather than X ray to visualize a fetus in the uterus?

2. If a child swallows a pin, which technique would most likely be used to detect the exact location of the pin? Why?

3. In an autopsy (examination of organs and tissues to determine the cause of death), what types of anatomy would be observed and which anatomical methods would most likely be used?

Review Activities

1. Distinguish between anatomy and physiology.

2. Provide three examples to illustrate how the structure and function of body parts are related.

3. Name three major subdivisions of anatomy.

4. Distinguish between macroscopic and microscopic structures.

5. Explain how the study of body parts is organized in systematic anatomy.

6. Explain why regional anatomy is of special interest to physicians and surgeons.

7. Distinguish between cytology and histology.

8. Define *embryology*.

9. Name five noninvasive methods for visualizing internal structures.

10. Describe the images produced by light and dissecting microscopes.

11. Compare the images produced by a transmission and a scanning electron microscope.

12. Explain how X-ray and photographic film can be used to visualize internal body parts.

13. Explain the advantages of using computed tomography over ordinary X-ray techniques to visualize internal parts.

14. Describe the kinds of body parts that can be studied using ultrasonography.

15. Explain how radioactive isotopes can be used to study internal body parts.

16. Explain how *magnetic resonance imaging* differs from other forms of imaging.

17. Explain why anatomic terms usually are latinized.

18. Provide three examples to illustrate how some anatomic terms are descriptive.

19. Explain why anatomists found it necessary to prepare standardized lists of anatomic terms such as the *Nomina Anatomica*.

REFERENCE PLATES

The Human Organism

The following series of illustrations shows the major organs of the human torso. The first plate illustrates the anterior surface and reveals the superficial muscles on one side. Each subsequent plate exposes some deeper organs, including those in the thoracic, abdominal, and pelvic cavities.

The purpose of chapters 5–17 of this textbook is to describe the organ systems of the human organism in some detail. As you read them, you may want to refer to these plates to help yourself visualize the locations of various organs and the three-dimensional relationships that exist between them.

PLATE 1
Human female torso with a view of the anterior surface on one side and the superficial muscles exposed on the other side. (m. stands for muscle; v. stands for vein.)

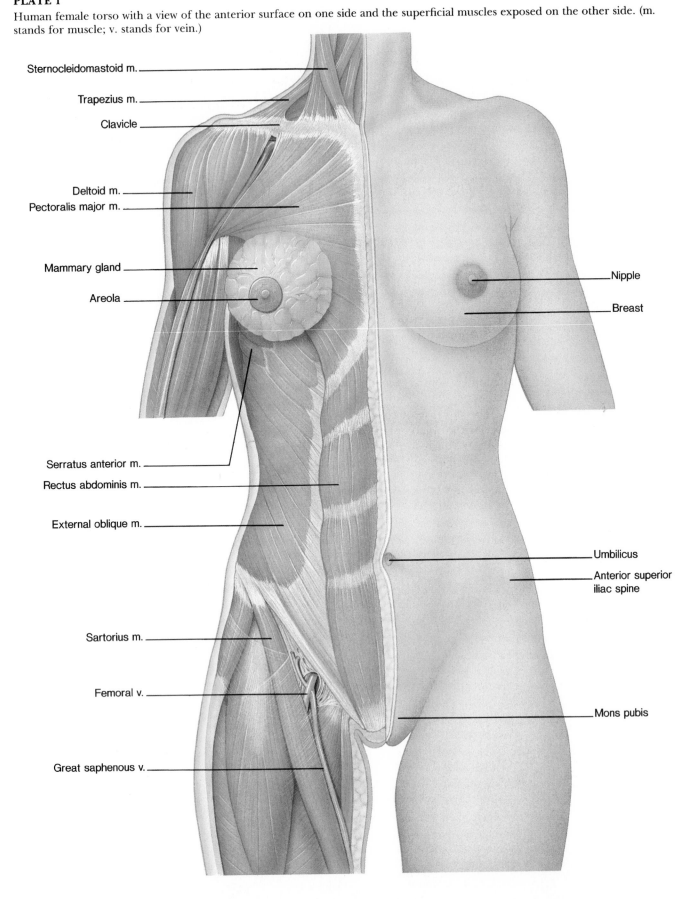

Sternocleidomastoid m.

Trapezius m.

Clavicle

Deltoid m.

Pectoralis major m.

Mammary gland

Areola

Serratus anterior m.

Rectus abdominis m.

External oblique m.

Sartorius m.

Femoral v.

Great saphenous v.

Nipple

Breast

Umbilicus

Anterior superior iliac spine

Mons pubis

PLATE 2
Human male torso with the deeper muscle layers exposed. (a. stands for artery; n. stands for nerve.)

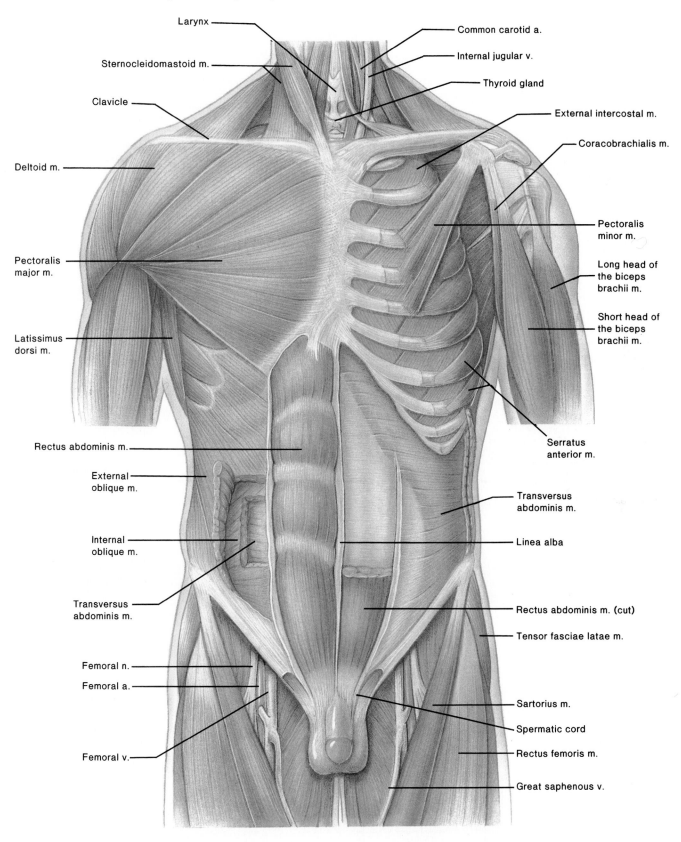

Larynx

Common carotid a.

Internal jugular v.

Sternocleidomastoid m.

Thyroid gland

Clavicle

External intercostal m.

Coracobrachialis m.

Deltoid m.

Pectoralis
minor m.

Long head of
the biceps
brachii m.

Pectoralis
major m.

Short head of
the biceps
brachii m.

Latissimus
dorsi m.

Rectus abdominis m.

Serratus
anterior m.

External
oblique m.

Transversus
abdominis m.

Internal
oblique m.

Linea alba

Transversus
abdominis m.

Rectus abdominis m. (cut)

Tensor fasciae latae m.

Femoral n.

Femoral a.

Sartorius m.

Spermatic cord

Femoral v.

Rectus femoris m.

Great saphenous v.

PLATE 3
Human male torso with the deep muscles removed and the abdominal viscera exposed.

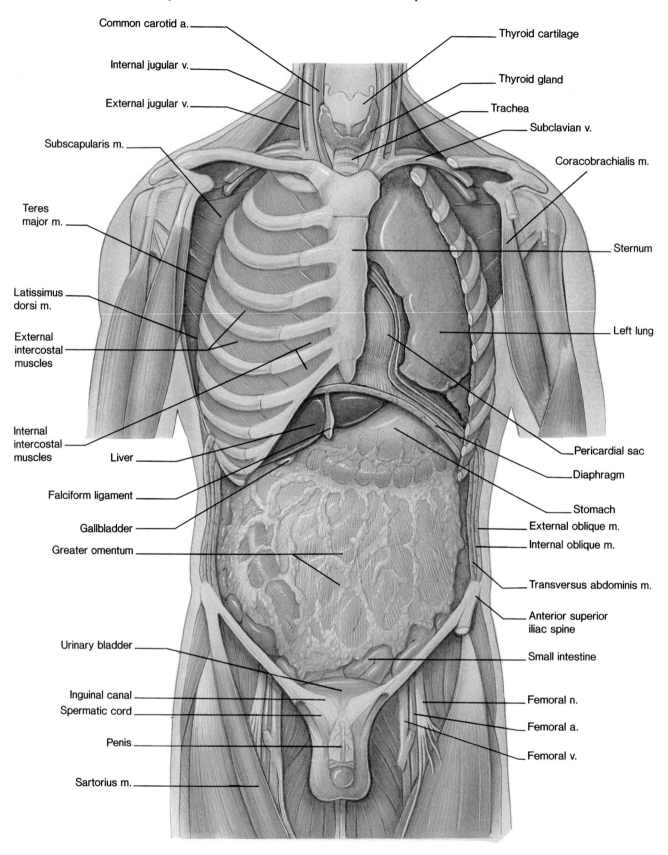

Common carotid a.

Internal jugular v.

External jugular v.

Subscapularis m.

Teres major m.

Latissimus dorsi m.

External intercostal muscles

Internal intercostal muscles

Liver

Falciform ligament

Gallbladder

Greater omentum

Urinary bladder

Inguinal canal

Spermatic cord

Penis

Sartorius m.

Thyroid cartilage

Thyroid gland

Trachea

Subclavian v.

Coracobrachialis m.

Sternum

Left lung

Pericardial sac

Diaphragm

Stomach

External oblique m.

Internal oblique m.

Transversus abdominis m.

Anterior superior iliac spine

Small intestine

Femoral n.

Femoral a.

Femoral v.

PLATE 4
Human male torso with the thoracic and abdominal viscera exposed.

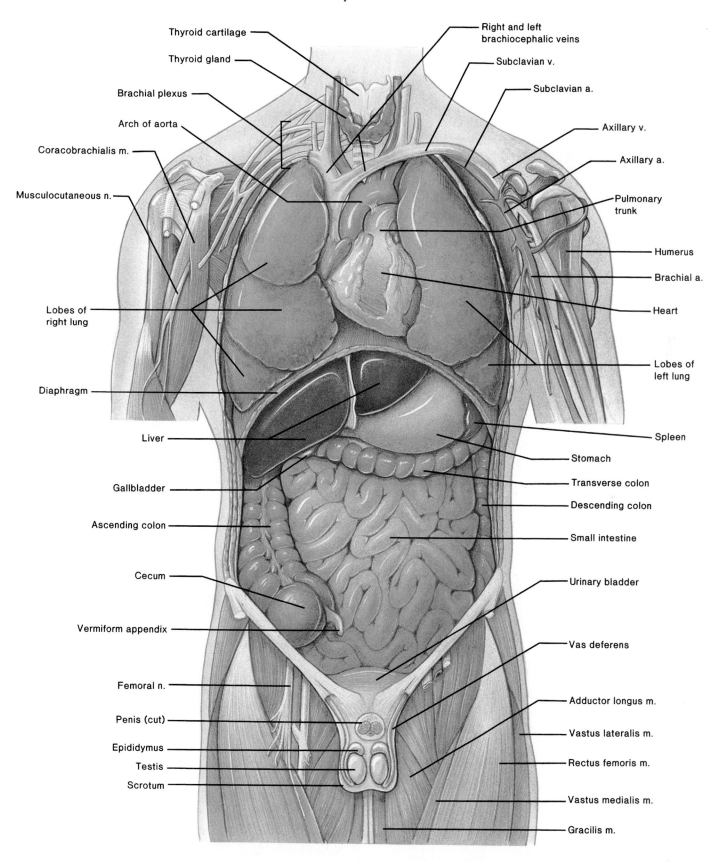

Thyroid cartilage

Thyroid gland

Brachial plexus

Arch of aorta

Coracobrachialis m.

Musculocutaneous n.

Lobes of right lung

Diaphragm

Liver

Gallbladder

Ascending colon

Cecum

Vermiform appendix

Femoral n.

Penis (cut)

Epididymus

Testis

Scrotum

Right and left brachiocephalic veins

Subclavian v.

Subclavian a.

Axillary v.

Axillary a.

Pulmonary trunk

Humerus

Brachial a.

Heart

Lobes of left lung

Spleen

Stomach

Transverse colon

Descending colon

Small intestine

Urinary bladder

Vas deferens

Adductor longus m.

Vastus lateralis m.

Rectus femoris m.

Vastus medialis m.

Gracilis m.

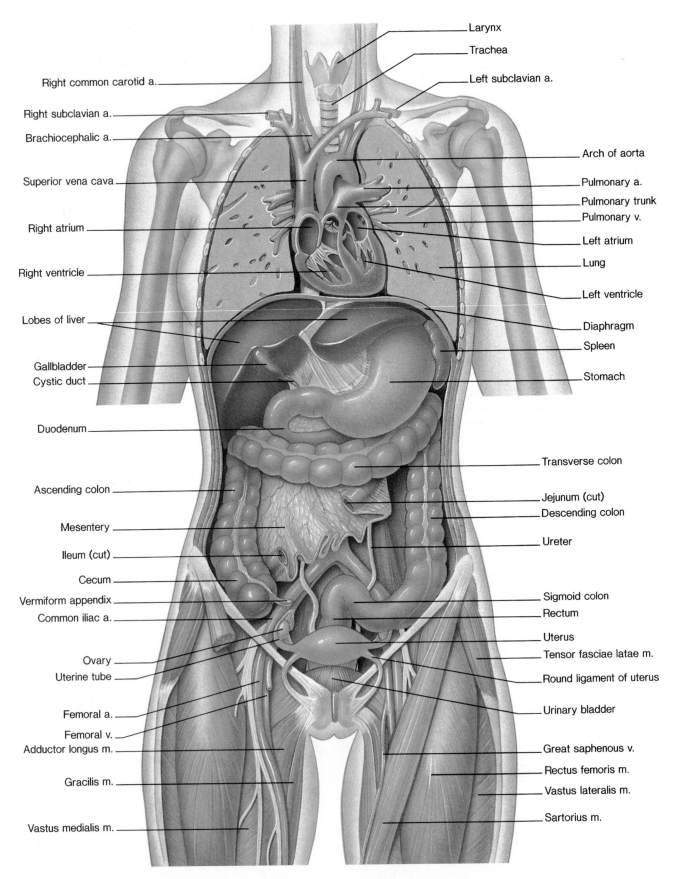

Larynx

Trachea

Left subclavian a.

Right common carotid a.

Right subclavian a.

Brachiocephalic a.

Arch of aorta

Superior vena cava

Pulmonary a.

Pulmonary trunk

Pulmonary v.

Right atrium

Left atrium

Lung

Right ventricle

Left ventricle

Lobes of liver

Diaphragm

Spleen

Gallbladder

Stomach

Cystic duct

Duodenum

Transverse colon

Ascending colon

Jejunum (cut)

Descending colon

Mesentery

Ureter

Ileum (cut)

Cecum

Sigmoid colon

Vermiform appendix

Rectum

Common iliac a.

Uterus

Tensor fasciae latae m.

Ovary

Round ligament of uterus

Uterine tube

Urinary bladder

Femoral a.

Femoral v.

Great saphenous v.

Adductor longus m.

Rectus femoris m.

Vastus lateralis m.

Gracilis m.

Sartorius m.

Vastus medialis m.

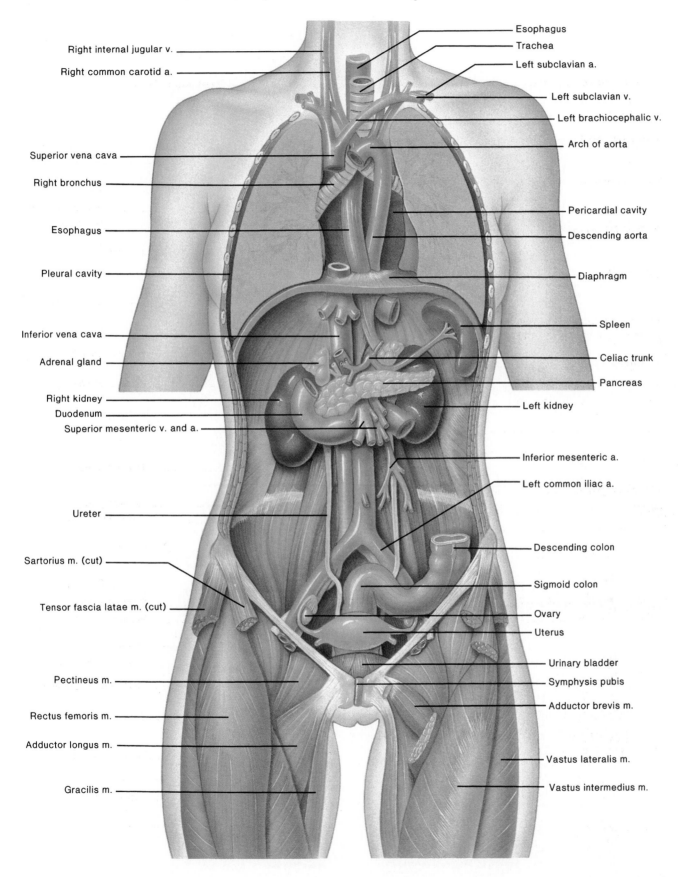

Right internal jugular v.

Right common carotid a.

Superior vena cava

Right bronchus

Esophagus

Pleural cavity

Inferior vena cava

Adrenal gland

Right kidney
Duodenum
Superior mesenteric v. and a.

Ureter

Sartorius m. (cut)

Tensor fascia latae m. (cut)

Pectineus m.

Rectus femoris m.

Adductor longus m.

Gracilis m.

Esophagus
Trachea
Left subclavian a.
Left subclavian v.
Left brachiocephalic v.
Arch of aorta
Pericardial cavity
Descending aorta
Diaphragm

Spleen
Celiac trunk
Pancreas

Left kidney

Inferior mesenteric a.

Left common iliac a.

Descending colon

Sigmoid colon

Ovary
Uterus

Urinary bladder
Symphysis pubis
Adductor brevis m.

Vastus lateralis m.

Vastus intermedius m.

PLATE 7
Human female torso with the thoracic, abdominal, and pelvic visceral organs removed.

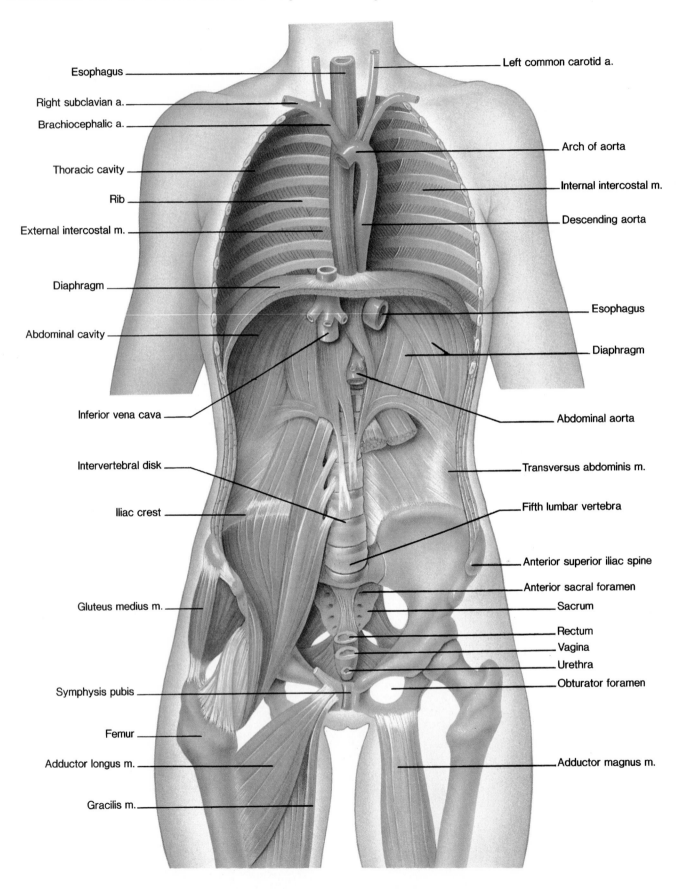

Esophagus

Right subclavian a.

Brachiocephalic a.

Thoracic cavity

Rib

External intercostal m.

Diaphragm

Abdominal cavity

Inferior vena cava

Intervertebral disk

Iliac crest

Gluteus medius m.

Symphysis pubis

Femur

Adductor longus m.

Gracilis m.

Left common carotid a.

Arch of aorta

Internal intercostal m.

Descending aorta

Esophagus

Diaphragm

Abdominal aorta

Transversus abdominis m.

Fifth lumbar vertebra

Anterior superior iliac spine

Anterior sacral foramen

Sacrum

Rectum

Vagina

Urethra

Obturator foramen

Adductor magnus m.

CHAPTER 2

Body Organization and Terminology

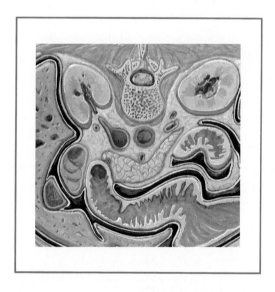

In chapter 2, a discussion of the ways complex human bodies are organized provides a beginning for the study of human anatomy. This chapter also introduces a special set of terms used to describe the major body parts.

Chapter Outline

Introduction

Levels of Organization

Organization of the Human Body
  Body Cavities
  Thoracic and Abdominopelvic
    Membranes
  Organ Systems

Anatomical Terminology
  Relative Position
  Body Sections
  Body Regions

Some Medical and Applied Sciences

Chapter Objectives

After you have studied this chapter, you should be able to

1. Explain what is meant by levels of organization.

2. Describe the location of the major body cavities.

3. List the organs located in each body cavity.

4. Name the membranes associated with the thoracic and abdominopelvic cavities.

5. Name the major organ systems of the body and list the organs associated with each.

6. Describe the general functions of each organ system.

7. Properly use the terms that describe relative positions, body sections, and body regions.

8. Complete the review activities at the end of this chapter. Note that the items are worded in the form of specific learning objectives. You may want to refer to them before reading the chapter.

Aids to Understanding Words

append-, to hang something: *append*icular—pertaining to arms and legs.

ax-, *ax*is: axial—pertaining to central portion of the body, including the head and trunk.

cardi-, heart: peri*cardi*um—membrane that surrounds the heart.

cran-, helmet: *cran*ial—pertaining to the portion of the skull that surrounds the brain.

dors-, back: *dors*al—a position toward the back of the body.

nas-, nose: *nas*al—pertaining to the nose.

orb-, circle: *orb*ital—pertaining to the portion of skull that encircles an eye.

pariet-, wall: *pariet*al membrane—membrane that lines the wall of a cavity.

pelv-, basin: *pelv*ic cavity—basin-shaped cavity enclosed by pelvic bones.

peri-, around: *peri*cardial membrane—membrane that surrounds the heart.

pleur-, rib: *pleur*al membrane—membrane that encloses the lungs within the rib cage.

viscera-, organs: *viscera*l—referring to the internal organs of the body.

Introduction

Early investigators focused their attention on larger body structures, for they were limited in their ability to observe small parts. Studies of small parts had to wait for the invention of magnifying lenses and microscopes. Once these tools were available, scientists discovered that larger body structures were made up of smaller parts, which, in turn, were composed of even smaller ones.

Levels of Organization

Today, scientists recognize that all materials, including those that comprise the human body, are composed of chemicals. These substances are made up of tiny, invisible particles called **atoms,** which are commonly bound together to form larger particles, called **molecules;** small molecules may be combined to form larger molecules, called **macromolecules.**

Within the human organism, the basic unit of structure and function is a microscopic part called a **cell.** Although individual cells vary in size, shape, and specialized functions, all have certain traits in common. For instance, all cells contain tiny parts called **organelles,** which carry on specific activities. These organelles are composed of macromolecules, such as proteins, carbohydrates, lipids, and nucleic acids.

Cells are organized into layers or masses that have common functions. Such a group of cells constitutes a **tissue.** Groups of different tissues form **organs**—complex structures with specialized functions—and groups of organs are arranged into **organ systems.** Organ systems make up an **organism.** Thus, various body parts occupy different levels of organization. Furthermore, body parts vary in complexity from one level to the next. That is, atoms are less complex than molecules, molecules are less complex than organelles, organelles are less complex than cells, cells are less complex than tissues, tissues are less complex than organs, organs are less complex than organ systems, and organ systems are less complex than the whole organism (figure 2.1).

FIGURE 2.1

A human body is composed of parts within parts, which vary in complexity.

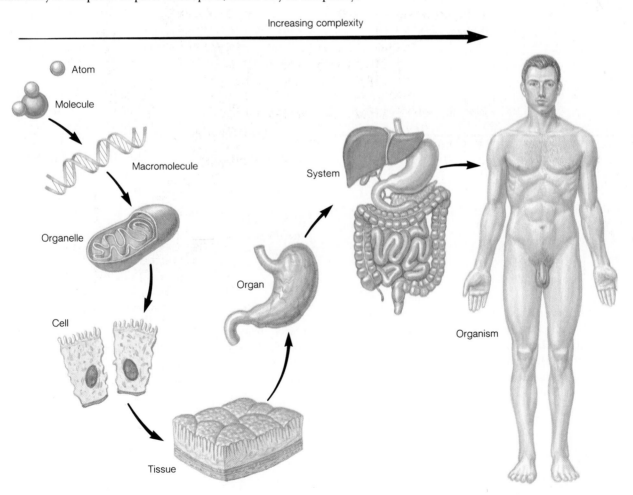

Increasing complexity

Atom

Molecule

Macromolecule

Organelle

System

Organ

Cell

Organism

Tissue

Chart 2.1 Linear measurements used with various levels of organization

Measurement (abbreviation)	Equivalent measure	Level of organization where most used	Example
Nanometer (nm)	.001 μm	Molecule, organelle	Protein molecule = 2–10 nm; ribosome diameter = 25 nm
Micrometer (μm)	.001 mm	Cell	Red blood cell diameter = 7.5 μm; egg cell diameter = 140 μm
Millimeter (mm)	1,000 μm	Tissue	Epidermis of skin = 1.4 mm (thickness)
Centimeter (cm)	10 mm	Organ	Trachea length = 12.5 cm; stomach length = 25–30 cm
Meter (m)	100 cm	Organ, organism	Small intestine length = 3.0 m; human height = 1.78 m

Chart 2.1 demonstrates some of the linear measurements used with various levels of organization. Additional measurements are described in Appendix A.

Chapters 3–5 discuss these levels of organization in more detail. Chapter 3 deals with organelles and cellular structures and functions; chapter 4 describes tissues; and chapter 5 presents membranes as examples of organs, and the skin and its accessory organs as an example of an organ system. Beginning with chapter 6, the structure and functions of each organ system are described in detail.

1. How can the human body be used to illustrate the idea of levels of organization?
2. What is an organism?
3. How do body parts that occupy different levels of organization vary in complexity?

Organization of the Human Body

The human organism is a complex structure composed of many parts. Major features of the human body include various cavities, a set of membranes, and a group of organ systems.

Body Cavities

The human organism can be divided into an **axial portion,** which includes the head, neck, and trunk, and an **appendicular portion,** which includes the upper and lower extremities. Within the axial portion there are two major cavities—a **posterior (dorsal) cavity** and a larger **anterior (ventral) cavity.** These cavities are spaces between the body wall and internal organs. The organs contained within such cavities are called *visceral organs.* The posterior cavity can be subdivided into two parts—the **cranial cavity,** which houses the brain; and the **vertebral canal,** which contains the spinal cord and is surrounded by sections of the backbone (vertebrae). The anterior cavity consists of a **thoracic cavity** and an **abdominopelvic cavity.** These major body cavities are shown in figure 2.2 and reference plate 7.

The **thoracic cavity** is separated from the lower abdominopelvic cavity by a broad, thin muscle called the *diaphragm.* When at rest, this muscle curves upward into the thorax like a dome. When it contracts during inhalation, it presses down upon the abdominal visceral organs. The wall of the thoracic cavity is composed of skin, skeletal muscles, and various bones. The viscera within it include the lungs and a region between the lungs, called the *mediastinum.* The mediastinum separates the thorax into two compartments that contain the right and left lungs. The remaining thoracic viscera—heart, esophagus, trachea, and thymus gland—are located within the mediastinum.

The abdominopelvic cavity, which includes an upper abdominal portion and a lower pelvic portion, extends from the diaphragm to the floor of the pelvis. Its wall consists primarily of skin, skeletal muscles, and bones. The visceral organs within the **abdominal cavity** include the stomach, liver, spleen, gallbladder, and most of the small and large intestines.

The **pelvic cavity** is the portion of the abdominopelvic cavity enclosed by the pelvic bones. The upper margin of these bones forms the *pelvic brim,* which is the boundary between the abdominal and pelvic cavities. The pelvic cavity contains the terminal end of the large intestine, urinary bladder, and internal reproductive organs.

FIGURE 2.2
Major body cavities as viewed from (*a*) the side and (*b*) the front.

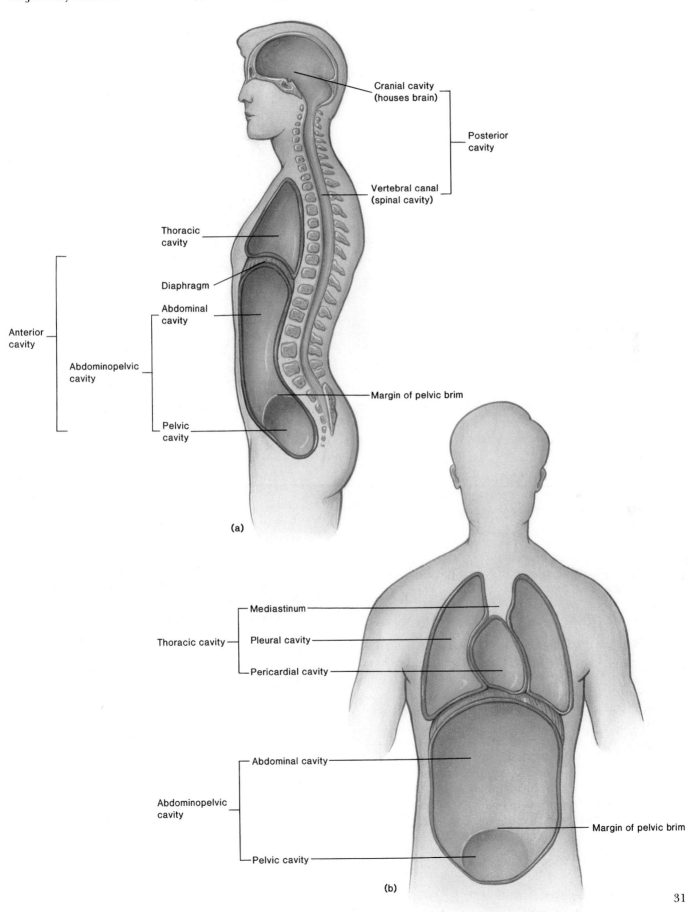

(a)

(b)

FIGURE 2.3

Cavities within the head include the oral, nasal, orbital, and middle ear cavities, and several sinuses.

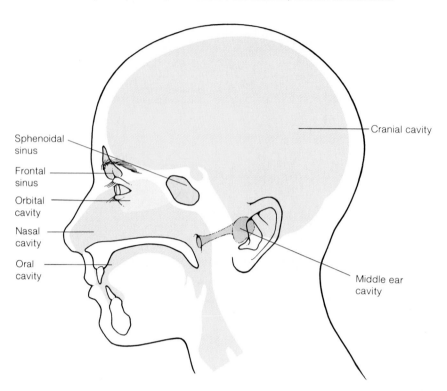

In addition to the relatively large anterior and posterior body cavities, there are several smaller cavities within the head. They include the following:

1. *Oral cavity,* containing the teeth and tongue.
2. *Nasal cavity,* located within the nose and divided into right and left portions by a nasal septum. Eight air-filled sinuses are connected to the nasal cavity.
3. *Orbital cavities,* containing the eyes and associated skeletal muscles and nerves.
4. *Middle ear cavities,* containing the three middle ear bones (figure 2.3).

Thoracic and Abdominopelvic Membranes

The thoracic and abdominopelvic cavities have *membranes* associated with them. These membranes are thin, flexible, sheetlike structures that line the insides of cavities and cover the outsides of organs.

The thoracic cavity is lined with **pleural membranes.** The walls of the right and left thoracic compartments, which contain the lungs, are lined with a membrane called the *parietal pleura.* This membrane folds back to cover the lungs themselves and here it is called the *visceral pleura.* (Note: *parietal* refers to the membrane attached to the wall of a cavity, and *visceral* refers to one that is deeper and is associated with an internal organ, such as a lung.)

The parietal and visceral pleura are separated by a thin film of fluid (serous fluid) that they secrete. Although there is normally no actual space between these membranes, the potential space between them is called the *pleural cavity.*

The heart, which is located in the broadest portion of the mediastinum, is surrounded by **pericardial membranes.** A thin *visceral pericardium* (epicardium) covers the heart's surface. It folds back upon itself to form the *parietal pericardium.* The potential space between these membranes is called the *pericardial cavity* and contains a small amount of serous fluid. Figure 2.4 and plate 54 show the membranes associated with the heart and lungs.

In the abdominopelvic cavity, the lining membranes are called **peritoneal membranes.** A *parietal peritoneum* lines the wall, and a *visceral peritoneum* covers each organ in the abdominal cavity. The potential space between these membranes is called the *peritoneal cavity* (figures 2.5 and 2.6 and plate 56).

---

1. What is meant by the term *visceral organ?*
2. What organs occupy the posterior cavity? The anterior cavity?
3. Name the cavities of the head.
4. Describe the membranes associated with the thoracic and abdominopelvic cavities.

FIGURE 2.4

Transverse section through the thorax reveals the serous membranes associated with the heart and lungs.

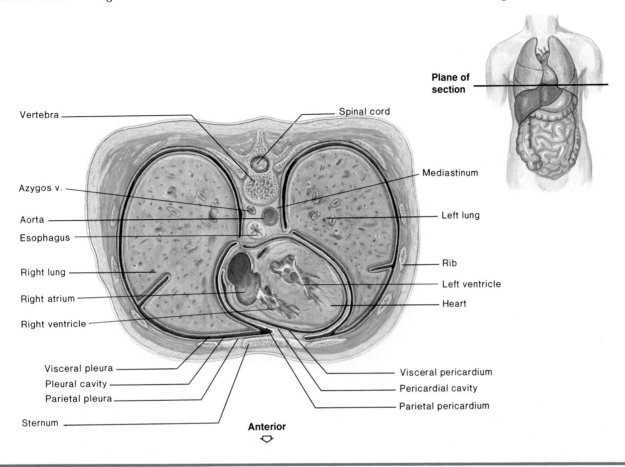

- Vertebra
- Spinal cord
- Azygos v.
- Mediastinum
- Aorta
- Left lung
- Esophagus
- Right lung
- Rib
- Right atrium
- Left ventricle
- Right ventricle
- Heart
- Visceral pleura
- Pleural cavity
- Parietal pleura
- Visceral pericardium
- Pericardial cavity
- Sternum
- Parietal pericardium

Anterior

FIGURE 2.5

Transverse section through the abdomen at the level of the stomach.

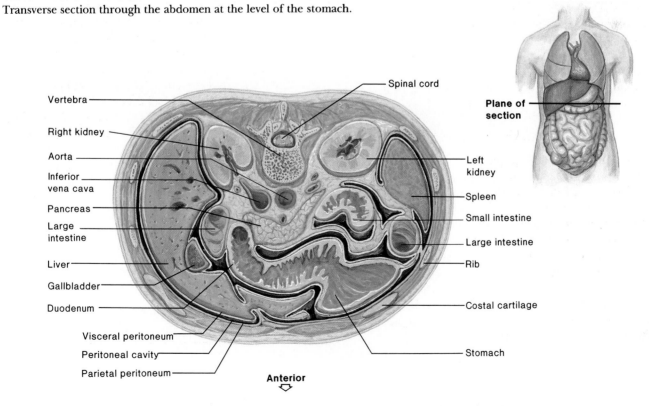

- Vertebra
- Spinal cord
- Right kidney
- Aorta
- Left kidney
- Inferior vena cava
- Spleen
- Pancreas
- Small intestine
- Large intestine
- Large intestine
- Liver
- Rib
- Gallbladder
- Duodenum
- Costal cartilage
- Visceral peritoneum
- Peritoneal cavity
- Parietal peritoneum
- Stomach

Anterior

Body Organization and Terminology   33

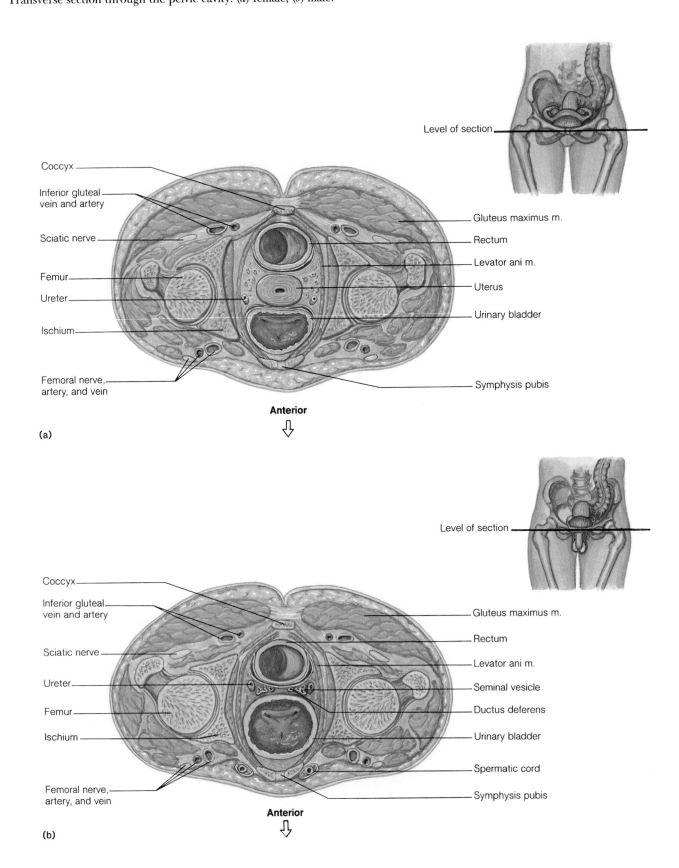

Level of section

Coccyx

Inferior gluteal
vein and artery

Sciatic nerve

Femur

Ureter

Ischium

Femoral nerve,
artery, and vein

Gluteus maximus m.

Rectum

Levator ani m.

Uterus

Urinary bladder

Symphysis pubis

Anterior

(a)

Level of section

Coccyx

Inferior gluteal
vein and artery

Sciatic nerve

Ureter

Femur

Ischium

Femoral nerve,
artery, and vein

Gluteus maximus m.

Rectum

Levator ani m.

Seminal vesicle

Ductus deferens

Urinary bladder

Spermatic cord

Symphysis pubis

Anterior

(b)

Organ Systems

The human organism consists of several organ systems. Each of these systems includes a set of interrelated organs that work together to provide specialized functions. As you read about each organ system, you may want to consult the illustrations of the human torso provided in reference plates 1–7 and locate some of the features listed in the descriptions.

Body Covering

Organs of the **integumentary system** include the skin and various accessory organs such as the hair, nails, sweat glands, and sebaceous glands. These parts protect underlying tissues, help regulate body temperature, house a variety of sensory receptors, and synthesize certain cellular products (figure 2.7). The integumentary system is discussed in chapter 5.

Support and Movement

Organs of the skeletal and muscular systems function to support and move body parts (figure 2.8).

The **skeletal system** consists of the bones as well as the ligaments and cartilages, which bind bones together at joints. These parts provide frameworks and protective shields for softer tissues, serve as attachments for muscles,

and act together with muscles when body parts move. Tissues within bones also function to produce blood cells and store minerals.

Muscles are organs of the **muscular system.** By contracting and pulling their ends closer together, they provide the forces that cause body movements. They also function in maintaining posture and are the main source of body heat. The skeletal and muscular systems are discussed in chapters 6, 7, and 8.

Integration and Coordination

For the body to act as a unit, its parts must be integrated and coordinated. That is, their activities must be controlled and adjusted. This is the general function of the nervous and endocrine systems (figure 2.9).

The **nervous system** consists of the brain, spinal cord, nerves, and sense organs. Nerve cells within these organs use signals called *nerve impulses* to communicate with one another and with muscles and glands. Each impulse produces a relatively short-term effect on the part it influences. Some nerve cells act as specialized sensory receptors that can detect changes occurring inside and outside the body. Others receive impulses transmitted from these sensory units and interpret and act on the information received. Still others carry impulses from the brain or spinal cord to muscles or glands and stimulate these parts to contract or to secrete various products. The nervous system is discussed in chapters 9 and 10.

FIGURE 2.7

The integumentary system forms the body covering.

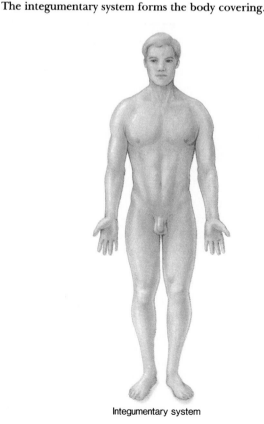

Integumentary system

FIGURE 2.8

Organ systems associated with support and movement.

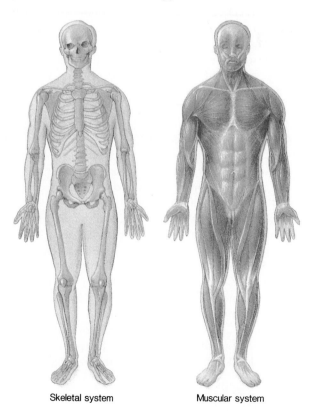

Skeletal system   Muscular system

FIGURE 2.9
Organ systems associated with integration and coordination.

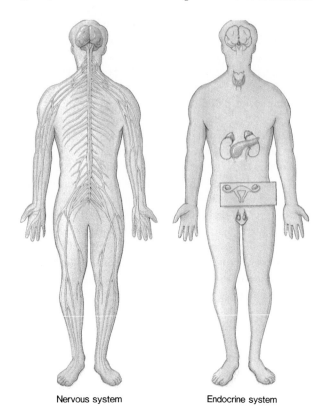

Nervous system   Endocrine system

The **endocrine system** includes all glands that secrete *hormones*. The hormones, in turn, travel away from the glands in body fluids such as blood. Usually a particular hormone affects only a particular group of cells, which is called its *target tissue*. The effect of a hormone is to alter the target tissue.

Organs of the endocrine system include the pituitary, thyroid, parathyroid, and adrenal glands, as well as the pancreas, ovaries, testes, pineal gland, thymus gland, and placenta. They are discussed in chapter 11.

Processing and Transporting

Organs of several systems are involved with processing and transporting nutrients, oxygen, and various wastes. Organs of the digestive system, for example, receive foods from outside the body. Then, they convert food molecules into simpler forms that can pass through cell membranes and thus be absorbed. Materials that are not absorbed are eliminated by being transported back to the outside.

The **digestive system** includes the mouth, tongue, teeth, salivary glands, pharynx, esophagus, stomach, liver, gallbladder, pancreas, small intestine, and large intestine. This system is discussed in chapter 12.

Organs of the **respiratory system** provide for the intake and output of air, and for exchange of gases between the blood and air. More specifically, oxygen passes

from air within the lungs into the blood, and carbon dioxide leaves the blood and enters the air. The nasal cavity, pharynx, larynx, trachea, bronchi, and lungs are parts of this system, which is discussed in chapter 13.

The **cardiovascular system** includes the heart, arteries, veins, and capillaries. The heart functions as a muscular pump that forces blood through the blood vessels. The blood serves as a fluid for transporting gases, nutrients, and hormones, and carries wastes. It carries oxygen from the lungs and nutrients from the digestive organs to all body cells, where these substances are used. Blood also transports hormones from various endocrine glands to their target tissues and transports wastes from body cells to the excretory organs, where the wastes are removed from the blood and released to the outside. The cardiovascular system is discussed in chapter 14.

The **lymphatic system** is sometimes considered part of the cardiovascular system. It is composed of the lymphatic vessels, lymph fluid, lymph nodes, thymus gland, and spleen. This system transports some of the fluid from the spaces within tissues (tissue fluid) back to the blood stream and carries certain absorbed food molecules away from digestive organs. Lymphatic organs also aid in defending the body against infections by removing particles, such as microorganisms, from tissue fluid and by supporting the activities of certain cells (lymphocytes) that produce immunity by reacting against specific disease-causing agents. The lymphatic system is discussed in chapter 15.

The **urinary system** consists of the kidneys, ureters, urinary bladder, and urethra. The kidneys remove various wastes from blood, and assist in maintaining water and electrolyte balance. The product of these activities is urine. Other portions of the urinary system are concerned with storing urine and transporting it to the outside of the body. The urinary system is discussed in chapter 16.

Sometimes the urinary system is called the excretory system. However, excretion, or waste removal, is also a function of the respiratory, digestive, and integumentary systems.

The systems associated with processing and transporting are shown in figure 2.10.

Reproduction

Reproduction is the process of producing offspring (progeny). Cells reproduce when they divide and give rise to new cells. The **reproductive system** of an organism, however, is involved with the production of new organisms. (See chapter 17.)

The male reproductive system includes the scrotum, testes, epididymides, vasa deferentia, seminal vesicles, prostate gland, bulbourethral glands, urethra, and penis. These parts are concerned with producing and maintaining the male sex cells, or sperm cells. They also function to transfer these cells from their site of origin into the female reproductive tract.

FIGURE 2.10
Organ systems associated with processing and transporting.

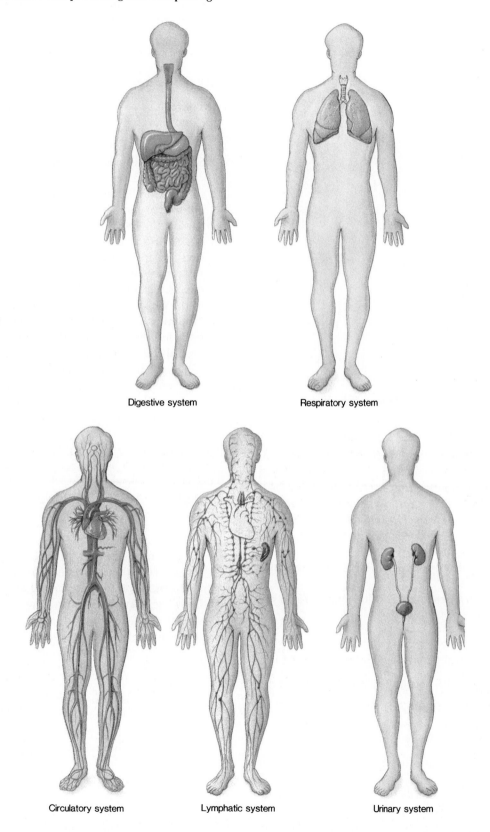

Digestive system

Respiratory system

Circulatory system

Lymphatic system

Urinary system

FIGURE 2.11
Organ systems associated with reproduction.

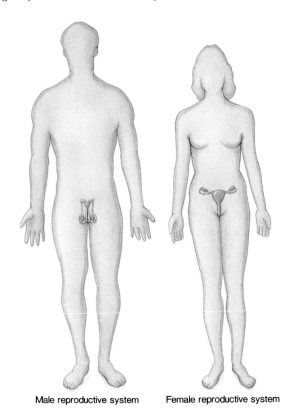

Male reproductive system   Female reproductive system

The female reproductive system consists of the ovaries, uterine tubes, uterus, vagina, clitoris, and vulva. These organs produce and maintain female sex cells, or egg cells, receive the male cells, and transport the male and female cells within the female system. The female system also provides for the support and development of embryos and functions in the birth process.

Figure 2.11 illustrates female and male reproductive systems.

Chart 2.2 summarizes features of the major organ systems.

1. Name the major organ systems, and list the organs of each system.
2. Describe the general functions of each organ system.

Anatomical Terminology

To communicate with each other more effectively, investigators over the ages have developed a set of terms with precise meanings. Some of these terms concern the relative positions of body parts, others refer to imaginary planes along which cuts may be made, and still others describe various regions of the body.

When such terms are used, it is assumed that the body is in the **anatomical position;** that is, it is standing erect, the face is forward, and the arms are at the sides, with the palms forward.

Relative Position

Terms of relative position are used to describe the location of one body part with respect to another. They include the following:

1. **Superior** means a part is above another part, or closer to the head. (The thoracic cavity is superior to the abdominopelvic cavity.)
2. **Inferior** means situated below another part, or toward the feet. (The neck is inferior to the head.)
3. **Anterior** (or ventral) means toward the front. (The eyes are anterior to the brain.)
4. **Posterior** (or dorsal) is the opposite of anterior; it means toward the back. (The pharynx is posterior to the oral cavity.)
5. **Medial** relates to an imaginary midline dividing the body into equal right and left halves. A part is medial if it is closer to this line than another part. (The nose is medial to the eyes.)

Terms such as *medial* and *lateral aspect* are often used to describe a view from the medial or lateral side. Thus, the medial aspect of a structure would show the medial surface.

6. **Lateral** means toward the side with respect to the imaginary midline. (The ears are lateral to the eyes.) **Bilateral** refers to two sides. (The human body has bilateral construction in that it has two similar sides.) **Ipsilateral** pertains to the same side (the spleen and the descending colon are ipsilateral), while **contralateral** refers to the opposite side (the spleen and the gallbladder are contralateral).
7. **Proximal** is used to describe a part that is closer to a point of attachment or closer to the trunk of the body than another part. (The elbow is proximal to the wrist; the duodenum is the proximal portion of the small intestine.)
8. **Distal** is the opposite of proximal. It means a particular body part is farther from the point of attachment or farther from the trunk than another part. (The fingers are distal to the wrist; the ileum is the distal portion of the small intestine.)

Chart 2.2 Organ systems		
Organ system	**Major organs**	**Major functions**
Integumentary	Skin, hair, nails, sebaceous glands	Protect tissues, regulate body temperature, support sensory structures
Skeletal	Bones, ligaments, cartilage	Provide framework, protect soft tissues, provide attachments for muscles, produce blood cells, store minerals
Muscular	Muscles	Cause movements, maintain posture, produce body heat
Nervous	Brain, spinal cord, nerves, sense organs	Detect changes, receive and interpret sensory information, stimulate muscles and glands
Endocrine	Pituitary, thyroid, parathyroid, adrenal glands, pancreas, ovaries, testes, and other glands that secrete hormones	Control activities of body structures
Digestive	Mouth, pharynx, esophagus, stomach, liver, gallbladder, pancreas, small and large intestines	Receive, break down, and absorb food; eliminate unabsorbed material
Respiratory	Nasal cavity, pharynx, larynx, trachea, bronchi, lungs	Intake and output of air, exchange of gases between air and blood
Cardiovascular	Heart, arteries, veins, capillaries	Pump blood through blood vessels and transport substances throughout body
Lymphatic	Lymphatic vessels, lymph nodes, thymus, spleen	Return tissue fluid to blood vessels, carry certain absorbed food molecules, defend the body against infection
Urinary	Kidneys, ureters, urinary bladder, urethra	Remove wastes from blood, maintain water and electrolyte balance, store and transport urine
Reproductive	Male: scrotum, testes, epididymides, vasa deferentia, seminal vesicles, prostate gland, bulbourethral glands, urethra, penis	Produce and maintain sperm cells, transfer sperm cells into female reproductive tract
	Female: ovaries, uterine tubes, uterus, vagina, clitoris, vulva	Produce and maintain egg cells; receive and transport sperm cells; support development of an embryo and function in birth process

9. **Superficial** means situated near the surface. (The epidermis is the superficial layer of skin.) **Peripheral** also means outward or away from the center. It is used to describe the location of certain blood vessels and nerves. (The nerves that branch from the brain and spinal cord are peripheral nerves.)

10. **Deep** is used to describe parts that are more internal. (The dermis is the deep layer of skin.)

Body Sections

To observe the relative locations and arrangements of internal parts, it is necessary to cut or section the body along various planes (figures 2.12 and 2.13). The following terms are used to describe such planes and sections:

1. **Sagittal.** This refers to a lengthwise cut that divides the body into right and left portions. If a sagittal section passes along the midline and divides the body into equal parts, it is called *median* (midsagittal).

2. **Transverse** (or *horizontal*) refers to a cut that divides the body into superior and inferior portions.

FIGURE 2.12

To observe internal parts, the body may be sectioned along various planes.

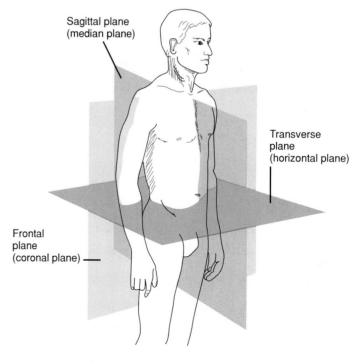

Sagittal plane (median plane)

Transverse plane (horizontal plane)

Frontal plane (coronal plane)

Body Organization and Terminology   39

FIGURE 2.13

A human brain sectioned along (*a*) the sagittal plane, (*b*) the transverse plane, and (*c*) the frontal plane.

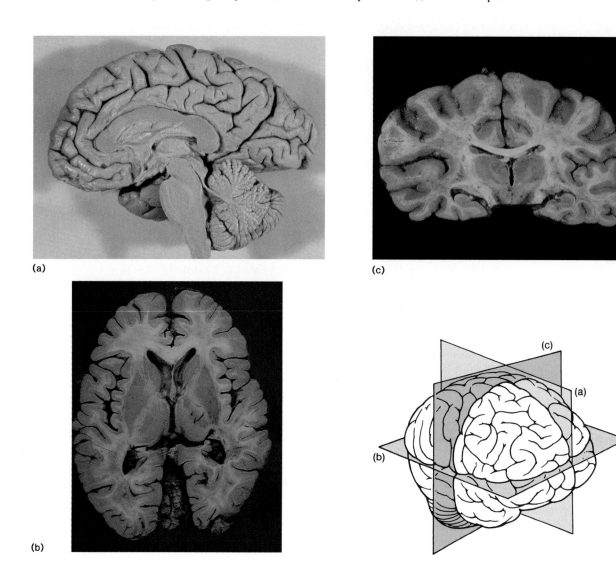

(a)

(c)

(b)

FIGURE 2.14

Cylindrical parts may be cut in (*a*) cross section, (*b*) oblique section, or (*c*) longitudinal section.

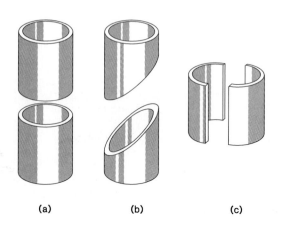

(a)   (b)   (c)

3. **Frontal** (or *coronal*) refers to a section that divides the body into anterior and posterior portions.

Sometimes an elongated organ such as a blood vessel is sectioned. In this case, a cut across the structure is called a *cross section*, a lengthwise cut is called a *longitudinal section*, and an angular cut is called an *oblique section* (figure 2.14).

Body Regions

A number of terms are used to designate various body regions. The abdominal area, for example, is subdivided into the following nine regions, as shown in figure 2.15:

1. **Epigastric region:** upper middle portion.
2. **Left** and **right hypochondriac regions:** on each side of the epigastric region.
3. **Umbilical region:** central portion.

FIGURE 2.15

The abdominal area is subdivided into nine regions. How do the names of these regions describe their locations?

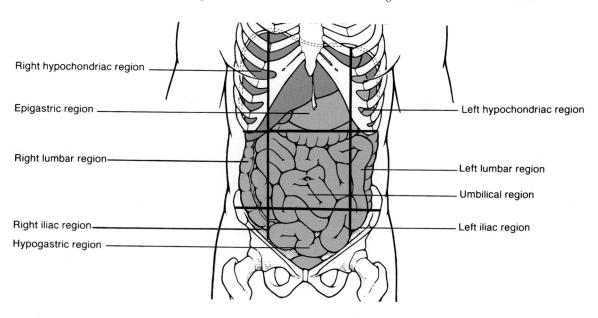

Right hypochondriac region

Epigastric region

Right lumbar region

Right iliac region

Hypogastric region

Left hypochondriac region

Left lumbar region

Umbilical region

Left iliac region

FIGURE 2.16

The abdominal area may be subdivided into four quadrants.

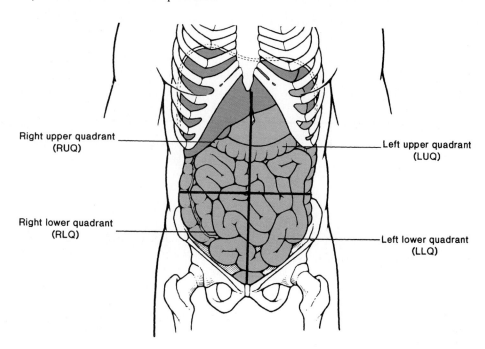

Right upper quadrant (RUQ)

Right lower quadrant (RLQ)

Left upper quadrant (LUQ)

Left lower quadrant (LLQ)

4. **Left** and **right lumbar regions:** on each side of the umbilical region.
5. **Hypogastric region:** lower middle portion.
6. **Left** and **right iliac regions:** on each side of the hypogastric region.

These nine regions are created by planes through surface landmarks.

1. One horizontal plane just inferior to the rib cage.
2. One horizontal plane just inferior to the tops of the hip bones.
3. Two vertical planes through the nipples.

Another method of designating abdominal regions is to divide the area into four quadrants by passing two perpendicular lines through the umbilicus (navel). Figure 2.16 illustrates these quadrants.

FIGURE 2.17

Some terms used to describe body regions: (*a*) anterior regions; (*b*) posterior regions.

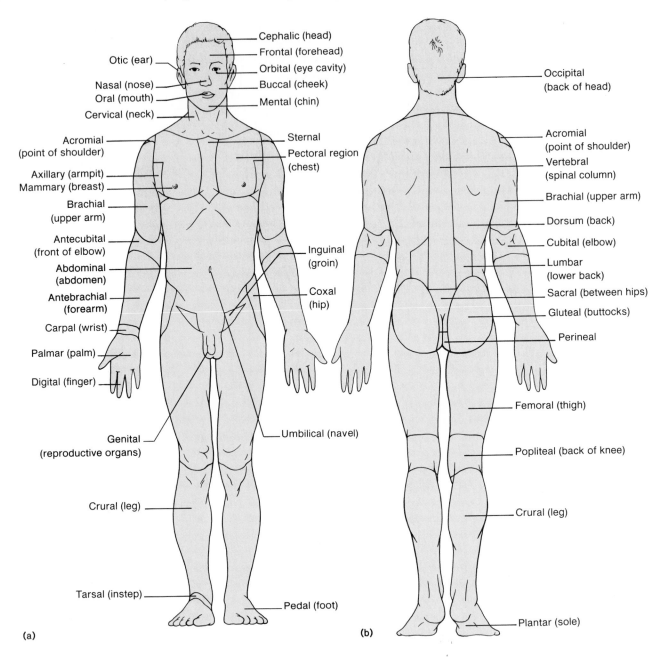

(a)

(b)

Other terms commonly used to indicate regions of the body include the following (figures 2.17 and 2.18 illustrate some of these regions):

Abdominal (ab-dom′ĭ-nal) the region between the thorax and pelvis.

Acromial (ah-kro′me-al) the point of the shoulder.

Antebrachial (an″te-bra′ke-al) the forearm.

Antecubital (an″te-ku′bĭ-tal) the space in front of the elbow.

Axillary (ak′sĭ-ler″e) the armpit.

Brachial (bra′ke-al) the upper arm.

Buccal (buk′al) the cheek.

Calcaneal (kal-ka′ne-al) the heel bone.

Carpal (kar′pal) the wrist.

Celiac (se′le-ak) the abdomen.

Cephalic (sĕ-fal′ik) the head.

Cervical (ser′vĭ-kal) the neck.

Clavicular (kla-vik′u-lar) the area over the clavicles (collar bones).

FIGURE 2.18
Some terms used to describe body regions: (*a*) anterior regions; (*b*) posterior regions.

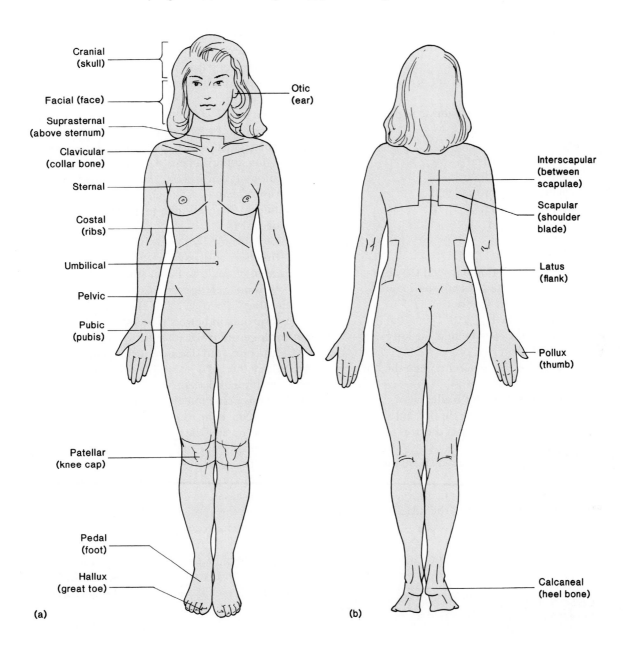

Cranial (skull)
Facial (face)
Otic (ear)
Suprasternal (above sternum)
Clavicular (collar bone)
Sternal
Costal (ribs)
Umbilical
Pelvic
Pubic (pubis)
Patellar (knee cap)
Pedal (foot)
Hallux (great toe)

(a)

Interscapular (between scapulae)
Scapular (shoulder blade)
Latus (flank)
Pollux (thumb)
Calcaneal (heel bone)

(b)

Costal (kos′tal) the ribs.
Coxal (kok′sal) the hip.
Cranial (kra′ni-al) the part of the skull that encloses the brain.
Crural (krōōr′al) the leg.
Cubital (ku′bǐ-tal) the elbow.
Digital (dij′ǐ-tal) the finger.
Dorsum (dor′sum) the back.
Facial (fa′shel) the face.

Femoral (fem′or-al) the thigh.
Frontal (frun′tal) the forehead.
Genital (jen′i-tal) the reproductive organs.
Gluteal (gloo′te-al) the buttocks.
Hallux (hal′uks) the great toe.
Infrascapular (in″fra-skap′u-lar) the area below the scapula (shoulder blade).
Inguinal (ing′gwi-nal) the depressed area of the abdominal wall near the thigh (groin).

Interscapular (in″ter-skap′u-lar) the area between the scapulae.

Latus (la′tus) the outer side between the ribs and upper border of the pelvis (flank).

Lumbar (lum′bar) the region of the lower back between the ribs and the pelvis (loin).

Mammary (mam′er-e) the breast.

Mental (men′tal) the chin.

Nasal (na′zal) the nose.

Occipital (ok-sip′ĭ-tal) the lower posterior region of the head.

Oral (o′ral) the mouth.

Orbital (or′bi-tal) the eye cavity.

Otic (o′tik) the ear.

Palmar (pahl′mar) the palm of the hand.

Patellar (pa-tel′ar) the kneecap.

Pectoral (pek′tor-al) the chest.

Pedal (ped′l) the foot.

Pelvic (pel′vik) the pelvis.

Perineal (per″ĭ-ne′al) the region between the anus and the external reproductive organs (perineum).

Plantar (plan′tar) the sole of the foot.

Pollux (pol′eks) the thumb.

Popliteal (pop″lĭ-te′al) the area behind the knee.

Pubic (pu′bik) the pubis.

Sacral (sa′kral) the posterior region between the hip bones.

Scapular (skap′u-lar) the shoulder blade.

Sternal (ster′nal) the middle of the thorax, anteriorly.

Supraclavicular (su″pra-kla-vik′u-lar) the area above the clavicle (collar bones).

Suprasternal (su″pra-ster′nal) the area above the sternum.

Tarsal (tahr′sal) the instep of the foot.

Temporal (tem″por-al) the region of the head in front of the ear and over the zygomatic arch.

Umbilical (um-bil′ĭ-kal) the navel.

Vertebral (ver′te-bral) the spinal column.

---

1. Describe the anatomical position.
2. Using the appropriate terms, describe the relative positions of several body parts.
3. Describe three types of sections.
4. Identify the nine regions of the abdomen.

Some Medical and Applied Sciences

cardiology (kar″de-ol′o-je) branch of medical science dealing with the heart and heart diseases.

cytology (si-tol′o-je) study of the structure, function, and diseases of cells.

dentistry (den′tis-tre) branch of medicine dealing with the care of teeth and associated structures of the oral cavity.

dermatology (der″mah-tol′o-je) study of skin and its diseases.

endocrinology (en″do-krĭ-nol′o-je) study of hormones, hormone-secreting glands, and diseases involving them.

epidemiology (ep″ĭ-de″me-ol′o-je) study of infectious diseases, their distribution within a population and their control.

gastroenterology (gas″tro-en″ter-ol′o-je) study of the stomach and intestines, and diseases involving these organs.

geriatrics (jer″e-at′riks) branch of medicine dealing with elderly persons and their medical problems.

gerontology (jer″on-tol′o-je) study of the process of aging and problems of elderly persons.

gynecology (gi″nĕ-kol′o-je) study of the female reproductive system and its diseases.

hematology (hem″ah-tol′o-je) study of blood and blood diseases.

histology (his-tol′o-je) study of the structure and function of tissues.

immunology (im″u-nol′o-je) study of the body's resistance to disease.

neonatology (ne″o-na-tol′o-je) study and treatment of disorders in newborn infants.

nephrology (nĕ-frol′o-je) study of the structure, function, and diseases of the kidneys.

neurology (nu-rol′o-je) study of the nervous system in health and disease.

nuclear medicine (nu′kle-ar med′ĭ-sin) branch of medicine concerned with the use of radiation.

obstetrics (ob-stet′riks) branch of medicine dealing with pregnancy and childbirth.

oncology (ong-kol′o-je) study of tumors.

ophthalmology (of″thal-mol′o-je) study of the eye and eye diseases.

orthopedics (or″tho-pe′diks) branch of medicine dealing with the muscular and skeletal systems, and problems of these systems.

otolaryngology (o″to-lar″in-gol′o-je) study of the ear, throat, and larynx, and diseases of these parts.

pathology (pah-thol′o-je) study of body changes produced by diseases.

pediatrics (pe″de-at′riks) branch of medicine dealing with children and their diseases.

pharmacology (fahr″mah-kol′o-je) study of drugs and their uses in the treatment of diseases.

podiatry (po-di′ah-tre) study of the care and treatment of the feet.

psychiatry (si-ki′ah-tre) branch of medicine dealing with the mind and its disorders.

radiology (ra″de-ol′o-je) study of X rays and radioactive substances as well as their uses in diagnosing and treating disease.

toxicology (tok″sĭ-kol′o-je) study of poisonous substances and their effects upon body parts.

urology (u-rol′o-je) branch of medicine dealing with the kidneys and urinary system, and their diseases.

Chapter Summary

Introduction (page 29)

Levels of Organization (page 29)
The body is composed of parts that occupy different levels of organization.

1. All material substances are composed of atoms that unite to form molecules.
2. Organelles contain aggregates of large molecules.
3. Cells, which are composed of organelles, are the basic units of structure and function within the body.
4. Cells are organized into layers or masses called tissues.
5. Tissues are organized into organs, which are arranged into organ systems, constituting the organism.
6. These parts vary in complexity progressively from one level to the next.

Organization of the Human Body (page 30)
1. Body cavities
   a. The axial portion of the body contains the posterior (dorsal) and anterior (ventral) cavities.
      (1) The posterior cavity includes the cranial and vertebral cavities.
      (2) The anterior cavity includes the thoracic and abdominopelvic cavities, which are separated by the diaphragm.
   b. The organs within a body cavity are called visceral organs.
   c. Other body cavities include the oral, nasal, orbital, and middle ear cavities.
2. Thoracic and abdominopelvic membranes
   a. Thoracic membranes
      (1) Pleural membranes line the thoracic cavity and cover the lungs.
      (2) Pericardial membranes surround the heart and cover its surface.
      (3) The pleural and pericardial cavities are potential spaces between these membranes.
   b. Abdominopelvic membranes
      (1) Peritoneal membranes line the abdominopelvic cavity and cover the organs inside.
      (2) The peritoneal cavity is a potential space between these membranes.
3. Organ systems
   The human organism consists of several organ systems. Each system includes a set of interrelated organs with specific functions.
   a. The integumentary system provides the body covering that protects underlying tissues, regulates body temperature, houses sensory receptors, and synthesizes various cellular substances.
   b. The skeletal system, composed of bones, ligaments, and cartilages, provides frameworks, protective shields, and attachments for muscles; it also produces blood cells and stores inorganic salts.
   c. The muscular system includes the muscles of the body and is responsible for body movements and maintenance of posture.
   d. The nervous system consists of the brain, spinal cord, nerves, and sense organs; nerve cells receive nerve impulses and interpret and act on these impulses by causing muscles or glands to respond.
   e. The endocrine system consists of glands that secrete hormones. Hormones help regulate body activities. It includes the pituitary, thyroid, parathyroid, and adrenal glands; the pancreas, ovaries, testes, pineal gland, thymus gland, and placenta.
   f. The digestive system organs receive food, convert food molecules into forms that can pass through cell membranes, and eliminate the materials that are not absorbed.
   g. The respiratory system provides for the intake and output of air, and for the exchange of gases between the blood and the air. It includes the airways and lungs.
   h. The cardiovascular system includes the heart, which pumps blood, and arteries, veins, and capillaries, which carry blood to and from body parts.
   i. The lymphatic system is composed of lymphatic vessels, lymph nodes, lymph, the thymus gland, and the spleen. It transports lymph from tissue spaces to the blood stream, carries lipids from the digestive organs, and aids in defending the body against infections.
   j. The urinary system includes the kidneys, ureters, urinary bladder, and urethra. It filters wastes from the blood and helps maintain fluid and electrolyte balance.
   k. The reproductive systems are concerned with the production of new organisms.
      (1) The male reproductive system organs produce, maintain, and transport male sex cells.
      (2) The female reproductive system organs produce, maintain, and transport female sex cells, and function in childbirth.

Anatomical Terminology (page 38)
Terms with precise meanings are used to help investigators communicate effectively.

1. Relative position: These terms are used to describe the location of one part with respect to another part.
2. Body sections: Body sections are planes along which the body may be cut to observe the relative locations and arrangements of internal parts.
3. Body regions: Various body regions are designated by special terms.

Clinical Application of Knowledge

1. Suppose two individuals are afflicted with benign (noncancerous) tumors that produce symptoms because they occupy space and crowd adjacent organs. If one of these persons has the tumor in the anterior cavity and the other has it in the posterior cavity, which would be likely to develop symptoms first? Why?
2. When a woman is pregnant, what changes would occur in the relative sizes of the abdominal and pelvic portions of the abdominopelvic cavity?

3. Inhaling involves flattening of the diaphragm. How would this alter the size and shape of the thoracic and abdominal cavities?

4. If a patient complained of a "stomachache" and pointed to the umbilical region as the site of the discomfort, what organs located in this region might be the source of the pain?

Review Activities

Part A

1. Explain what is meant by levels of organization.
2. List the levels of organization within the human.
3. Distinguish between the axial and appendicular portions of the body.
4. Distinguish between the posterior and anterior body cavities, and name the smaller cavities that occur within each.
5. Explain what is meant by a *visceral organ.*
6. Describe the mediastinum.
7. Describe the location of the oral, nasal, orbital, and middle ear cavities.
8. Distinguish between a parietal and a visceral membrane.
9. Name the major organ systems, and describe the general functions of each.
10. List the major organs that comprise each organ system.
11. Name the body cavity in which each of the following organs is located:
    a. Stomach
    b. Heart
    c. Brain
    d. Liver
    e. Trachea
    f. Rectum
    g. Spinal cord
    h. Esophagus
    i. Spleen
    j. Urinary bladder

12. Write complete sentences using each of the following terms correctly:
    a. Superior
    b. Inferior
    c. Anterior
    d. Posterior
    e. Medial
    f. Lateral
    g. Ipsilateral
    h. Contralateral
    i. Proximal
    j. Distal
    k. Superficial
    l. Peripheral
    m. Deep

13. Prepare a sketch of a human body, and use lines to indicate each of the following sections:
    a. Sagittal
    b. Median
    c. Transverse
    d. Frontal

14. Prepare a sketch of the abdominal area and indicate the location of each of the following regions:
    a. Epigastric
    b. Umbilical
    c. Hypogastric
    d. Hypochondriac
    e. Lumbar
    f. Iliac

Part B

Provide the common name for the region to which each of the following terms pertains:

    a. Acromial
    b. Antebrachial
    c. Axillary
    d. Buccal
    e. Celiac
    f. Clavicular
    g. Coxal
    h. Cranial
    i. Crural
    j. Femoral
    k. Gluteal
    l. Inguinal
    m. Mental
    n. Occipital
    o. Orbital
    p. Palmar
    q. Pectoral
    r. Pedal
    s. Perineal
    t. Plantar
    u. Popliteal
    v. Sacral
    w. Sternal
    x. Tarsal
    y. Temporal
    z. Vertebral

CHAPTER 3

The Cell

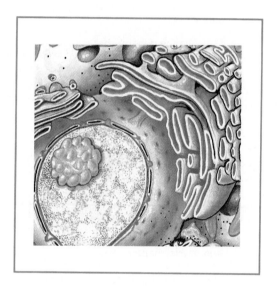

The human body is composed entirely of cells, products of cells, and various fluids. These cells represent the basic structural units of the body; they are the building blocks from which all larger parts are formed. They are also the functional units, because whatever a body part can do is the result of activities within its cells.

Cells account for the shape, organization, and construction of the body and carry on its life processes. In addition, they can reproduce and thus provide the new cells needed for growth, development, and the replacement of worn and injured tissues.

Chapter Outline

Chapter Objectives

After you have studied this chapter, you should be able to

1. Explain how cells differ from one another.

2. Describe the general characteristics of a composite cell.

3. Explain the functions of a cell membrane.

4. Describe each kind of cytoplasmic organelle and explain its function.

5. Describe the cell nucleus and its parts.

6. Describe the life cycle of a cell.

7. Explain how a cell reproduces.

8. Complete the review activities at the end of this chapter. Note that the items are worded in the form of specific learning objectives. You may want to refer to them before reading the chapter.

Aids to Understanding Words

chromo-, color: *chromo*some—dark-staining structures within the nucleus of a cell.

cyt-, cell: *cyt*oplasm—fluid that occupies the space between the cell membrane and nuclear envelope.

endo-, within: *endo*plasmic reticulum—network of membranes within cytoplasm.

inter-, between: *inter*phase—stage that occurs between mitotic divisions of a cell.

lys-, to break up: *lys*osome—organelle that contains chemicals capable of breaking up cell structures.

mit-, thread: *mit*osis—process during which threadlike chromosomes appear within a cell.

nucl-, kernel: *nucl*eus—central structure within a cell.

-plasm, matter: cyto*plasm*—fluid that occupies the space between the cell membrane and nuclear envelope.

reticulum, net: endoplasmic *reticulum*—network of membranes within cytoplasm.

-som, body: ribo*som*e—tiny, spherical organelle.

syn-, together: *syn*thesis—process by which substances are united to form a new type of substance.

vesic-, bladder: *vesic*le—small sac containing material from a cell.

Introduction

It is estimated that an adult human body consists of about 75 trillion cells. These **cells** have much in common, yet those in different tissues vary in a number of ways. For example, they vary considerably in size.

Cell sizes are measured in units called *micrometers*. A micrometer equals 1/1000th of a millimeter and is symbolized μm. Measured in micrometers, a human egg cell is about 140 μm in diameter and is just barely visible to an unaided eye. This is large when compared to a red blood cell, which is about 7.5 μm in diameter, or the most common white blood cells, which vary from 10–12 μm in diameter. On the other hand, smooth muscle cells can be between 20–500 μm long (figure 3.1).

Cells also vary in shape, and typically their shapes are closely related to their functions (figure 3.2). For instance, nerve cells often have long, threadlike extensions that transmit nerve impulses from one part of the body to another. The epithelial cells that line the inside of the mouth shield underlying cells. These protective cells are thin, flattened, and tightly packed, somewhat like the tiles of a floor. Muscle cells, which function to pull parts closer together, are slender and rodlike, with their ends attached to the parts they move.

FIGURE 3.1

Cells vary considerably in size. (*a*) Red blood cell, 7.5 μm in diameter; (*b*) white blood cell, 10–12 μm in diameter; (*c*) human egg cell, 140 μm in diameter; (*d*) smooth muscle cell, 50–500 μm in length.

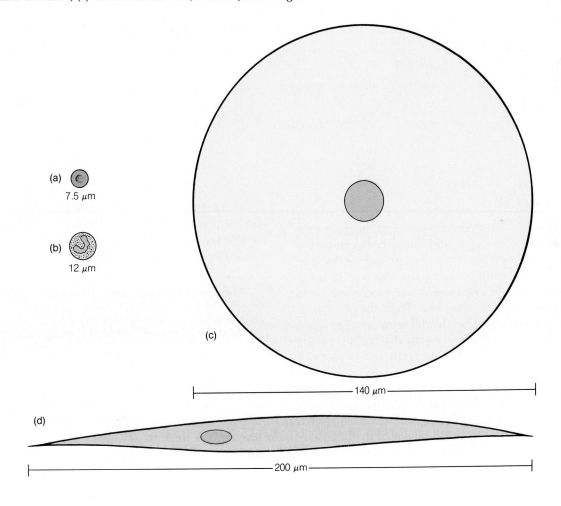

FIGURE 3.2
Cells vary in structure and function. (*a*) A nerve cell transmits impulses from one body part to another; (*b*) epithelial cells protect underlying cells; and (*c*) muscle cells pull parts closer together.

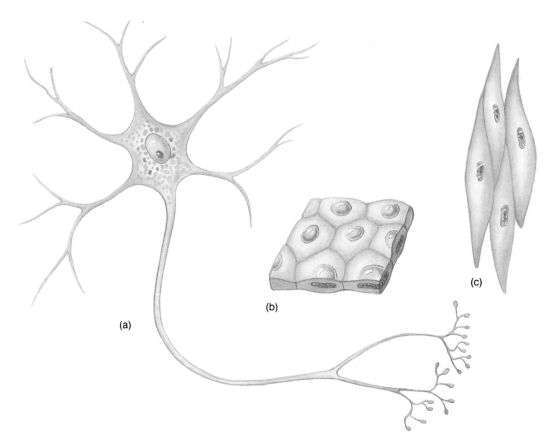

(a)

(b)

(c)

A Composite Cell

It is not possible to describe a typical cell, because cells vary so greatly in size, shape, and function. For purposes of discussion, however, it is convenient to imagine that one exists. Such a cell would contain parts observed in many kinds of cells, even though some of these cells lack parts included in the imagined structure. Thus, the cell shown in figure 3.3 and described in the following sections is not real. Instead, it is a *composite cell*—one that includes many known cell structures. In specialized cells, one or more of these structures are emphasized.

Commonly, a cell consists of two major parts—the nucleus and the cytoplasm. The *nucleus* is the innermost part and is enclosed by a thin, double-layered membrane called a *nuclear envelope*. The *cytoplasm* is a mass of fluid that surrounds the nucleus and is itself encircled by a *cell membrane* (or a cytoplasmic membrane).

Within the cytoplasm are specialized cellular parts called *cytoplasmic organelles*. These organelles perform specific functions necessary for cell survival. The nucleus directs the overall activities of the cell.

1. Give two examples to illustrate that the shape of a cell is related to its function.
2. Name the two major parts of a cell.
3. What are the general functions of these two parts?

Cell Membrane

The cell membrane is the outermost limit of a cell, but it is more than a simple envelope surrounding the cellular contents. It is an actively functioning part of the living material, and many important reactions take place on its surfaces.

FIGURE 3.3
A composite cell. (Note that the organelles of this composite cell are not drawn to scale.)

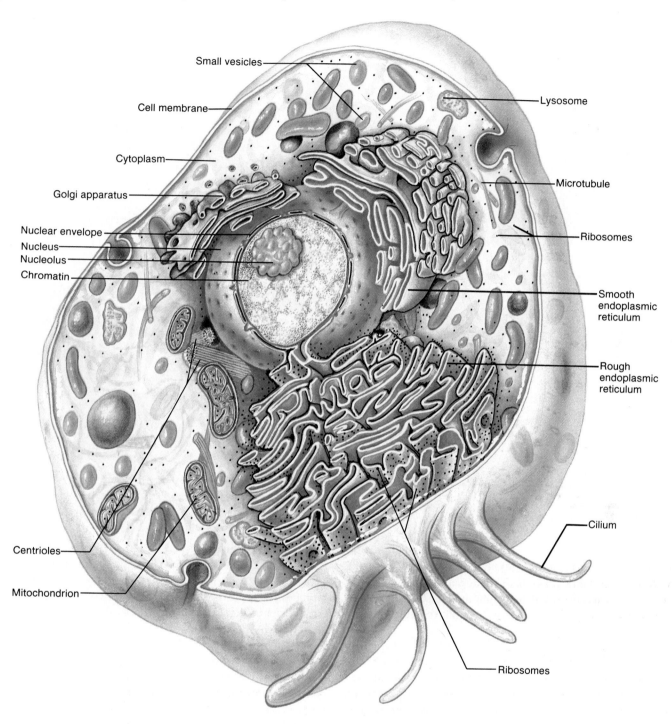

Small vesicles

Cell membrane

Cytoplasm

Golgi apparatus

Nuclear envelope

Nucleus

Nucleolus

Chromatin

Centrioles

Mitochondrion

Lysosome

Microtubule

Ribosomes

Smooth endoplasmic reticulum

Rough endoplasmic reticulum

Cilium

Ribosomes

FIGURE 3.4

(a) The cell membrane consists of two layers, which can be seen in this transmission electron micrograph (×250,000). (b) Pore-forming particles are scattered throughout the membrane.

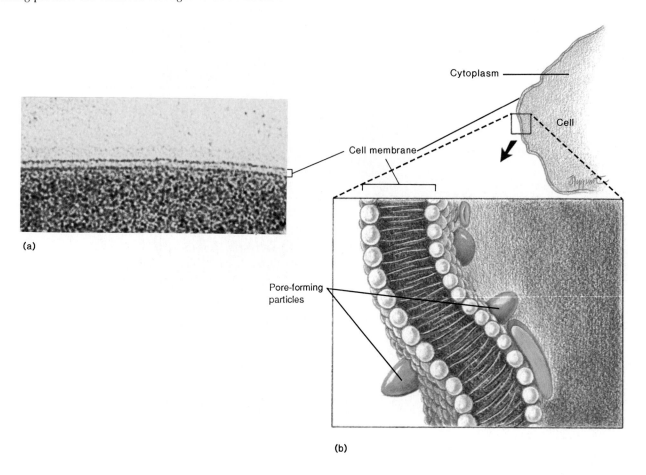

(a)

(b)

General Characteristics

The cell membrane is extremely thin—visible only with the aid of an electron microscope—but it is flexible and somewhat elastic. It consists of two layers and many pore-forming particles (figure 3.4). It typically has a complex surface with many outpouchings and infoldings that provide extra surface area. The membrane quickly seals minute breaks, but if it is extensively damaged, the cell contents escape, and the cell dies.

In addition to maintaining the wholeness of the cell, the membrane controls the entrance and exit of substances. That is, it allows some substances to pass through the membrane and excludes others. This occurs through pores. A membrane that functions in this manner is called *selectively permeable.*

Intercellular Junctions

Many cells, such as blood cells, are not in direct contact with one another, because fluid-filled space (intercellular space) separates them. In other cases, however, the cells are tightly packed, and their cell membranes are commonly connected by **intercellular junctions.** In one type,

called a *tight junction,* the membranes of adjacent cells converge and become fused together. This fusion surrounds the cell like a belt, and the junction closes the intercellular space between the cells. Cells that form sheetlike layers, such as those that line the inside of the digestive tube, often are joined by tight junctions. These junctions prevent substances from moving out of the tube between the cells.

Other intercellular junctions that function to hold cells together in sheets are adhesion belts and desmosomes. *Adhesion belts* create bands around cells and hold the cells together. *Desmosomes* serve to rivet or "spot weld" adjacent cells. Microfilaments in cells become attached to the desmosomes, strengthening them and forming a reinforced structural unit.

Cells such as heart muscle fibers and bone cells are interconnected by tubular channels called *gap junctions.* These channels link the cytoplasm of adjacent cells and allow the cells to exchange certain small molecules (figure 3.5).

Chart 3.1 summarizes the functions and gives examples of locations of the intercellular junctions.

FIGURE 3.5

(a) Many cells are joined by intercellular junctions. (b–d) Transmission electron micrographs of three types of intercellular junctions: (b) desmosome (×60,000); (c) tight junction (×182,272); and (d) gap junction.

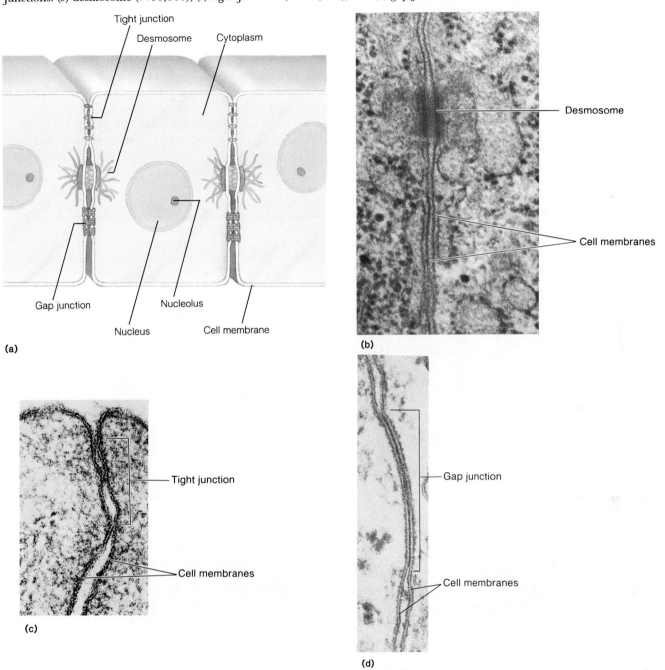

(a)

(b)

(c)

(d)

Chart 3.1 Types of intercellular junctions

Type	Function	Location
Tight junction	Close intercellular space between cells	Epithelial cells lining small intestine
Desmosome	Bind cells together	Epithelial cells of skin; heart muscle
Adhesion belt	Bind cells in sheets	Epithelial cells of skin and intestine
Gap junction	Form tubular channels between cells	Nerve cells, heart muscle, bone cells, and epithelial cells

Cytoplasm

When viewed through a light microscope, **cytoplasm** usually appears as a structureless substance with specks scattered throughout. However, a transmission electron microscope, which produces much greater magnification and resolution, reveals that cytoplasm contains networks of membranes and other organelles suspended in a clear liquid (cytosol).

The activities of a cell occur largely in its cytoplasm, where food molecules are received, processed, and used. In other words, cytoplasm is where the following **cytoplasmic organelles** play specific roles.

1. **Endoplasmic reticulum.** The endoplasmic reticulum (ER) is a complex network of interconnected membranes that form flattened sacs, elongated canals, and fluid-filled vesicles. This membranous network is connected to the nuclear envelope. Thus, endoplasmic reticulum is widely distributed through the cytoplasm. It functions as a tubular communication system through which molecules can be transported from one cell part to another.

The endoplasmic reticulum also plays a role in the synthesis of protein and other molecules.

FIGURE 3.6

(*a*) A transmission electron micrograph of rough endoplasmic reticulum (×100,000). (*b*) Rough endoplasmic reticulum has ribosomes attached to its surface, while (*c*) smooth endoplasmic reticulum lacks ribosomes. (*d*) A transmission electron micrograph of smooth endoplasmic reticulum.

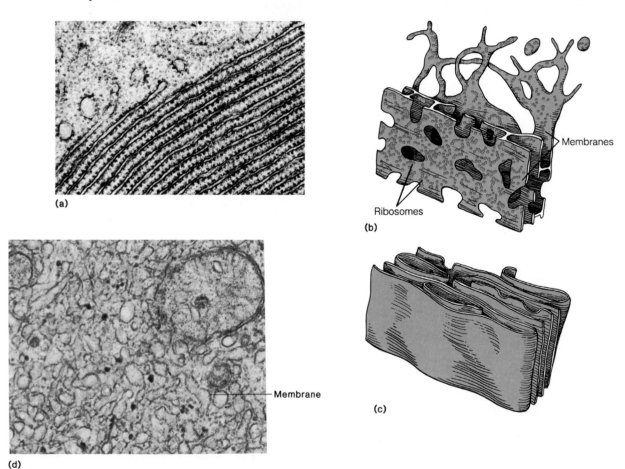

(a)

(d)

Membranes

Ribosomes

(b)

(c)

Membrane

Commonly, for example, its outer membranous surface has numerous tiny, spherical organelles, called **ribosomes,** attached to it. These particles cause the endoplasmic reticulum to have a textured appearance when visualized using an electron microscope. For this reason such endoplasmic reticulum is called *rough ER.* Endoplasmic reticulum, which lacks ribosomes, is called *smooth ER* (figure 3.6).

The ribosomes of rough endoplasmic reticulum synthesize proteins. The resulting molecules may be transported through tubules of the endoplasmic reticulum and then to the Golgi apparatus for further processing. Although rough endoplasmic reticulum is present in most cells, a large amount is found in certain pancreas cells (acinar cells), white blood cells (lymphocytes), and immature egg cells. Smooth endoplasmic reticulum, on the other hand, is involved in manufacturing various molecules, including certain hormones. Most cells contain little smooth endoplasmic reticulum. Cells that contain large amounts of smooth ER include liver cells, testis cells, and cells of the adrenal cortex.

2. **Ribosomes.** Although many ribosomes are attached to membranes of the endoplasmic reticulum, others occur as free particles scattered throughout the cytoplasm. These tiny, spherical particles function in the synthesis of protein molecules.

3. **Golgi apparatus.** The Golgi apparatus is usually located near the nucleus. It is composed of a stack of six or more flattened, membranous sacs called *cisternae.* The apparatus is involved in refining, "packaging," and delivering proteins synthesized by the ribosomes associated with the endoplasmic reticulum. (See figure 3.7.)

The proteins arrive at the Golgi apparatus enclosed in tiny sacs (vesicles) composed of membrane from the endoplasmic reticulum, which fuse with the membrane of the Golgi apparatus. The proteins then pass from layer to layer through the Golgi stacks and are modified chemically. When they reach the outermost layer, the altered proteins are packaged in bits of Golgi apparatus membrane that bud off and form transport vesicles. Such a vesicle may then move to the cell membrane, where it fuses with the membrane and releases its contents to the outside as a secretion. Other vesicles may transport membrane and proteins to various membranous organelles within the cell (figure 3.10). Note that although membrane is first assembled in the endoplasmic reticulum, portions of this membrane may then be transferred to the Golgi apparatus. From there, some of the membrane may move into the cytoplasm as part of a vesicle.

1. What is meant by a selectively permeable membrane?
2. Describe the types of intercellular junctions.
3. What are the functions of the endoplasmic reticulum?
4. Describe how the Golgi apparatus functions.

4. **Mitochondria.** Mitochondria are elongated, fluid-filled sacs 2–5 μm long that often move about slowly in the cytoplasm. Unlike other membranous organelles, mitochondria can divide to form new mitochondria.

FIGURE 3.7

(*a*) A transmission electron micrograph of a Golgi apparatus (×36,000). (*b*) The Golgi apparatus consists of membranous sacs that are continuous with the endoplasmic reticulum.

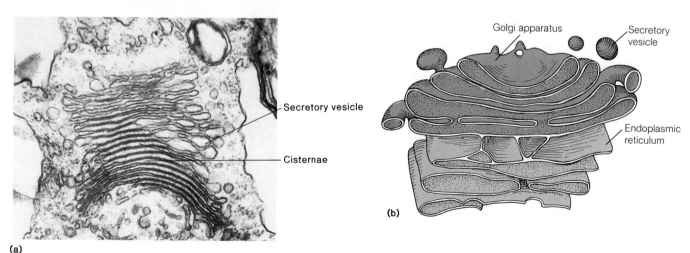

Golgi apparatus

Secretory vesicle

Secretory vesicle

Cisternae

Endoplasmic reticulum

(a)

(b)

FIGURE 3.8

(*a*) A transmission electron micrograph of a mitochondrion (×79,000). (*b*) Cristae form shelflike partitions within this saclike organelle.

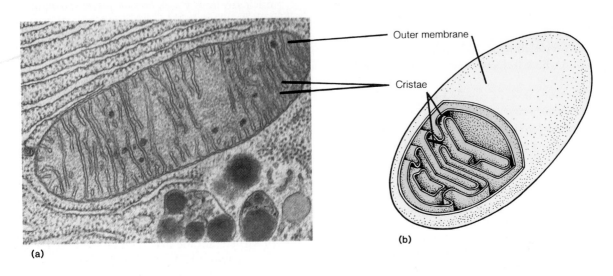

FIGURE 3.9

In this transmission electron micrograph, lysosomes appear as membranous sacs (×14,137).

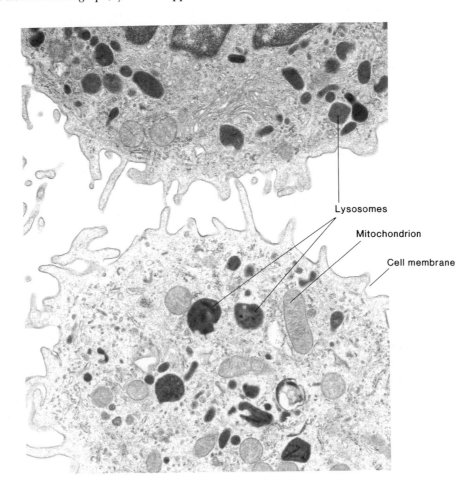

The membrane of a mitochondrion has two layers—an outer membrane and an inner membrane. The inner membrane is folded extensively to form shelflike partitions called *cristae*. Mitochondria control some of the chemical reactions by which energy is released from food. The mitochondria also function in transforming this energy into a chemical form that is usable by various cell parts. For this reason mitochondria are sometimes called the "powerhouses" of cells (figure 3.8).

5. **Lysosomes.** Lysosomes are sometimes difficult to identify because their shapes vary so greatly. However, they commonly appear as tiny, membranous sacs (figure 3.9). These sacs contain powerful chemicals that are capable of breaking down nutrients and foreign particles that enter cells. Certain white blood cells, for example, can engulf bacteria that are then digested by the lysosomes. Consequently, white blood cells help prevent bacterial infections. Such scavenger cells may also engulf dead or injured body cells and digest them. The organelles are then replaced with newly formed organelles. The lysosomal membrane is itself continually being replenished by vesicles coming from the Golgi apparatus. (See figure 3.10.)

Lysosomal digestive activity seems to be responsible for decreasing the size of body tissues at certain times. Such regression in size occurs in the maternal uterus following the birth of an infant, in the maternal breasts after the weaning of an infant, and in skeletal muscles during prolonged periods of inactivity.

6. **Peroxisomes.** Peroxisomes are membranous sacs that resemble lysosomes in size and shape. They occur most commonly in cells of the liver and kidneys, and contain substances that break down certain toxic chemicals, such as hydrogen peroxide.

7. **Vesicles.** Vesicles (vacuoles) are membranous sacs that vary in size. They may be formed by an action of the cell membrane in which a portion of the membrane folds inward and pinches off. As a result, a tiny bubblelike vesicle, containing some liquid or solid material that was outside the cell a moment before, appears in the cytoplasm (figure 3.10). Vesicles also may be formed from the Golgi apparatus during secretion of cell products.

FIGURE 3.10

A portion of cell membrane folds inward to form a vesicle. (*a*) Vesicles are also formed by the endoplasmic reticulum and (*b*) the Golgi apparatus. (*c, d*) Vesicles are moved between various organelles and the cell membrane.

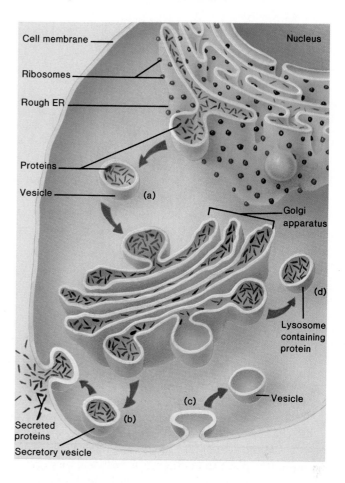

8. **Microfilaments** and **microtubules.** Two types of thin, threadlike structures found within the cytoplasm are microfilaments and microtubules.

Microfilaments are tiny rods arranged in meshworks or bundles. They cause various kinds of cellular movements. In muscle cells, for example, they are highly developed as *myofibrils*, which help these cells to shorten, or contract. In other cells, microfilaments are usually associated with the inner surface of the cell membrane and seem to aid in cell movement (figure 3.11).

Microtubules are long, slender tubes with a diameter two to three times greater than microfilaments. They are usually stiff, forming an

FIGURE 3.11

Bundles of microfilaments function in various types of cell movements.

Microfilaments   Microtubule

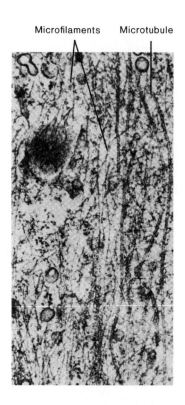

FIGURE 3.12

Microtubules help maintain the shape of a cell by forming an "internal skeleton" within the cytoplasm.

Cell membrane   Ribosome   Endoplasmic reticulum

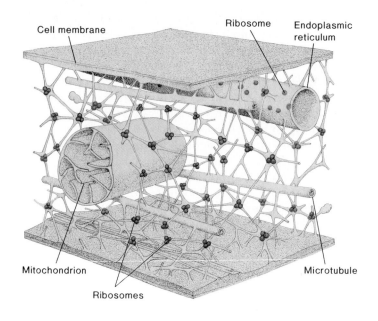

Mitochondrion   Ribosomes   Microtubule

"internal skeleton" within a cell, which helps maintain the shape of the cell or its parts (figure 3.12). For example, microtubules provide support to the structures called cilia and flagella.

Microtubules also aid in moving organelles from one place to another. For instance, they are involved in the movement of vesicles and other membranous organelles. Most microtubules are formed in an area called the centrosome.

9. **Centrosome.** A centrosome (central body) is a region in the cytoplasm near the Golgi apparatus and nucleus. It is nonmembranous and consists of two hollow cylinders called *centrioles,* which, in turn, contain microtubules. The centrioles usually lie at right angles to each other and function in cell reproduction. During this process, the centriole pairs move away from one another and take positions on either side of the nucleus. There they aid in distributing structures called chromosomes, which carry inherited information to the newly forming cells (figure 3.13). Centrioles also function

in initiating the formation of hairlike cellular projections called cilia and flagella.

10. **Cilia** and **flagella.** Cilia and flagella are motile processes that extend outward from the surfaces of certain cells. They are structurally similar and differ mainly in their length and in the number present. Both contain a constant number of microtubules arranged in a distinct pattern.

Cilia occur in large numbers on the free surfaces of some cells. Each cilium is a tiny, hairlike structure about 10 μm long and is attached just beneath the cell membrane to a modified centriole called a *basal body.* Cilia are arranged in precise patterns, and they have a "to-and-fro" type of movement. This movement is coordinated so that rows of cilia beat one after the other, creating a wave of motion that sweeps across the ciliated surface. This action propels fluids, such as mucus, over the surface of certain tissues, such as those that form the lining of the respiratory tubes. (See figure 3.14.)

FIGURE 3.13

(a) A transmission electron micrograph of the two centrioles in a centrosome (×142,000). (b) Note that the centrioles lie at right angles to one another.

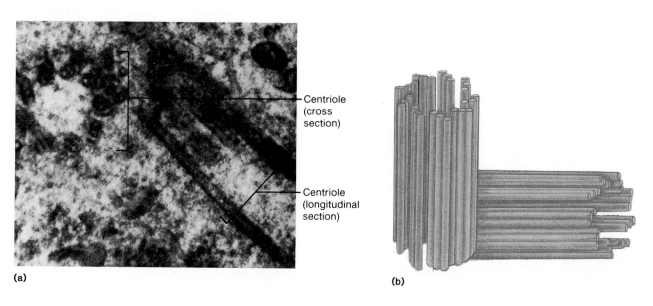

(a)

(b)

FIGURE 3.14

(a) Cilia (arrows) are common on the surface of certain cells that form the inner lining of respiratory tubes. (b) Each cilium has a "to-and-fro" movement. (c) An electron micrograph of a cross section of a basal body (×10,000).

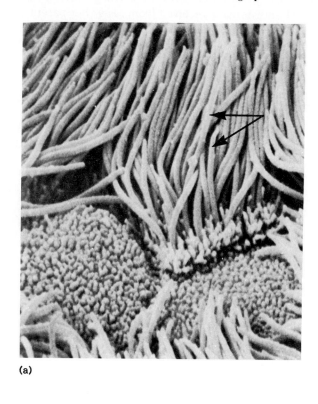

(a)

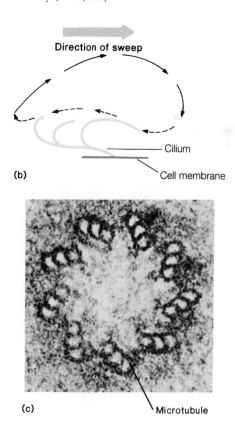

(b)

(c)

Flagella are considerably longer than cilia, and usually there is only a single flagellum on a cell. These projections have an undulating, wavelike motion that begins at the base of a flagellum. The tail of a sperm cell, for example, is a flagellum that causes the sperm's swimming movement. (See figure 3.15.)

In addition to these functional organelles, cytoplasm may contain masses of lifeless chemical substances called *inclusions*. Most commonly, inclusions consist of cellular products that remain in a cell only temporarily. Examples of inclusions are various stored nutrients and pigments.

1. Why are mitochondria sometimes called the "powerhouses" of cells?
2. Trace the pathways of vesicles formed by the endoplasmic reticulum.
3. Describe the functions of microfilaments and microtubules.
4. Distinguish between organelles and inclusions.

Cell Nucleus

A **nucleus** is a cellular organelle that is usually located near the center of the cell's cytoplasm. It is a relatively large, usually spherical structure that directs the activities of the cell.

The nucleus is enclosed in a double-layered *nuclear envelope* that consists of an inner and an outer membrane. These two membranes have a narrow space between them, but are joined at various places that surround relatively large openings, or "pores." The pores in the nuclear envelope allow certain dissolved substances to move between the nucleus and the cytoplasm (figure 3.16).

The nucleus contains a fluid (nucleoplasm) in which other structures float. These structures include the following:

1. *Nucleolus.* A nucleolus ("little nucleus") is a small, dense body. It has no surrounding membrane and is formed in specialized regions of certain chromosomes. It functions in the production of ribosomes. Once ribosomes are formed, they migrate through the pores in the nuclear envelope and enter the cytoplasm. The nuclei of cells that synthesize large amounts of protein, such as those of glands, may contain especially large nucleoli.
2. *Chromatin.* Chromatin consists of loosely coiled fibers present in the nuclear fluid. When the cell begins to undergo the reproductive process, these fibers become more tightly coiled into tiny, rodlike *chromosomes.*

Chromatin fibers are composed mainly of DNA (*deoxyribonucleic acid*) molecules that contain the genetic information of the cell. This information is a set of instructions that directs the cell to make specific structures and to carry out its life processes. The *genetic information* of each individual is received from his or her parent's sex cells, and as a person develops from a fertilized egg cell, the information is passed from cell to cell during cell division.

Chart 3.2 summarizes the structures and functions of the cellular organelles.

FIGURE 3.15

(*a*) Scanning electron micrograph of human sperm cells (×4,000). Flagella form the tails of these cells; (*b*) a flagellum moves with a wavelike motion.

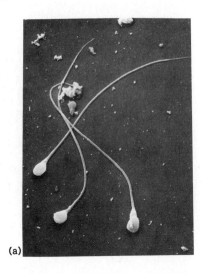

(a)

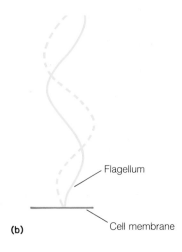

(b)

Flagellum

Cell membrane

FIGURE 3.16

(a) A transmission electron micrograph of a cell nucleus (×8,000). It contains a nucleolus and masses of chromatin.
(b) The nuclear envelope is porous and allows substances to pass between the nucleus and the cytoplasm.

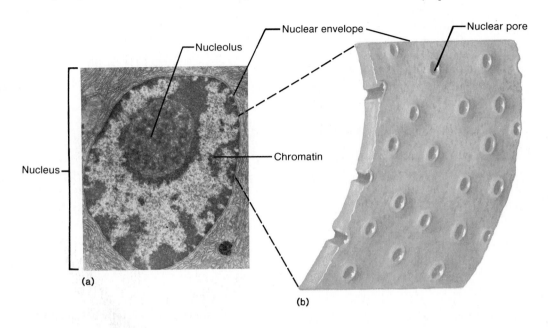

(a)

(b)

Chart 3.2 Structures and functions of cellular organelles

Organelles	Structure	Function	Figure
Cell membrane	Double-layered membrane with pores.	Maintains wholeness of cell and controls passage of materials in and out of cell.	3.4
Endoplasmic reticulum	Network of interconnected membrane forming sacs and canals.	Transports materials within the cell, provides attachment for ribosomes; forms new membrane.	3.6
Ribosomes	Globular particles.	Synthesize proteins.	3.3
Golgi apparatus	Group of flattened, membranous sacs.	Packages protein molecules for secretion.	3.7
Mitochondria	Membranous sacs with inner partitions.	Release energy from food molecules and transform energy into usable form.	3.8
Lysosomes	Membranous sacs.	Contain chemicals capable of digesting substances that enter cells.	3.9
Peroxisomes	Membranous vesicles.	Contain chemicals that break down toxic substances.	
Vesicles	Membranous sacs.	Transport substances between membranous organelles.	3.10
Microfilaments and microtubules	Thin rods and tubules.	Provide support to cytoplasm, help move substances and organelles within the cytoplasm, and produce cell movement.	3.11, 3.12
Centrosome	Nonmembranous structure composed of two rodlike centrioles.	Helps distribute chromosomes to new cells during cell reproduction and initiates formation of microtubules.	3.13
Cilia and flagella	Hairlike projections attached to basal bodies beneath cell membrane.	Propel fluids over cellular surface and enable sperm cells to move.	3.14, 3.15
Nuclear envelope	Porous double membrane that separates nuclear contents from cytoplasm.	Maintains wholeness of the nucleus and controls passage of materials between nucleus and cytoplasm.	3.16
Nucleolus	Dense, nonmembranous body within nucleus.	Forms ribosomes.	3.16
Chromatin	Fibers in nucleus.	Contains genetic information for carrying on life processes.	3.16

Although the effects of aging on cells are poorly understood, studies of aged tissues indicate that certain organelles may be altered with time. For example, within the nucleus, chromatin and chromosomes may show changes such as clumping, shrinking, or fragmenting, and the number and size of nucleoli may increase. In the cytoplasm, mitochondria may undergo changes in shape and number, and the Golgi apparatus may become fragmented. Some inclusions tend to accumulate in the cytoplasm, while others tend to disappear.

1. How are the nuclear contents separated from the cytoplasm of a cell?
2. What is the function of the nucleolus?
3. What is chromatin?

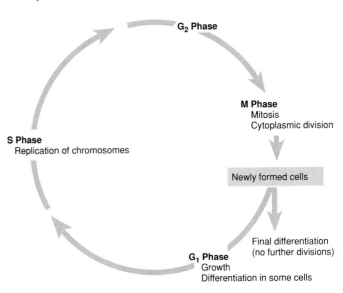

FIGURE 3.17
Life cycle of a cell.

Life Cycle of a Cell

The series of changes that a cell undergoes from the time it is formed until it reproduces is called its *life cycle* (figure 3.17). Superficially, this cycle seems rather simple—a newly formed cell grows for a time and then divides in half to form two new cells, which, in turn, may grow and divide. Yet the details of the cycle are quite complex, involving mitosis, cytoplasmic division, interphase, and differentiation.

Mitosis

Cell reproduction involves the dividing of a cell into two portions and includes two separate processes: (1) division of the nuclear parts, which is called **mitosis** (karyokinesis), and (2) division of the cytoplasm (cytokinesis). Another type of cell division called meiosis that occurs during the maturation of sex cells is described in chapter 17.

Division of the nuclear parts by mitosis is, of necessity, very precise, because the nucleus contains information in the chromosomes that "tells" cell parts how to carry on life processes. Each new cell resulting from mitosis must have a copy of this information in order to survive. Thus, the chromosomes of the parent cell must be replicated, and the resulting sets must be distributed equally to the offspring cells. Once this has been accomplished, the cytoplasm and its parts can be divided.

Although mitosis is often described in stages, the process is really a continuous one without marked changes between one step and the next (figure 3.18). The idea of stages is useful, however, to indicate the sequence in which major events occur. These stages include the following:

1. **Prophase.** One of the first indications that a cell is going to reproduce is the appearance of *chromosomes*. These structures form from chromatin in the nucleus, as fibers of chromatin condense into tightly coiled, rodlike parts. Sometime earlier (during interphase) the chromosomes became replicated, and consequently each is composed of two identical portions (chromatids). These parts are temporarily fastened together by a region on each called a *centromere* (kinetochore). (See figure 3.19.)

   The centrioles of the centrosome replicate just before the onset of mitosis. During prophase, the two newly formed pairs of centrioles move to opposite sides of the cytoplasm. Soon the nuclear envelope and the nucleolus disappear. Microtubules are assembled from proteins in the cytoplasm, and these structures become associated with the centrioles and chromosomes (figures 3.20 and 3.21). A spindle-shaped group of microtubules (spindle fibers) forms between the centrioles as they move apart.

2. **Metaphase.** The chromosomes are lined up in an orderly fashion about midway between the centrioles, as a result of microtubule activity. Spindle fibers become attached to the centromeres of the chromosomes so that a microtubule accompanying one pair of centrioles is attached to one side of a centromere and a microtubule accompanying the other pair of centrioles is attached to the other side (figure 3.22).

FIGURE 3.18
Mitosis is a continuous process during which the nuclear parts of a cell are divided into two equal portions. After reading about mitosis, identify the phases of the process and the cell parts included in this diagram.

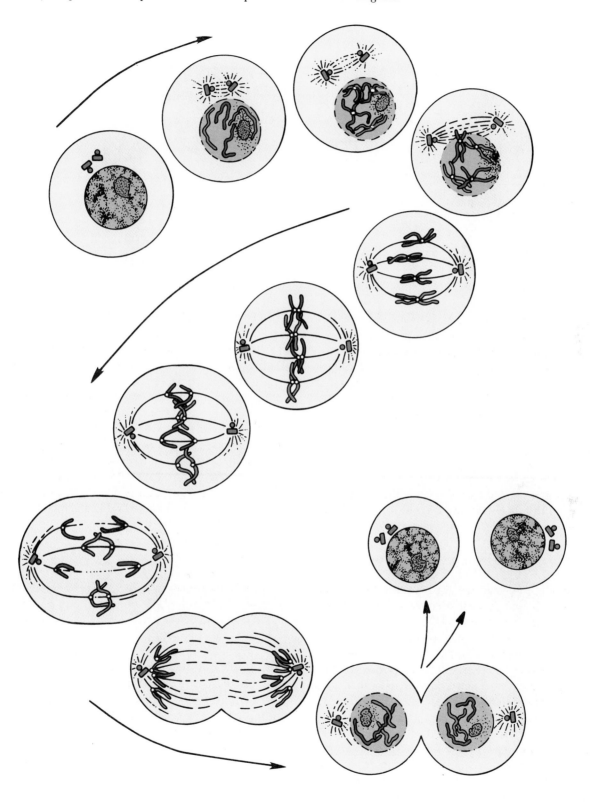

FIGURE 3.19

(a) A chromosome condenses from chromatin. Each replicated chromosome includes two chromatids that are joined at the centromere; (b) transmission electron micrograph of a human chromosome (×33,824); (c) a typical human cell contains 46 chromosomes.

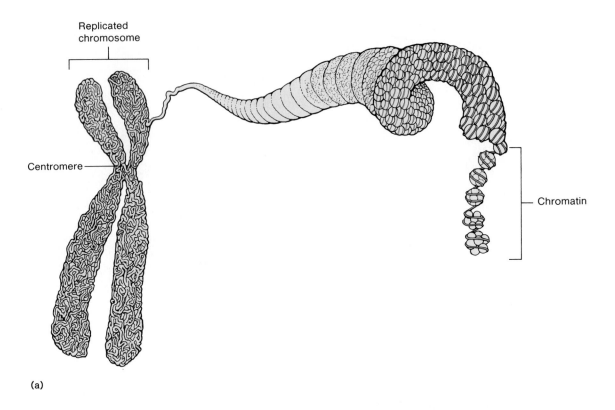

(a)

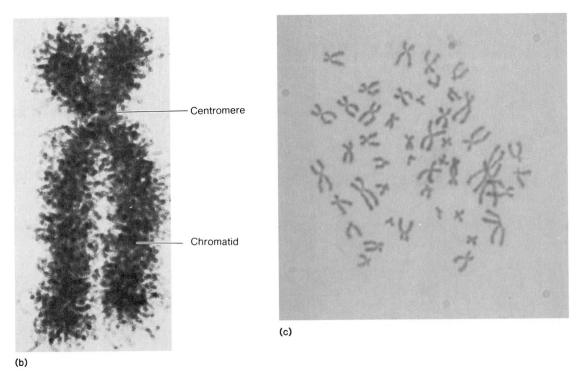

(b)

(c)

FIGURE 3.20

(a) In early prophase, chromosomes form from chromatin in the nucleus, and the centrioles move to opposite sides of the cell. (b) Light micrograph of a cell in early prophase (×250).

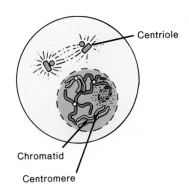

(a)

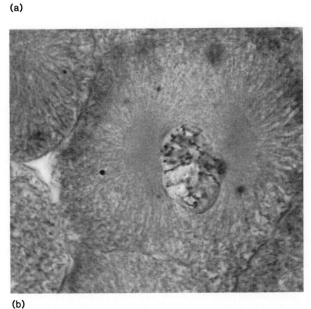

(b)

FIGURE 3.21

(a) Later in prophase, the nuclear envelope and nucleolus disappear. (b) A micrograph of a cell in late prophase.

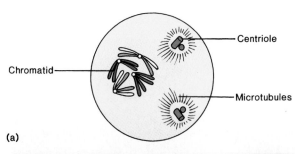

(a)

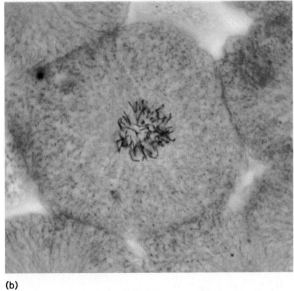

(b)

FIGURE 3.22

(a) In metaphase, the chromosomes become lined up midway between the centrioles. (b) A micrograph of a cell in metaphase (×250).

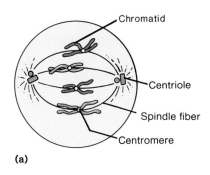

(a)

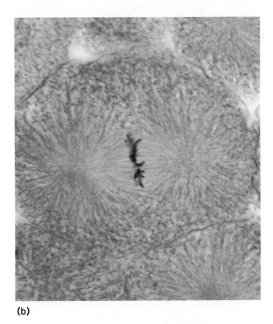

(b)

The Cell   65

FIGURE 3.23

(*a*) In anaphase, the centromeres divide, and the spindle fibers that have become attached to them pull the chromosome parts toward the centrioles. (*b*) A micrograph of a cell in anaphase (×250).

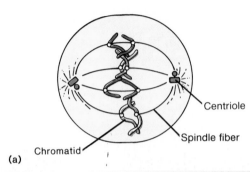

Centriole

Spindle fiber

Chromatid

(a)

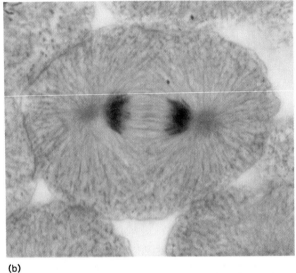

(b)

FIGURE 3.24

(*a*) In telophase, the chromosomes elongate to become chromatin threads, and the cytoplasm begins to divide. (*b*) A micrograph of a cell in telophase (×250).

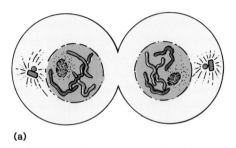

(a)

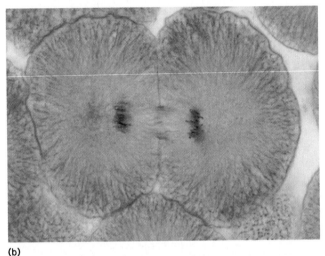

(b)

3. **Anaphase.** Soon the centromeres of the chromosomes separate, and the chromatids become individual chromosomes. The separated chromosomes now move in opposite directions, and once again the movement seems to result from microtubule activity. In this case, the spindle fibers appear to shorten and pull their attached chromosomes toward the centrioles at opposite sides of the cell (figure 3.23).

4. **Telophase.** The final stage of mitosis is said to begin when the chromosomes complete their migration toward the centrioles. It is much like prophase, but in reverse. As the chromosomes approach the centrioles, the chromosomes begin to elongate and change from rodlike into threadlike structures. A nuclear envelope forms around each chromosome set, and nucleoli appear within the newly formed nuclei. Finally, the spindle fibers disappear (figure 3.24). Telophase is accompanied by cytoplasmic division in which the cytoplasm is split into two portions.

Chart 3.3 summarizes the phases of mitosis.

Chart 3.3 Major events in mitosis

Stage	Major events
Prophase (fig. 3.21)	Chromatin condenses into chromosomes; centrioles move to opposite sides of cytoplasm; nuclear envelope and nucleolus disappear; microtubules appear and become associated with centrioles and chromosomes.
Metaphase (fig. 3.22)	Chromosomes become arranged midway between the centrioles; spindle fibers from the centrioles become attached to the centromeres of each chromosome.
Anaphase (fig. 3.23)	Centromeres separate, and chromatids become separated; spindle fibers shorten and pull individual chromosomes toward centrioles.
Telophase (fig. 3.24)	Chromosomes elongate and form chromatin threads; nuclear envelopes appear around each chromosome set; nucleoli appear; spindle fibers disappear.

Cytoplasmic Division

Cytoplasmic division (cytokinesis) begins when the cell membrane starts to constrict during anaphase and continues to constrict through telophase. This process involves the musclelike contraction of a ring of microfilaments. These filaments are assembled from the cytoplasm and are attached to the inner surface of the cell membrane. This contractile ring is positioned at right angles to the microtubules that pulled the chromosomes to opposite ends of the cell during mitosis. As the ring pinches inward, it separates the two newly formed nuclei and divides about half of the cytoplasmic organelles into each of the new cells.

Although the newly formed cells may differ slightly in size and number of cytoplasmic parts, they have identical chromosomes and thus contain identical information. Except for size, they are copies of the parent cell (figure 3.25).

Interphase

Interphase can be divided into three phases and lasts until the cell begins to undergo mitosis (figure 3.17).

Newly formed cells enter the *G_1 phase*, during which they begin growing and carrying out cellular activities. This requires that the young cells obtain nutrients and use them in the manufacture of new living materials and in the synthesis of many vital compounds. In the cytoplasm, new ribosomes, lysosomes, mitochondria, and membranes are formed. In many cells, the G_1 phase is followed by the *S phase*, when the chromosomes are replicated. A cell that

FIGURE 3.25
Following mitosis, the cytoplasm of the parent cell is divided into two portions as seen in these scanning electron micrographs. (a) ×3,750; (b) ×3,750; (c) ×3,190.

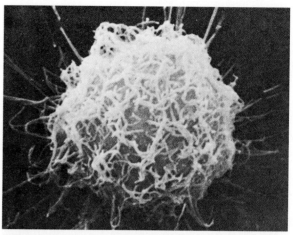

(a)

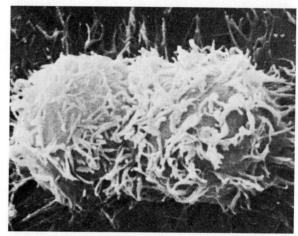

(b)

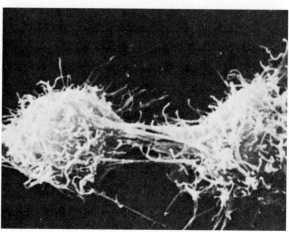

(c)

FIGURE 3.26

(a) Interphase lasts until a cell begins to undergo mitosis. (b) A micrograph of a cell in interphase (×250).

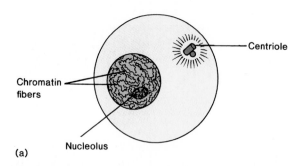

(a)

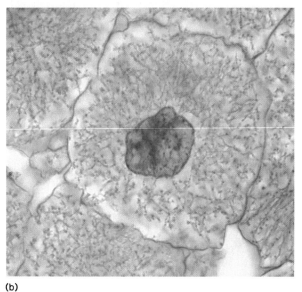

(b)

has entered the S phase has begun the preparations for mitosis. Following the S phase, the cell enters a *G₂ phase* in which the final preparations are made for cell division. The G₂ phase and interphase end when mitosis begins (figure 3.26).

Many kinds of body cells are constantly growing, reproducing, and increasing the number of cells that are present. Such activity is responsible for the growth and development of an embryo into a child, and a child into an adult. It also is necessary for replacing cells that have relatively short life spans and cells that are continually worn out or lost due to injury or disease.

Skin cells, blood-forming cells, and cells that line the intestine reproduce continually throughout life. Those that compose some organs, such as the liver, seem to reproduce until a particular number of cells is present, and then they cease reproducing. Interestingly, if the number of liver cells is reduced by injury or surgery, the remaining cells are stimulated to reproduce again. Still other cells, such as nerve cells, do not reproduce as they become mature; therefore, damage to nerve cells is likely to result in permanent loss of nerve function.

Cell Differentiation

Because all body cells are formed by mitosis and contain the same genetic information, they might be expected to look and act alike; obviously, they do not.

A human begins life as a single cell—a fertilized egg cell. This cell reproduces by mitosis to form two new cells; they, in turn, divide into four cells, the four become eight, and so forth. Then, sometime during development, the cells begin to *specialize.* That is, they develop special structures or begin to function in different ways. Some become skin cells, others become bone cells, and still others become nerve cells (figure 3.27).

The process by which cells develop different characteristics in structure and function is called **differentiation.** In this process, cells use portions of their genetic information and form specialized cellular parts. Cells of many kinds are produced, and each kind carries on specialized functions; for example, layers of flattened skin cells protect underlying tissues, red blood cells carry oxygen, and nerve cells transmit impulses. Each type of cell somehow helps the others and aids in the survival of the organism.

Differentiated cells are continually wearing out and must be replaced with new cells. Replacement cells can form by the division of differentiated cells, or by the division of undifferentiated *stem cells.* For example, when liver cells die, other differentiated liver cells divide and form new replacement liver cells. However, when blood cells or intestinal lining cells die, the division of stem cells forms replacements. When these stem cells divide, some of the newly formed cells remain as stem cells, while others differentiate into mature blood cells or intestinal lining cells that do not divide. Consequently, there is always a group of stem cells available to produce new replacement cells in these tissues.

1. Why is it important that the division of nuclear materials during mitosis be so precise?
2. Describe the events that occur during mitosis.
3. How do cells vary in their rates of reproduction?
4. Name the process by which some cells become muscle cells and others become nerve cells.

FIGURE 3.27

During development, the numerous body cells are produced from a single fertilized egg cell by mitosis. As these cells undergo differentiation, they become different kinds of cells that carry on specialized functions.

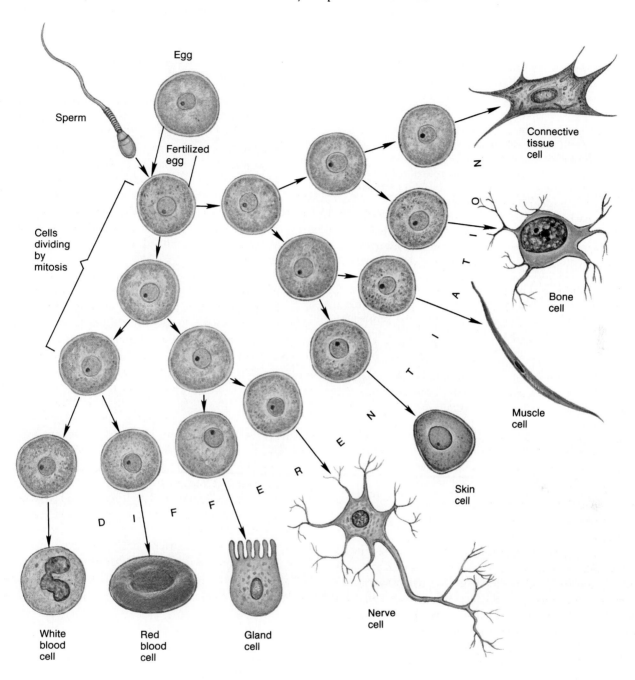

Cancer

Cancer is a disease that can occur in many different tissues. It results from changes in cells that allow them to avoid some of the normal control mechanisms. Cancerous conditions have certain common characteristics, including the following:

1. **Hyperplasia** (hi″per-pla′zĭ-ă). Hyperplasia is the uncontrolled reproduction of cells. Although the rate of reproduction among cancer cells is usually unchanged, they are not responsive to normal controls on cell numbers. As a result, cancer cells eventually give rise to very large cell populations.

2. **Anaplasia** (an-a-pla′zĭ-ă). The word anaplasia is used to describe the appearance of abnormalities in cellular structure. Cancer cells have larger nuclei and nucleoli than noncancer cells. Typically, cancer cells resemble undifferentiated or immature cells. That is, they fail to develop the specialized structure of the kind of cell they represent. Also, they fail to function in expected ways. Certain white blood cells, for example, normally function in resisting bacterial infections. When cells of this type become cancerous, they do not function effectively, and the cancer patient becomes more subject to infectious diseases. Cancer cells also are likely to form disorganized masses rather than to become arranged in orderly groups like normal cells (figure 3.28).

3. **Metastasis** (mĕ-tas′tă-sis). Metastasis is a tendency to spread. Normal cells are usually cohesive; that is, they are bound together in groups of similar kinds. Cancer cells often become detached from their cellular mass and usually become rounded. These cells may then be carried away from their place of origin to establish new cancerous growths in other parts of the body. Metastasis is the characteristic most closely associated with the word *malignant,* which suggests a power to threaten life. This characteristic is often used to distinguish a cancerous growth from a noncancerous (benign) one.

Increasing evidence indicates that the cause or causes of cancer are complex. Among the factors that may be involved are exposure to various chemicals or to harmful radiation or virus infections. These agents cause changes in chromosome structure that affect the regulation of cell division. Two or more such changes may be needed to cause a cancer.

When untreated, cancer cells eventually accumulate in large numbers. They may damage normal cells by effectively competing with them for nutrients. At the same time, cancer cells may invade vital organs and interfere with their functions, obstruct important passageways, or penetrate blood vessels and cause internal bleeding.

FIGURE 3.28

(*a*) Cancer cells, such as these from the human cervix, develop larger nuclei than normal cells (×40). (*b*) Cancer cells form disorganized masses, such as in this section of cervix. The cancer cells stain darker (×130).

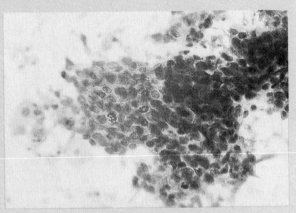

(a)

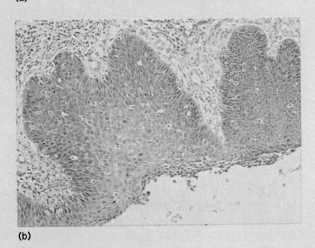

(b)

If detected in its early stages, a cancerous growth may be removed surgically. At other times, cancers are treated with radiation or drugs (chemotherapy), or some combination of surgery and treatments. The drugs most commonly used act on the structure of chromosomes or on the formation of microtubules, affecting the rapidly reproducing normal cells as well as those of cancer cells. This effect on normal cells is responsible for many of the side effects of drugs used to treat cancers.

Chapter Summary

Introduction (page 49)
Cells vary considerably in size, shape, and function. The shapes of cells are closely related to their functions.

A Composite Cell (page 50)
1. A cell includes a nucleus, cytoplasmic organelles, cytoplasm, and a cell membrane.
2. Cytoplasmic organelles perform specific vital functions, but the nucleus controls the overall activities of the cell.
3. Cell membrane
   a. The cell membrane acts as a selectively permeable passageway that controls the movements of substances between the cell and its surroundings.
   b. Some cells are connected by means of specialized intercellular junctions called tight junctions, adhesion belts, desmosomes, and gap junctions.
4. Cytoplasm
   a. Cytoplasm contains networks of membranes and organelles suspended in fluid.
   b. Endoplasmic reticulum is a network of membranes that provides a tubular communication system and an attachment for ribosomes.
   c. Ribosomes are particles that function in protein synthesis.
   d. The Golgi apparatus is composed of a stack of flattened, membranous sacs that package proteins for secretion and transport to other organelles.
   e. Mitochondria are membranous sacs that are involved with releasing energy from food molecules and transforming energy into a usable form.
   f. Lysosomes are membranous sacs containing digestive chemicals that can destroy substances that enter cells.
   g. Peroxisomes are membranous vesicles that destroy toxic chemicals.
   h. Vesicles are membranous sacs formed from the cell membrane, endoplasmic reticulum, and Golgi apparatus.
   i. Microfilaments and microtubules are threadlike processes that aid cellular movements, and provide support and stability to cytoplasm.
   j. The centrosome is a nonmembranous structure, consisting of two centrioles, that aids in the distribution of chromosomes during cell reproduction.
   k. Cilia and flagella are motile processes that extend outward from some cell surfaces.
      (1) Cilia are numerous, tiny, hairlike parts that serve to move fluids across cell surfaces.
      (2) Flagella are longer processes; the tail of a sperm cell is a flagellum that enables the cell to swim.
   l. Cytoplasm may contain nonliving cellular products such as nutrients and pigments called inclusions.
5. Cell nucleus
   a. The nucleus is enclosed in a double-layered nuclear envelope that controls the movement of substances between the nucleus and cytoplasm.
   b. A nucleolus is a dense body that functions in the production of ribosomes.
   c. Chromatin is composed of loosely coiled fibers that become chromosomes during cell reproduction.

Life Cycle of a Cell (page 62)
1. The life cycle of a cell includes mitosis, cytoplasmic division, interphase, and differentiation.
2. Mitosis
   a. Mitosis (karyokinesis) is the division and distribution of chromosomes during cell reproduction.
   b. The stages of mitosis include prophase, metaphase, anaphase, and telophase.
3. Cytoplasmic division (cytokinesis) is a process by which cytoplasm is divided into two portions following mitosis.
4. Interphase
   a. Interphase is the stage in the life cycle when a cell grows and forms new organelles, such as mitochondria, lysosomes, and ribosomes.
   b. It terminates when the cell begins to undergo mitosis.
   c. Cellular reproductive capacities vary greatly.
5. Cell differentiation involves the development of specialized structures and functions. In some tissues, differentiated cells reproduce while in other tissues, cells are replenished from stem cells.

Clinical Application of Knowledge

1. A person who has been exposed to excessive amounts of X ray may develop a decreased white blood cell number and an increased susceptibility to infections. In what way are these effects related?
2. Certain drugs used to treat cancer interfere with the formation of microtubules. This, in turn, decreases the rate of mitosis in cancer and other cells. Explain the relationship between these effects.
3. The smooth endoplasmic reticulum of liver cells is involved with the breakdown of certain drugs, such as phenobarbitol. When the drug is taken regularly, the amount of smooth endoplasmic reticulum in the cells increases. When the drug is discontinued, the extra smooth endoplasmic reticulum is removed. Which cell organelle would most likely destroy the endoplasmic reticulum?
4. Individuals suffering from malnutrition develop enlarged mitochondria (megamitochondria) in their heart and liver cells. What technique might be used to observe these changes?
5. In a process called a biopsy, a small sample of a tissue is removed and examined with a light microscope. How might malignant cells be distinguished from benign cells?

Review Activities

Part A

1. Use specific examples to illustrate how cells vary in size.
2. Describe how the shapes of nerve, epithelial, and muscle cells are related to their functions.
3. Name the two major portions of a cell and describe their relationship to one another.
4. Discuss the structure and functions of a cell membrane.
5. Define *selectively permeable*.
6. Describe four kinds of intercellular junctions.
7. Name the cell structures that are membranous.
8. Explain how new sections are added to the cell membrane.
9. Name the cell structures that are composed of microtubules.
10. Define *inclusion*.
11. Describe the structure of the nucleus and the functions of its parts.
12. List the phases in the life cycle of a cell.
13. Name the two processes included in cell reproduction.
14. Describe the major events of mitosis.
15. Explain what happens during interphase.
16. Define *differentiation*.
17. Explain the function of stem cells.

Part B

Match the organelle in column I with its description in column II.

I	II
1. endoplasmic reticulum	A. series of flattened sacs
2. ribosome	B. short, hairlike processes from cell surface
3. Golgi apparatus	C. includes centrioles
4. mitochondrion	D. may be attached to ER or found in cytoplasm
5. lysosome	E. forms the tail of a sperm cell
6. peroxisome	F. small, hollow tube
7. vesicle	G. interconnected membranous canals
8. microtubule	H. transports molecules to cell membrane
9. centrosome	I. destroys toxic chemicals
10. cilia	J. double membrane structure, transfers energy
11. flagella	K. membranous sac that destroys worn cell parts

C H A P T E R 4

Tissues

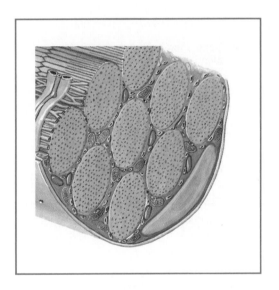

Cells, the basic units of structure and function within the human organism, are organized into groups and layers called tissues. Each type of tissue is composed of similar cells that are specialized to carry on particular functions. For example, epithelial tissues form protective coverings and function in secretion and absorption; connective tissues provide support for softer body parts and bind structures together; muscle tissues are responsible for producing body movements; and nerve tissue is specialized to conduct impulses that help control and coordinate body activities.

Chapter Outline

Chapter Objectives

After you have studied this chapter, you should be able to

1. Describe the general characteristics and functions of epithelial tissue.

2. Name the types of epithelium and identify an organ in which each type is found.

3. Explain how glands are classified.

4. Describe the general characteristics of connective tissue.

5. Describe the major cell types and fibers of connective tissue.

6. List the types of connective tissue.

7. Describe the major functions of each type of connective tissue.

8. Distinguish between the three types of muscle tissue.

9. Describe the general characteristics and functions of nerve tissue.

10. Complete the review activities at the end of this chapter. Note that the items are worded in the form of specific learning objectives. You may want to refer to them before reading the chapter.

Aids to Understanding Words

adip-, fat: *adip*ose tissue—tissue that stores fat.

chondro-, cartilage: *chondro*cyte—a cartilage cell.

-cyt, cell: osteo*cyte*—a bone cell.

epi-, upon: *epi*thelial tissue—tissue that covers all free body surfaces.

-glia, glue: neuro*glia*—cells that bind nerve tissue together.

inter-, between: *inter*calated disk— band located between the ends of adjacent cardiac muscle cells.

neuro-, nerve: *neuro*n—a nerve cell.

osseo-, bone: *osseo*us tissue—bone tissue.

phag-, to eat: macro*phag*e—a large cell that engulfs and destroys foreign and damaged cells.

pseudo-, false: *pseudo*stratified epithelium—tissue whose cells appear to be arranged in layers, but actually are not.

squam-, scale: *squam*ous epithelium— tissue whose cells appear flattened or scalelike.

strat-, layer: *strat*ified epithelium— tissue whose cells occur in layers.

stria-, groove: *stria*ted muscle—tissue whose cells are characterized by alternating light and dark cross-markings.

Introduction

In all complex organisms, cells are organized into layers or groups called **tissues.** Although the cells of different tissues vary in size, shape, arrangement, and function, those within a tissue are quite similar.

Usually tissue cells are separated by nonliving, intercellular materials that the cells secrete. These intercellular materials vary in composition from one tissue to another and may take the form of solids, semisolids, or liquids. For example, bone tissue cells are separated by a solid substance, while blood tissue cells are separated by a liquid.

The tissues of the human body include four major types: *epithelial, connective, muscle,* and *nerve.* These tissues are organized into organs that have specialized functions.

---

1. What is a tissue?
2. List four major types of tissues.

Epithelial Tissues

General Characteristics

Epithelial tissues are widespread throughout the body. They cover most body surfaces—inside and out—and they are the major tissues of glands.

Since epithelium covers organs, forms the inner lining of body cavities, and lines hollow organs, it always has a free surface—one that is exposed to the outside or to an open space internally. The underside of this tissue is anchored by desmosomes to a thin, nonliving layer called the *basement membrane* (basement lamina). This basement membrane serves a supporting function and is also attached to underlying connective tissue. It is formed by both the epithelial and connective tissues.

Before they can metastasize, cancer cells must cross the basement membrane associated with the epithelial linings of blood and lymph vessels. The cancer cells secrete a chemical that digests the basement membrane, creating breaks in it. This allows malignant cells to enter a vessel and be carried away by the moving blood or lymph inside.

As a rule, epithelial tissues lack blood vessels. However, they are nourished by substances that move from underlying connective tissues, which are well supplied with blood vessels.

Although cells of some tissues have limited abilities to reproduce, those of epithelium reproduce readily. Injuries to epithelium are likely to heal rapidly as cells divide and produce new cells to replace lost or damaged ones. For example, both skin cells and cells that line the stomach and intestines are continually being damaged and replaced.

Epithelial cells are tightly packed, and there is little intercellular material between them. Often they are attached to one another by several types of intercellular junctions (see chapter 3). Consequently, these cells are effective protective barriers in such structures as the outer layer of skin and inner lining of the mouth. Other epithelial functions include secretion, absorption, excretion, and sensory reception.

Epithelial tissues are classified according to the specialized shapes, arrangements, and functions of their cells. For example, epithelial tissues that are composed of single layers of cells are called *simple,* those with many layers of cells are said to be *stratified,* those with thin, flattened cells are called *squamous,* those with cube-shaped cells are called *cuboidal,* and those with elongated cells are called *columnar.* In the following descriptions, note that the free surfaces of various epithelial cells are modified in ways that reflect their specialized functions.

Simple Squamous Epithelium

Simple squamous epithelium consists of a single layer of thin, flattened cells. These cells fit tightly together, somewhat like floor tiles, and their nuclei are usually broad and thin (figure 4.1).

As a rule, substances pass rather easily through this type of tissue, and it occurs commonly where substances move across a membrane. For instance, simple squamous epithelium lines the air sacs of the lungs, where oxygen and carbon dioxide are exchanged. It also forms walls of capillaries, lines the insides of blood and lymph vessels, and forms the surface layer of membranes that line body cavities. However, because it is so thin and delicate, simple squamous epithelium can be damaged relatively easily.

Simple Cuboidal Epithelium

Simple cuboidal epithelium consists of a single layer of cube-shaped cells. These cells usually have centrally located spherical nuclei (figure 4.2).

This tissue covers the ovaries, lines the kidney tubules, and lines ducts of various glands such as the salivary glands, pancreas, and liver. In the kidneys, simple cuboidal epithelium functions in secretion and absorption, while in glands it is concerned with secretion of glandular products.

Simple Columnar Epithelium

The cells of **simple columnar epithelium** are elongated; that is, they are longer than they are wide. This tissue is composed of a single layer of cells whose nuclei are usually located deep in the cell near the basement membrane (figure 4.3).

Simple columnar epithelium occurs in linings of the uterus and various organs of the digestive tract, including the stomach and intestines. Because its cells are elongated,

FIGURE 4.1

(a) Simple squamous epithelium consists of a single layer of tightly packed flattened cells. (b) In this micrograph (×250), the cells are viewed on the flattened surface of the tissue; (c) cells are viewed from the edge.

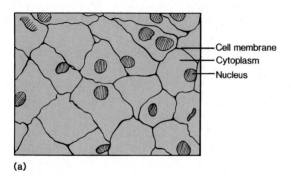

(a)

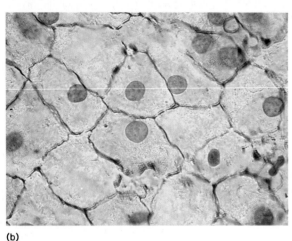

(b)

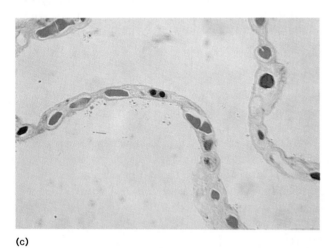

(c)

FIGURE 4.2

(a) Simple cuboidal epithelium consists of a single layer of tightly packed, cube-shaped cells. (b) Note the single layer of simple cuboidal cells in this micrograph (×250).

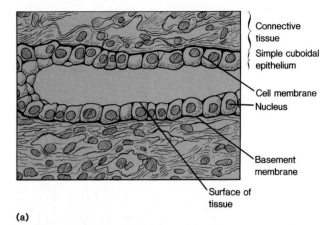

(a)

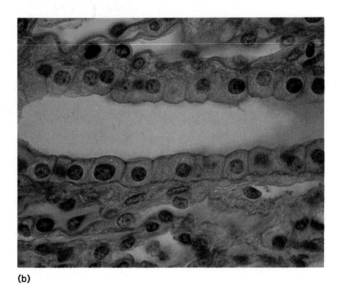

(b)

They function to increase the surface of the cell membrane where it is exposed to substances being absorbed, such as in the small intestine (figure 4.4).

Typically, specialized, flask-shaped glandular cells are scattered among the columnar cells of this tissue. These cells, called *goblet cells,* secrete a protective fluid called mucus onto the free surface of the tissue (see figure 4.3).

Pseudostratified Columnar Epithelium

The cells of **pseudostratified columnar epithelium** appear stratified or layered, but they are not. The layered effect occurs because their nuclei are located at two or more levels within the cells of the tissue. However, the cells, which vary in shape, all reach the basement membrane, even though some of them may not contact the free surface.

this tissue is relatively thick, providing protection for underlying tissues. It also functions in secretion of digestive fluids and in absorption of nutrient molecules that result from the digestion of foods.

Columnar (and some cuboidal) cells, whose principal function is absorption, often have numerous minute, cylindrical processes extending from their cell surfaces. These processes, called *microvilli,* measure 0.5–1.0 μm in length.

FIGURE 4.3

(*a*) Simple columnar epithelium consists of a single layer of elongated cells. (*b*) Light micrograph (×400).

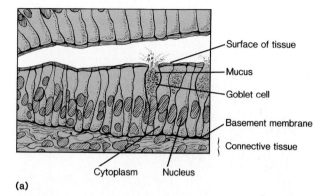

(a)

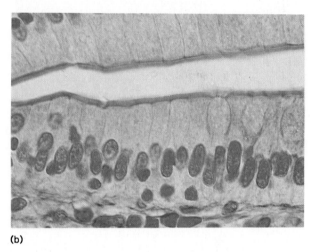

(b)

FIGURE 4.4

A scanning electron micrograph of microvilli, which occur on the exposed surfaces of some columnar (and cuboidal) epithelial cells.

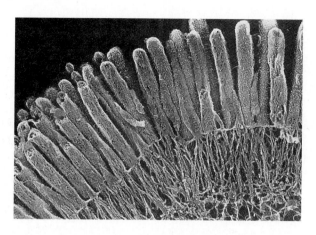

FIGURE 4.5

(*a*) Pseudostratified columnar epithelium appears stratified, because the nuclei of various cells are located at different levels. (*b*) What features of the tissue can you identify in this micrograph (×500)?

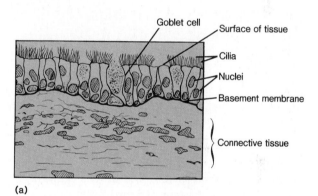

(a)

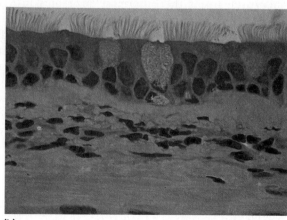

(b)

These cells commonly possess *cilia* (see figure 3.14), which measure 7–10 μm in length. They extend from the free surfaces of the cells, and move constantly. Goblet cells also are scattered throughout this tissue, and the mucus they secrete is swept along by the activity of the cilia (figure 4.5).

Pseudostratified columnar epithelium is found lining passages of the respiratory system and in various tubes of the reproductive systems. In respiratory passages, the mucus-covered linings are sticky and tend to trap particles of dust and microorganisms that enter with air. The cilia move the mucus and the trapped particles upward and out of the airways. In the reproductive tubes, cilia aid in moving sex cells from one region to another.

Stratified Squamous Epithelium

Stratified squamous epithelium consists of many layers of cells, making this tissue relatively thick. Only the cells near the free surface, however, are likely to be flattened. Those in deeper layers, where cellular reproduction occurs, are usually cuboidal or columnar. As the newer cells grow,

FIGURE 4.6

(a) Stratified squamous epithelium consists of many layers of cells. (b) In this micrograph, note how the cells near the surface of the tissue have become flattened (×67).

FIGURE 4.7

(a) Micrograph of transitional epithelium (×100). (b) This tissue is thicker when the organ wall is contracted; (c) the tissue appears thinner when the wall is stretched.

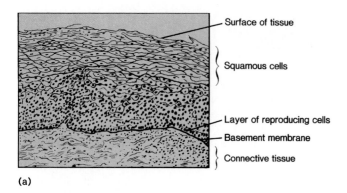

(a)

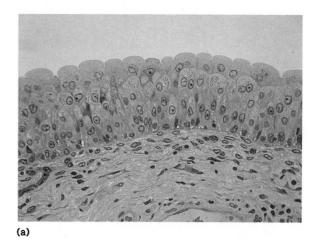

(a)

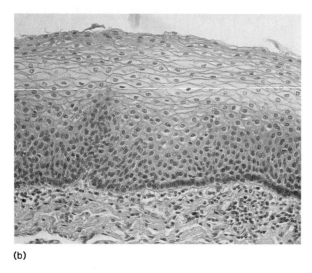

(b)

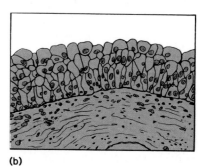

(b)

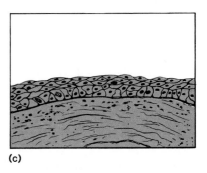

(c)

older ones are pushed farther and farther outward, and they tend to become flattened (figure 4.6).

This tissue forms the outermost layer of skin (epidermis). As older cells are pushed outward, they accumulate a protein called *keratin,* become hardened, and die. This action produces a covering of dry, tough, protective material, which prevents water from escaping underlying tissues and various microorganisms from entering.

Stratified squamous epithelium also lines the mouth cavity, throat, vagina, and anal canal. In these parts, the tissue is not keratinized; it stays moist, and cells on its free surfaces remain alive.

Transitional Epithelium

Transitional epithelium (uroepithelium) is specialized to undergo changes in response to increased tension. It forms the inner lining of the urinary bladder and passageways of the urinary system. When the wall of one of these organs is contracted, the tissue consists of several layers of cu-

boidal cells; however, when the organ is distended, the cell layers are stretched and appear to contain only a few layers of cells (figure 4.7).

In addition to providing an expandable lining, transitional epithelium forms a barrier that helps prevent contents of the urinary tract from moving through the walls of its passageways.

Certain specialized epithelial cells function as sense receptors in the mouth and ear. (See chapter 10.)

Chart 4.1 summarizes the characteristics of the different types of epithelial tissue.

Chart 4.1 Epithelial tissues

Type	Function	Location	Figure
Simple squamous epithelium	Allows movement of substances through membrane	Air sacs of lungs, walls of capillaries, linings of blood and lymph vessels	4.1
Simple cuboidal epithelium	Secretion, absorption	Surface of ovaries, linings of kidney tubules, and linings of ducts of various glands	4.2
Simple columnar epithelium	Protection, secretion, absorption	Linings of uterus and tubes of the digestive tract	4.3
Pseudostratified columnar epithelium	Protection, secretion, movement of mucus and cells	Linings of respiratory passages and various tubes of the reproductive system	4.5
Stratified squamous epithelium	Protection	Outer layer of skin, linings of mouth cavity, throat, vagina, and anal canal	4.6
Transitional epithelium	Distensibility, protection	Inner lining of urinary bladder and passageways of urinary tract	4.7

A cancer originating in epithelium is called a carcinoma, and it is estimated that up to 90% of all human cancers are of this type. Most carcinomas begin on surfaces that contact the external environment, such as skin, linings of the airways in the respiratory tract, or linings of the stomach or intestines in the digestive tract. This observation suggests that the more common cancer-causing agents may not penetrate tissues very deeply.

1. List the general characteristics of epithelial tissue.
2. Explain how epithelial tissues are classified.
3. Describe the structure of each type of epithelium.
4. Describe the special functions of each type of epithelium.

Glandular Epithelium

Glandular epithelium is composed of cells that are specialized to produce and secrete various substances into ducts or into body fluids. Such glandular cells are usually found within columnar or cuboidal epithelium, and one or more of these cells constitutes a **gland.** Glands that secrete their products into ducts that open onto some internal or external surface are called **exocrine glands.** Those that secrete into tissue fluid or blood are called **endocrine glands.** (Endocrine glands are discussed in chapter 11.)

An exocrine gland may consist of a single epithelial cell (unicellular gland), such as a mucus-secreting goblet cell, or it may be composed of many cells (multicellular gland). In turn, the multicellular forms can be subdivided structurally into two groups—simple and compound glands.

A *simple gland* communicates with the surface by means of an unbranched duct, and a *compound gland* has a branched duct. These two types of glands can be further classified according to the shapes of their secretory portions. Thus, those that consist of epithelial-lined tubes are called *tubular glands;* those whose terminal portions form saclike dilations are called *alveolar glands.* Figure 4.8 illustrates several types of exocrine glands.

Chart 4.2 summarizes the types of exocrine glands, lists their characteristics, and provides an example of each type.

Glandular secretions are classified according to whether they consist of cellular products or portions of glandular cells. Glands that release fluid cellular products through cell membranes without loss of cytoplasm are called *merocrine glands.* Those of an intermediate type that lose small portions of their glandular cell bodies during secretion are called *apocrine glands.* Glands that release entire cells filled with secretory products are called *holocrine glands* (figure 4.9). Chart 4.3 summarizes these glands and their secretions.

Most secretory cells are merocrine, and they can be further subdivided as either *serous cells* or *mucous cells.* The secretion of serous cells is typically watery and is called *serous fluid.* Such cells are common in glands of the digestive tract and secrete digestive chemicals. Mucous cells secrete the thicker fluid called *mucus.* This substance is secreted abundantly from inner linings of the digestive and respiratory tubes.

1. Distinguish between exocrine and endocrine glands.
2. How are exocrine glands classified?
3. Distinguish between a serous cell and a mucous cell.

FIGURE 4.8
Structural types of exocrine glands.

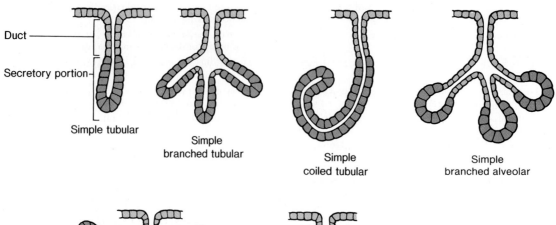

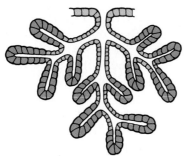

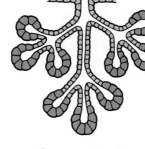

Compound tubular   Compound alveolar

Chart 4.2 Types of exocrine glands

Type	Characteristics	Example
Unicellular glands	A single secretory cell	Mucus-secreting goblet cell (see figure 4.3)
Multicellular glands	Gland consists of many cells	
Simple glands	Glands communicate with surface by means of unbranched ducts	
1. Simple tubular gland	Straight, tubelike gland that opens directly onto surface; no duct present	Intestinal glands of small intestine (see figure 12.3)
2. Simple coiled tubular gland	Long, coiled, tubelike gland; long duct	Eccrine (sweat) glands of skin (see figure 5.11)
3. Simple branched tubular gland	Branched, tubelike gland; duct short or absent	Mucous glands in small intestine (see figure 12.3)
4. Simple branched alveolar gland	Secretory portions of gland expand into saclike compartments arranged along duct	Sebaceous gland of skin (see figure 5.8)
Compound glands	Glands communicate with surface by means of branched ducts	
1. Compound tubular gland	Secretory portions are coiled tubules, usually branched	Bulbourethral glands of male (see figure 17.1)
2. Compound alveolar gland	Secretory portions are irregularly branched tubules with numerous saclike outgrowths	Salivary glands (see figure 12.11)

FIGURE 4.9
(a) Merocrine glands release fluid without a loss of cytoplasm; (b) apocrine glands lose small portions of their cell bodies during secretion; and (c) holocrine glands release entire cells filled with secretory products.

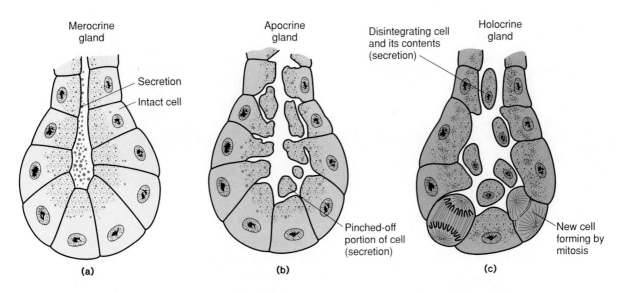

Chart 4.3 Types of glandular secretions		
Type	**Description of secretion**	**Example**
Merocrine glands	A fluid cellular product that is released through the cell membrane	Salivary glands, pancreatic glands, certain sweat glands of the skin
Apocrine glands	Cellular product and portions of the free ends of glandular cells that are pinched off during secretion	Mammary glands, certain sweat glands of the skin
Holocrine glands	Entire cells that are laden with secretory products	Sebaceous glands of the skin

Connective Tissues

General Characteristics

Connective tissues occur throughout the body and represent the most abundant type of tissue by weight. They bind structures together, provide support and protection, serve as frameworks, fill spaces, store fat, produce blood cells, provide protection against infections, and help repair tissue damage.

Connective tissue cells are usually farther apart than epithelial cells, and they have an abundance of intercellular material, or *matrix*, between them. This matrix consists of *fibers* and a *ground substance* whose consistency varies from fluid to semisolid to solid.

Connective tissue cells are able to reproduce. In most cases, they have good blood supplies and are well nourished. Although some connective tissues, such as bone and cartilage, are quite rigid, loose connective tissue, adipose connective tissue, and fibrous connective tissue are more flexible.

Major Cell Types

Connective tissues contain a variety of cell types. Some of them are called resident cells because they are usually present in relatively stable numbers. These include fibroblasts, macrophages, and mast cells. Another group known as wandering cells temporarily appears in the tissues, usually in response to an injury or infection. Wandering cells include several types of white blood cells.

The **fibroblast** is the most common kind of resident cell in connective tissues. It is relatively large and usually star-shaped. Fibroblasts function to produce fibers by secreting protein in the intercellular matrix of connective tissues (figure 4.10).

Macrophages (histiocytes) are almost as numerous as fibroblasts in some connective tissues. They are usually attached to fibers but can become detached and actively move about. Macrophages are specialized to engulf and destroy foreign and damaged body cells. Because they function as

FIGURE 4.10

A scanning electron micrograph of fibroblasts (×5,000). What is the function of this type of cell?

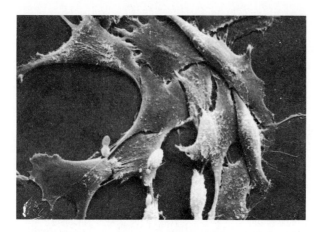

FIGURE 4.11

Macrophages are common in connective tissues where they function as scavenger cells. In this scanning electron micrograph, a macrophage is seen engulfing two cells (×5,600).

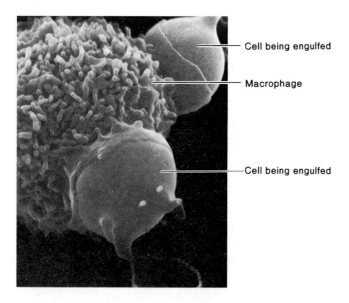

Cell being engulfed

Macrophage

Cell being engulfed

scavenger cells that can clear foreign particles from tissues, macrophages represent an important defense against infectious agents (figure 4.11). They also remove dead and damaged cells during the process of cell replacement following an injury.

Mast cells are relatively large cells that contain many vesicles. They are widely distributed in connective tissues and are usually located near blood vessels. They release substances important for the defense against foreign cells and particles (figure 4.12).

FIGURE 4.12

A transmission electron micrograph of a mast cell (×4,000).

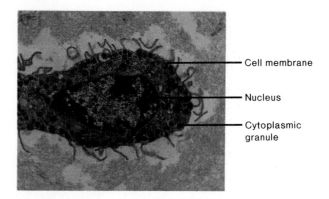

Cell membrane

Nucleus

Cytoplasmic granule

Connective Tissue Fibers

Three types of connective tissue fibers are produced by fibroblasts: *collagenous fibers, elastic fibers,* and *reticular fibers.*

Collagenous fibers are relatively thick, threadlike parts composed of the protein collagen, which is the major structural protein of the body. These fibers are grouped in long, parallel bundles, and they are flexible but only slightly elastic. More importantly, they have great tensile strength—that is, they are capable of resisting considerable pulling force. Thus, collagenous fibers are important components of body parts that hold structures together.

When collagenous fibers are present in abundance, the tissue containing them is called dense connective tissue. Such a tissue appears white, and for this reason collagenous fibers are sometimes called white fibers. Loose connective tissue, on the other hand, is sparsely supplied with collagenous fibers.

Elastic fibers are composed of bundles of microfibrils embedded in a protein called elastin. These fibers tend to be branched and form complex networks in various tissues. They have less strength than collagenous fibers, but they are very elastic. That is, they are easily stretched or deformed and will resume their original lengths and shapes when the force acting upon them is removed. They are common in body parts that are normally subjected to stretching, such as the vocal cords and various air passages of the respiratory system. Elastic fibers are sometimes called yellow fibers, because tissues amply supplied with them appear yellowish. (See figure 4.13.)

Reticular fibers are very thin fibers composed of collagen. They are highly branched and form delicate supporting networks in tissues, such as the spleen, thymus, and liver.

When skin is exposed to sunlight excessively, both of its connective tissue fibers tend to lose their elasticity, and the skin becomes increasingly stiff and leathery. In time, the skin may sag and wrinkle. On the other hand, skin of a healthy, well-nourished person that remains covered usually shows much less change.

FIGURE 4.13
Scanning electron micrograph of (*a*) collagenous fibers (×65,600) and (*b*) elastic fibers. How do these fibers differ?

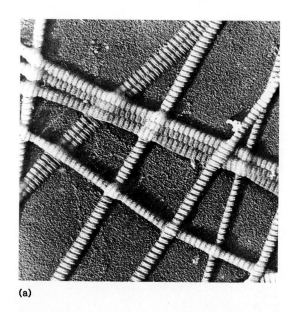

(a)

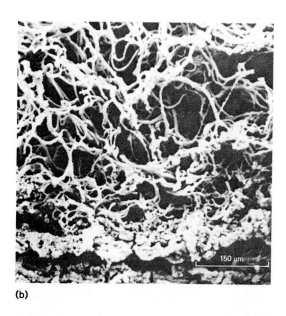

(b)

1. What are the general characteristics of connective tissue?
2. What are the major types of resident cells in connective tissue?
3. What is the primary function of fibroblasts?
4. What are the characteristics of collagen and elastin?

Loose Connective Tissue

Loose connective tissue forms delicate, thin membranes throughout the body. Cells of this tissue, which are mainly fibroblasts, are located some distance apart and are separated by a gel-like ground substance that contains many collagenous and elastic fibers (figure 4.14). This tissue binds skin to underlying organs and fills spaces between muscles. It lies beneath most layers of epithelium, where its numerous blood vessels provide nourishment for nearby epithelial cells.

Adipose Tissue

Adipose tissue, commonly called fat, is a specialized form of loose connective tissue. Certain cells within loose connective tissue (adipocytes) store fat in droplets within their cytoplasm. At first these cells resemble fibroblasts, but as they accumulate fat, they become enlarged and rounded, and their nuclei are pushed to one side (figure 4.15). When they occur in such large numbers that other cell types are crowded out, they form adipose tissue.

Adipose tissue is found beneath the skin and in spaces between muscles. It also occurs around the kidneys, behind the eyeballs, in certain abdominal membranes, on the surface of the heart, and around various joints.

Adipose tissue serves as a protective cushion for joints and some organs, such as the kidneys. It also functions as a heat insulator beneath the skin and it stores energy in fat molecules.

FIGURE 4.14

(*a*) Loose connective tissue contains numerous fibroblasts that produce collagenous and elastic fibers. (*b*) Micrograph of loose connective tissue (×250).

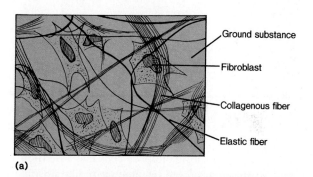

Ground substance

Fibroblast

Collagenous fiber

Elastic fiber

(a)

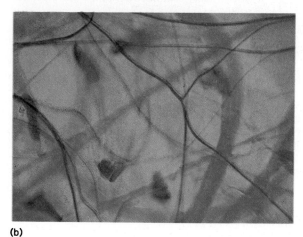

(b)

Tissues   83

FIGURE 4.15

(a) Adipose tissue cells contain large fat droplets that cause the nuclei to be pushed close to their cell membranes. (b) Note the nucleus indicated by the arrow in this micrograph (×250).

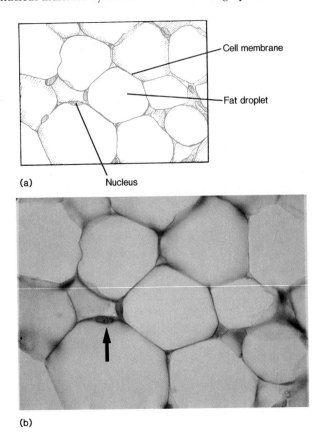

(a)

- Cell membrane
- Fat droplet
- Nucleus

(b)

FIGURE 4.16

(a) Fibrous connective tissue consists largely of tightly packed collagenous fibers. (b) The collagenous fibers are stained red in this micrograph (×100).

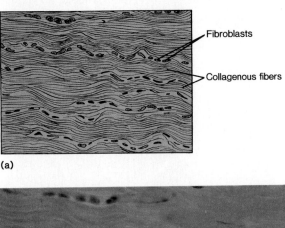

(a)

- Fibroblasts
- Collagenous fibers

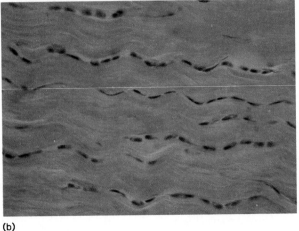

(b)

Because excess food substances are likely to be converted to fat and stored, the amount of adipose tissue present in the body is usually related to a person's diet. During a period of fasting, adipose cells may lose their fat droplets, shrink in size, and become more like fibroblasts again.

Infants and young children usually have a continuous layer of adipose tissue just beneath the skin. This layer gives their bodies the rounded appearance of well-nourished youngsters. In adults, this subcutaneous fat tends to become thinner in some regions and thicker in others. For example, in males it usually thickens in the upper back, upper arms, lower back, and buttocks; in females it is more likely to develop in the breasts, buttocks, and upper legs.

Fibrous Connective Tissue

Fibrous connective tissue is a dense tissue that contains many closely packed, thick, collagenous fibers and a fine network of elastic fibers. It has relatively few cells, almost all of which are fibroblasts (figure 4.16).

Since collagenous fibers are very strong, this type of tissue can withstand pulling forces, and it often binds body parts together. For example, *tendons,* which connect muscles to bones, and *ligaments,* which connect bones to bones at joints, are composed largely of fibrous connective tissue. In these structures, parallel bundles of collagen fibers are arranged in groups. Thus, tendons and ligaments can withstand the greatest stress in the directions of these fibers. Fibrous connective tissue also occurs in the protective white layer of the eyeball and in deeper portions of the skin. However, in these areas, the collagen fibers run in all directions and can therefore withstand stress in many directions.

The blood supply to fibrous connective tissue is relatively poor, so tissue repair occurs slowly. This is why a sprain, which involves damage to tissues surrounding a joint, may take considerable time to heal.

Elastic Connective Tissue

Elastic connective tissue consists mainly of yellow, elastic fibers arranged in parallel strands or in branching networks. Spaces between the fibers contain collagenous fibers and fibroblasts.

FIGURE 4.17
Micrograph of elastic tissue (×100).

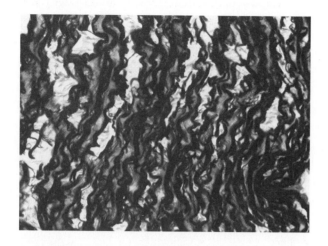

FIGURE 4.18
Micrograph of reticular tissue (×110).

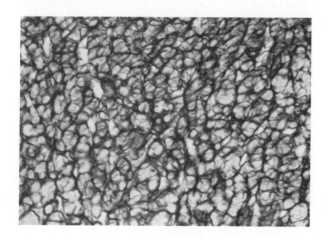

This tissue occurs in the layers within walls of various hollow internal organs, including the larger arteries, some portions of the heart, and the larger airways. It is also found in certain ligaments. It imparts an elastic quality to these structures. (See figure 4.17.)

Reticular Connective Tissue

Reticular connective tissue is composed of thin reticulin (similar to collagen) fibers arranged in a three-dimensional network. It functions as supporting tissue in the walls of certain internal organs, such as the liver, spleen, bone marrow, and various lymphatic organs. (See figure 4.18.)

1. How is loose connective tissue related to adipose tissue?
2. What are the functions of adipose tissue?
3. How can fibrous, elastic, and reticular connective tissues be distinguished?

FIGURE 4.19
(a) Hyaline cartilage cells (chondrocytes) are located in lacunae surrounded by intercellular material containing very fine collagenous fibers. (b) Micrograph of hyaline cartilage (×250).

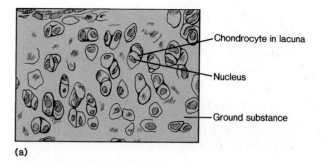

(a)

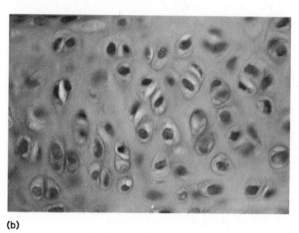

(b)

Cartilage

Cartilage is one of the rigid connective tissues. It supports parts, provides frameworks and attachments, protects underlying tissues, and forms structural models for many developing bones.

The matrix of cartilage is abundant and is composed largely of fibers embedded in a gel-like ground substance. Cartilage cells, or *chondrocytes,* occupy small chambers called *lacunae,* and thus are completely surrounded by matrix.

As a rule, a cartilaginous structure is enclosed in a covering of fibrous connective tissue called the *perichondrium.* Although cartilage tissue lacks a direct blood supply, there are blood vessels in the perichondrium that surround it. The cartilage cells obtain nutrients from these vessels. This lack of a direct blood supply is related to the slow rate of cellular reproduction and repair that is characteristic of cartilage.

There are three kinds of cartilage, and each kind contains a different type of intercellular material. Hyaline cartilage has very fine collagenous fibers in its matrix; elastic cartilage contains a dense network of elastic fibers; and fibrocartilage contains many large collagenous fibers.

Hyaline cartilage (figure 4.19), the most common type of cartilage, looks somewhat like milk glass. It occurs on the ends of bones in many joints, in the soft part of the

FIGURE 4.20

(a) Elastic cartilage contains many elastic fibers in its intercellular material. (b) Micrograph of elastic cartilage (×100).

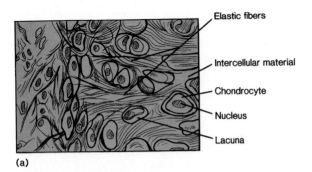

Elastic fibers

Intercellular material

Chondrocyte

Nucleus

Lacuna

(a)

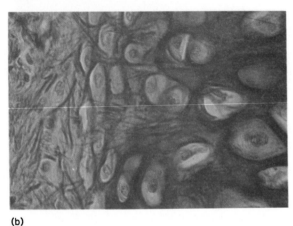

(b)

FIGURE 4.21

(a) Fibrocartilage contains many large collagenous fibers in its intercellular material. (b) Micrograph of fibrocartilage (×195).

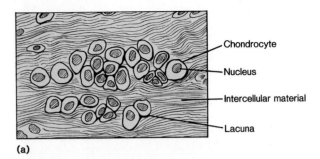

Chondrocyte

Nucleus

Intercellular material

Lacuna

(a)

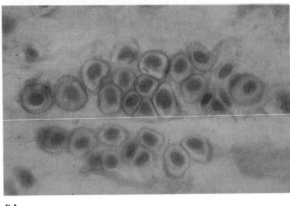

(b)

nose, and in the supporting rings of the respiratory passages. In an embryo, many of the skeletal parts are formed at first of hyaline cartilage, which is later replaced by bone. Hyaline cartilage also plays an important role in the growth of most bones and in repair of bone fractures. (See chapter 6.)

Elastic cartilage (figure 4.20) is more flexible than hyaline cartilage because it contains many elastic fibers in its matrix. It provides the framework for the external ears and parts of the larynx.

Fibrocartilage (figure 4.21), a very tough tissue, contains many collagenous fibers. It often serves as a shock absorber for structures that are subjected to pressure. For example, fibrocartilage forms pads (intervertebral disks) between the individual parts of the backbone. It also forms protective cushions between bones in the knees, and between bones in the pelvic girdle.

Bone

Bone (osseous tissue) is the most rigid of the connective tissues. Its hardness is due largely to the presence of minerals in its intercellular matrix. This intercellular material also contains a considerable amount of collagen, whose fibers provide flexible reinforcement for the mineral components of bone.

Bone provides an internal support for body structures. It protects vital parts in the cranial and thoracic cavities, and serves as an attachment for muscles. Some bone also contains red marrow, which forms blood cells. Bone matrix stores various minerals.

Bone matrix is deposited in thin layers called *lamellae,* which most commonly are arranged in concentric patterns around tiny longitudinal tubes called *osteonic* (Haversian) *canals.* Bone cells, or *osteocytes,* are located in lacunae, rather evenly spaced between the lamellae. Consequently, they too are arranged in patterns of concentric circles. In a bone, the osteocytes and lamellae form a cylindrical shaped unit called an **osteon** (Haversian system). Many of these units cemented together form the substance of bone (figure 4.22).

Each osteonic canal contains a blood vessel, so that every bone cell is fairly close to a nutrient supply. In addition, the bone cells have numerous cytoplasmic processes that extend outward and pass through minute tubes in the matrix called *canaliculi.* These cellular processes are attached to the membranes of nearby cells by gap junctions (see chapter 3). As a result, materials can move rapidly between blood vessels and bone cells. Thus, in spite of its inert appearance, bone is a very active tissue. When it is injured, bone heals much more rapidly than cartilage.

FIGURE 4.22

(*a*) Bone matrix is deposited in concentric layers around osteonic canals. (*b*) What features of the tissue can you identify in this micrograph (×160)? (*c*) Transmission electron micrograph of an osteocyte.

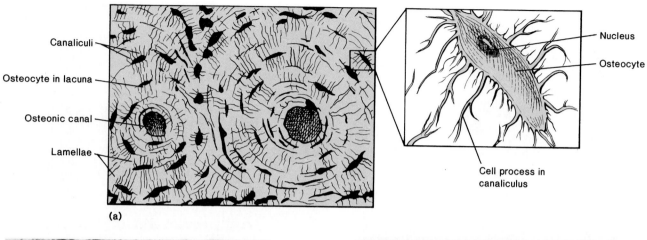

(a)

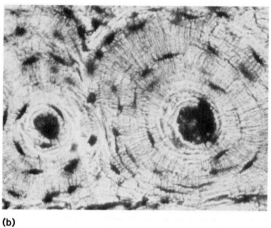

(b)

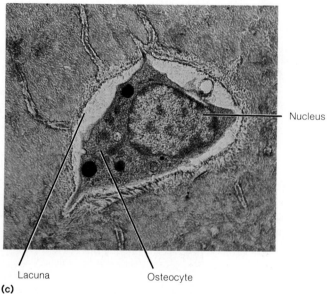

(c)

Blood

Blood is composed of cells that are suspended in a fluid intercellular matrix called *blood plasma*. These cells include *red blood cells, white blood cells,* and cellular fragments called *platelets* (figure 4.23). Most blood cells are formed by red marrow (hematopoietic tissue) within the hollow parts of various bones (figure 4.23).

After birth, all of the blood cells develop from red bone marrow. Red marrow gives rise to *hemocytoblasts* (stem cells). (See figure 4.24.). These cells may then differentiate in various ways to form the different types of blood cells. Hormones and other factors normally regulate the rate of blood cell production. Figure 4.25 illustrates the stages in development of blood cells.

Red blood cells, or *erythrocytes,* are tiny, biconcave disks that are thin near their centers and thicker around their rims. This special shape is related to the red cell's function of transporting gases, in that it provides an increased surface area through which gases can move (figure 4.26).

Although red blood cells have nuclei during their early stages of development, these nuclei are lost as the cells mature. This characteristic, like the shape of a red blood cell, seems to be related to the function of transporting oxygen. Since their nuclei are missing, red blood cells are unable to reproduce, and with age the red blood cells become less and less active. The average life span of a red blood cell is about 120 days, and a large number of these cells are removed from circulation each day by the liver and spleen.

FIGURE 4.23

(a) Blood tissue consists of an intercellular fluid in which red blood cells, white blood cells, and platelets are suspended.
(b) Micrograph of human blood cells (×640).

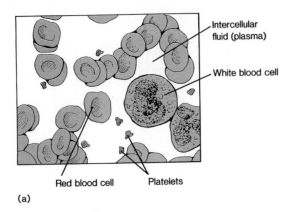

Intercellular
fluid (plasma)

White blood cell

Red blood cell   Platelets

(a)

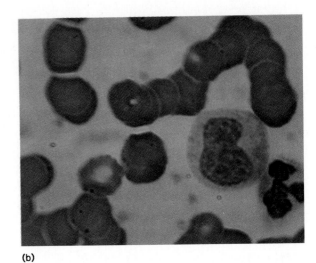

(b)

FIGURE 4.24

Hemocytoblasts in red bone marrow (×640).

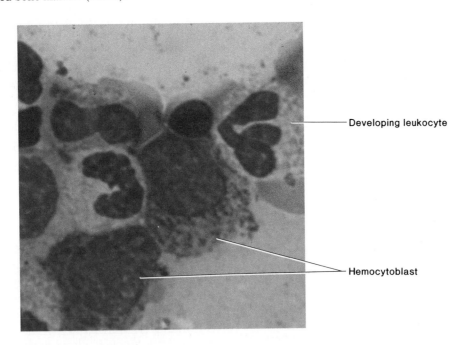

Developing leukocyte

Hemocytoblast

White blood cells, or *leukocytes,* function primarily to defend the body against microorganisms. Normally, five types of white cells can be found in circulating blood. They are distinguished by size, nature of their cytoplasm, shape of their nuclei, and their staining characteristics. For example, some types have granular cytoplasm and make up a group called *granulocytes.* Others lack cytoplasmic granules and are called *agranulocytes.*

Each granulocyte is typically about twice the size of a red cell. Members of this group include three types of white cells—*neutrophils, eosinophils,* and *basophils.*

Neutrophils are characterized by the presence of fine cytoplasmic granules that stain pinkish in neutral stain. The nucleus of a neutrophil is lobed and consists of two to five parts connected by thin strands of chromatin. For this

FIGURE 4.25

Origin and development of blood cells.

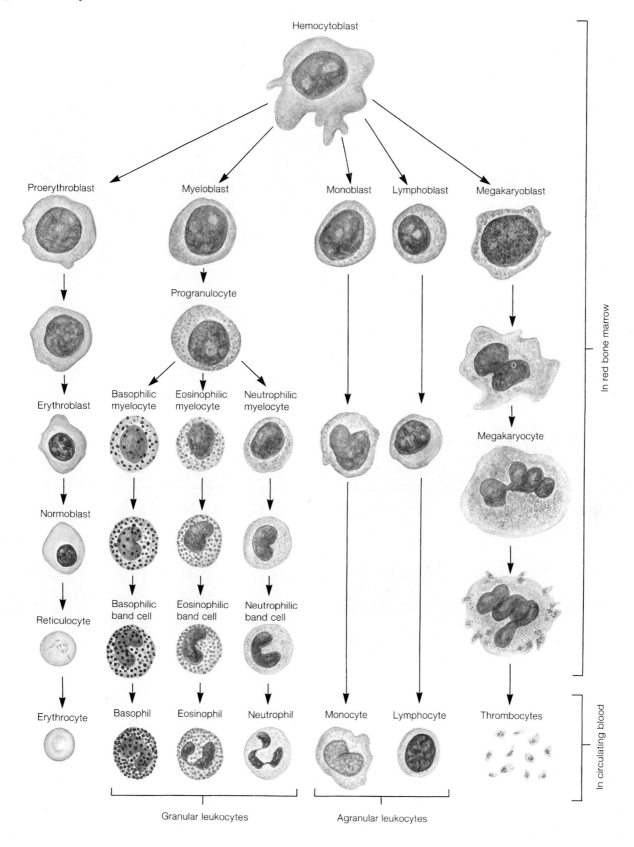

Hemocytoblast

Proerythroblast Myeloblast Monoblast Lymphoblast Megakaryoblast

Progranulocyte

Erythroblast Basophilic myelocyte Eosinophilic myelocyte Neutrophilic myelocyte

Normoblast

Reticulocyte Basophilic band cell Eosinophilic band cell Neutrophilic band cell

Megakaryocyte

Erythrocyte Basophil Eosinophil Neutrophil Monocyte Lymphocyte Thrombocytes

Granular leukocytes

Agranular leukocytes

In red bone marrow

In circulating blood

FIGURE 4.26
(a) How is the biconcave shape of a red blood cell related to its function? (b) Scanning electron micrograph (false color) of human red blood cells.

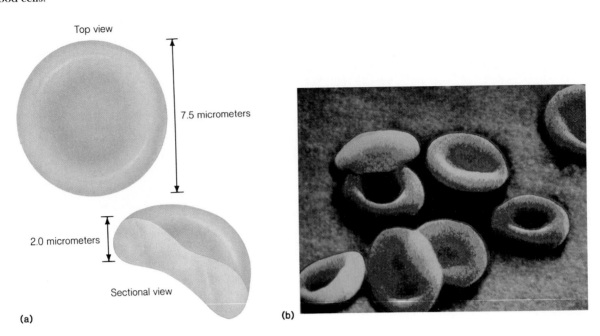

Top view

7.5 micrometers

2.0 micrometers

Sectional view

(a)

(b)

FIGURE 4.27
A neutrophil has a lobed nucleus with two to five parts ($\times 400$).

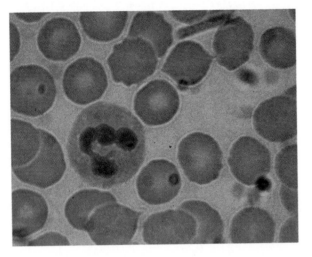

FIGURE 4.28
An eosinophil is characterized by the presence of red-staining cytoplasmic granules.

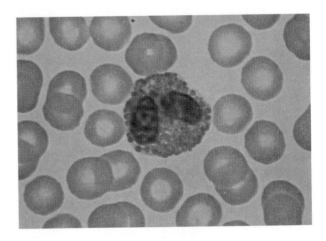

reason, neutrophils are also called polymorphonuclear leukocytes, which means their nuclei take many forms (figure 4.27).

Eosinophils contain coarse, uniformly sized cytoplasmic granules that stain deep red in acid stain. The nucleus usually has only two lobes (bilobed) (figure 4.28).

Basophils are similar to eosinophils in size and in the shape of their nuclei. However, they have fewer, more irregularly shaped cytoplasmic granules that stain deep blue in basic stain (figure 4.29).

FIGURE 4.29

A basophil has cytoplasmic granules that stain deep blue (×563).

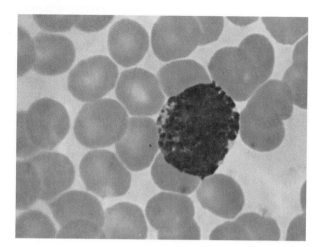

FIGURE 4.30

A monocyte is the largest type of blood cell (×640).

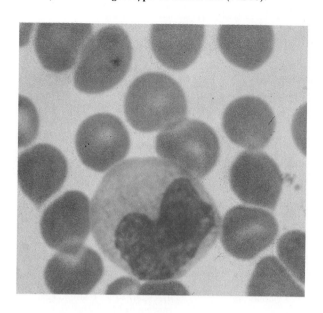

Leukocytes of the agranulocyte group include *monocytes* and *lymphocytes.*

Monocytes are the largest cells found in blood, having diameters two to three times greater than red cells. Their nuclei vary in shape and are described as round, kidney-shaped, oval, or lobed (figure 4.30).

Although large *lymphocytes* are sometimes found in blood, usually they are only slightly larger than red cells. Typically, a lymphocyte contains a relatively large, round nucleus with a thin rim of cytoplasm surrounding it (figure 4.31). Lymphocytes usually complete their development in lymphatic organs.

Platelets, or *thrombocytes,* are not complete cells. They arise from very large cells in red bone marrow, called *megakaryocytes.* These cells give off tiny cytoplasmic fragments, and as they detach and enter the circulation, they become platelets (figure 4.23). Each platelet is a round disk that lacks a nucleus and is much smaller than a red blood cell.

Chart 4.4 summarizes the characteristics of blood cells and platelets.

FIGURE 4.31

The lymphocyte (arrow) contains a large, round nucleus; a neutrophil has a lobed nucleus (on the right) (×640).

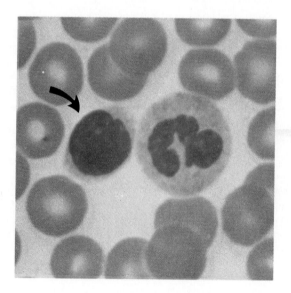

Chart 4.4 Cellular components of blood

Component	Description	Number present	Function
Red blood cell (erythrocyte)	Biconcave disk without nucleus	4,000,000 to 6,000,000 per mm	Transports oxygen and carbon dioxide
White blood cells (leukocytes)		5,000 to 10,000 per mm	Aids in defense against infections by microorganisms
Granulocytes	About twice the size of red cells, cytoplasmic granules present		
1. Neutrophil	Nucleus with two to five lobes, cytoplasmic granules stain pink in neutral stain	54%–62% of white cells present	Engulfs and destroys relatively small particles
2. Eosinophil	Nucleus bilobed, cytoplasmic granules stain red in acid stain	1%–3% of white cells present	Helps break down foreign substances, break down clots and remove products of immune reactions
3. Basophil	Nucleus lobed, cytoplasmic granules stain blue in basic stain	Less than 1% of white cells present	Releases substances that aid immune reactions
Agranulocytes	Cytoplasmic granules absent		
1. Monocyte	Two to three times larger than red cell, nuclear shape varies from round to kidney-shaped	3%–9% of white cells present	Engulfs and destroys relatively large particles
2. Lymphocyte	Only slightly larger than red cell, nucleus nearly fills cell	25%–33% of white cells present	Produces substances that act against foreign particles
Platelet (thrombocyte)	Cytoplasmic fragment	130,000 to 360,000 per mm	Helps control blood loss from broken vessels

A CLINICAL APPLICATION

Leukemia

Leukemia is a form of cancer characterized by an uncontrolled production of specific types of leukocytes. There are two major types of leukemia. *Myeloid leukemia* results from an abnormal production of granulocytes by the red bone marrow, while *lymphoid leukemia* is accompanied by increased formation of lymphocytes from lymph nodes. In both types, the cells produced usually fail to mature into functional cells. Thus, even though large numbers of neutrophils may be formed in myeloid leukemia, these cells have little ability to destroy bacteria, and the patient has a lowered resistance to infections.

Eventually, the cells responsible for the overproduction of leukocytes tend to spread from the bone marrow or lymph nodes to other parts, and as a result white blood cells are produced abnormally in tissues throughout the body. As with other forms of cancer, the leukemic cells finally appear in such great numbers that they crowd out the normal, functioning cells. For example, leukemic cells originating in red bone marrow may invade other regions of the bone, weakening its structure and stimulating pain receptors. Also, as the normal red marrow is crowded out, the patient is likely to develop deficiencies of red blood cells (anemia) and blood platelets (thrombocytopenia).

Anemia results in a reduced oxygen-carrying capacity of the blood. The lack of platelets usually is reflected in an increasing tendency to bleed.

Leukemias also are classified as *acute* or *chronic*. An acute condition appears suddenly, the symptoms progress rapidly, and death occurs in a few months when the condition is untreated. Chronic forms begin more slowly and may remain undetected for many months. Without treatment, life expectancy is about three years.

The greatest success in treatment has been achieved with acute lymphoid leukemia, which is the most common cancerous condition in children. This treatment usually involves counteracting the side effects of the condition, such as anemia, blood loss, and an increased susceptibility to infections, as well as administering chemotherapeutic drugs.

Although acute lymphoid leukemia may occur at any age, the chronic form usually occurs after 50 years of age. Acute myeloid leukemia also may occur at any age, but it is more frequent in adults; chronic myeloid leukemia is primarily a disease of adults between 20 and 50 years of age.

Chart 4.5 Connective tissues

Type	Function	Location	Figure
Loose connective tissue	Binds organs together, holds tissue fluids	Beneath the skin, between muscles, beneath most epithelial layers	4.14
Adipose tissue	Protection, insulation, and storage of energy in fat	Beneath the skin, around the kidneys, behind the eyeballs, on the surface of the heart	4.15
Fibrous connective tissue	Binds organs together	Tendons, ligaments, skin	4.16
Elastic connective tissue	Provides elastic quality	In walls of arteries, airways, and certain ligaments	4.17
Reticular connective tissue	Support	Walls of liver, spleen, and lymphatic organs	4.18
Hyaline cartilage	Support, protection, provides framework	Ends of bones, nose, and rings in walls of respiratory passages	4.19
Elastic cartilage	Support, protection, provides framework	Framework of external ear and part of the larynx	4.20
Fibrocartilage	Support, protection	Between bony parts of backbone, pelvic girdle, and knee	4.21
Bone	Support, protection, provides framework, stores minerals, produces blood cells	Bones of skeleton	4.22
Blood	Transports substances, fights infection	Within blood vessels and spaces between cells	4.23
Reticuloendothelial tissue	Destroys foreign particles	Blood, lungs, brain, bone marrow, lymph organs	4.11

Reticuloendothelial Tissue

Reticuloendothelial tissue is composed of a variety of specialized cells that are widely scattered throughout the body. As a group, these cells function to ingest and destroy foreign particles, such as microorganisms, that may invade the body. Thus, they are particularly important in defending the body against infection.

Reticuloendothelial cells include types found in the blood, lungs, brain, bone marrow, spleen, liver, and lymph glands. The most common ones, however, are *macrophages*. Typically, a macrophage remains in a fixed position until it "senses" a foreign particle. Then, the macrophage becomes motile, moves toward the invader, and may engulf and destroy it. Once the invader has been destroyed, the macrophage may become fixed again (figure 4.11).

Chart 4.5 lists the characteristics of the major types of connective tissues.

1. Describe the general characteristics of cartilage.
2. Explain why injured bone heals more rapidly than injured cartilage.
3. What are the components of blood?
4. What do the cells of reticuloendothelial tissue have in common?

Muscle Tissues

General Characteristics

Muscle tissues are contractile—their elongated cells, or *muscle fibers,* can change shape by becoming shorter and thicker. As they contract, the fibers pull at their attached ends and cause body parts to move. The three types of muscle tissue are skeletal muscle, smooth muscle, and cardiac muscle.

Skeletal Muscle Tissue

Skeletal muscle tissue (figure 4.32) is found in muscles that usually are attached to bones and can be controlled by conscious effort. For this reason, the tissue is often called *voluntary muscle.*

Each cell, or muscle fiber, is a thin, elongated cylinder with rounded ends. Just beneath its cell membrane or *sarcolemma,* the cytoplasm, or *sarcoplasm,* of the fiber contains many small, oval nuclei and mitochondria. Also, within the sarcoplasm are numerous threadlike *myofibrils* that lie parallel to one another (figure 4.33). The myofibrils contain thick and thin filaments (microfilaments). The arrangement of these filaments produces the characteristic light and dark *striations* of muscle fibers (figure 4.34).

FIGURE 4.32

(a) Skeletal muscle tissue is composed of striated muscle fibers that contain many nuclei. (b) Micrograph of skeletal muscle tissue (×250).

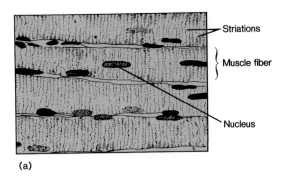

(a)

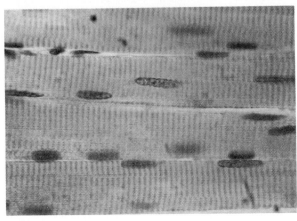

(b)

FIGURE 4.33

A single skeletal muscle fiber.

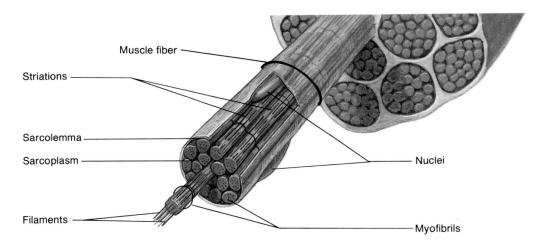

During embryonic development, skeletal muscle cells form from the fusion of cells called myoblasts. In an adult skeletal muscle, a few myoblasts remain as satellite cells. These are flattened, inactive cells lying on the surface of skeletal muscle fibers. If muscle cells are damaged, the satellite cells may divide to form new myoblasts that fuse and form new skeletal muscle cells.

Within the cytoplasm of a muscle fiber is the *sarcoplasmic reticulum*. It is a specialized type of smooth endoplasmic reticulum. Another set of membranous channels called *transverse tubules* (T-tubules) extends inward from the cell surface and passes all the way through the fiber. Each of these tubules contains fluid from outside the cell. Enlarged portions of the sarcoplasmic reticulum called *cisternae* lie on either side of a transverse tubule, and both of these structures function in muscle cell contraction (figure 4.35).

FIGURE 4.34

(a) A skeletal muscle fiber contains numerous myofibrils, each consisting of units called sarcomeres (b). (c) Note the bands of striations in this transmission electron micrograph of myofibrils.

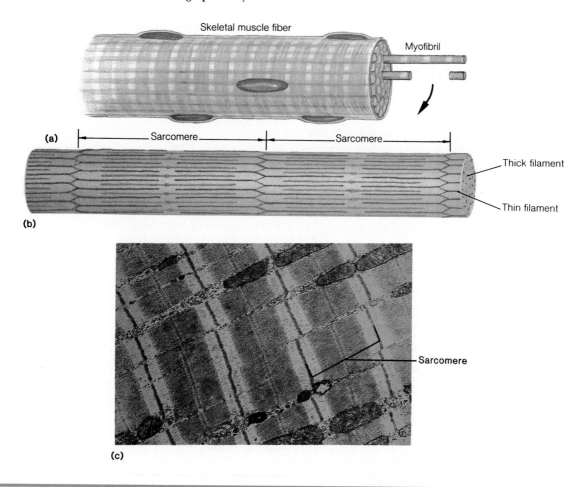

Skeletal muscle fiber

Myofibril

(a)

Sarcomere

Sarcomere

(b)

Thick filament

Thin filament

Sarcomere

(c)

FIGURE 4.35

Within the sarcoplasm of a skeletal muscle fiber are a network of sarcoplasmic reticulum and a system of transverse tubules.

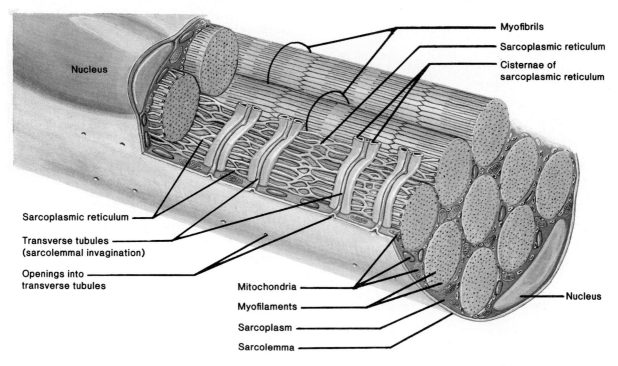

Nucleus

Myofibrils

Sarcoplasmic reticulum

Cisternae of sarcoplasmic reticulum

Sarcoplasmic reticulum

Transverse tubules (sarcolemmal invagination)

Openings into transverse tubules

Mitochondria

Myofilaments

Sarcoplasm

Sarcolemma

Nucleus

Smooth Muscle Tissue

Smooth muscle tissue (figure 4.36) is called smooth because its cells lack striations. Unlike skeletal muscle, smooth muscle usually cannot be stimulated to contract by conscious efforts. Thus, it is a type of *involuntary muscle.*

Smooth muscle cells are shorter than those of skeletal muscle, and they have single, centrally located nuclei. These cells are elongated with tapering ends. They lack transverse tubules and their sarcoplasmic reticula are not well developed.

There are two major types of smooth muscles. In one type, called *multiunit smooth muscle,* the muscle fibers are less organized and occur as separate fibers rather than in sheets. Smooth muscle of this type is found in irises of the eyes and in walls of blood vessels.

The second type of smooth muscle is called *visceral smooth muscle.* It is composed of sheets of spindle-shaped cells that are in close contact and possess gap junctions

between one another. These cells are positioned so the thick portion of each cell is next to the thin parts of adjacent cells. Visceral smooth muscle is the more common type and is found in walls of hollow visceral organs such as the stomach, intestines, urinary bladder, and uterus. Usually there are two layers of smooth muscle in the walls of these organs. The fibers of the outer coat are directed longitudinally, while those of the inner coat are arranged circularly. These layers are responsible for the changes in size and shape that occur in visceral organs as they carry on their special functions.

Cardiac Muscle Tissue

Cardiac muscle tissue occurs only in the heart. Its cells, which are striated, are joined end to end. The resulting fibers are branched and interconnected in complex networks. Each cell has a single nucleus, well-developed sarcoplasmic reticulum, a system of transverse tubules, and many mitochondria.

Opposing ends of cardiac muscle cells are separated by specialized areas of cell membrane called *intercalated disks.* These disks contain many gap junctions (see chapter 3) that help to hold adjacent cells together and allow muscle impulses to travel from cell to cell (figure 4.37).

Cardiac muscle, like smooth muscle, is controlled involuntarily, and, in fact, can continue to function without being stimulated by nerve impulses. This tissue is responsible for pumping blood through the heart chambers and into blood vessels.

Chart 4.6 summarizes the general characteristics of muscle tissues.

FIGURE 4.36

(*a*) Smooth muscle tissue is formed of spindle-shaped cells, each containing a single nucleus. (*b*) Note the nuclei in this micrograph (×250).

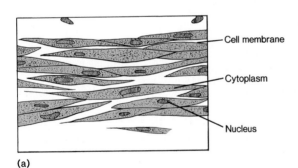

Cell membrane

Cytoplasm

Nucleus

(a)

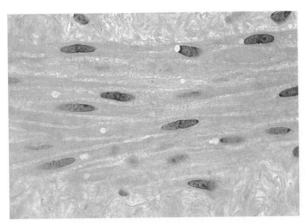

(b)

The cells of different tissues vary greatly in their abilities to reproduce. For example, the epithelial cells of skin and inner lining of the digestive tube, and the connective tissue cells that form blood cells in bones are reproducing continuously. However, skeletal and cardiac muscle cells and nerve cells do not seem to reproduce at all after becoming differentiated.

Fibroblasts respond rapidly to injuries by reproducing and becoming active in fiber production. Therefore, they are often the principal agents of repair in tissues that have limited abilities to regenerate themselves. For instance, cardiac muscle tissue typically degenerates in the regions damaged by a heart attack. Such tissue may be replaced by connective tissue built by fibroblasts, which later appears as a scar.

1. List the general characteristics of muscle tissue.
2. Distinguish between skeletal, smooth, and cardiac muscle tissue.

FIGURE 4.37

(a) How is this cardiac muscle tissue similar to skeletal muscle? How is it similar to smooth muscle? (b) Note the intercalated disks in this micrograph (×400). (c) Intercalated disks (arrow) of cardiac muscle, shown in this transmission electron micrograph, hold adjacent cells together.

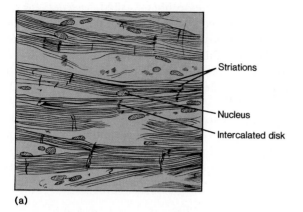

Striations

Nucleus

Intercalated disk

(a)

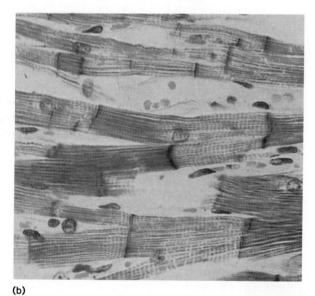

(b)

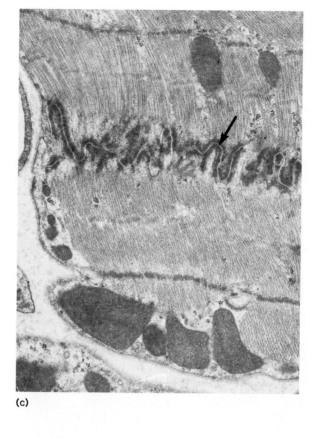

(c)

Nerve Tissue

Nerve tissue is found in the brain, spinal cord, and peripheral nerves. The basic cells of this tissue are called *nerve cells,* or *neurons,* and they are among the more highly specialized body cells. Neurons are sensitive to changes in their surroundings. They respond by transmitting nerve impulses along cellular extensions to other neurons or to muscles or glands.

A neuron includes a *cell body* and tubular *nerve fibers* extending from it. The cell body contains mitochondria,

	Chart 4.6 Types of muscle tissue		
	Skeletal	**Smooth**	**Cardiac**
Major location	Skeletal muscles	Walls of hollow visceral organs	Wall of heart
Major function	Movement of bones at joints, maintenance of posture	Movement of visceral organs	Pumping action of heart
Cellular characteristics			
Striations	Present	Absent	Present
Nucleus	Multiple nuclei	Single nucleus	Single nucleus
Special features	Transverse tubule system well developed	Lacks transverse tubules	Transverse tubule system well developed, adjacent cells separated by intercalated disks
Mode of control	Voluntary	Involuntary	Involuntary

FIGURE 4.38

(*a*) Neurons in nerve tissue function to transmit impulses to other neurons or to muscles or glands. (*b*) What features of a neuron can you identify in this micrograph (×450)?

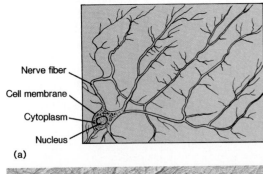

Nerve fiber

Cell membrane

Cytoplasm

Nucleus

(a)

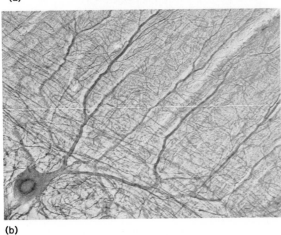

(b)

lysosomes, a Golgi apparatus, and many cytoplasmic inclusions. Near the center of the cell body there is a large spherical nucleus. This nucleus, however, does not undergo mitosis after the nervous system has completed development; consequently, mature neurons seem to be incapable of reproducing (figure 4.38).

Two kinds of nerve fibers, called *dendrites* and *axons*, extend from the cell bodies of most neurons. Although a neuron usually has many dendrites, it has a single axon.

As a result of the extremely complex patterns by which neurons are connected with each other and with other body parts, they are able to coordinate and regulate many body functions.

In addition to neurons, nerve tissue contains *neuroglial cells*. These cells support and bind the components of nerve tissue together, destroy foreign particles, and supply nutrients to neurons by connecting them to blood vessels. A more detailed discussion of nerve tissue is found in chapter 9.

1. Describe the general characteristics of nerve tissue.
2. Distinguish between neurons and neuroglial cells.

An organ is composed of two or more types of tissues. Figure 4.39 is a micrograph illustrating the arrangement of tissues in skin.

FIGURE 4.39

The tissues that comprise the skin (×25).

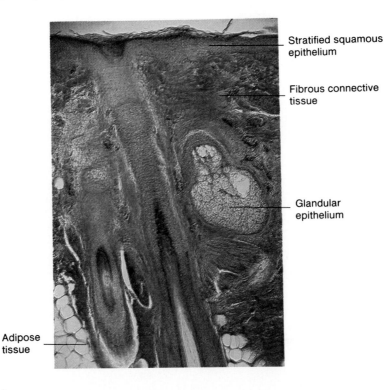

Stratified squamous epithelium

Fibrous connective tissue

Glandular epithelium

Adipose tissue

Chapter Summary

Introduction (page 75)

Cells are arranged in layers or groups called tissues. Cells are separated by intercellular materials whose composition varies from solid to liquid. Four major types of human tissues are epithelial tissue, connective tissue, muscle tissue, and nerve tissue.

Epithelial Tissues (page 75)

1. General characteristics
   a. Epithelial tissue covers all free body surfaces and is the major tissue of glands.
   b. Epithelium is anchored to a basement membrane, which is, in turn, attached to underlying connective tissue. Epithelial tissue lacks blood vessels, contains little intercellular material, and is replaced continuously.
   c. It functions in protection, secretion, absorption, excretion, and sensory reception.
2. Simple squamous epithelium
   a. This tissue consists of a single layer of thin, flattened cells through which substances pass rather easily.
   b. It functions in the exchange of gases in the lungs and lines blood vessels, lymph vessels, and various membranes within the thorax and abdomen.
3. Simple cuboidal epithelium
   a. This tissue consists of a single layer of cube-shaped cells.
   b. It carries on secretion and absorption in the kidneys and various glands.
4. Simple columnar epithelium
   a. This tissue is composed of elongated cells whose nuclei are located near the basement membrane.
   b. It lines the uterus and digestive tract, where it functions in protection, secretion, and absorption.
   c. Absorbing cells often possess microvilli.
   d. This tissue usually contains goblet cells that secrete mucus.
5. Pseudostratified columnar epithelium
   a. This tissue appears stratified because the nuclei are located at different levels within the cells.
   b. Its cells may have cilia, which function to move mucus or cells over the surface of the tissue.
   c. It lines various tubes of the respiratory and reproductive systems.
6. Stratified squamous epithelium
   a. This tissue is composed of many cell layers.
   b. It protects underlying cells from harmful environmental effects.
   c. It covers the skin and lines the mouth, throat, vagina, and anal canal.
7. Transitional epithelium
   a. This tissue is specialized to undergo distension.
   b. It occurs in the walls of various organs of the urinary tract.
   c. It helps prevent the contents of the urinary passageways from moving outward.
8. Glandular epithelium
   a. Glandular epithelium is composed of cells that are specialized to secrete substances.
   b. One or more cells can constitute a gland.
      (1) Exocrine glands secrete into ducts.
      (2) Endocrine glands secrete into tissue fluid or blood.
   c. Glands are classified according to the arrangement of their cells.
      (1) Simple glands have unbranched ducts.
      (2) Compound glands have branched ducts.
      (3) Tubular glands consist of simple epithelial-lined tubes.
      (4) Alveolar glands consist of saclike dilations connected to the surface by narrow ducts.
   d. Exocrine glands are classified according to the composition of their secretions.
      (1) Merocrine glands secrete watery fluids without loss of cytoplasm. Most secretory cells are merocrine.
         (a) Serous cells secrete watery fluid.
         (b) Mucous cells secrete mucus.
      (2) Apocrine glands lose portions of their cells during secretion.
      (3) Holocrine glands release cells filled with secretory products.

Connective Tissues (page 81)

1. General characteristics
   a. Connective tissue connects, supports, protects, provides frameworks, fills spaces, stores fat, produces blood cells, provides protection against infection, and helps repair tissues.
   b. Connective tissue cells usually are some distance apart, and they have considerable intercellular material between them.
   c. The intercellular matrix consists of fibers and ground substance.
2. Major cell types
   a. Fibroblasts produce collagenous and elastic fibers.
   b. Macrophages engulf and destroy foreign cells.
   c. Mast cells release substances that aid immune reactions.
3. Connective tissue fibers
   a. Collagenous fibers are composed of collagen and have great tensile strength.
   b. Elastic fibers are composed of microfibrils embedded in elastin and are very elastic.
   c. Reticular fibers are very fine collagenous fibers.
4. Loose connective tissue
   a. This tissue forms thin membranes between organs and binds them together.
   b. It is found beneath the skin and between muscles.
   c. It contains tissue fluids in intercellular spaces.
5. Adipose tissue
   a. Adipose tissue is a specialized form of loose connective tissue that stores energy as fat, provides a protective cushion, and functions as a heat insulator.
   b. It is found beneath the skin, in certain abdominal membranes, and around the kidneys, heart, and various joints.

6. Fibrous connective tissue
    a. This tissue is composed largely of strong, collagenous fibers that bind parts together.
    b. It is found in tendons, ligaments, eyes, and skin.
7. Elastic connective tissue
    a. This tissue is composed mainly of elastic fibers.
    b. It imparts an elastic quality to the walls of certain hollow internal organs.
8. Reticular connective tissue
    a. This tissue consists largely of thin, branched collagenous fibers.
    b. It supports the walls of the liver, spleen, and lymphatic organs.
9. Cartilage
    a. Cartilage provides support and framework for various parts.
    b. Its intercellular material is largely composed of fibers and a gel-like ground substance.
    c. It lacks a direct blood supply and is slow to heal following an injury.
    d. Cartilaginous structures are usually enclosed in a perichondrium, which contains blood vessels.
    e. Major types are hyaline cartilage, elastic cartilage, and fibrocartilage.
    f. Cartilage occurs at the ends of various bones, in the ear, in the larynx, and in pads between bones of the backbone, pelvic girdle, and knees.
10. Bone
    a. The intercellular matrix of bone contains minerals and collagen.
    b. Its cells are arranged in concentric circles around osteonic canals and are interconnected by canaliculi.
    c. It is an active tissue that heals rapidly following an injury.
11. Blood
    a. Blood is composed of cells suspended in fluid.
    b. The cells are formed by red marrow in the hollow parts of certain bones.
    c. Characteristics of red blood cells
        (1) Red blood cells are biconcave disks that lack nuclei.
    d. Types of white blood cells
        (1) White blood cells function to defend the body against infections by microorganisms.
        (2) Granulocytes include neutrophils, eosinophils, and basophils.
        (3) Agranulocytes include monocytes and lymphocytes.
    e. Blood platelets are fragments of giant cells that leave bone marrow and enter the circulation.
12. Reticuloendothelial tissue
    a. This tissue is composed of a variety of cells that are widely distributed throughout the body tissues.
    b. It defends the body against invasion by microorganisms.

Muscle Tissues (page 93)
1. General characteristics
    a. Muscle tissue is contractile tissue that moves parts attached to it.
    b. Three types are skeletal, smooth, and cardiac muscle tissues.
2. Skeletal muscle tissue
    a. Muscles containing this tissue are usually attached to bones and are controlled by conscious effort.
    b. Skeletal muscle fibers
        (1) Each skeletal muscle cell has numerous nuclei.
        (2) The cytoplasm contains mitochondria, a sarcoplasmic reticulum, transverse tubules, and myofibrils.
        (3) Striations are produced by the arrangement of thick and thin filaments.
        (4) Transverse tubules extend from the cell membrane into the cytoplasm.
3. Smooth muscle tissue
    a. This tissue is found in walls of hollow internal organs and usually functions involuntarily.
    b. Smooth muscle cells contain filaments, lack transverse tubules and striations, and the sarcoplasmic reticula are not well developed.
    c. Types include multiunit smooth muscle and visceral smooth muscle.
4. Cardiac muscle tissue
    a. This tissue is found only in the heart.
    b. Cells are joined by intercalated disks and arranged in branched, interconnecting networks.
    c. Cells have single nuclei, well-developed sarcoplasmic reticula, transverse tubules, and many mitochondria.
    d. Cardiac muscle tissue is controlled by involuntary activity.

Nerve Tissue (page 97)
1. Nerve tissue is found in the brain, spinal cord, and peripheral nerves.
2. Neurons
    a. Neurons are sensitive to changes and respond by transmitting nerve impulses to other neurons or to other body parts.
    b. The cell body of a neuron contains a nucleus and other organelles usually found in cells.
    c. Dendrites and axons are nerve fibers that extend from the cell body.
    d. They function in coordinating and regulating body activities.
    e. Neuroglial cells function to bind and support nerve tissue, destroy foreign particles, and connect neurons to blood vessels.

Clinical Application of Knowledge

1. The sweeping action of the ciliated epithelium that lines respiratory passages is inhibited by excessive exposure to tobacco smoke and airborne pollutants. What special problems is this likely to create?
2. Vitamin A deficiency causes nonkeratinized epithelium to become keratinized. What would be the results of such a change in this tissue?
3. Joints, such as the elbow, shoulder, and knee, contain considerable amounts of cartilage and fibrous connective tissue. How is this related to the fact that joint injuries are often very slow to heal?
4. A group of disorders called collagenous diseases are characterized by the deterioration of connective tissues. Why would you expect such diseases to produce widely varying symptoms?
5. Since nerve cells cannot divide, which cells would you expect to produce the most tumors in the nerve tissue?

Review Activities

Part A
1. Define *tissue*.
2. Name the four major types of tissue found in the human body.
3. Describe the general characteristics of epithelial tissue.
4. Distinguish between a simple epithelium and a stratified epithelium.
5. Explain how the structure of simple squamous epithelium is related to its function.
6. Name an organ in which each of the epithelial tissues is found, and give the function of the tissue in each case.
7. Define *gland*.
8. Distinguish between an exocrine gland and an endocrine gland.
9. Explain how glands are classified according to the structure of their ducts and the arrangement of their cells.
10. Explain how glands are classified according to the nature of their cellular secretions.
11. Distinguish between a serous cell and a mucous cell.
12. Describe the general characteristics of connective tissue.
13. Describe three major types of connective tissue cells.
14. Distinguish between collagenous fibers and elastic fibers.
15. Explain how adipose tissue forms from connective tissue.
16. Describe the functions of adipose tissue.
17. Distinguish between elastic and reticular connective tissues.
18. Explain why injured fibrous connective tissue and cartilage are usually slow to heal.
19. Name the major types of cartilage, and describe their differences and similarities.
20. Describe how bone cells are arranged in bone tissue.
21. Explain how nutrients are supplied to bone cells.
22. Describe the cellular components of blood.
23. Define *reticuloendothelial tissue*.
24. Describe the general characteristics of muscle tissue.
25. Distinguish between skeletal, smooth, and cardiac muscle tissues.
26. Describe the general characteristics of nerve tissue.
27. Distinguish between neurons and neuroglial cells.

Part B
Match the features in column I to the tissues in column II.

I	II
1. basement membrane	A. epithelial tissue
2. macrophage	B. connective tissue
3. collagen fibers	C. muscle tissue
4. striated cells	D. nerve tissue
5. osteon	
6. dendrites	
7. microvilli	
8. matrix	
9. holocrine gland	
10. chondrocyte	

CHAPTER 5

Membranes and the Integumentary System

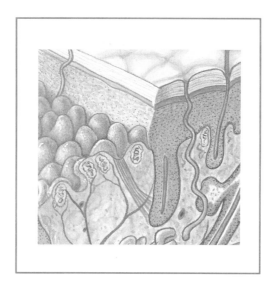

The previous chapters dealt with the lower levels of organization within the human organism—tissues, cells, and cellular organelles.

Chapter 5 explains how tissues are grouped to form organs and how organs comprise organ systems. In this explanation, various membranes, including the skin, are used as examples of organs. Because skin acts with hair follicles, sebaceous glands, and sweat glands to provide a variety of vital functions, these organs together constitute the integumentary organ system.

Chapter Outline

Chapter Objectives

After you have studied this chapter, you should be able to

1. Describe four major types of membranes.

2. Describe the structure of the various layers of skin.

3. List the general functions of each layer of the skin.

4. Describe the accessory organs associated with skin.

5. Explain the functions of each accessory organ.

6. Complete the review activities at the end of this chapter. Note that the items are worded in the form of specific learning objectives. You may want to refer to them before reading the chapter.

Aids to Understanding Words

alb-, white: *alb*ino—condition characterized by a lack of pigment.

cut-, skin: sub*cut*aneous—beneath the skin.

derm-, skin: *derm*is—inner layer of the skin.

epi-, upon: *epi*dermis—outer layer of the skin.

follic-, small bag: hair *follic*le—tubelike depression in which a hair develops.

kerat-, horn: *kerat*in—protein produced as epidermal cells die and harden.

melan-, black: *melan*in—dark pigment produced by certain cells.

por-, channel: *por*e—opening by which a sweat gland communicates to the skin surface.

seb-, grease: *seb*aceous gland—gland that secretes an oily substance.

Introduction

Two or more kinds of tissues grouped together and performing specialized functions constitute an organ. Thus, the thin, sheetlike structures called membranes, composed of epithelium and connective tissue, which cover body surfaces and line body cavities, are organs. One of these membranes, the cutaneous membrane, together with various accessory organs makes up the **integumentary system.**

Types of Membranes

The four major types of membranes are: *serous, mucous, cutaneous,* and *synovial.* Usually these structures are relatively thin. Serous, mucous, and cutaneous membranes are composed of epithelial tissue and some underlying connective tissue; synovial membranes are composed entirely of various connective tissues.

Serous membranes line body cavities that lack openings to the outside. They form the inner linings of the thorax and abdomen, and they cover the organs within these cavities. A serous membrane consists of a layer of simple squamous epithelium (mesothelium) and a thin layer of loose connective tissue. It secretes watery *serous fluid,* which helps to lubricate the surfaces of the membrane. (See figures 2.4 and 2.5.)

Mucous membranes line cavities and tubes that open to the outside of the body. These include the oral and nasal cavities, and tubes of the digestive, respiratory, urinary, and reproductive systems. A mucous membrane consists of epithelium overlying a layer of loose connective tissue; however, the type of epithelium varies with the location of the membrane. For example, stratified squamous epithelium lines the oral cavity, pseudostratified columnar epithelium lines part of the nasal cavity, and simple columnar epithelium lines the small intestine. Specialized cells within a mucous membrane secrete *mucus,* which lubricates and protects these membranes.

The **cutaneous membrane** is an organ of the integumentary system and is more commonly called *skin.* It is described in detail in the following section of this chapter.

Synovial membranes form the inner linings of joint cavities between the ends of bones at freely movable joints (synovial joints). These membranes usually include fibrous connective tissue overlying loose connective tissue and adipose tissue. They secrete a thick, colorless *synovial fluid* into the joint cavity, which lubricates the ends of bones within the joint. (Synovial joints are described in chapter 7.)

Skin and Its Tissues

Skin is one of the larger and more versatile organs. For example, it functions as a protective covering that prevents many harmful substances, including microorganisms, from entering the body. At the same time, it retards the loss of water from deeper tissues. Skin helps regulate body temperature, houses sensory receptors, synthesizes various chemicals, and excretes small quantities of waste substances. Also, people are recognized (and their ages often judged) by characteristics of their skin.

Skin includes two distinct layers of tissues. The outer layer, called **epidermis,** is composed of stratified squamous epithelium. The inner layer, or **dermis,** is thicker than the epidermis, and includes a variety of tissues, such as fibrous connective tissue, epithelial tissue, smooth muscle tissue, nerve tissue, and blood (figure 5.1). These two layers of the skin are separated by a *basement membrane,* which is anchored to the dermis by short fibers.

Beneath the dermis are masses of loose connective and adipose tissues that bind the skin to underlying organs. They form the **subcutaneous layer.**

1. Name four types of membranes and explain how they differ.
2. List the general functions of skin.
3. Name the tissue(s) found in the outer and inner layers of the skin.

Epidermis

Because the epidermis is composed of epithelium, it lacks blood vessels. However, the deeper cells of the epidermis, which are near the dermis, are nourished by dermal blood vessels and are capable of reproducing. They form a layer called *stratum basale* (stratum germinativum), in which the cells divide and grow. As they enlarge, these newer cells push the older epidermal cells away from the dermis toward the outer skin surface. The farther the cells travel, the poorer their nutrient supply becomes, and in time they die.

Meanwhile, the membranes of the older cells (keratinocytes) become thickened and develop numerous desmosomes that fasten them to adjacent cells. At the same time, the cells begin to undergo a hardening process called **keratinization,** during which strands of tough, fibrous, waterproof protein called *keratin* develop within the cell. As a result, many layers of tough, tightly packed dead cells accumulate in the outer portion of the epidermis. This outermost layer is called **stratum corneum,** and the dead cells that compose it are continually lost from the surface.

The structural organization of epidermis varies from region to region. For example, it is most highly developed on the palms of the hands and soles of the feet, and may be 0.8 to 1.4 mm thick. In these areas, five layers of epidermis can be distinguished. They include *stratum basale* (stratum germinativum or basal cell layer), which is the deepest layer; *stratum spinosum,* a relatively thick layer; *stratum granulosum,* a granular layer (this layer may be missing in areas where the epidermis is thin); *stratum lucidum* (this layer may be absent where the epidermis is thin); and *stratum corneum,* a fully keratinized layer. The cells of

FIGURE 5.1

A section of skin. Why is the skin considered to be an organ?

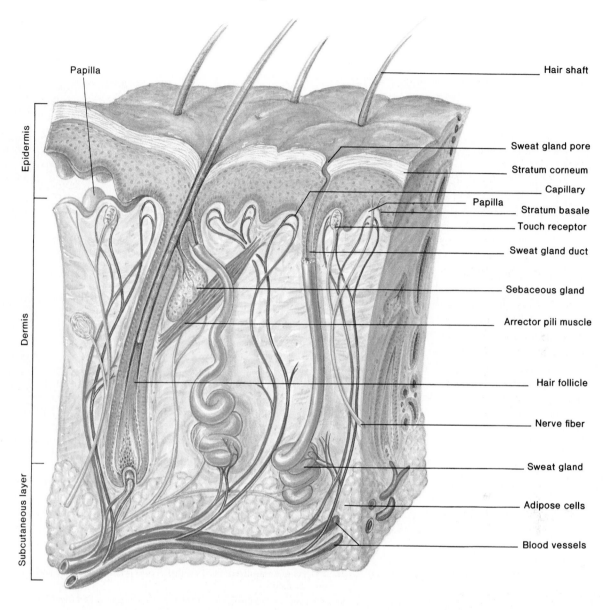

Papilla

Epidermis

Dermis

Subcutaneous layer

Hair shaft

Sweat gland pore

Stratum corneum

Capillary

Papilla

Stratum basale

Touch receptor

Sweat gland duct

Sebaceous gland

Arrector pili muscle

Hair follicle

Nerve fiber

Sweat gland

Adipose cells

Blood vessels

these layers are characterized by changes they undergo as they are pushed toward the surface (figure 5.2).

In other body regions, the epidermis is usually much thinner, averaging 0.07 to 0.12 mm. Chart 5.1 summarizes the characteristics of each layer of epidermis.

In healthy skin, production of epidermal cells is closely balanced with loss of stratum corneum, so that skin seldom wears away completely. In fact, the rate of cellular reproduction tends to increase in regions where skin is being rubbed or pressed regularly. This response causes the growth of calluses on the palms and soles as well as the development of corns on the toes when poorly fitting shoes rub the skin excessively.

FIGURE 5.2
(*a*) The various layers of the epidermis are characterized by changes that occur in cells as they are pushed toward the surface of the skin. (*b*) Which layers of the epidermis can you identify in this micrograph from the palm of the hand (×150)?

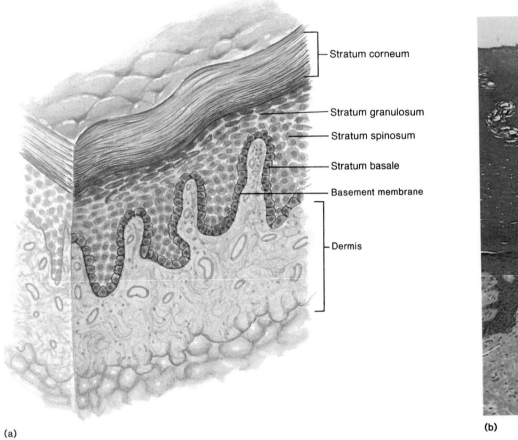

(a)

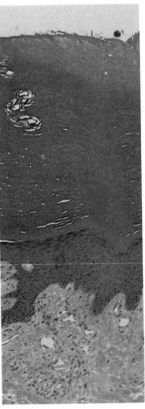

(b)

Chart 5.1 Layers of the epidermis

Layer	Location	Characteristics
Stratum corneum (horny layer)	Outermost layer	Many layers of keratinized, dead epithelial cells that are flattened and nonnucleated
Stratum lucidum	Beneath stratum corneum	Several layers of flattened, clear cells that are closely packed together
Stratum granulosum	Beneath stratum corneum and stratum lucidum	Three to five layers of flattened granular cells that contain shrunken fibers of keratin and shriveled nuclei
Stratum spinosum	Beneath stratum granulosum	Many layers of cells with centrally located, large oval nuclei and developing fibers of keratin; cells becoming flattened
Stratum basale (basal cell layer)	Deepest layer	A single row of cuboidal or columnar cells that undergo mitosis; this layer also includes pigment-producing melanocytes

FIGURE 5.3

Melanocytes (arrows) that occur mainly in the deeper layers of the epidermis produce the pigment called melanin (×160).

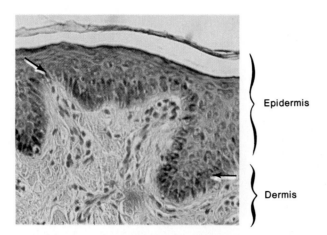

Epidermis

Dermis

FIGURE 5.4

(a) Transmission electron micrograph of a melanocyte with pigment-containing granules (×10,000); (b) a melanocyte includes pigment-containing extensions that pass between nearby epidermal cells.

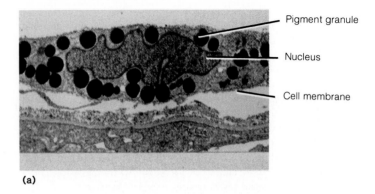

Pigment granule

Nucleus

Cell membrane

(a)

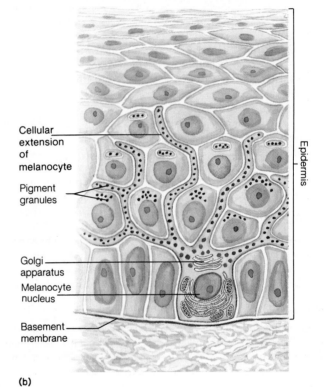

Cellular extension of melanocyte

Pigment granules

Golgi apparatus

Melanocyte nucleus

Basement membrane

Epidermis

(b)

Because blood vessels in the dermis supply nutrients to the epidermis, any interference with blood flow is likely to result in death of epidermal cells. For example, when a person lies in one position for a prolonged time, weight of the body pressing against the bed interferes with the skin's blood supply. If cells die, tissues begin to break down (necrosis) and a pressure ulcer (also called decubitus ulcer, or bedsore) may appear.

Pressure ulcers usually occur in skin overlying bony projections, such as on the hip, heel, elbow, or shoulder. These ulcers often can be prevented by changing body position frequently or by massaging the skin to stimulate blood flow in regions associated with bony prominences. In the case of a paralyzed person who cannot feel pressure or respond to it by shifting position, special care must be taken to frequently turn the body in order to prevent pressure ulcers from developing.

A diet containing necessary nutrients and an adequate intake of fluids also helps to prevent this condition.

The epidermis has important protective functions. It shields the moist underlying tissues against excessive water loss, mechanical injury, and the effects of harmful chemicals. When it is unbroken, epidermis also prevents the entrance of many disease-causing microorganisms. *Melanin* is a dark pigment that occurs in the epidermis and is produced by specialized cells known as **melanocytes.** It absorbs light energy, and in this way helps to protect deeper cells from the damaging effects of ultraviolet rays of sunlight.

Melanocytes are found in the deepest portion of the epidermis (figure 5.3) and in underlying connective tissue of the dermis. Although they are the only cells that can produce melanin, the pigment may also be found in nearby epidermal cells. This happens because melanocytes have long, cellular extensions that pass upward between neighboring epidermal cells, and they can transfer granules of

melanin into these other cells by a process called *cytocrine secretion* (figure 5.4). Consequently, nearby epidermal cells may contain more melanin than the melanocytes.

1. Explain how the epidermis is organized.
2. What factors help prevent loss of body fluids through skin?
3. What is the function of melanin?

Skin Cancer

Skin cancer is most likely to arise from nonpigmented epithelial cells within the deep layer of the epidermis or from pigmented melanocytes. Skin cancers originating from epithelial cells are called *cutaneous carcinomas* (basal cell carcinoma or squamous cell carcinoma); those arising from melanocytes are known as *cutaneous melanomas* (melanocarcinomas or malignant melanomas).

Cutaneous carcinomas represent the most common type of skin cancer, and they occur most frequently in members of light-skinned populations who are over forty years of age. These cancers seem to be caused by the effects of the ultraviolet portion of sunlight on the chromosomes (DNA) of epithelial cells, and they usually appear in persons who are exposed to sunlight regularly. Thus, the incidence of cutaneous carcinoma is increased in persons who have spent considerable amounts of time outdoors—farmers, sailors, athletes, sunbathers, and so forth.

Cutaneous carcinoma often develops from hard, dry, scaly growths (lesions) that have reddish bases. Such lesions may be either flat or raised above the surface, and they adhere firmly to the skin, appearing most often on the neck, face, and scalp. Fortunately, cutaneous carcinomas are typically slow growing and can usually be cured completely by surgical removal or radiation treatment.

Because cutaneous melanomas develop from melanocytes, they are pigmented with melanin. Such lesions often have a variety of colored areas—variegated brown, black, gray, or blue—that are arranged haphazardly. They usually have irregular margins rather than smooth, regular outlines (figure 5.5).

Cutaneous melanomas may appear in young adults as well as in older ones, and seem to be caused by relatively short, intermittent exposure to high-intensity sunlight. Thus, the incidence of melanoma is increased in persons who generally stay indoors but occasionally sustain blistering sunburns during weekend activities or vacations.

Cutaneous melanomas occur most often in light-skinned persons, particularly those whose skin tends to burn rather than tan. They usually appear in the skin of the trunk, especially the back, or in the skin of the limbs. Such a lesion may arise from

FIGURE 5.5
A cutaneous (malignant) melanoma.

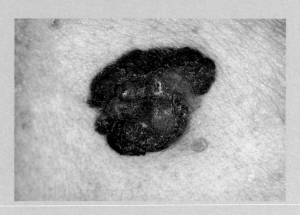

normal appearing skin or from a mole (nevus). Typically, the lesion enlarges by spreading through the skin horizontally, but eventually it may thicken and grow downward into the skin, invading the deeper tissues as well. If the melanoma is removed surgically while it is in its horizontal growth phase, its growth may be arrested. Once it has thickened and spread into the deeper tissues, however, it becomes difficult to treat, and the survival rate for persons with this form of cancer is very low.

For reasons that are not well understood, the incidence of melanoma within the U.S. population has been increasing rapidly for the past twenty years. To reduce the chances of occurrence, it is advisable to avoid exposing the skin to high-intensity sunlight and other sources of ultraviolet light. Whenever people are exposed to such radiation, they should wear protective clothing or use sunscreening lotions with high protective factors. In addition, such individuals should examine their skin regularly, and any unusual lesions—particularly those undergoing changes in color, shape, or surface texture—should be examined by a physician.

Dermis

The surface between the epidermis and dermis is usually uneven, because the epidermis has ridges projecting inward and the dermis has fingerlike *papillae* passing into the spaces between the ridges (see figure 5.1).

The dermis binds the epidermis to underlying tissues. It is composed largely of fibrous connective tissue that includes tough collagenous fibers and elastic fibers surrounded by a gel-like ground substance. Networks of these fibers give skin toughness and elasticity. The dermis can be divided into an upper *papillary layer* and a lower *reticular layer*. The collagenous and elastic fibers are thinner in the papillary layer (figure 5.1). On the average, the dermis is 1.0 to 2.0 mm thick; however, it may be as thin as 0.5 mm or less on the eyelids, or as thick as 3.0 mm on the soles of the feet.

Dermis also contains muscle fibers. In some regions, such as in the skin that encloses the testes (scrotum), there are numerous smooth muscle cells that can cause the skin to wrinkle when they contract. Other smooth muscles in the dermis are associated with accessory organs such as hair follicles and various glands. Many striated muscle fibers are anchored in the dermis of the skin of the face. They help produce the voluntary movements associated with facial expressions.

As was discussed, dermal blood vessels supply nutrients to deep living layers of the epidermis, as well as to dermal cells. These vessels also play an important role in the regulation of body temperature. When body heat production is excessive, the brain signals the dermal blood vessels to dilate. More blood enters them and some of the heat escapes to the outside. If heat is lost excessively, as may occur in a very cold environment, the dermal blood vessels are stimulated to constrict. This reduces the flow of heat-carrying blood through the skin and helps reduce heat loss.

Numerous nerve fibers are scattered throughout the dermis. Some of them (motor fibers) carry impulses to dermal muscles and glands, causing these structures to react. Others (sensory fibers) carry impulses away from specialized sensory receptors, such as touch, temperature, and pain receptors, located within the dermis (figure 5.1). Sensory receptors are discussed in chapter 10.

Hair follicles, sebaceous glands, and sweat glands also occur at various depths in the dermis. These parts, composed of epithelial tissue, are discussed in subsequent sections of this chapter.

Subcutaneous Layer

As was mentioned, the subcutaneous layer (hypodermis) lies beneath the dermis and consists largely of loose connective and adipose tissues (see figure 5.1). Collagenous and elastic fibers of this layer are continuous with those of the dermis, and although most of the fibers run parallel to the surface, they may travel in all directions. As a result, no sharp boundary exists between the dermis and the subcutaneous layer.

Adipose tissue of the subcutaneous layer functions as a heat insulator—helping to conserve body heat and impeding the entrance of heat from the outside. The amount of adipose tissue varies greatly with each individual's nutritional condition. It also varies in thickness from one region to another—for example, it is usually quite thick over the abdomen, but absent altogether in the eyelids.

The subcutaneous layer also contains the major blood vessels that supply the skin. Branches of these vessels form a network (rete cutaneum) between the dermis and subcutaneous layer. They, in turn, give off smaller vessels that supply the dermis above and the underlying adipose tissue.

1. What kinds of tissues make up the dermis?
2. What are the functions of these tissues?
3. What are the functions of the subcutaneous layer?

Accessory Organs of the Skin

Hair Follicles

Hair is present on all skin surfaces except the palms, soles, lips, nipples, and various parts of the external reproductive organs; however, it is not always well developed. For example, hair on the forehead and anterior surface of the arm is very fine.

Each hair develops from a group of epidermal cells at the base of a tubelike depression called a **hair follicle.** This follicle extends from the surface into the dermis and is occupied by the *root* of the hair. Epidermal cells at its base receive nourishment from dermal blood vessels that occur in a projection of connective tissue (dermal papilla) at the deep end of the follicle. As these epidermal cells divide and grow, older cells are pushed toward the surface. The cells that move upward and away from the nutrient supply become keratinized and die. Their remains constitute the structure of a developing hair, whose shaft extends outward from the skin's surface. In other words, a hair is composed of dead epidermal cells (figures 5.6 and 5.7).

FIGURE 5.6

(*a*) A hair grows from the base of a hair follicle when epidermal cells undergo cell division and older cells move outward and become keratinized. (*b*) What features can you identify in this micrograph of a hair follicle?

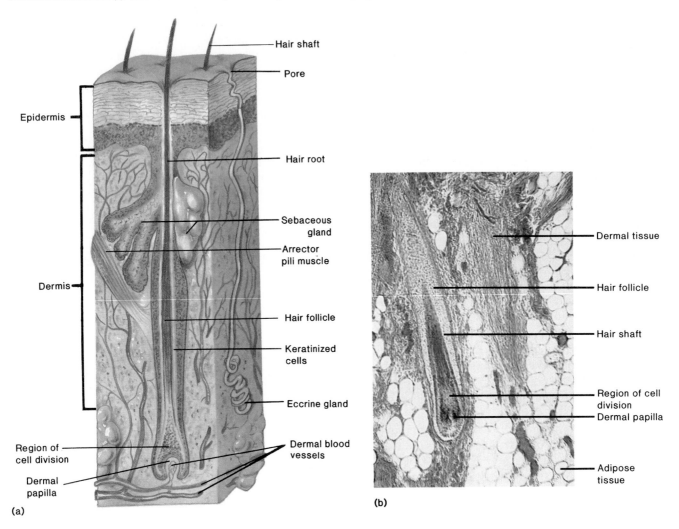

(a)

(b)

FIGURE 5.7

A scanning electron micrograph of a hair emerging from the epidermis.

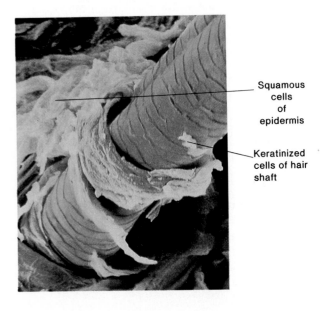

Usually a hair grows for a time and then undergoes a resting period during which it remains anchored in its follicle. Later, a new hair begins to grow from the base of the follicle, and the old hair is pushed outward and drops off. Sometimes, however, hairs are not replaced. When this occurs in the scalp, the result is baldness (alopecia). Baldness is usually inherited and is most likely to occur in males.

Hair color, like skin color, is determined by the type and amount of pigment produced by epidermal melanocytes. In the case of hair, the melanocytes are located at the deep end of the hair follicles. For example, dark hair contains an abundance of melanin, while blond hair contains an intermediate quantity; white hair lacks melanin. Bright red hair contains an iron pigment that does not occur in hair of any other color. A mixture of pigmented and unpigmented hair usually appears gray.

A bundle of smooth muscle cells, forming the **arrector pili muscle** (figure 5.1), is attached to each hair follicle. This muscle is positioned so that a short hair within the follicle stands on end when the muscle contracts. If a person is emotionally upset or very cold, nerve impulses may stimulate arrector pili muscles to contract, causing goose flesh, or goose bumps. Each hair follicle also has one or more sebaceous glands associated with it.

Sebaceous Glands

Sebaceous glands (figure 5.1) contain groups of specialized epithelial cells and are usually associated with hair follicles. They are holocrine glands and their cells produce globules of a fatty material that accumulates, causing the cells to swell and burst. (See chapter 4.) The resulting mixture of fatty material and cellular debris is called *sebum*.

Sebum is secreted into hair follicles through short ducts and helps to keep the hairs and skin soft, pliable, and relatively waterproof (figure 5.8).

Sebaceous glands are scattered throughout the skin, except on the palms and soles, where they are lacking. In some regions, such as on the lips, in the corners of the mouth, and on various parts of the external reproductive organs, sebaceous glands open directly to the surface rather than being connected to hair follicles.

A disorder of sebaceous glands is responsible for the condition called acne (acne vulgaris), which is common in adolescents. In this condition, the glands become overactive in some body regions. At the same time, their ducts may become plugged, and the glands may be surrounded by small, red elevations containing blackheads (comedones) or pimples (pustules).

Nails

Nails are protective coverings on the ends of the fingers and toes. Each nail consists of a *nail plate* over a surface of skin called the *nail bed*. The nail plate is produced by specialized epithelial cells that are continuous with epithelium of the skin. The whitish, thickened, half-moon region (*lunula*) at the base of a nail plate is its most active growing region. Epithelial cells in this region reproduce, and the newly formed cells undergo keratinization. This gives rise to tiny, horny scales that become part of the nail plate, pushing it forward over the nail bed. In time, the plate extends beyond the end of the nail bed and with normal use is gradually worn away (figure 5.9).

FIGURE 5.8
Sebaceous glands secrete sebum through short ducts into a hair follicle (shown here in cross section) (×175).

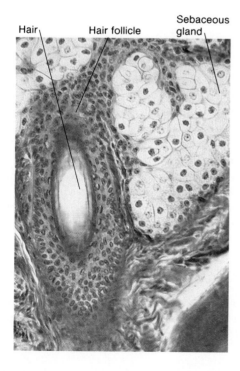

FIGURE 5.9
A nail is produced by epithelial cells that reproduce and undergo keratinization in the lunula region of the nail.

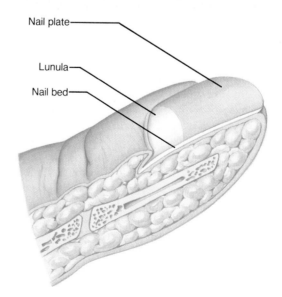

FIGURE 5.10
How do the functions of eccrine sweat glands and apocrine sweat glands differ?

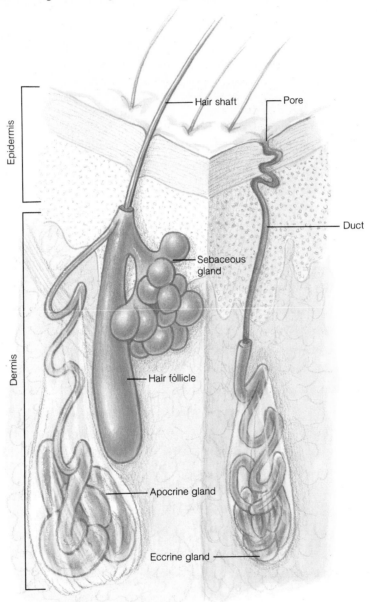

Sweat Glands

Sweat glands (figure 5.1) occur in nearly all regions of skin, but are most numerous in the palms and soles. Each gland consists of a tiny tube that originates as a ball-shaped coil in the dermis or subcutaneous layer. The coiled portion of the gland is closed at its deep end and is lined with sweat-secreting epithelial cells.

Certain sweat glands, the *apocrine glands,* respond to emotional stress. Apocrine secretions typically have odors, and the glands are considered to be scent glands. They begin to function at puberty and can cause some skin regions to become moist when a person is emotionally upset, frightened, or experiencing pain. They also become active when a person is sexually stimulated. In adults, apocrine glands are most numerous in the armpits (axillary regions), groin, and around the nipples. They are usually associated with hair follicles.

Other sweat glands, the *eccrine glands,* are not connected to hair follicles. They function throughout life by responding to elevated body temperature due to environmental heat or physical exercise. These glands are common on the forehead, neck, and back, where they produce profuse sweating on hot days and when a person is physically active. They are also responsible for the moisture that may appear on the palms and soles when a person is emotionally stressed.

Fluid secreted by the eccrine glands is carried away by a tubular part that opens at the surface as a pore. Although it is mostly water, the fluid contains small quantities of salts and certain wastes. Thus, secretion of sweat is, to a limited degree, an excretory function (figures 5.10 and 5.11).

With advancing age, there is a reduction in sweat gland activity, and in the very old, sweat glands may be replaced by fibrous tissues. Similarly, there is a decrease in sebaceous gland activity with age, so that the skin of elderly people tends to be dry and lack oils.

1. Explain how a hair forms.
2. What is the function of arrector pili muscles?
3. What is the function of sebaceous glands?
4. How does the composition of a fingernail differ from that of a hair?
5. Describe the structure and functions of the sweat glands.

FIGURE 5.11

FIGURE 5.11
The tubular portion of the eccrine gland in this micrograph opens on the surface of the skin.

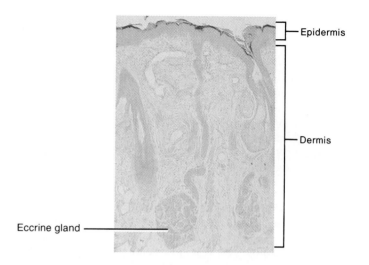

Epidermis

Dermis

Eccrine gland

NORMAL VARIATION

Skin Color

Skin color, like hair color, is due largely to the presence or absence of pigment produced by epidermal melanocytes. The amount of pigment synthesized by these cells is influenced by inherited and environmental factors.

Regardless of racial origin, all humans possess about the same concentrations of melanocytes in their skin. Differences in skin coloration are due largely to inherited differences in the amount of melanin these cells produce. Individuals whose melanocytes produce a relatively large amount of pigment have dark skin, while those whose melanocytes form less pigment have lighter complexions. The granules of very dark skin tend to occur singly and are relatively large; those in lighter skin tend to occur in clusters of 2–4 granules and are somewhat smaller. Still other individuals have defective melanocytes, and their cells are unable to manufacture melanin. As a consequence, their skin remains nonpigmented, producing a condition called *albinism* (figure 5.12).

Environmental factors such as sunlight, ultraviolet light from sun lamps, or X rays also affect skin color. These factors cause existing melanin to darken rapidly, and they stimulate melanocytes to produce more pigment and transfer it to nearby epidermal cells within a few days. This is why sunbathing results in skin tanning. Unless the exposure to sunlight is continued, however, the tan is eventually lost, as pigmented epidermal cells become keratinized and are worn away.

FIGURE 5.12
An albino lacks the ability to produce the skin pigment melanin because of the presence of a mutant gene.

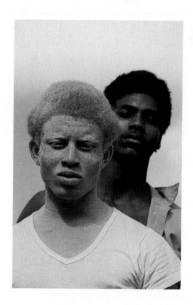

Burns and Wound Healing

As with other types of injuries, the skin's response to a burn depends upon the amount of damage it sustains. For example, if the skin is only slightly burned from a minor sunburn, the skin may become warm and reddened (erythema) as a result of dermal blood vessel dilation. This response may be accompanied by mild swelling, and, in time, the surface layer of skin may be shed. Such a burn that involves injury to the epidermis alone is called a *superficial partial-thickness,* or first degree, *burn.* Healing of the injury usually occurs within a few days to two weeks, and there is no scarring of the skin.

A burn that involves destruction of some epidermis as well as some underlying dermis is called a *deep partial-thickness,* or second degree, *burn.* In this condition, fluid escapes from damaged dermal blood vessels, and as the fluid accumulates beneath the outer layer of epidermal cells, blisters appear. The injured region becomes moist and firm, and it may appear dark red to waxy white. Such a burn most commonly occurs as a result of exposure to hot objects, hot liquids, flames, or burning clothing.

The healing of a deep partial-thickness burn involves accessory organs of the skin that survive the injury because they are located in deeper portions of the dermis. These organs, which include hair follicles, sweat glands, and sebaceous glands, contain epithelial cells. During healing, these cells may be able to grow out onto the surface of the dermis, spread over it, and form a new epidermis. In time, recovery usually is complete, and scar tissue does not develop unless an infection occurs.

A burn that destroys the epidermis, dermis, and the accessory organs of the skin is called a *full-thickness,* or third degree, *burn.* In this instance, the injured skin becomes dry and leathery, and its color may vary from red to black to white.

A full-thickness burn usually occurs as a result of immersion in hot liquids, prolonged exposure to hot objects, flames, or corrosive chemicals. Since most of the epithelial cells in the affected region are likely to be destroyed, spontaneous healing can occur only by the growth of epithelial cells inward from its margin. If the injury is large, treatment may involve removing a thin layer of skin from an unburned region of the body. This skin is usually stretched with a skin expanding device so that it will cover a larger area and then transplanted to the injured area to speed healing. This procedure is called an *autograft.*

If the burn is too extensive to allow removal of skin from the patient, cadaveric skin from a skin bank or various skin substitutes may be used to cover the injury. In this case, the transplant is called a *homograft,* and it serves as a temporary covering that decreases the size of the wound, helps to prevent infection, and aids in preserving deeper tissues. In time, after healing has begun, the temporary covering may be removed and replaced with an autograft, as skin becomes available in areas that have healed. However, the healing of wounds using grafts is likely to be accompanied by extensive scarring.

Various skin substitutes also may be used to temporarily cover extensive burns. An artificial membrane made of silicone or polyurethane and collagen fibers has been used as a temporary graft. In other cases, pieces of an individual's skin may be removed and the cells cultured in the laboratory. The cells are provided with nutrients and substances that stimulate mitosis. The cells reproduce rapidly, forming sheets of new skin that can then be grafted over burned areas.

The process by which damaged skin heals depends on the extent of the injury. If a break in the skin is shallow, epithelial cells along its margin are stimulated to reproduce more rapidly than usual, and the newly formed cells simply fill the gap.

If the injury extends into the dermis or subcutaneous layer, blood vessels are broken, and the blood that escapes forms a clot in the wound. The blood clot forms a scab that covers and protects the underlying tissues. Before long, fibroblasts migrate into the injured region and begin forming new collagen fibers. These fibers tend to bind the edges of the wound together. The closer the edges of the wound, the sooner the gap can be filled. This is one reason for suturing or otherwise closing a large break in the skin.

As the healing process continues, blood vessels send out new branches that grow into the area beneath the scab. Macrophages remove dead cells and other debris. Eventually, the damaged tissues are replaced, and the scab sloughs off. If the wound is extensive, the newly formed connective tissue may appear on the surface as a scar.

In large, open wounds, the healing process may be accompanied by the formation of *granulations* that develop in the exposed tissues as small, rounded masses. Each of these granulations consists of a new branch of a blood vessel and a cluster of collagen-secreting fibroblasts that are being nourished by the vessel. In time, some of the blood vessels are resorbed, and the fibroblasts migrate away, leaving a scar that is composed largely of collagenous fibers. Figure 5.13 shows the stages in the healing of a wound.

FIGURE 5.13

(a) If normal skin is (b) injured deeply, (c) blood escapes from dermal blood vessels, and (d) a blood clot soon forms. (e) The blood clot and dried tissue fluid form a scab that protects the damaged region. (f) Later, blood vessels send out branches, and fibroblasts migrate into the area. (g) The fibroblasts produce new connective tissue fibers, and when the skin is largely repaired, the scab sloughs off.

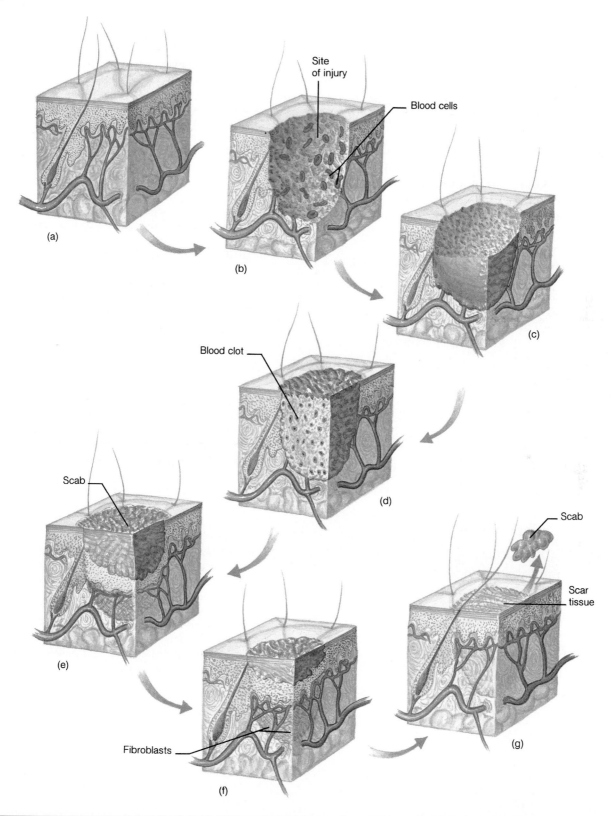

Common Skin Disorders

acne (ak′ne) a disease of the sebaceous glands accompanied by blackheads and pimples.

alopecia (al″o-pe′she-ah) loss of hair.

birthmark (berth′ mark) vascular tumor involving the skin and subcutaneous tissues that is visible at birth or soon after.

cyst (sist) a liquid-filled sac or capsule.

keloid (ke′loid) an elevated, enlarging, fibrous scar usually initiated by an injury.

mole (mōl) a fleshy skin tumor (nevus) that usually is pigmented; colors range from yellow to brown or black.

seborrhea (seb″o-re′ah) a disease characterized by hyperactivity of the sebaceous glands and accompanied by greasy skin and dandruff.

ulcer (ul′ser) an open sore.

wart (wort) a flesh-colored raised area caused by a virus infection.

Chapter Summary

Introduction (page 104)
Organs are composed of two or more kinds of tissues. The skin together with its accessory organs constitutes the integumentary system.

Types of Membranes (page 104)
1. Serous membranes
   a. Serous membranes are organs that line body cavities lacking openings to the outside.
   b. They are composed of epithelium and loose connective tissue.
   c. They secrete watery serous fluid, which lubricates membrane surfaces.
2. Mucous membranes
   a. Mucous membranes are organs that line cavities and tubes opening to the outside.
   b. They are composed of various kinds of epithelium and loose connective tissue.
   c. They secrete mucus, which protects the membrane.
3. The cutaneous membrane is the external body covering commonly called the skin.
4. Synovial membranes
   a. Synovial membranes are organs that line joint cavities.
   b. They are composed of fibrous connective tissue overlying loose connective tissue and adipose tissue.
   c. They secrete synovial fluid that lubricates the ends of bones at joints.

Skin and Its Tissues (page 104)
Skin functions as a protective covering, aids in regulating body temperature, houses sensory receptors, synthesizes various chemicals, and excretes wastes. It is composed of an epidermis and a dermis, which are separated by a basement membrane with a subcutaneous layer beneath.

1. Epidermis
   a. The epidermis is a layer composed of stratified squamous epithelium, which lacks blood vessels.
   b. The deepest layer, called stratum basale, contains cells undergoing mitosis.
   c. Epidermal cells undergo keratinization as they are pushed toward the surface.
   d. The outermost layer, the stratum corneum, is composed of dead epidermal cells.
   e. The production of epidermal cells is balanced with the rate at which they are lost.
   f. Epidermis functions to protect underlying tissues against water loss, mechanical injury, and the effects of harmful chemicals.
   g. Melanin protects underlying cells from the effects of ultraviolet light.
   h. Melanocytes transfer melanin to nearby epidermal cells.
2. Dermis
   a. The dermis is a layer composed largely of fibrous connective tissue that binds the epidermis to underlying tissues.
   b. It also contains muscle fibers, blood vessels, and nerve fibers.
   c. Dermal blood vessels supply nutrients to all skin cells and help regulate body temperature.
   d. Nerve tissue is scattered through the dermis.
      (1) Some dermal nerve fibers carry impulses to muscles and glands of the skin.
      (2) Other dermal nerve fibers are associated with various sensory receptors in the skin.
3. Subcutaneous layer
   a. The subcutaneous layer is composed of loose connective tissue and adipose tissue.
   b. Adipose tissue helps to conserve body heat.
   c. This layer contains blood vessels that supply the skin and underlying adipose tissue.

Accessory Organs of the Skin (page 109)
1. Hair follicles
   a. Hair occurs in nearly all regions of the skin.
   b. Each hair develops from epidermal cells at the base of a tubelike hair follicle.
   c. As newly formed cells develop and grow, older cells are pushed toward the surface and undergo keratinization.
   d. A hair usually grows for a while, undergoes a resting period, and is then replaced by a new hair.
   e. Hair color is determined by the type and amount of pigment in its cells.
   f. A bundle of smooth muscle cells and one or more sebaceous glands are attached to each hair follicle.
2. Sebaceous glands
   a. Sebaceous glands secrete sebum, which helps keep skin and hair soft and waterproof.
   b. In some regions, they open directly to the skin surface.

3. Nails
   a. Nails are protective covers on the ends of fingers and toes.
   b. They are produced by epidermal cells that undergo keratinization.
4. Sweat glands
   a. Sweat glands are located in nearly all regions of the skin.
   b. Each gland consists of a coiled tube.
   c. Apocrine glands respond to emotional stress, while eccrine glands respond to elevated body temperature.
   d. Sweat is primarily water, but also contains salts and waste products.

Clinical Application of Knowledge

1. In the disease called cystic fibrosis, there is an overproduction of mucus in the airways of the lungs. The condition called pleurisy results in decreased production of serous fluid within the pleural cavity. What would be the consequences of each of these disorders?
2. After a full-thickness burn, which of the skin functions would be lost in the injured area?
3. A premature infant typically lacks subcutaneous adipose tissue. How do you think this factor influences such an infant's ability to regulate its body temperature?
4. When the epidermis is destroyed by a burn, new epidermis forms from the edges of the burn and from hair follicles in the dermis. Explain how epidermis can be formed from hair follicles.

5. When the skin is exposed to excessive friction, a portion of the epidermis may be pulled away from the connection to the dermis. The result is called a blister. Which skin functions would be lost in the area of such an injury?
6. Typically, a superficial partial-thickness burn is more painful than one involving deeper tissues. How would you explain this observation?

Review Activities

1. Explain why a membrane is an organ.
2. Define *integumentary system.*
3. Distinguish between serous and mucous membranes.
4. Compare the functions of serous fluid and mucus.
5. Relate the functions of serous fluid and mucus to the locations of serous and mucous membranes.
6. List six functions of skin.
7. Distinguish between the epidermis and the dermis.
8. Explain what happens to epidermal cells as they undergo keratinization.
9. List the layers of the epidermis.
10. Describe the function of melanocytes and explain why epidermal cells may contain melanin.
11. Describe the structure of the dermis.
12. Explain how dermal blood vessels function in body temperature regulation.
13. Review the functions of dermal nerve tissue.
14. Describe the structure and function of the subcutaneous layer.
15. Distinguish between a hair and a hair follicle.
16. Review how hair color is determined.
17. Explain the function of sebaceous glands.
18. Describe how nails are formed.
19. Distinguish between apocrine and eccrine glands.

U N I T 2
Support and Movement

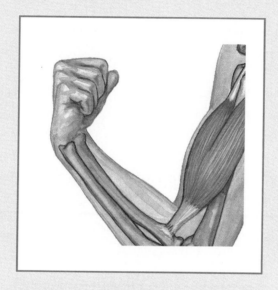

The chapters of unit 2 deal with structures of the skeletal and muscular systems. They describe how organs of the skeletal system support and protect other body parts, and how they function with organs of the muscular system to enable body parts to move. These chapters also describe how skeletal structures carry out functions such as the formation of blood and the storage of minerals.

6
The Skeletal System

7
Joints of the Skeletal System

8
The Muscular System

CHAPTER 6

The Skeletal System

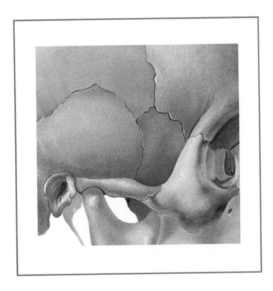

Bones of the skeleton are composed of several kinds of tissues, and thus they are organs of the *skeletal system.*

Because bones are rigid structures, they provide support and protection for softer tissues, and they act together with skeletal muscles to make body movements possible. They also house the tissue that produces blood cells, and they store minerals.

Shapes of individual bones are closely related to their functions. Projections provide places for attachments of muscles, tendons, and ligaments; openings serve as passageways for blood vessels and nerves; and the ends of bones are modified to form joints with other bones.

Chapter Outline

Chapter Objectives

After you have studied this chapter, you should be able to

1. Classify bones according to their shapes and name an example from each group.

2. Describe the general structure of a long bone and list the functions of its parts.

3. Distinguish between intramembranous and endochondral bones. Explain how such bones grow and develop.

4. Discuss the major functions of bones.

5. Distinguish between the axial and appendicular skeletons, and name the major parts of each.

6. Locate and identify the bones and major features of bones that comprise the skull, vertebral column, thoracic cage, pectoral girdle, upper limb, pelvic girdle, and lower limb.

7. Complete the review activities at the end of this chapter. Note that the items are worded in the form of specific learning objectives. You may want to refer to them before reading the chapter.

Aids to Understanding Words

ax-, an axis: *ax*ial skeleton—upright portion of the skeleton that supports the head, neck, and trunk.

-blast, budding or developing: osteo*blast*—cell that forms bone tissue.

carp-, wrist: *carp*als—wrist bones.

-clast, broken: osteo*clast*—cell that breaks down bone tissue.

condyl-, knob: *condyl*e—a rounded, bony process.

corac-, beak: *corac*oid process—beaklike process of the scapula.

cribr-, sieve: *cribr*iform plate—portion of the ethmoid bone with many small, sievelike openings.

crist-, ridge: *crist*a galli—a bony ridge that projects upward into the cranial cavity.

fov-, pit: *fov*ea capitis—a pit in the head of a femur.

gladi-, sword: *gladi*olus—middle portion of the bladelike sternum.

glen-, joint socket: *glen*oid cavity—a depression in the scapula that articulates with the head of a humerus.

inter-, between: *inter*vertebral disk—a structure located between adjacent vertebrae.

intra-, inside: *intra*membranous bone—bone that forms within sheetlike masses of connective tissue.

meat-, passage: auditory *meat*us—canal of the temporal bone that leads inward to parts of the ear.

odont-, tooth: *odont*oid process—a toothlike process of the second cervical vertebra.

poie-, making: hemato*poie*sis—process by which blood cells are formed.

Introduction

An individual bone is composed of a variety of tissues, including bone tissue, cartilage, fibrous connective tissue, blood, and nerve tissue. Because so much nonliving material is present in the matrix of bone tissue, the whole organ may appear to be inert. A bone, however, contains very active, living tissues.

Bone Structure

Although various bones of the skeletal system differ greatly in size and shape, they are similar in their structure, development, and functions.

Classification of Bones

Bones can be classified according to their shapes: long, short, flat, or irregular (figure 6.1).

1. **Long bones** have long longitudinal axes and expanded ends. Examples are the arm and leg bones.
2. **Short bones** are somewhat cubelike, with their lengths and widths roughly equal. Bones of the wrists and ankles are examples of this type.

3. **Flat bones** are platelike structures with broad surfaces, such as the ribs, scapulae, and bones of the skull.
4. **Irregular bones** have a variety of shapes and are usually connected to several other bones. Irregular bones include vertebrae that comprise the backbone and many of the facial bones.

In addition to these four groups of bones, some authorities recognize a fifth group called *round,* or *sesamoid, bones.* Members of this group are usually small, and they often occur within tendons adjacent to joints, where tendons undergo compression. The kneecap (patella) is an example of a very large sesamoid bone.

Parts of a Long Bone

To describe the structure of bone, the femur, a long bone in the upper leg, will be used as an example (figure 6.2). At each end of such a bone there is an expanded portion

FIGURE 6.1

(*a*) A femur of the leg is a long bone, (*b*) a tarsal bone of the ankle is a short bone, (*c*) a parietal bone of the skull is a flat bone, (*d*) a vertebra of the backbone is an irregular bone, and (*e*) the patella of the knee is a round bone.

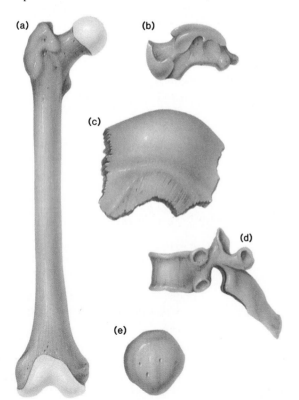

FIGURE 6.2

Major parts of a long bone.

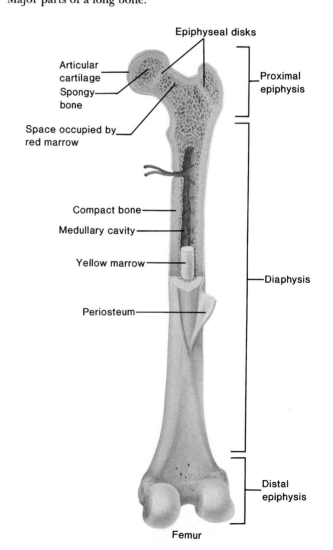

called an **epiphysis** (plural, **epiphyses**), which articulates (or forms a joint) with another bone. On its outer surface, the articulating portion of the epiphysis is coated with a layer of hyaline cartilage called **articular cartilage.** The shaft of the bone, which is located between the epiphyses, is called the **diaphysis.** The diaphysis contains small holes called *nutrient foramina* through which blood vessels enter the bone.

Except for the articular cartilage on its ends, the bone is completely enclosed by a tough, vascular covering of fibrous tissue called the **periosteum.** This membrane is firmly attached to the bone, and the periosteal fibers are continuous with various ligaments and tendons that are connected to the bone. The periosteum also functions in formation and repair of bone tissue.

Each bone has a shape closely related to its functions. Bony projections called *processes,* for example, provide sites for the attachment of ligaments and tendons; grooves and openings serve as passageways for blood vessels and nerves; and a depression of one bone might articulate with a process of another.

The wall of the diaphysis is composed of tightly packed tissue called **compact bone** (cortical bone). This type of bone is solid, strong, and resistant to bending.

The epiphyses, on the other hand, are composed largely of **spongy bone** (cancellous bone) with thin layers of compact bone on their surfaces. Spongy bone consists of numerous branching bony plates called **trabeculae.** Irregular interconnecting spaces occur between these plates and help reduce the weight of bone (figure 6.2). Spongy bone provides strength and its bony plates are most developed in regions of the epiphyses that are subjected to the forces of compression.

Both compact and spongy tissues usually are present in each bone. Short, flat, and irregular bones typically consist of a mass of spongy bone that is either covered by a thin layer of compact bone or sandwiched between plates of compact bone.

Compact bone in the diaphysis of a long bone forms a rigid tube with a hollow chamber called the **medullary cavity.** This cavity is continuous with the spaces of spongy bone. All of these areas are lined with a thin membrane called the **endosteum** and are filled with a specialized type of soft connective tissue called **marrow** (figure 6.3).

Microscopic Structure

In compact bone, osteocytes and layers of matrix clustered concentrically around an osteonic canal form a cylinder-shaped unit called an *osteon* (Haversian system). Many of these units cemented together form the substance of compact bone. (See chapter 4.)

Each osteonic canal contains small blood vessels (usually capillaries) and nerves, surrounded by some loose connective tissue. Blood in these vessels provides nourishment for bone cells associated with the osteonic canal.

FIGURE 6.3

Photographs of a long bone. (*a*) Proximal epiphysis, sectioned longitudinally; (*b*) diaphysis, sectioned longitudinally; (*c*) distal epiphysis.

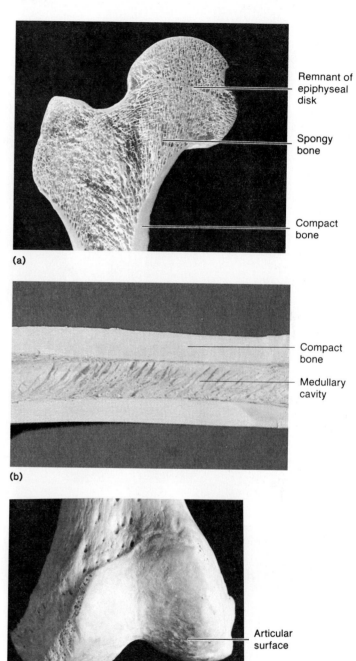

(a)

(b)

(c)

Osteonic canals travel longitudinally through bone tissue. They are interconnected by transverse *communicating canals* (Volkmann's canals). These canals contain larger blood vessels by which vessels in the osteonic canals communicate with the surface of the bone and medullary cavity (figure 6.4).

FIGURE 6.4

(*a*) Compact bone is composed of osteons cemented together. (*b*) What features do you recognize in this scanning electron micrograph of a single osteon in compact bone (about ×1,300)?
R. G. Kessel and R. H. Kardon, *Tissues and Organs: A Text Atlas of Scanning Electron Microscopy,* © 1979, W. H. Freeman & Co.

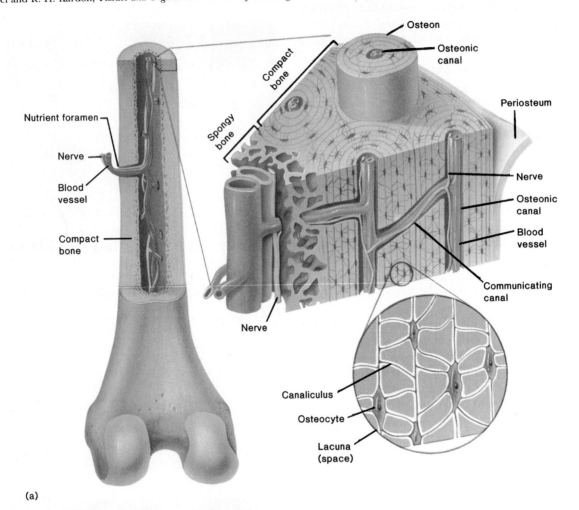

(a)

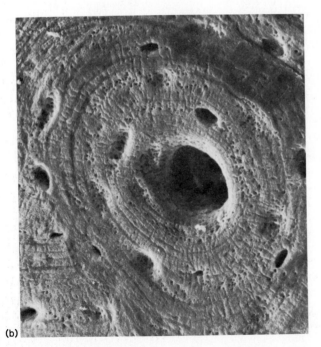

(b)

Spongy bone is also composed of osteocytes and bone matrix. However, the bone cells are not arranged around osteonic canals. Instead, the cells are found within the trabeculae, and they send cellular processes through canaliculi to the surface of the trabeculae. There the cells obtain nutrients from blood vessels in the marrow.

1. Explain how bones are classified.
2. List five major parts of a long bone.
3. How do compact and spongy bone differ in structure?
4. Describe the microscopic structure of compact and spongy bone.

Bone Development and Growth

Parts of the skeletal system begin to form during the first few weeks of prenatal development, and bony structures continue to grow and develop into adulthood. Bones form by replacement of existing connective tissue in one of two

FIGURE 6.5
The tissues of this miscarried fetus (about 14 weeks old) have been cleared, and the developing bones have been stained selectively.

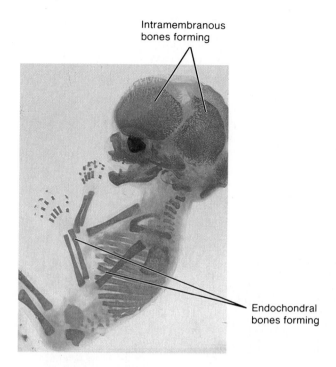

Intramembranous bones forming

Endochondral bones forming

ways. Some first appear between sheetlike layers of connective tissues, and are called intramembranous bones. Others begin as masses of cartilage that are later replaced by bone tissue. They are called endochondral bones (figure 6.5).

Intramembranous Bones

Examples of **intramembranous bones** are the broad, flat bones of the skull. During their development (osteogenesis), membranelike layers of primitive connective tissues appear at the sites of the future bones. These layers are supplied with dense networks of blood vessels, and some of the connective tissue cells become arranged around these vessels. These primitive cells enlarge and differentiate into bone-forming cells called **osteoblasts,** which, in turn, deposit bony matrix around themselves. As a result, spongy bone is produced in all directions of the blood vessels within the layers of primitive connective tissues. Later, some spongy bone may be converted to compact bone, as spaces become filled with bone matrix.

As development continues, osteoblasts may become completely surrounded by matrix, and in this manner they become secluded within lacunae. At the same time, matrix enclosing the cellular processes of osteoblasts gives rise to canaliculi. Once they are isolated in lacunae, bone cells are called **osteocytes.**

Cells of primitive connective tissue that persist outside the developing bone give rise to the periosteum. Osteo-

blasts on the inside of the periosteum create a layer of compact bone over the surface of the newly formed spongy bone.

This process of forming an intramembranous bone by replacement of connective tissue is called *intramembranous ossification*. Chart 6.1 lists the major steps of the process.

Endochondral Bones

Most bones of the skeleton are **endochondral bones.** Their development proceeds from masses of hyaline cartilage with shapes similar to future bony structures. These cartilaginous models grow rapidly for a time, and then begin to undergo extensive changes. For example, cartilage cells enlarge and increase the sizes of their respective lacunae. This is accompanied by destruction of the surrounding matrix, and soon the cartilage cells die and degenerate.

About the same time, a periosteum forms from connective tissue that encircles the developing structure, and as the cartilage breaks down, blood vessels and undifferentiated connective tissue cells invade the disintegrating tissue. Some invading cells differentiate into osteoblasts and begin to form spongy bone in the spaces previously occupied by cartilage.

This process of forming an endochondral bone by replacement of hyaline cartilage is called *endochondral ossification*. The major steps of this process are listed in chart 6.1.

Chart 6.1 Major steps in bone development

Intramembranous ossification

1. Membranelike layers of primitive connective tissue appear at sites of future bones.
2. Primitive connective tissue cells become arranged around blood vessels in these layers.
3. Connective tissue cells differentiate into osteoblasts, which form spongy bone.
4. Osteoblasts become osteocytes when they are completely surrounded by bony matrix.
5. Connective tissue on the surface of each developing structure forms a periosteum.

Endochondral ossification

1. Masses of hyaline cartilage form models of future bones.
2. Cartilage tissue breaks down and disappears.
3. Blood vessels and differentiating osteoblasts from periosteum invade the disintegrating tissue.
4. Osteoblasts form spongy bone in space occupied by cartilage.

Growth of an Endochondral Bone

In a long bone, replacement of hyaline cartilage by bony tissue begins in the center of the diaphysis. This region is called the *primary ossification center,* and bone develops from it toward the ends of the cartilaginous structure. Meanwhile, osteoblasts from the periosteum deposit a thin layer

FIGURE 6.6

(*a*) The cartilaginous cells of an epiphyseal disk are arranged in four layers, each of which may be several cells thick. (*b*) A micrograph of an epiphyseal disk. What features can you identify?

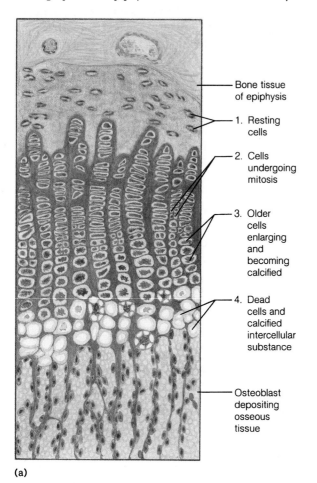

— Bone tissue of epiphysis

1. Resting cells

2. Cells undergoing mitosis

3. Older cells enlarging and becoming calcified

4. Dead cells and calcified intercellular substance

— Osteoblast depositing osseous tissue

(a)

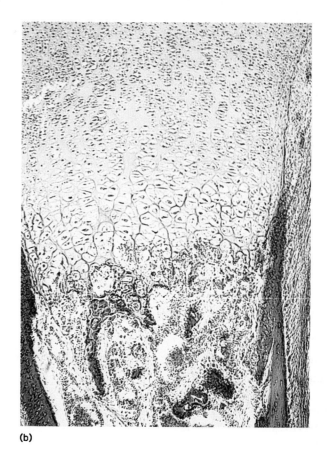

(b)

of compact bone around the primary ossification center by intramembranous ossification. The epiphyses of the developing bone remain cartilaginous and continue to grow. Later, secondary ossification centers appear in the epiphyses, and spongy bone forms in all directions from them. As spongy bone is deposited in the diaphysis and in the epiphysis, a band of cartilage called the **epiphyseal disk** is left between the two ossification centers.

Cartilaginous cells of an epiphyseal disk are arranged in four layers, each of which may be several cells thick, as shown in figure 6.6. The first layer, closest to the end of the epiphysis, is composed of resting cells. Although these cells are not actively participating in the growing process, this layer anchors the epiphyseal disk to the bony tissue of the epiphysis.

The second layer contains rows of numerous young cells that are undergoing mitosis. As new cells are produced, and as intercellular material is formed around them, the cartilaginous disk thickens.

The rows of older cells, which are left behind when new cells appear, form the third layer. These cells enlarge and cause the epiphyseal disk to thicken even more. Consequently, length of the entire bone increases. At the same time, calcium accumulates in the intercellular matrix adjacent to the oldest of the cartilaginous cells, and as the matrix becomes calcified, cells begin to die.

The fourth layer of the epiphyseal disk is quite thin and is composed largely of dead cells and calcified intercellular substance.

In time, the calcified matrix is broken down by the action of large, multinucleated cells called **osteoclasts.** These large cells originate by the fusion of several white blood cells (monocytes). Osteoclasts secrete substances that dissolve the calcium portion of the matrix, and at the same time the lysosomes digest the collagen fibers. After the matrix is removed, bone-building osteoblasts invade the region and deposit bone tissue in place of the cartilage.

FIGURE 6.7

(a–f) Major stages in the development of an endochondral bone.

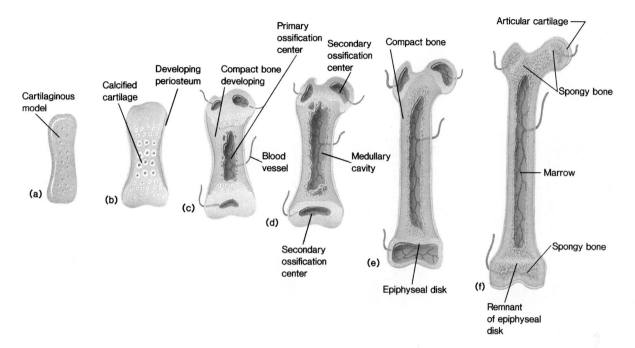

A long bone will continue to grow in length while cartilaginous cells of the epiphyseal disk are active. However, once ossification centers of the diaphysis and epiphyses come together, and the epiphyseal disks become ossified, growth in length is no longer possible in that end of the bone.

A developing bone grows in thickness as compact bone is deposited on the outside, just beneath the periosteum. As this compact bone is forming on the surface, other bone tissue is being eroded away on the inside by osteoclasts. The space that is produced becomes the medullary cavity in the diaphysis, which later fills with marrow.

Bone in the central regions of the epiphyses remains spongy, and hyaline cartilage on the ends of the epiphyses persists throughout life as articular cartilage. Figure 6.7 illustrates stages in the development and growth of an endochondral bone. Chart 6.2 lists ages at which various bones become ossified.

It is possible to determine whether a child's long bones are still growing by examining an X-ray film to see if epiphyseal disks are present (figure 6.8). If a disk is damaged as a result of a fracture before it becomes ossified, elongation of the long bone may cease prematurely, or if growth continues, it may be uneven. For this reason, injuries to the epiphyses of a young person's bones are of special concern. On the other hand, an epiphysis is sometimes altered surgically in order to equalize growth of bones that are developing at very different rates.

Chart 6.2 Ossification timetable

Age	Occurrence
Third month of prenatal development	Ossification in long bones beginning.
Fourth month	Most primary ossification centers have appeared in diaphyses of bones.
Birth to 5 years	Secondary ossification centers appear in epiphyses.
5 to 12 years in females; 5 to 14 years in males	Ossification spreads rapidly from ossification centers and various bones are becoming ossified.
17 to 20 years	Bones of upper limbs and scapulae become completely ossified.
18 to 23 years	Bones of lower limbs and coxal bones become completely ossified.
23 to 25 years	Bones of sternum, clavicles, and vertebrae become completely ossified.
By 25 years	Nearly all bones are completely ossified.

Bone Reorganization

Once a bone has formed, it does not become inactive. Instead, its tissue is continually broken down and reformed. This process is called *bone remodeling*, and it continues throughout a person's life. In bone remodeling, osteoclasts resorb bone matrix and form small canals (figure 6.9). Blood vessels (capillaries) grow into these spaces and osteoblasts line the canals. The osteoblasts secrete new layers of matrix, thus forming new osteons.

FIGURE 6.8

The presence of epiphyseal disks (arrows) in a child's femur and tibia are indications that the bones are still growing in length.

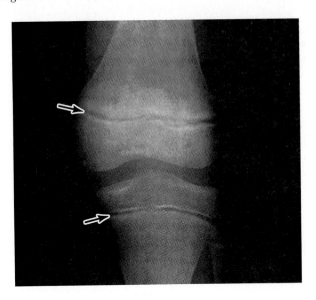

FIGURE 6.9

A scanning electron micrograph of an osteoclast (×5,625). (Oc = osteoclast; HL = lacuna; CF = collagen fiber.)
R. G. Kessel and R. H. Kardon, *Tissues and Organs: A Text Atlas of Scanning Electron Microscopy,* © 1979, W. H. Freeman & Co.

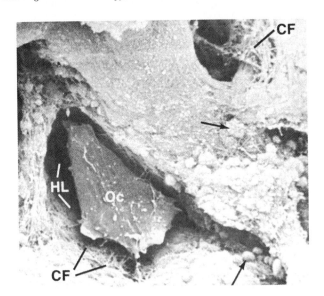

FIGURE 6.10

When teeth are lost, bone remodeling alters the shape of the jaws. This is the skull of an elderly person.

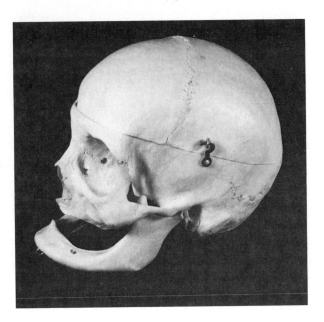

Physical stress has a stimulating effect on bone formation and remodeling. For example, when skeletal muscles contract, they pull at their attachments on bones, and the resulting stress stimulates bone tissue to thicken and strengthen (hypertrophy). Conversely, with lack of exercise, the same bone tissue undergoes a wasting process and tends to become thinner and weaker (atrophy). This is why the bones of athletes are usually stronger and heavier than those of nonathletes. It is also the reason that bones of casted limbs may decrease in size.

Bone remodeling also is responsible for changes in the shape of the jaw when teeth are lost. The presence and use of teeth normally create stress on jaws and their normal shape is maintained. When teeth are lost, however, remodeling takes place and it alters the shape of the bones. (See figure 6.10.)

1. Describe the development of an intramembranous bone.
2. Explain how an endochondral bone develops.
3. List the steps in the growth of a long bone.
4. How does physical stress affect bone structure?

Fractures

Although a fracture may involve injury to cartilaginous structures, it is usually defined as a break in a bone. A fracture can be classified according to its cause and the nature of the break sustained. For example, a break due to injury is a *traumatic fracture*, while one resulting from disease is a *spontaneous*, or *pathologic, fracture*.

If a broken bone is exposed to the outside by an opening in the skin, the injury is termed a *compound fracture*. Such a fracture is accompanied by the added danger of infection, since microorganisms almost surely enter through broken skin. On the other hand, if the break is protected by uninjured skin, it is called a *simple fracture*. Figure 6.11 shows several types of traumatic fractures.

Repair of a Fracture

Whenever a bone is broken, blood vessels within the bone and its periosteum are ruptured, and the periosteum is likely to be torn. Blood escaping from broken vessels spreads through the damaged area and soon forms a blood clot, or *hematoma*. As vessels in surrounding tissues dilate, those tissues become swollen and inflamed.

Within days or weeks, the hematoma is invaded by developing blood vessels and large numbers of osteoblasts originating from the periosteum. Osteoblasts multiply rapidly in the regions close to new blood vessels, building spongy bone nearby. Fibroblasts produce masses of fibrocartilage in regions further from a blood supply.

FIGURE 6.11
Various types of traumatic fractures.

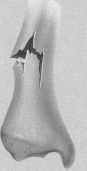 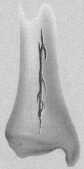 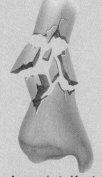

A *greenstick* fracture is incomplete, and the break occurs on the convex surface of the bend in the bone.

A *fissured* fracture involves an incomplete longitudinal break.

A *comminuted* fracture is complete and results in several bony fragments.

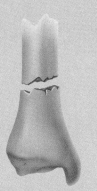 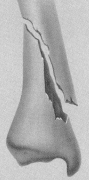 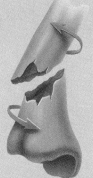

A *transverse* fracture is complete, and the break occurs at a right angle to the axis of the bone.

An *oblique* fracture occurs at an angle other than a right angle to the axis of the bone.

A *spiral* fracture is caused by twisting a bone excessively.

Continued on next page

Meanwhile, other cells begin to remove the blood clot as well as any dead or damaged cells in the affected area. Osteoclasts also appear and resorb bone fragments, thus aiding in "cleaning up" debris.

In time, a large amount of fibrocartilage fills the gap between the ends of broken bone, and this mass is termed a *cartilaginous callus*. The callus is later replaced by bone tissue in much the same way that hyaline cartilage of a developing endochondral bone is replaced. That is, the cartilaginous callus is broken down, the area is invaded by blood vessels and osteoblasts, and the space is filled with a *bony callus*.

Usually more bone is produced at the site of a healing fracture than is needed to replace damaged tissues. However, osteoclasts are able to remove the excess, and the final result of the repair process is a bone shaped very much like the original one. Figure 6.12 shows the steps in the healing of a fracture.

The rate at which a fracture is repaired depends on several factors. For instance, if the ends of broken bone are close together, healing is more rapid than if they are far apart. This is the reason for setting fractured bones (also called reduction of a fracture) and for using casts or metal pins (internal fixation) to keep broken ends together. Also, some bones naturally heal more rapidly than others. Long bones of the arms, for example, may heal in half the time required by long bones of the legs. Furthermore, as age increases, so does the time required for healing.

FIGURE 6.12
Major steps in the repair of a fracture.

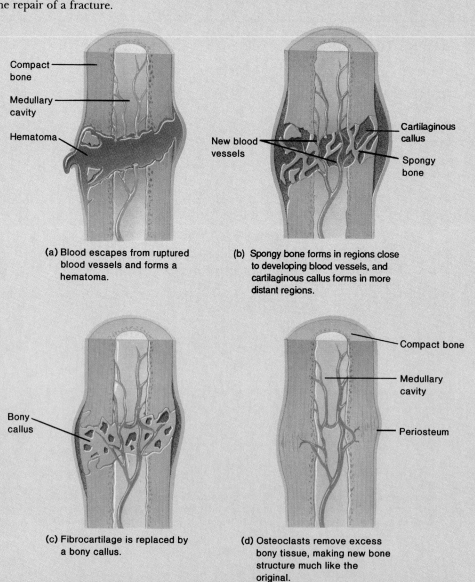

(a) Blood escapes from ruptured blood vessels and forms a hematoma.

(b) Spongy bone forms in regions close to developing blood vessels, and cartilaginous callus forms in more distant regions.

(c) Fibrocartilage is replaced by a bony callus.

(d) Osteoclasts remove excess bony tissue, making new bone structure much like the original.

Functions of Bones

Skeletal parts provide shape, support, and protection for body structures. They also act as levers that aid body movements, house tissues that produce blood cells, and store various minerals.

Support and Protection

Bones give shape to structures such as the head, face, thorax, and limbs. They also provide support and protection. For example, bones of the feet, legs, pelvis, and backbone support the weight of the body. Bones of the skull protect the eyes, ears, and brain. Those of the rib cage and shoulder girdle protect the heart and lungs, while bones of the pelvic girdle protect the lower abdominal and internal reproductive organs.

Body Movements

Whenever limbs or other body parts are moved, bones and muscles function together as simple mechanical devices called **levers.** Such a lever has four basic components: (*a*) a rigid bar or rod, (*b*) a pivot or fulcrum on which the bar turns, (*c*) an object or weight that is moved, and (*d*) a force that supplies energy for the movement of the bar.

A playground seesaw is a lever. The board of the seesaw serves as a rigid bar that rocks on a pivot near its center. The person on one end of the board represents the weight that is moved, while the person at the opposite end supplies the force needed for moving the board and its rider.

There are three kinds of levers, and they differ in the arrangements of their parts, as shown in figure 6.13. A *first-class lever* is one whose parts are arranged like those of the seesaw. Its pivot is located between the weight and force,

FIGURE 6.13

Three types of levers: (*a*) a first-class lever is used in a pair of scissors, (*b*) a second-class lever is used in a wheelbarrow, and (*c*) a third-class lever is used in a pair of forceps.

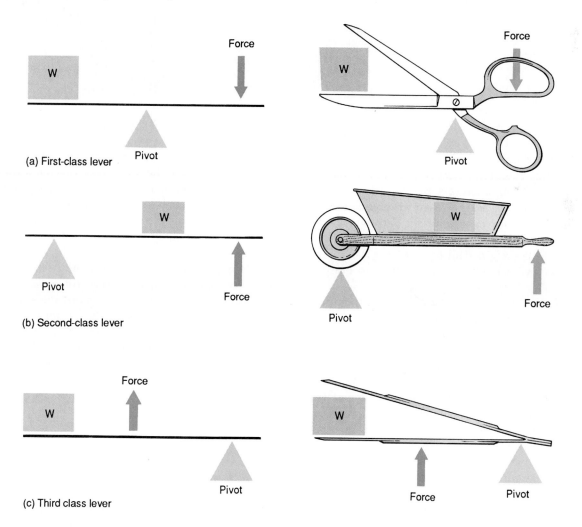

(a) First-class lever

(b) Second-class lever

(c) Third class lever

FIGURE 6.14

(a) When the arm is bent at the elbow, a third-class lever is employed; (b) when the arm is straightened at the elbow, a first-class lever is used.

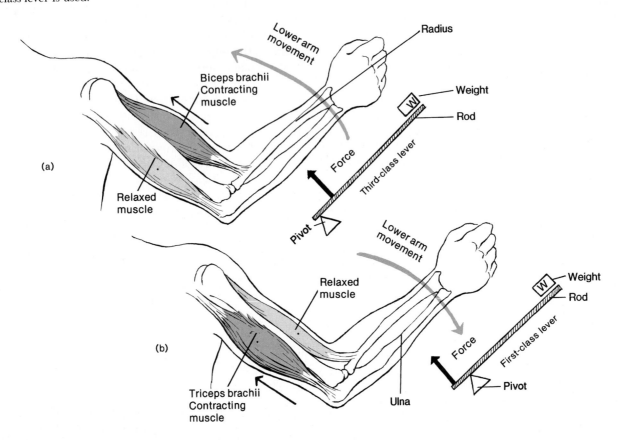

making the sequence of parts weight-pivot-force. Other examples of first-class levers are scissors and hemostats (devices used to clamp blood vessels).

The parts of a *second-class lever* are arranged in the sequence pivot-weight-force, as in a wheelbarrow.

The parts of a *third-class lever* are arranged in the sequence pivot-force-weight. This type of lever is employed when eyebrow tweezers or forceps are used to grasp an object.

The actions of bending and straightening the arm at the elbow, for example, involve bones and muscles functioning together as levers, as illustrated in figure 6.14. When the arm is bent (flexion), the lower arm bones represent the rigid bar, the elbow joint is the pivot, the hand is the weight that is moved, and the force is supplied by muscles on the anterior side of the upper arm. One of these muscles, the biceps brachii, is attached by a tendon to a projection (radial tuberosity) on the radius bone in the lower arm, a short distance below the elbow. Since the parts of this lever are arranged in the sequence pivot-force-weight, it is an example of a third-class lever.

When the arm is straightened at the elbow (extension), lower arm bones again serve as a rigid bar, the hand is the weight, and the elbow joint is the pivot. However, this time the force is supplied by the triceps brachii, a muscle located on the posterior side of the upper arm. A tendon of this muscle is attached to a projection (olecranon process) of the ulna bone at the point of the elbow. Thus, the parts of the lever are arranged weight-pivot-force—a first-class lever.

Although many lever arrangements occur throughout the skeletal-muscular systems, they are not always easy to identify. Nevertheless, these levers provide advantages in performing movements. The parts of some levers, such as those that function in moving the limbs, are arranged in ways that produce rapid motions, while others, such as those that move the head, aid in maintaining posture with minimal effort.

Blood Cell Formation

The process of blood cell formation is called **hematopoiesis.** Very early in life this process occurs in a structure called a yolk sac, which lies outside the body of a human embryo. (See chapter 18.) Later in development, blood cells are manufactured in the liver and spleen, and still later they are formed in marrow of various bones.

Osteoporosis

Osteoporosis is a disorder of the skeletal system in which there is excessive loss of bone matrix. This disorder is associated with the aging process. Within the affected bones, trabeculae tend to be lost (figure 6.15). Consequently, the bones develop spaces and canals, and as these enlarge they fill with fibrous and fatty tissues. Such bones are easily fractured and may break spontaneously because they are no longer able to support body weight. For example, a person with osteoporosis may suffer a spontaneous fracture of the upper leg bone (femur) at the hip or the collapse of sections of the backbone (vertebrae). Similarly, the distal portion of a lower arm bone (radius) near the wrist may fracture as a result of a minor stress.

Osteoporosis is responsible for a large proportion of fractures occurring in persons over forty-five years of age. Although it may affect persons of either gender, it is most common in thin, light-complexioned females after menopause.

Factors that increase the risk of osteoporosis include low intake of dietary calcium and lack of physical exercise (particularly during the early growing years), and in females, a decrease in the blood concentration of the sex hormone called estrogen. (This hormone is produced by the ovaries, which cease to secrete estrogen at menopause.) Heavy use of alcohol or tobacco also seems to increase the risk. In addition, some people may have a genetic tendency for developing this condition.

Fortunately, osteoporosis may be prevented if steps are taken early enough. It is known, for example, that bone mass usually reaches a maximum at about age thirty-five. Thereafter, bone loss may exceed bone formation in both males and females. To reduce such loss, people in their mid-twenties and older are advised to ensure that their calcium intake is adequate and engage in some type of regular exercise in which their bones support their body weight, such as walking or jogging. Additionally, postmenopausal women may require estrogen replacement therapy, which should be carried out under the supervision of a physician. As a rule, women have about 30% less bone than men; after menopause, women typically lose bone mass twice as fast as men do.

Confirming that a patient is developing osteoporosis is sometimes difficult. An X-ray film, for example, may not reveal a decrease in bone density until 20% to 30% of the bone tissue has been lost. Various noninvasive diagnostic techniques, however, can detect rapid changes in bone mass. These include the use of a scanner, called a *densitometer,* that measures the density of the wrist bones; and *quantitative computed tomography,* which can be used to visualize the density of other bones (see chapter 1).

In other cases, a bone sample may be removed, usually from a hip bone, in order to directly assess the condition of the bone tissue. Such a biopsy may also be used to judge the effectiveness of the treatment for bone disease.

FIGURE 6.15
Scanning electron micrographs of: (*a*) normal bone, and (*b*) bone from a person with osteoporosis.

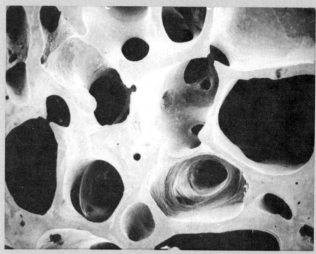
(a)

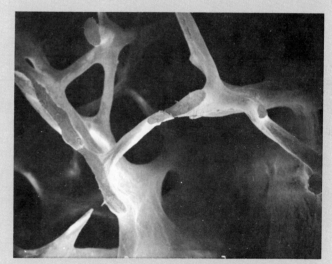
(b)

Marrow is a soft, netlike mass of connective tissue found within medullary cavities of long bones, in irregular spaces of spongy bone, and in larger osteonic canals of compact bone.

There are two kinds of marrow—red and yellow. *Red marrow* functions in the formation of all blood cells and platelets. It occupies the cavities of most bones in an infant. With age, however, more and more of it is replaced by *yellow marrow* that functions as fat storage tissue and is inactive in blood cell production.

In an adult, red marrow is found primarily in spongy bone of the skull, ribs, sternum, clavicles, vertebrae, and pelvis. If the blood cell supply is deficient, some yellow marrow may revert into red marrow and become active in blood cell production.

Storage of Minerals

As mentioned in chapter 4, intercellular matrix of bone tissue contains both collagen and minerals. Actually, the minerals are responsible for about 70% of the matrix by weight, and are mostly in the form of tiny crystals of a type of calcium phosphate called *hydroxyapatite.*

Calcium is needed for a number of vital body processes. When a low blood calcium level exists, osteoclasts are stimulated to break down bone tissue and calcium is released from the intercellular matrix into the blood. On the other hand, if the blood calcium level is high, osteo-clast activity is inhibited and osteoblasts are stimulated to form bone tissue. As a result, excess calcium is stored in the matrix. The regulation of osteoclast and osteoblast activity is controlled by hormones produced in the endocrine glands.

---

1. Name three major functions of bones.
2. Explain how body parts of the arm form a first-class lever; a third-class lever.
3. What minerals are normally stored in bone tissue?

Organization of the Skeleton

Number of Bones

Although the number of bones in a human skeleton is often reported to be 206, the actual number varies from person to person. Some people lack certain bones, while others have extra ones. For example, the flat bones of the skull usually grow together and become tightly joined along irregular lines called **sutures.** Occasionally extra bones called *sutural bones* (wormian bones) develop in these sutures (figure 6.16). Also, extra small, round sesamoid bones may develop in tendons, where they function to reduce friction in places where tendons pass over bony prominences (see chart 6.3).

FIGURE 6.16

(*a*) Sutural bones are extra bones that sometimes develop in sutures between the flat bones of the skull; (*b*) photograph of sutural bones.

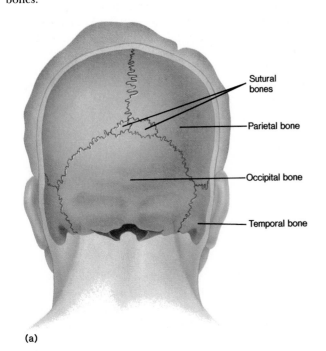

(a)

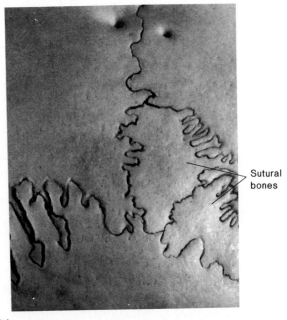

(b)

Chart 6.3 Bones of the adult skeleton

1. Axial Skeleton
   a. Skull   22 bones
      cranial bones
         frontal (1)
         parietal (2)
         occipital (1)
         temporal (2)
         sphenoid (1)
         ethmoid (1)

      facial bones
         maxilla (2)
         palatine (2)
         zygomatic (2)
         lacrimal (2)
         nasal (2)
         vomer (1)
         inferior nasal concha (2)

      mandible (1)
   b. Middle ear bones   6 bones
      malleus (2)
      incus (2)
      stapes (2)
   c. Hyoid   1 bone
      hyoid bone (1)
   d. Vertebral column   26 bones
      cervical vertebra (7)
      thoracic vertebra (12)
      lumbar vertebra (5)
      sacrum (1)
      coccyx (1)
   e. Thoracic cage   25 bones
      rib (24)
      sternum (1)
2. Appendicular Skeleton
   a. Pectoral girdle   4 bones
      scapula (2)
      clavicle (2)
   b. Upper limbs   60 bones
      humerus (2)
      radius (2)
      ulna (2)
      carpal (16)
      metacarpal (10)
      phalanx (28)
   c. Pelvic girdle   2 bones
      coxal bone (2)
   d. Lower limbs   60 bones
      femur (2)
      tibia (2)
      fibula (2)
      patella (2)
      tarsal (14)
      metatarsal (10)
      phalanx (28)

                    Total   206 bones

Divisions of the Skeleton

For purposes of study, it is convenient to divide the skeleton into two major portions—an axial skeleton and an appendicular skeleton (figure 6.17).

The **axial skeleton** consists of the bony and cartilaginous parts that support and protect organs of the head, neck, and trunk. These parts include the following:

1. **Skull.** The skull is composed of the *cranium* (brain case) and the *facial bones.*

2. **Hyoid bone.** The hyoid (hi'oid) bone is located in the neck between the lower jaw and larynx. It does not articulate with any other bones, but is fixed in position by muscles and ligaments. The hyoid bone supports the tongue and serves as an attachment for certain muscles that help move the tongue and function in swallowing. It can be felt approximately a finger's width above the anterior prominence of the larynx. The hyoid bone includes a body, two lesser cornua, and two greater cornua (sing. cornu). (See figure 6.18.)

3. **Vertebral column.** The vertebral column, or backbone, consists of many vertebrae separated by cartilaginous *intervertebral disks.* This column forms the central axis of the skeleton. Near its distal end, several vertebrae are fused to form the sacrum, which is part of the pelvis. A small, rudimentary tailbone called the **coccyx** is attached to the end of the sacrum.

4. **Thoracic cage.** The thoracic cage protects organs of the thorax and upper abdomen. It is composed of twelve pairs of ribs that articulate posteriorly with thoracic vertebrae. It also includes the **sternum** (ster'num), or breastbone, to which most of the ribs are attached anteriorly.

The **appendicular skeleton** consists of bones of the limbs and the bones that anchor the limbs to the axial skeleton. It includes the following:

1. **Pectoral girdle.** The pectoral girdle is formed by a scapula (scap'u-lah), or shoulder blade, and a **clavicle** (klav'i-k'l), or collarbone, on both sides of the body. The pectoral girdle connects bones of the arms to the axial skeleton and aids in arm movements.

2. **Upper limbs** (arms). Each upper limb consists of a **humerus** (hu'mer-us), or upper arm bone, and two lower arm bones—a **radius** (ra'de-us) and an **ulna** (ul'nah). These three bones articulate with each other at the elbow joint. At the distal end of the radius and ulna, there are eight **carpals** (kar'pals), or wrist bones. Bones of the palm are called **metacarpals,** and finger bones are called **phalanges** (fah-lan'jēz).

3. **Pelvic girdle.** The pelvic girdle is formed by two **coxal** (kok'sal), or **innominate** (i-nom'ĭ-nāt), **bones** (hip bones), which are attached to each other anteriorly and to the sacrum posteriorly. They connect bones of the legs to the axial skeleton and, with the sacrum and coccyx, form the pelvis, which protects the lower abdominal and internal reproductive organs.

FIGURE 6.17
Major bones of the skeleton. (*a*) Anterior view; (*b*) posterior view. (Note that the axial and appendicular portions are distinguished with color.)

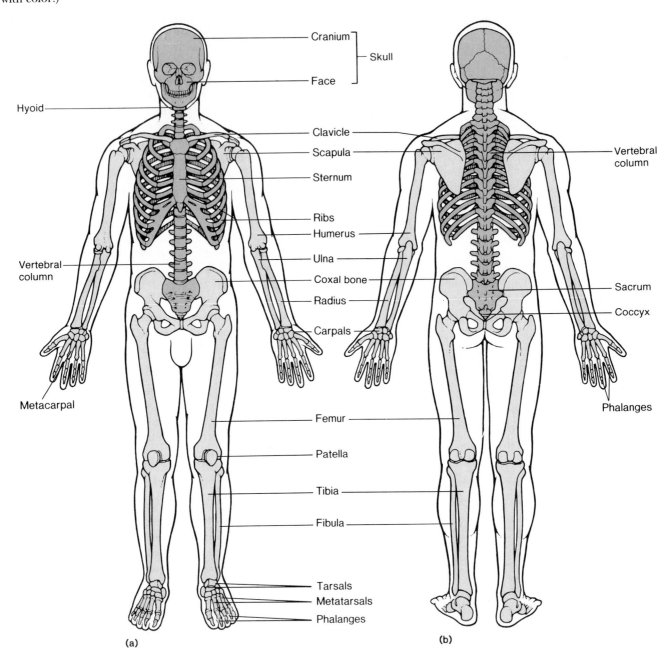

(a) (b)

4. **Lower limbs** (legs). Each lower limb consists of a **femur** (fe′mur), or thigh bone, and two lower leg bones—a large **tibia** (tib′e-ah), or shinbone, and a slender **fibula** (fib′u-lah), or calf bone. These three bones articulate with each other at the knee joint, where the **patella** (pah-tel′ah), or kneecap, covers the anterior surface. At the distal ends of the tibia and fibula, there are seven **tarsals** (tahr′sals), or ankle bones. Bones of the foot are called **metatarsals,** and those of the toes (like the fingers) are called **phalanges.** Chart 6.4 defines some terms used to describe skeletal structures.

FIGURE 6.18
The hyoid bone supports the tongue and serves as an attachment for muscles that move the tongue and function in swallowing.

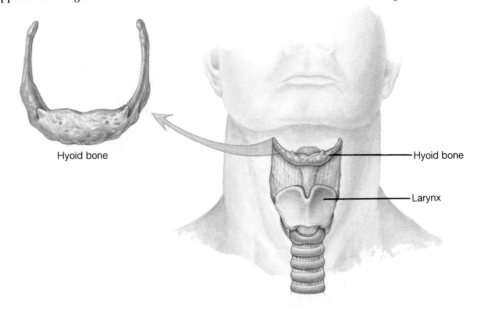

Hyoid bone

Hyoid bone

Larynx

Chart 6.4 Terms used to describe skeletal structures

Term	Definition	Example
Condyle (kon′dĭl)	A rounded process that usually articulates with another bone	Occipital condyle of the occipital bone (figure 6.22)
Crest (krest)	A narrow, ridgelike projection	Iliac crest of the ilium (figure 6.56)
Epicondyle (ep″ĭ-kon′dĭl)	A projection situated above a condyle	Medial epicondyle of the humerus (figure 6.51)
Facet (fas′et)	A small, nearly flat surface	Facet of a thoracic vertebra (figure 6.39)
Fissure (fish′-ūr)	A cleft or groove	Inferior orbital fissure in the orbit of the eye (figure 6.20)
Fontanel (fon″tah-nel′)	A soft spot in the skull where membranes cover the space between bones	Anterior fontanel between the frontal and parietal bones (figure 6.34)
Foramen (fo-ra′men)	An opening through a bone that usually serves as a passageway for blood vessels, nerves, or ligaments	Foramen magnum of the occipital bone (figure 6.22)
Fossa (fos′ah)	A relatively deep pit or depression	Olecranon fossa of the humerus (figure 6.51)
Fovea (fo′ve-ah)	A tiny pit or depression	Fovea capitis of the femur (figure 6.61)
Head (hed)	An enlargement on the end of a bone	Head of the humerus (figure 6.51)
Linea (lin′e-ah)	A narrow ridge	Linea aspera of the femur (figure 6.61)
Meatus (me-a′tus)	A tubelike passageway within a bone	External auditory meatus of the ear (figure 6.21)
Process (pros′es)	A prominent projection on a bone	Mastoid process of the temporal bone (figure 6.21)
Ramus (ra′mus)	A structure given off from another larger one	Ramus of the mandible
Sinus (si′nus)	A cavity within a bone	Frontal sinus of the frontal bone (figure 6.26)
Spine (spīn)	A sharp projection	Spine of the scapula (figure 6.48)
Suture (su′chur)	An interlocking line of union between bones	Lambdoidal suture between the occipital and parietal bones (figure 6.21)
Trochanter (tro-kan′ter)	A relatively large process	Greater trochanter of the femur (figure 6.61)
Tubercle (tu′ber-kl)	A small, knoblike process	Tubercle of a rib (figure 6.45)
Tuberosity (tu″bĕ-ros′ĭ-te)	A knoblike process usually larger than a tubercle	Radial tuberosity of the radius (figure 6.52)

FIGURE 6.19

Anterior view of the skull.

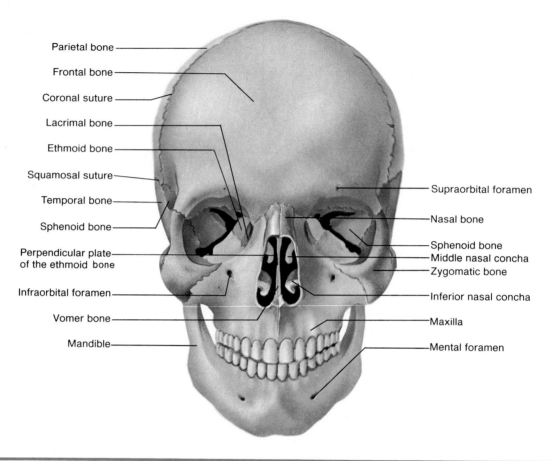

Parietal bone

Frontal bone

Coronal suture

Lacrimal bone

Ethmoid bone

Squamosal suture

Temporal bone

Sphenoid bone

Perpendicular plate
of the ethmoid bone

Infraorbital foramen

Vomer bone

Mandible

Supraorbital foramen

Nasal bone

Sphenoid bone

Middle nasal concha

Zygomatic bone

Inferior nasal concha

Maxilla

Mental foramen

FIGURE 6.20

The orbit of the eye includes both cranial and facial bones.

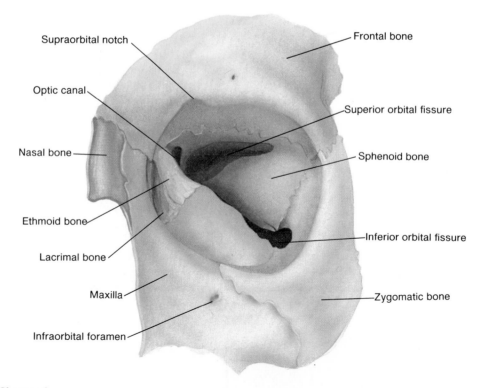

Supraorbital notch

Optic canal

Nasal bone

Ethmoid bone

Lacrimal bone

Maxilla

Infraorbital foramen

Frontal bone

Superior orbital fissure

Sphenoid bone

Inferior orbital fissure

Zygomatic bone

The Skull

A human skull usually consists of twenty-two bones that, except for the lower jaw, are firmly interlocked along irregular lines called *sutures* (su'churz). Eight of these interlocked bones make up the cranium, and thirteen form the facial skeleton. The **mandible** (man'di-b'l), or lower jawbone, is a movable bone held to the cranium by ligaments (figures 6.19, 6.20, 6.21, and 6.22).

Cranium

The **cranium** (kra'ne-um) encloses and protects the brain, and its surface provides attachments for various muscles that make chewing and head movements possible. Some cranial bones contain air-filled cavities called *sinuses*, which are lined with mucous membranes and are connected by passageways to the nasal cavity. Sinuses reduce the weight of the skull and increase the intensity of the voice by serving as resonant sound chambers.

The eight bones of the cranium (chart 6.5) are as follows:

1. **Frontal bone.** The frontal (frun'tal) bone forms the anterior portion of the skull above the eyes and includes the forehead, part of the roof of the nasal cavity, and roofs of the orbits (bony sockets) of the eyes. On the upper margin of each orbit, the frontal bone is marked by a *supraorbital foramen* (or supraorbital notch in some skulls), through which blood vessels and nerves pass to tissues of the forehead. Within the frontal bone are two *frontal sinuses*, one above each eye near the midline. Although it is a single bone in adults, the frontal bone develops in two parts. These halves grow together and are usually completely fused by the fifth or sixth year of age.

2. **Parietal bones.** One parietal (pah-ri'ĕ-tal) bone is located on each side of the skull just behind the frontal bone. Each is shaped like a curved plate and has four borders. Together, the parietal bones form the bulging sides and roof of the cranium. They are joined at the midline along the *sagittal suture,* and they meet the frontal bone along the *coronal suture.*

FIGURE 6.21
Lateral view of the skull.

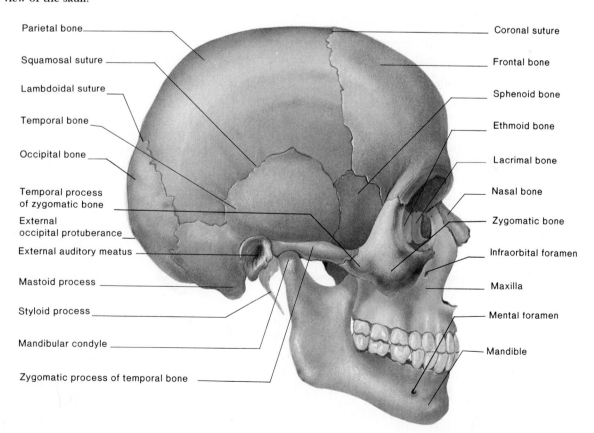

Parietal bone

Squamosal suture

Lambdoidal suture

Temporal bone

Occipital bone

Temporal process of zygomatic bone

External occipital protuberance

External auditory meatus

Mastoid process

Styloid process

Mandibular condyle

Zygomatic process of temporal bone

Coronal suture

Frontal bone

Sphenoid bone

Ethmoid bone

Lacrimal bone

Nasal bone

Zygomatic bone

Infraorbital foramen

Maxilla

Mental foramen

Mandible

The Skeletal System   139

FIGURE 6.22
Inferior view of the skull.

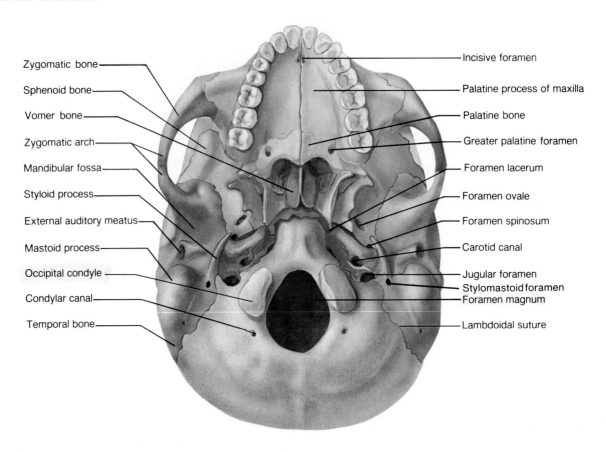

Zygomatic bone

Sphenoid bone

Vomer bone

Zygomatic arch

Mandibular fossa

Styloid process

External auditory meatus

Mastoid process

Occipital condyle

Condylar canal

Temporal bone

Incisive foramen

Palatine process of maxilla

Palatine bone

Greater palatine foramen

Foramen lacerum

Foramen ovale

Foramen spinosum

Carotid canal

Jugular foramen

Stylomastoid foramen

Foramen magnum

Lambdoidal suture

Chart 6.5 Cranial bones			
Name and number	**Description**	**Special features**	**Figure**
Frontal (1)	Forms forehead, roof of nasal cavity, and roofs of orbits	Supraorbital foramen, frontal sinuses	6.19
Parietal (2)	Form side walls and roof of cranium	Fused at midline along sagittal suture	6.21
Occipital (1)	Forms back of skull and base of cranium	Foramen magnum, occipital condyles	6.22
Temporal (2)	Form side walls and floor of cranium	External auditory meatus, mandibular fossa, mastoid process, styloid process, zygomatic process	6.23
Sphenoid (1)	Forms parts of base of cranium, sides of skull, and floors and sides of orbits	Sella turcica, sphenoidal sinuses	6.24
Ethmoid (1)	Forms parts of roof and walls of nasal cavity, floor of cranium, and walls of orbits	Cribriform plates, perpendicular plate, superior and middle nasal conchae, ethmoidal sinuses, crista galli	6.25

FIGURE 6.23

Lateral surface of the right temporal bone. What sensory structures are located within this bone?

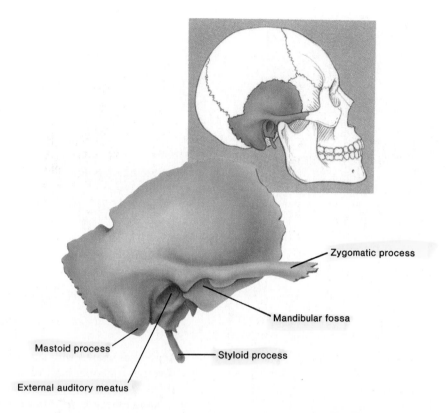

Zygomatic process

Mandibular fossa

Mastoid process

Styloid process

External auditory meatus

3. **Occipital bone.** The occipital (ok-sip'ĭ-tal) bone joins the parietal bones along the *lambdoidal* (lam'doid-al) *suture*. It forms the back of the skull and base of the cranium. There is a large opening on its lower surface called the *foramen magnum,* through which nerve fibers from the brain pass and enter the vertebral canal to become the spinal cord. Rounded processes called *occipital condyles,* located on each side of the foramen magnum, articulate with the first vertebra of the vertebral column. A posterior projection, the *external occipital protuberance,* can be felt in the midline on the back of the head.

4. **Temporal bones.** A temporal (tem'por-al) bone (figure 6.23) on each side of the skull joins the parietal bone along a *squamosal* (skwa-mo'sal) *suture*. The temporal bones form parts of the sides and the base of the cranium. Located near the inferior margin is an opening, the *external auditory meatus,* which leads inward to parts of the ear. The temporal bones also house the internal ear structures and have depressions called the *mandibular fossae* (glenoid fossae) that articulate with processes of the mandible. Below each external auditory meatus there are two projections—a rounded *mastoid process* and a long,

pointed *styloid process.* The mastoid process provides an attachment for certain muscles of the neck, and the styloid process serves as an anchorage for muscles associated with the tongue and pharynx. The hyoid bone is also attached to the styloid processes by ligaments. An opening near the mastoid process, the *carotid canal,* transmits the internal carotid artery, while an opening between the temporal and occipital bones, the *jugular foramen,* accommodates the jugular vein (figure 6.23). A *zygomatic process* projects anteriorly from the temporal bone in the region of the external auditory meatus. It joins the zygomatic bone and helps form the prominence of the cheek.

The mastoid process is of clinical interest because it may become infected. Tissues in this region of the temporal bone contain a number of interconnected air cells, lined with mucous membranes, that communicate with the middle ear. These spaces sometimes become inflamed when microorganisms spread from an infected middle ear (otitis media). The resulting mastoid infection, called *mastoiditis,* is of particular concern because the membranes that surround the brain are close by and may also become infected.

FIGURE 6.24

(*a*) The sphenoid bone as viewed from above; (*b*) posterior view.

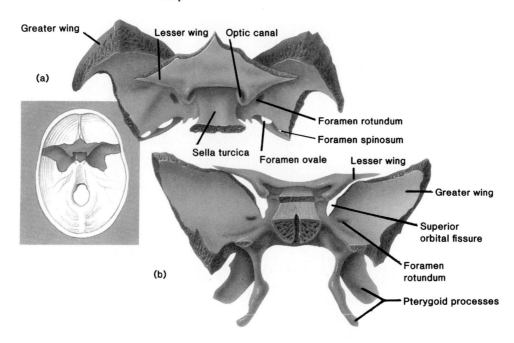

5. **Sphenoid bone.** The sphenoid (sfe'noid) bone (figure 6.24) is wedged between several other bones in the anterior portion of the cranium. It consists of a central part and two winglike structures that extend laterally toward each side of the skull. This bone helps form the base of the cranium, sides of the skull, and floors and sides of the orbits. Along the midline within the cranial cavity, a portion of the sphenoid bone rises up and forms a saddle-shaped mass called *sella turcica* (sel'ah tur'si-ka) (Turk's saddle). The depression of this saddle is occupied by the pituitary gland, which hangs from the base of the brain by a stalk. The *pterygoid processes* extend inferiorly from the central portion of the sphenoid bone and form part of the lateral wall of the nasal cavity.

The sphenoid bone also contains two *sphenoidal sinuses,* which lie side by side and are separated by a bony septum that projects downward into the nasal cavity.

6. **Ethmoid bone.** The ethmoid (eth'moid) bone (figure 6.25) is located in front of the sphenoid bone. It consists of two masses, one on each side of the nasal cavity, which are joined horizontally by thin *cribriform* (krib'rĭ-form) *plates*. These plates form part of the roof of the nasal cavity, and

nerves associated with the sense of smell pass through tiny openings (olfactory foramina) in them. Portions of the ethmoid bone also form sections of the cranial floor, orbital walls, and nasal cavity walls. A *perpendicular plate* projects downward in the midline from the cribriform plates to form most of the bony nasal septum.

Delicate scroll-shaped plates called the *superior nasal concha* (kong'kah) and *middle nasal concha* project inward from the lateral portions of the ethmoid bone toward the perpendicular plate. These bones, which are also called *turbinate bones,* support mucous membranes that line the nasal cavity. The mucous membranes, in turn, begin the processes of moistening, warming, and filtering air as it enters the respiratory tract. The lateral portions of the ethmoid bone contain many small air spaces, the *ethmoidal sinuses*. Various structures in the nasal cavity are shown in figure 6.26.

Projecting upward into the cranial cavity between the cribriform plates is a triangular process of the ethmoid bone called the *crista galli* (kris'tă gal'li) (cock's comb). This process serves as an attachment for membranes that enclose the brain. A view of the cranial cavity is shown in figure 6.27.

FIGURE 6.25

(a) Ethmoid bone viewed from above and (b) from behind.

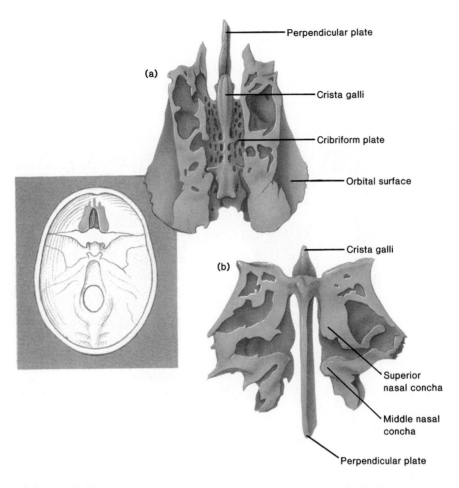

FIGURE 6.26

Lateral wall of the nasal cavity.

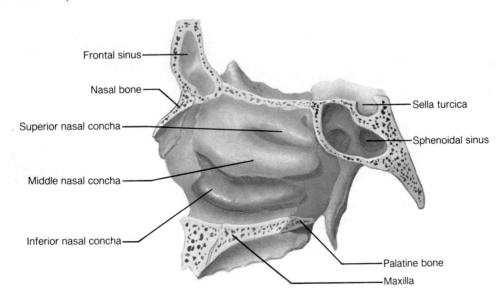

FIGURE 6.27
Floor of the cranial cavity viewed from above.

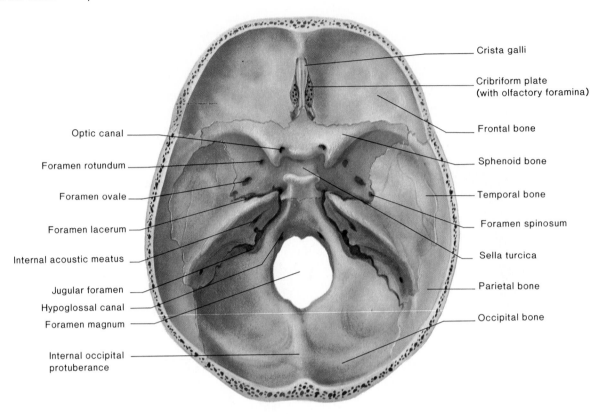

Crista galli

Cribriform plate
(with olfactory foramina)

Frontal bone

Sphenoid bone

Temporal bone

Foramen spinosum

Sella turcica

Parietal bone

Occipital bone

Optic canal

Foramen rotundum

Foramen ovale

Foramen lacerum

Internal acoustic meatus

Jugular foramen

Hypoglossal canal

Foramen magnum

Internal occipital
protuberance

Facial Skeleton

The **facial skeleton** consists of thirteen immovable bones and a movable lower jawbone. In addition to forming the basic shape of the face, these bones provide attachments for various muscles that move the jaw and control facial expressions.

The bones of the facial skeleton are as follows:

1. **Maxillary bones.** The maxillary (mak'si-ler"e) bones (pl. maxillae, mak-sil'e) form the upper jaw; together, they are the keystone of the face, for all other immovable facial bones articulate with them.

Portions of these bones comprise the anterior roof of the mouth (*hard palate*), floors of the orbits, and sides and floor of the nasal cavity. They also contain the sockets of the upper teeth. Inside the maxillae, lateral to the nasal cavity, are *maxillary sinuses* (antrums of Highmore). These spaces are the largest of the sinuses, and they extend from the floor of the orbits to the roots of the upper teeth. Figure 6.28 shows the locations of the maxillary

and other sinuses. See chart 6.6 for a summary of the sinuses.

During development, portions of the maxillary bones called *palatine processes* grow together and fuse along the midline to form the anterior section of the hard palate.

Chart 6.6 Sinuses of cranial and facial bones

Sinuses	Number	Location
Frontal sinuses	2	Frontal bone above each eye and near the midline
Sphenoidal sinuses	2	Sphenoid bone above the posterior portion of the nasal cavity
Ethmoidal sinuses	2 groups of small air cells	Ethmoid bone on either side of the upper portion of the nasal cavity
Maxillary sinuses	2	Maxillary bones lateral to the nasal cavity and extending from the floor of the orbits to the roots of the upper teeth

FIGURE 6.28
Location of the sinuses.

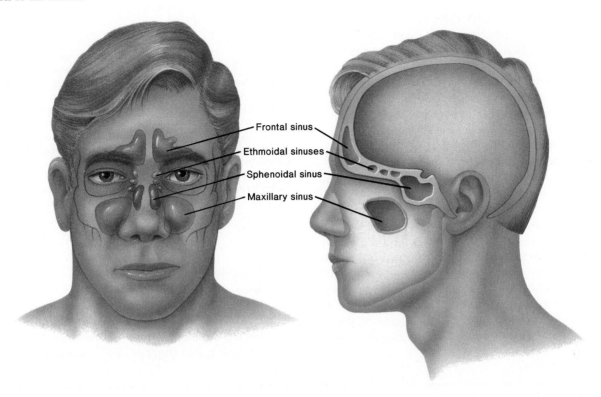

Frontal sinus
Ethmoidal sinuses
Sphenoidal sinus
Maxillary sinus

Sometimes fusion of the palatine processes of the maxillae is incomplete at the time of birth; the result is called a cleft palate. Infants with this deformity may have trouble suckling because of the opening that remains between the oral and nasal cavities.

The inferior border of each maxillary bone projects downward, forming an *alveolar* (al-ve′o-lar) *process.* Together these processes create a horseshoe-shaped *alveolar arch* (dental arch). Cavities (alveoli) in this arch are occupied by teeth, which are attached to these bony sockets by fibrous connective tissue (see chapter 12).

2. **Palatine bones.** The palatine (pal′ah-tīn) bones (figure 6.29) are located behind the maxillae. Each bone is roughly L-shaped. The horizontal portions serve as the posterior section of the hard palate and the floor of the nasal cavity. Perpendicular portions help form the lateral walls of the nasal cavity.

3. **Zygomatic bones.** The zygomatic (zi″go-mat′ik) bones (malar bones) are responsible for the prominences of the cheeks below and to the sides of the eyes. These bones also help form the lateral walls and floors of the orbits. Each bone has a *temporal process,* which extends posteriorly to join the zygomatic process of a temporal bone. Together these processes form a *zygomatic arch* (figures 6.21 and 6.22).

FIGURE 6.29
The horizontal portions of the palatine bones form the posterior section of the hard palate, and the perpendicular portions help form the lateral walls of the nasal cavity.

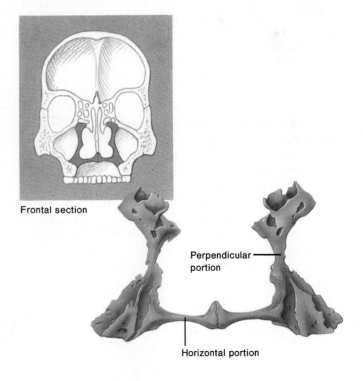

Frontal section

Perpendicular portion

Horizontal portion

4. **Lacrimal bones.** A lacrimal (lak'ri-mal) bone is a thin, scalelike structure located in the medial wall of each orbit between the ethmoid bone and maxillary bone. A groove in its anterior portion leads from the orbit to the nasal cavity, providing a pathway for a tube that carries tears from the eye to the nasal cavity.

5. **Nasal bones.** The nasal (na'zal) bones are long, thin, and nearly rectangular. They lie side by side and are fused at the midline, where they form the bridge of the nose. These bones serve as attachments for cartilaginous tissues that are largely responsible for the shape of the nose.

6. **Vomer bone.** The thin, flat vomer (vo'mer) bone is located along the midline within the nasal cavity. Posteriorly, it joins the perpendicular plate of the ethmoid bone, and along with the cartilage these form the nasal septum (figures 6.30 and 6.31).

7. **Inferior nasal conchae.** The inferior nasal conchae (kong'ke) are fragile, scroll-shaped bones attached to the lateral walls of the nasal cavity. They are the largest of the conchae and are positioned below the conchae of the ethmoid bone (see figures 6.19 and 6.26). Like the superior and middle conchae, the

inferior conchae provide support for mucous membranes within the nasal cavity that warm, moisten, and filter air.

The facial bones are sometimes broken or shattered as a result of an automobile accident in which the individual is thrown through the windshield. The impact of such an accident often damages the zygomatic, maxillary, and frontal bones. Three-dimensional CT scans are particularly useful for visualizing this type of injury. (See figure 1.16.) In cases where the facial bones are broken into many small fragments, the bones may be repaired by *reconstructive surgery.* In these procedures, extremely thin metal plates are bent to the desired shapes and then attached with small screws to undamaged bones. Small pieces of bone from locations such as the iliac crest, are then packed around the metal plates. With time, these pieces will grow and form new bone.

8. **Mandible.** The mandible (man'di̅-b'l), or lower jawbone, consists of a horizontal, horseshoe-shaped body with a flat *ramus* projecting upward at each end. The rami are divided into two processes—a posterior *mandibular condyle* and an anterior *coronoid process* (figure 6.32). The mandibular

FIGURE 6.30

Sagittal section of the skull.

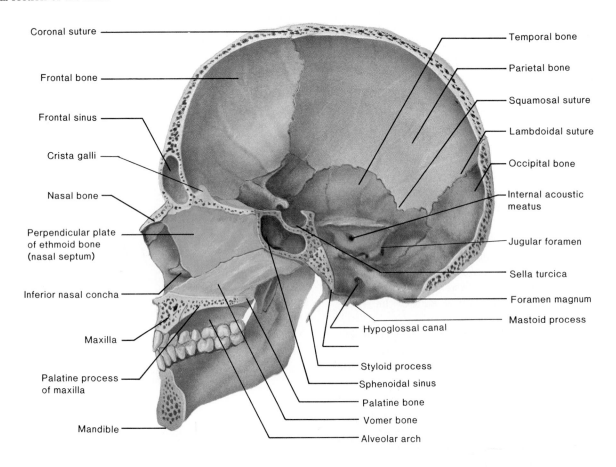

FIGURE 6.31
A frontal section of the skull (posterior view).

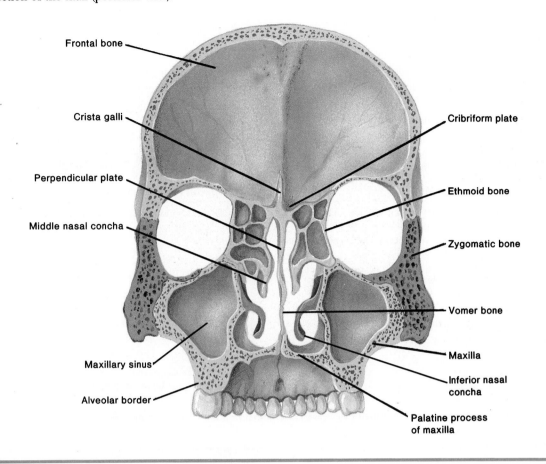

Frontal bone

Crista galli

Cribriform plate

Perpendicular plate

Ethmoid bone

Middle nasal concha

Zygomatic bone

Vomer bone

Maxilla

Maxillary sinus

Inferior nasal concha

Alveolar border

Palatine process of maxilla

FIGURE 6.32
(*a*) Lateral view of the mandible; (*b*) inferior lateral view.

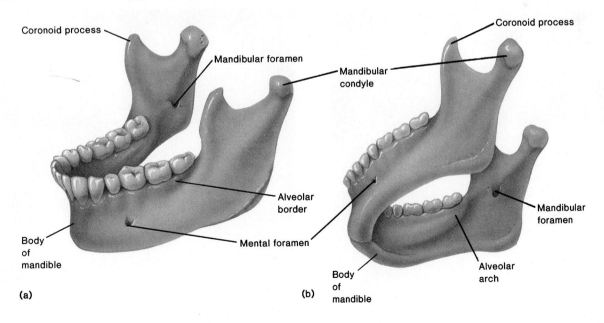

Coronoid process

Coronoid process

Mandibular foramen

Mandibular condyle

Alveolar border

Mandibular foramen

Body of mandible

Mental foramen

Body of mandible

Alveolar arch

(a)

(b)

condyles articulate with the mandibular fossae of the temporal bones, and the coronoid processes serve as attachments for muscles used in chewing. Other large chewing muscles are inserted on the lateral surfaces of the rami.

A curved bar of bone on the superior border of the mandible, the *alveolar border,* contains the hollow sockets that bear the lower teeth.

On the medial side of the mandible, near the center of each ramus, is a *mandibular foramen.* This opening admits blood vessels and a nerve, which supply roots of the lower teeth. Dentists commonly inject anesthetic into tissues near this foramen to temporarily block nerve impulse conduction and cause the teeth on that side of the jaw to become insensitive. Branches of these blood vessels and the nerve emerge from the mandible through the *mental foramen,* which opens on the outside near the point of the jaw. They supply tissues of the chin and lower lip.

Chart 6.7 Bones of the facial skeleton

Name and number	Description	Special features	Figure
Maxillary (2)	Form upper jaw, anterior roof of mouth, floors of orbits, and sides and floor of nasal cavity	Alveolar border, maxillary sinuses, palatine process	6.19
Palatine (2)	Form posterior roof of mouth, and floor and lateral walls of nasal cavity		6.29
Zygomatic (2)	Form prominences of cheeks, and lateral walls and floors of orbits	Temporal process	6.21
Lacrimal (2)	Form part of medial walls of orbits	Canal that leads from orbit to nasal cavity	6.20
Nasal (2)	Form bridge of nose		6.21
Vomer (1)	Forms part of nasal septum		6.22
Inferior nasal concha (2)	Extend into nasal cavity from its lateral walls		6.19
Mandible (1)	Forms lower jaw	Body, ramus, mandibular condyle, coronoid process, alveolar border, mandibular foramen, mental foramen	6.32

FIGURE 6.33

(*a*) X-ray films of the skull from the front and (*b*) from the side. What features of the cranium and facial skeleton do you recognize?

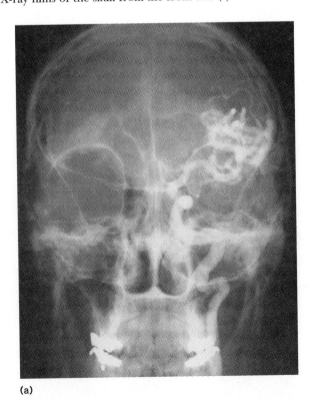

(a)

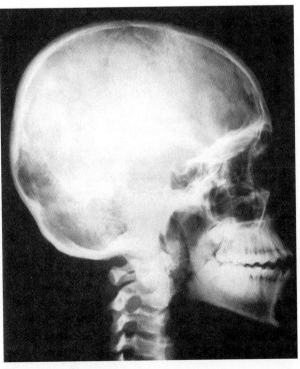

(b)

Chart 6.7 contains a descriptive summary of the fourteen facial bones. Various features of these bones can be seen in the X-ray films in figure 6.33.

Chart 6.8 lists the major openings (foramina) and passageways through bones of the skull, as well as their general locations and the structures they transmit.

Infantile Skull

At birth, the skull is incompletely developed, and the cranial bones are separated by fibrous membranes. These membranous areas are called **fontanels** (fon″tah-nelz′), or, more commonly, soft spots. They permit some movement between bones, so that the developing skull is partially compressible and can change shape slightly. This action, called *molding*, enables an infant's skull to pass more easily through the birth canal. Eventually the fontanels close as the cranial bones grow together. The posterior fontanel usually closes about two months after birth; the sphenoid (anterolateral) fontanel closes at about three months; the mastoid (posterolateral) fontanel closes near the end of the first year; and the anterior fontanel may not close until the middle or end of the second year (figure 6.34).

Other characteristics of an infantile skull include a relatively small face with a prominent forehead and large orbits. The jaw and nasal cavity are small, the sinuses are incompletely formed, and the frontal bone is in two parts. The skull bones are thin, but they are also somewhat flexible and thus are less easily fractured than adult bones.

Chart 6.8 Passageways through bones of the skull

Passageway	Location	Major structures transmitted
Carotid canal (figure 6.22)	Inferior surface of the temporal bone	Internal carotid artery, veins, and nerves
Condylar canal (figure 6.22)	Base of skull in occipital bone	Veins between the skull and the neck
Foramen lacerum (figure 6.22)	Floor of cranial cavity between temporal and sphenoid bones	Branch of pharyngeal artery (in life, opening is largely covered by fibrocartilage)
Foramen magnum (figure 6.22)	Base of skull in occipital bone	Nerve fibers between brain and spinal cord
Foramen ovale (figure 6.22)	Floor of cranial cavity in sphenoid bone	Mandibular division of trigeminal nerve and veins
Foramen rotundum (figure 6.24)	Floor of cranial cavity in sphenoid bone	Maxillary division of trigeminal nerve
Foramen spinosum (figure 6.24)	Floor of cranial cavity in sphenoid bone	Middle meningeal blood vessels and branch of mandibular nerve
Greater palatine foramen (figure 6.22)	Posterior portion of hard palate in palatine bone	Palatine blood vessels and nerves
Hypoglossal canal (figure 6.30)	Near margin of foramen magnum in occipital bone	Hypoglossal nerve
Incisive foramen (figure 6.22)	Anterior portion of hard palate	Nasopalatine nerves
Inferior orbital fissure (figure 6.20)	Floor of the orbit	Maxillary nerve and blood vessels
Infraorbital foramen (figure 6.20)	Below the orbit in maxillary bone	Infraorbital blood vessels and nerves
Internal acoustic meatus (figure 6.27)	Floor of cranial cavity in temporal bone	Branches of facial, vestibular, and cochlear nerves and blood vessels
Jugular foramen (figure 6.22)	Base of the skull between temporal and occipital bones	Glossopharyngeal, vagus and accessory nerves, and blood vessels
Mandibular foramen (figure 6.32)	Inner surface of ramus of mandible	Inferior alveolar blood vessels and nerves
Mental foramen (figure 6.32)	Near point of jaw in mandible	Mental nerve and blood vessels
Optic canal (figure 6.20)	Posterior portion of orbit in sphenoid bone	Optic nerve and ophthalmic artery
Stylomastoid foramen (figure 6.22)	Between styloid and mastoid processes	Facial nerve and blood vessels
Superior orbital fissure (figure 6.20)	Lateral wall of orbit	Oculomotor, trochlear, abducens, and ophthalmic division of trigeminal nerves
Supraorbital foramen (figure 6.19)	Upper margin of orbit in frontal bone	Supraorbital blood vessels and nerves

FIGURE 6.34

(a) Lateral view and (b) superior view of the infantile skull.

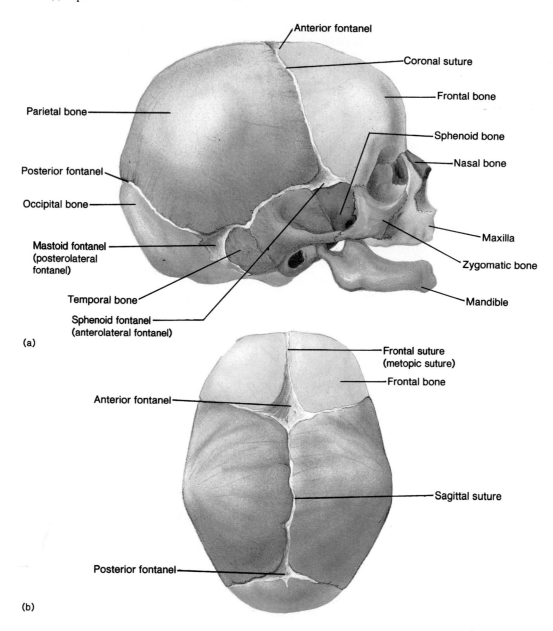

Anterior fontanel
Coronal suture
Frontal bone
Sphenoid bone
Nasal bone
Parietal bone
Posterior fontanel
Occipital bone
Maxilla
Mastoid fontanel (posterolateral fontanel)
Zygomatic bone
Mandible
Temporal bone
Sphenoid fontanel (anterolateral fontanel)

(a)

Frontal suture (metopic suture)
Frontal bone
Anterior fontanel
Sagittal suture
Posterior fontanel

(b)

In the infantile skull, the two parts of the developing frontal bone are separated in the midline by a frontal suture (metopic suture). This suture usually closes before the sixth year; however, in a small proportion of adult skulls, the frontal suture remains visible.

1. Locate and name each of the bones of the cranium.
2. Locate and name each of the facial bones.
3. Explain how an adult skull differs from that of an infant.

Vertebral Column

The **vertebral column** extends from the skull to the pelvis and forms the vertical axis of the skeleton. It is composed of many bony parts called **vertebrae.** These are separated by masses of fibrocartilage called *intervertebral disks* and are connected to one another by ligaments. The vertebral column supports the head and trunk of the body, yet is flexible enough to permit movements, such as bending forward, backward, or to the side, and turning or rotating on the central axis. It also protects the spinal cord, which passes through a *vertebral canal* formed by openings in the vertebrae.

FIGURE 6.35
The curved vertebral column consists of many vertebrae separated by intervertebral disks. (*a*) Lateral view; (*b*) posterior view.

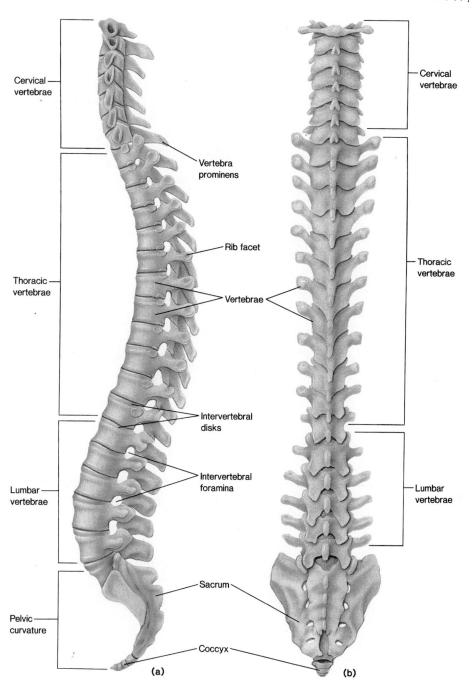

In an infant, there are thirty-three separate bones in the vertebral column. Five of these bones eventually fuse to form the sacrum, and four others join to become the coccyx. As a result, an adult vertebral column has twenty-six bones.

Normally, the vertebral column has four curvatures, which are associated with upright posture. The names of the curves correspond to the regions in which they occur, as shown in figure 6.35. The *thoracic* and *pelvic curvatures* are concave anteriorly and are called primary curves. The *cervical curvature* in the neck and *lumbar curvature* in the lower back are convex anteriorly and are called secondary curves.

FIGURE 6.36

(a) Lateral view of a typical vertebra; (b) adjacent vertebrae are joined at their articulating processes; (c) superior view of a typical thoracic vertebra.

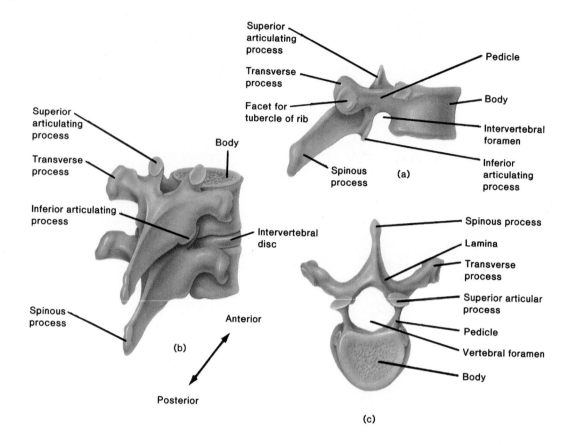

A Typical Vertebra

Although vertebrae in different regions of the vertebral column have special characteristics, they also have features in common. Thus, a typical vertebra (figure 6.36) has a drum-shaped body (centrum), which forms the thick, anterior portion of the bone. A longitudinal row of these vertebral bodies supports the weight of the head and trunk. Intervertebral disks, which separate adjacent vertebrae, are fastened to the roughened upper and lower surfaces of the bodies. These disks cushion and soften forces created by such movements as walking and jumping, which might otherwise fracture vertebrae or jar the brain.

Projecting posteriorly from each vertebral body are two short stalks called *pedicles* (ped'ĭ-klz), which form the sides of the *vertebral foramen*. Two plates called *laminae* (lam'ĭ-nē) arise from the pedicles and fuse in the back to become a *spinous process*. The pedicles, laminae, and spinous process together complete a bony *vertebral arch* around the vertebral foramen, through which the spinal cord passes.

Between the pedicles and laminae of a typical vertebra is a *transverse process*, which projects laterally and toward the back. Various ligaments and muscles are attached to the posterior spinous process and transverse processes. *Superior* and *inferior articulating processes* project from each

vertebral arch. These processes bear cartilage-covered facets that join each vertebra to the one above and the one below it.

On the inferior surfaces of the vertebral pedicles are notches that align to create openings called *intervertebral foramina* (in"ter-ver'tĕ-bral fo-ram'ĭ-nah). These openings provide passageways for spinal nerves that pass between adjacent vertebrae and connect to the spinal cord.

Athletes, such as gymnasts, basketball players, and pole vaulters, who repeatedly land on hard surfaces sometimes develop breaks or cracks in their vertebrae. These fractures commonly involve the articulating processes of the bones. Such a fracturing of a vertebra is called *spondylolysis*. It may be prevented by limiting the number of landings experienced during individual practice periods and by padding landing areas with floor mats.

Cervical Vertebrae

Seven **cervical vertebrae** comprise the bony axis of the neck. Although these are the smallest of the vertebrae, their bone tissues are denser than those in any other region of the vertebral column.

FIGURE 6.37

How do the structures of the (*a*) atlas and (*b*) axis function together to allow movement of the head? (*c*) Lateral view of the axis.

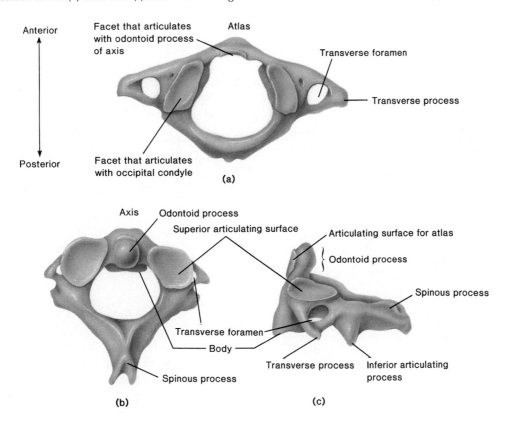

FIGURE 6.38
What features can you identify in this X-ray film of the neck?

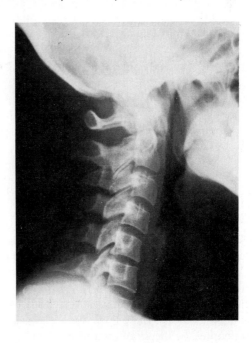

Transverse processes of cervical vertebrae are distinctive because they have *transverse foramina,* which serve as passageways for arteries leading to the brain. Also, the spinous processes of the second through fifth cervical vertebrae are uniquely forked (bifid). These processes provide attachments for various muscles.

The spinous process of the seventh vertebra is longer and protrudes beyond the other cervical spines. It is called the *vertebra prominens,* and because it can be felt through the skin, it is a useful landmark for locating other vertebral parts (figure 6.35).

Two of the cervical vertebrae, shown in figure 6.37, are of special interest. The first vertebra, or **atlas** (at'las), supports and balances the head. It has practically no body or spine and appears as a bony ring with two transverse processes. On its upper surface, the atlas has two kidney-shaped facets, which articulate with the occipital condyles of the skull.

The second cervical vertebra, or **axis** (ak'sis), bears a toothlike *odontoid process* (dens) on its body. This process projects upward and lies in the ring of the atlas. As the head is turned from side to side, the atlas pivots around the odontoid process. (See figure 6.38.)

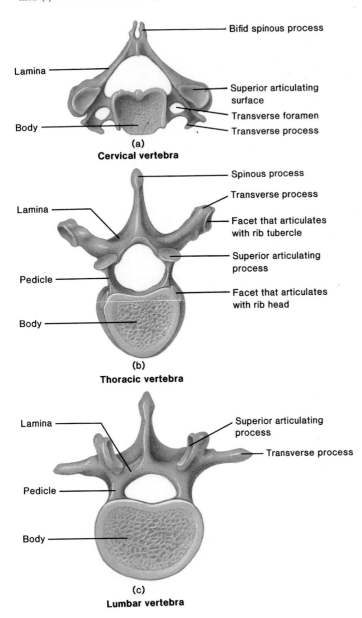

Bifid spinous process

Lamina

Superior articulating surface

Transverse foramen

Body

Transverse process

(a)
Cervical vertebra

Spinous process

Transverse process

Lamina

Facet that articulates with rib tubercle

Superior articulating process

Pedicle

Facet that articulates with rib head

Body

(b)
Thoracic vertebra

Lamina

Superior articulating process

Transverse process

Pedicle

Body

(c)
Lumbar vertebra

Thoracic Vertebrae

The twelve thoracic vertebrae are larger than those in the cervical region. Each vertebra has a long, pointed spinous process, which slopes downward, and facets on the sides of its body, which articulate with a rib.

Beginning with the third thoracic vertebra and moving downward, the bodies of these bones increase in size. Thus, they are adapted to the stress placed on them by the increasing amounts of body weight they bear.

Lumbar Vertebrae

There are five **lumbar vertebrae** in the small of the back (loins). The lumbars are adapted to support more weight than the vertebrae above them, and have larger and stronger bodies. The transverse processes of these vertebrae project laterally and backward while their short, thick spinous processes are directed nearly horizontally.

Figure 6.39 compares the structures of the cervical, thoracic, and lumbar vertebrae.

> Gymnasts, football players, and others who have their vertebral columns bent excessively and forcefully may experience the slipping of one vertebra over the one below it. This painful condition is called *spondylolisthesis*. It usually involves the fifth lumbar vertebra sliding forward over the body of the sacrum. The condition may be prevented by exercises designed to strengthen the back muscles associated with the vertebral column.

Sacrum

The **sacrum** (sa'krum) is a triangular structure at the base of the vertebral column. It is composed of five vertebrae that develop as separate structures but gradually become fused together between the eighteenth and thirtieth years. Spinous processes of these fused bones are represented by a ridge of *tubercles* that form the *median sacral crest*. To the sides of the tubercles are rows of openings, called *dorsal sacral foramina*, through which nerves and blood vessels pass (figure 6.40).

The sacrum is wedged between the coxal bones of the pelvis and is connected to them at its auricular surfaces by fibrocartilage of the *sacroiliac joints*. Weight of the body is transmitted to the legs through the pelvic girdle at these joints.

The sacrum forms the posterior wall of the pelvic cavity. The superior surface of the first sacral vertebra forms the *base* of the sacrum. The anterior margin of the base is called the *sacral promontory*. This projection can be felt during a vaginal examination and is used as a guide in determining the size of the pelvis. This measurement is helpful in estimating how easily an infant may be able to pass through a woman's pelvic cavity during birth.

Vertebral foramina of the sacral vertebrae form the *sacral canal*, which continues through the sacrum to an opening of variable size at the tip called the *sacral hiatus*. This foramen exists because the laminae of the last sacral vertebra are not fused. Four pairs of *pelvic sacral foramina* on the anterior surface of the sacrum provide passageways for nerves and blood vessels.

Coccyx

The **coccyx** (kok'siks), or tailbone, is the inferior portion of the vertebral column and is composed of four vertebrae that fuse together by age twenty-five. It is attached by lig-

FIGURE 6.40

(*a*) Anterior view of the sacrum and coccyx; (*b*) posterior view.

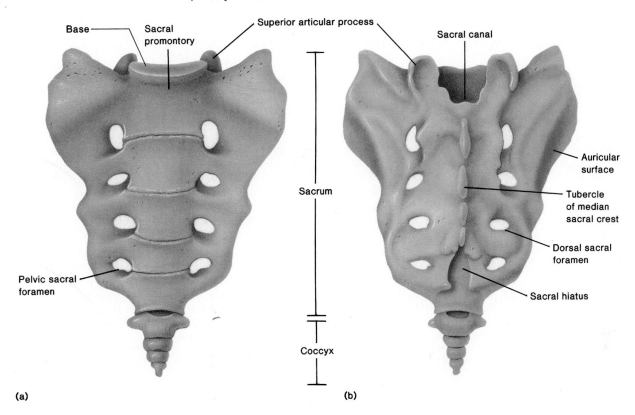

Chart 6.9 Bones of the vertebral column					
Bones	**Number**	**Special features**	**Bones**	**Number**	**Special features**
Cervical vertebrae	7	Transverse foramina; facets of atlas articulate with occipital condyles of skull; odontoid process of axis articulates with atlas; spinous processes of second through fifth vertebrae are bifid	Lumbar vertebrae	5	Large bodies; transverse processes that project backward at sharp angles; short, thick spinous processes directed nearly horizontally
			Sacrum	5 vertebrae fused into 1 bone	Dorsal sacral foramina, sacral promontory, sacral canal, sacral hiatus, auricular surfaces, pelvic sacral foramina
Thoracic vertebrae	12	Pointed spinous processes that slope downward; facets that articulate with ribs	Coccyx	4 vertebrae fused into 1 bone	

aments to the margins of the sacral hiatus. When a person is sitting, pressure is exerted upon the coccyx and it moves forward, acting somewhat like a shock absorber. Sitting down with great force sometimes causes the coccyx to be fractured or dislocated.

Chart 6.9 summarizes the bones of the vertebral column.

1. Describe the structure of the vertebral column.
2. Explain the difference between the vertebral column of an adult and that of an infant.
3. Describe a typical vertebra.
4. How do structures of cervical, thoracic, and lumbar vertebrae differ?

Some Disorders of the Vertebral Column

A common vertebral problem involves changes in the intervertebral disks. Each disk is composed of a tough, outer layer of fibrocartilage (anulus fibrosus) and an elastic central mass (nucleus pulposus). As a person ages, these disks tend to undergo degenerative changes in which central masses lose their firmness and outer layers become thinner, weaker, and develop cracks. Extra pressure, as when a person falls or lifts a heavy object, can break the outer layers of the disks and allow the central masses to squeeze out. Such a rupture may cause pressure on the spinal cord or on spinal nerves that branch from it. This condition—a *ruptured,* or *herniated, disk*—may cause back pain and numbness or loss of muscular function in parts innervated by the affected spinal nerves (figure 6.41).

Sometimes problems develop in the curvatures of the vertebral column because of poor posture, injury, or disease. For example, if an exaggerated thoracic curvature appears, the person develops rounded shoulders and a hunchback. This condition, called *kyphosis,* occasionally develops in adolescents who are active in strenuous athletic activities. Unless the problem is corrected before bone growth is complete, the vertebral column may be permanently deformed.

Sometimes the vertebral column develops an abnormal lateral curvature, so that one hip or shoulder is lower than the other. At the same time, the thoracic and abdominal organs may be displaced or compressed. This condition is called *scoliosis.* Although it most commonly develops without known cause in adolescent females, it also may accompany such diseases as poliomyelitis, rickets, or tuberculosis (figure 6.42).

If the vertebral column develops an accentuated lumbar curvature, the deformity is called *lordosis,* or swayback.

In addition to problems involving intervertebral disks and curvatures, the vertebral column is subject to degenerative diseases. For example, as a person ages the intervertebral disks tend to become smaller and more rigid, and the vertebral bodies are more likely to be fractured by compression. Consequently, the height of an elderly person may decrease, and the thoracic curvature of the vertebral column may be accentuated, causing the back to become bowed.

FIGURE 6.41
An MRI scan of a herniated lumbar disk (arrow).

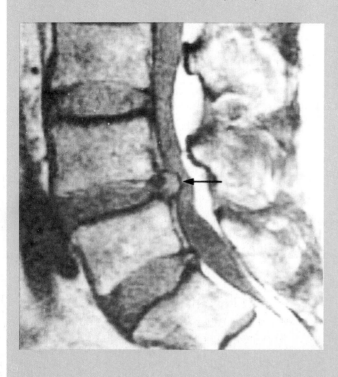

FIGURE 6.42
An X-ray film showing scoliosis, the lateral curvature of the vertebral column.

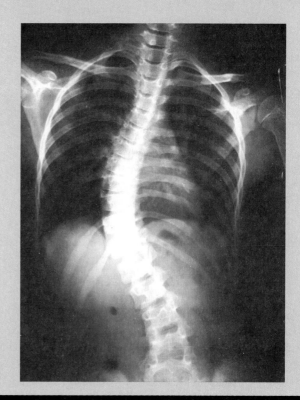

FIGURE 6.43

The thoracic cage includes the thoracic vertebrae, the sternum, the ribs, and the costal cartilages that attach the ribs to the sternum.

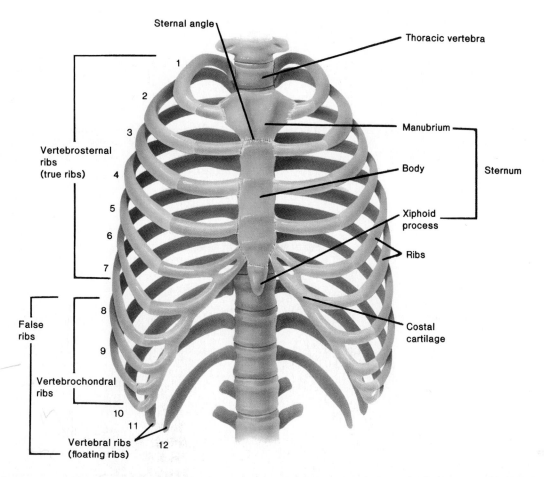

Thoracic Cage

The **thoracic cage** includes the ribs, thoracic vertebrae, sternum, and costal cartilages by which the ribs are attached to the sternum. These parts support the shoulder girdle and arms, protect visceral organs in the thoracic and upper abdominal cavities, and play a role in breathing (figures 6.43 and 6.44).

Ribs

Regardless of gender, each person usually has twelve pairs of ribs—one pair attached to each of the twelve thoracic vertebrae. Occasionally, however, some individuals develop extra ribs associated with their cervical or lumbar vertebrae.

The first seven rib pairs, called *vertebrosternal ribs* (true ribs), join the sternum directly by their costal cartilages. The remaining five pairs are called *vertebrochondral ribs* (false ribs) because their cartilages do not reach the sternum directly. Instead, the cartilages of the upper three vertebrochondral ribs join the cartilages of the ribs next above, while the last two rib pairs have no cartilaginous

FIGURE 6.44

X-ray film of the thoracic cage viewed from the front. Note the heart in the light region behind the sternum and above the diaphragm.

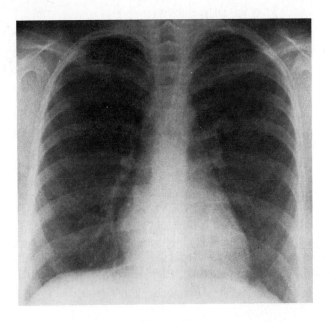

The Skeletal System   157

FIGURE 6.45

(a) A typical rib (posterior view); (b) articulations of a rib with a thoracic vertebra.

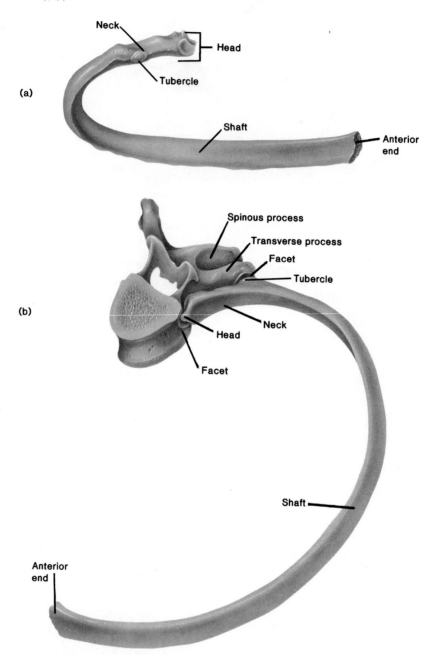

attachments to the sternum. These last two pairs (or sometimes the last three pairs) are often called *vertebral ribs* (floating ribs).

A typical rib (figure 6.45) has a long, slender *shaft* that curves around the chest and slopes downward. On its posterior end is an enlarged *head* by which the rib articulates with a facet on the body of its own vertebra and usually with the body of the next higher vertebra. The *neck* of the rib is a flattened region, lateral to the head, to which various ligaments are attached. Near the neck is a *tubercle,* which articulates with the transverse process of the vertebra.

Costal cartilages are composed of hyaline cartilage. They are attached to the anterior ends of the ribs and continue toward the sternum.

Sternum

The **sternum** (ster'num), or breastbone, is located along the midline in the anterior portion of the thoracic cage. It is a flat, elongated bone that develops in three parts—an upper *manubrium* (mah-nu'bre-um), a middle *body* (gladiolus), and a lower *xiphoid* (zif'oid) *process* that projects downward (figure 6.43).

The manubrium and body of the sternum lie in different planes, so that the line of union between them projects slightly forward. This projection, which occurs at the level of the second costal cartilage, is called the *sternal angle* (angle of Louis). It is commonly used as a landmark in locating particular ribs (figure 6.43).

1. What bones make up the thoracic cage?
2. Describe a typical rib.
3. What are the differences between true, false, and floating ribs?

A depression in the superior border of the manubrium is called the *jugular notch*. The sides of the manubrium and the body are notched where they articulate with costal cartilages. The manubrium also articulates with the clavicles by facets on its superior border. It usually remains as a separate bone until middle age or later, when it fuses to the body of the sternum.

The xiphoid process begins as a piece of cartilage. It slowly ossifies, and by middle age it is usually fused to the body of the sternum also.

Pectoral Girdle

The **pectoral** (pek′to-ral) **girdle** (shoulder girdle) is composed of four parts—two *clavicles* (collarbones) and two *scapulae* (shoulder blades). Although the word *girdle* suggests a ring-shaped structure, the pectoral girdle is an incomplete ring. It is open in the back between the scapulae, and its bones are separated in front by the sternum. The pectoral girdle supports the arms and serves as an attachment for several muscles that move the arms (figures 6.46 and 6.47).

Red marrow within spongy bone of the sternum functions in blood cell formation into adulthood. Since the sternum has a thin covering of compact bone and is easy to reach, samples of its blood-cell-forming tissue may be removed for use in diagnosing diseases. This procedure, a sternal puncture, involves suctioning (aspirating) some marrow through a hollow needle. (Marrow may also be removed from the iliac crest of a coxal bone.)

Chart 6.10 gives some examples of variations in the axial skeleton.

FIGURE 6.46

The pectoral girdle, to which the arms are attached, consists of a clavicle and a scapula on either side.

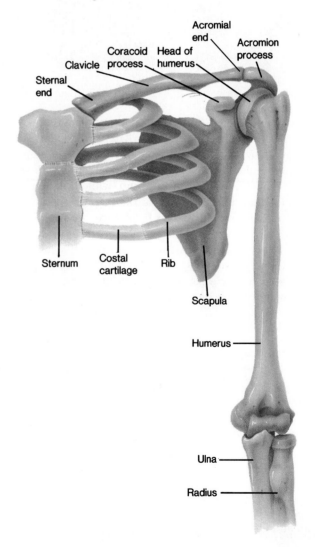

Chart 6.10	Normal variations in the axial skeleton
Skeletal part	**Variation**
Skull	There may be a suture between halves of the frontal bone in adults
	There may be size differences or absence of a sphenoidal sinus
	A third occipital condyle may be present
	There may be two mental foramina on each side of the mandible
Thoracic and lumbar vertebrae	There may be one extra or one less than usual number of vertebrae
Sacrum	Extra vertebra may be present, making sacrum longer
Coccyx	There may be three or five vertebrae in the coccyx
Ribs	An extra pair of ribs may be attached to seventh cervical vertebra
	An extra pair of ribs may be attached to first lumbar vertebra
	Tenth pair may be vertebral ribs
	Rarely, only eleven pairs of ribs are present

FIGURE 6.47

X-ray film of the right shoulder region, anterior view. What features can you identify?

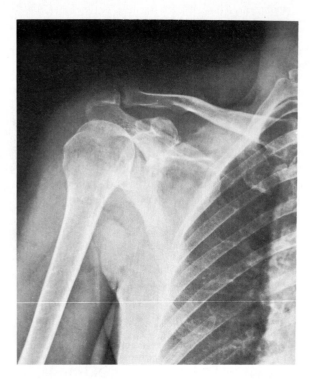

Clavicles

The **clavicles** (klav′ĭ-k′lz) are slender, rodlike bones with elongated S shapes (figure 6.46). They are located at the base of the neck and run horizontally between the sternum and the shoulders. The medial (or sternal) ends of the clavicles articulate with the manubrium, while the lateral (or acromial) ends join processes of the scapulae.

The clavicles act as braces for the freely movable scapulae, and thus help to hold the shoulders in place. They also provide attachments for muscles of the arms, chest, and back. Because of its elongated double curve, the clavicle is structurally weak. If compressed lengthwise due to abnormal pressure on the shoulder, it is likely to fracture.

Scapulae

The **scapulae** (skap′u-le) are broad, somewhat triangular bones located on either side of the upper back. They have flat bodies with concave anterior surfaces. The posterior surface of each scapula is divided into unequal portions by a spine. This spine leads to a *head*, which bears two processes—an *acromion* (ah-kro′me-on) *process*, which forms the tip of the shoulder, and a *coracoid* (kor′ah-koid) *process*, which curves forward and downward below the clavicle (figure 6.48). The acromion process articulates with a clavicle and provides attachments for muscles of the arm and chest. The coracoid process also provides attachments for arm and chest muscles.

On the head of the scapula, between the processes, is a depression called the *glenoid cavity*. It articulates with the head of the upper arm bone (humerus). On the superior border of the scapula, the *scapular notch* provides a passageway for nerves.

---

1. What bones form the pectoral girdle?
2. What is the function of the pectoral girdle?

Upper Limb

Bones of the upper limb form the framework of the arm, wrist, palm, and fingers. They also provide attachments for muscles and function in levers that move limb parts. These bones include a humerus, a radius, an ulna, and several carpals, metacarpals, and phalanges (figures 6.49 and 6.50).

Humerus

The **humerus** (hu′mer-us) (figure 6.51) is a heavy bone that extends from the scapula to the elbow. At its proximal end, it has a smooth, rounded *head* that fits into the glenoid cavity of the scapula. Just below the head, there are two processes—a *greater tubercle* on the lateral side and a *lesser tubercle* anteriorly. These tubercles provide attachments for muscles that move the arm at the shoulder. Between them is a narrow furrow, the *intertubercular groove* (bicipital groove), through which a tendon passes from a muscle in the upper arm (biceps brachii) to the shoulder.

A narrow groove along the lower margin of the head, called the *anatomical neck*, separates it from the tubercles. Just below the head and tubercles of the humerus is a tapering region called the *surgical neck*, so named because fractures commonly occur there. Near the middle of the bony shaft on the lateral side, there is a rough V-shaped area called the *deltoid tuberosity*. It provides an attachment for the muscle (deltoid) that raises the arm horizontally to the side.

At the distal end of the humerus, there are two smooth *condyles*—a knoblike *capitulum* (kah-pit′u-lum) on the lateral side and a pulley-shaped *trochlea* (trok′le-ah) on the medial side. The capitulum articulates with the radius at the elbow, while the trochlea joins the ulna.

Above the condyles on either side are *epicondyles*, which provide attachments for muscles and ligaments of the elbow. Between the epicondyles anteriorly there is a depression, the *coronoid* (kor′o-noid) *fossa*, that receives a process of the ulna (coronoid process) when the elbow is bent. Another depression on the posterior surface, the *olecranon* (o″-lek′ra-non) *fossa*, receives the olecranon process of the ulna when the arm is straightened at the elbow.

FIGURE 6.48

(*a*) Posterior surface of the scapula; (*b*) lateral view showing the glenoid cavity that articulates with the head of the humerus; (*c*) anterior surface.

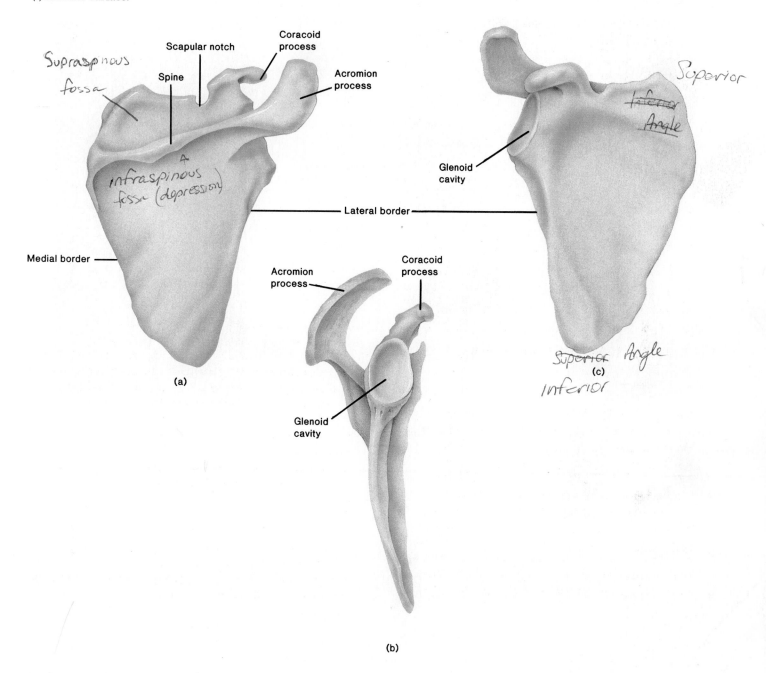

Supraspinous fossa

Scapular notch

Spine

Coracoid process

Acromion process

A

infraspinous fossa (depression)

Medial border

Lateral border

Glenoid cavity

Superior

Inferior Angle

Superior Angle

Inferior

(c)

(a)

Acromion process

Coracoid process

Glenoid cavity

(b)

FIGURE 6.49

Frontal view of the left arm (*a*) with the hand supinated and (*b*) with the hand pronated; (*c*) posterior view of the right elbow.

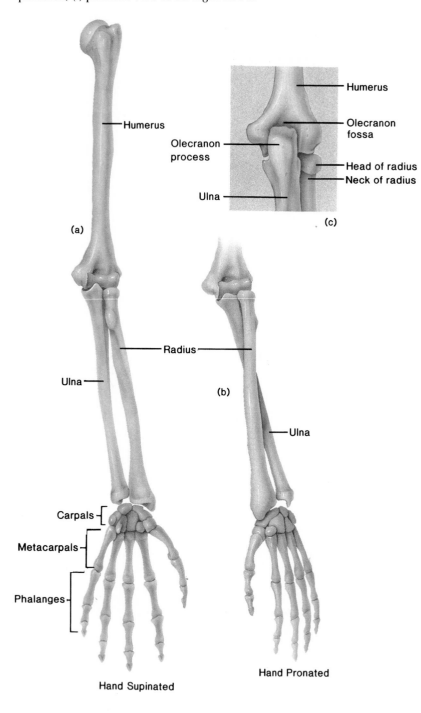

Humerus

Olecranon
process

Ulna

Humerus

Olecranon
fossa

Head of radius
Neck of radius

(c)

(a)

Radius

Ulna

(b)

Ulna

Carpals

Metacarpals

Phalanges

Hand Supinated

Hand Pronated

FIGURE 6.50

X-ray film of the left elbow and lower arm, viewed from the front.

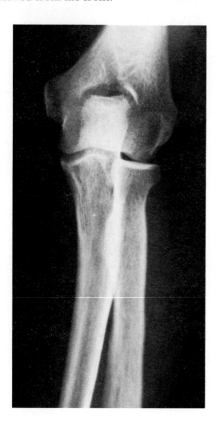

FIGURE 6.51

(a) Posterior surface and (b) anterior surface of the left humerus.

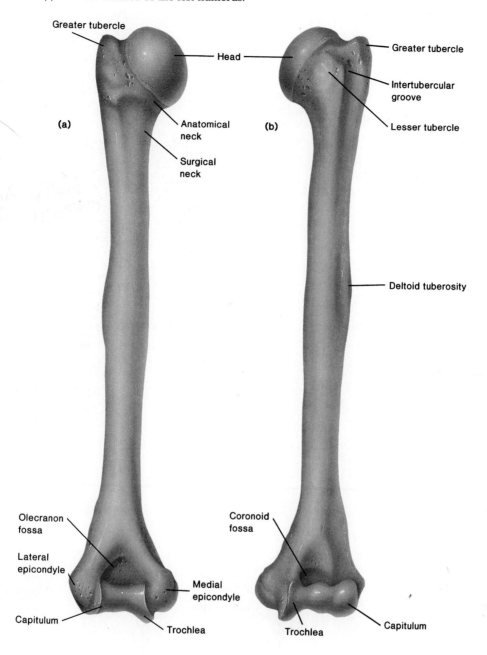

Radius

The **radius,** (ra′de-us) located on the thumb side of the lower arm, is somewhat shorter than its companion, the ulna (figure 6.52). The radius extends from the elbow to the wrist and crosses over the ulna when the hand is turned so that the palm faces backward.

A thick, disklike *head* at the proximal end of the radius articulates with the capitulum of the humerus and a notch

of the ulna (radial notch). This arrangement allows the radius to rotate freely.

On the radial shaft, just below the head, is a process called the *radial tuberosity.* It serves as an attachment for a muscle (biceps brachii) that bends the arm at the elbow. At the lower end of the radius, a lateral *styloid* (sti′loid) *process* provides attachments for ligaments of the wrist.

FIGURE 6.52

(*a*) The head of the radius articulates with the radial notch of the ulna, and the head of the ulna articulates with the ulnar notch of the radius; (*b*) lateral view of the head of the ulna.

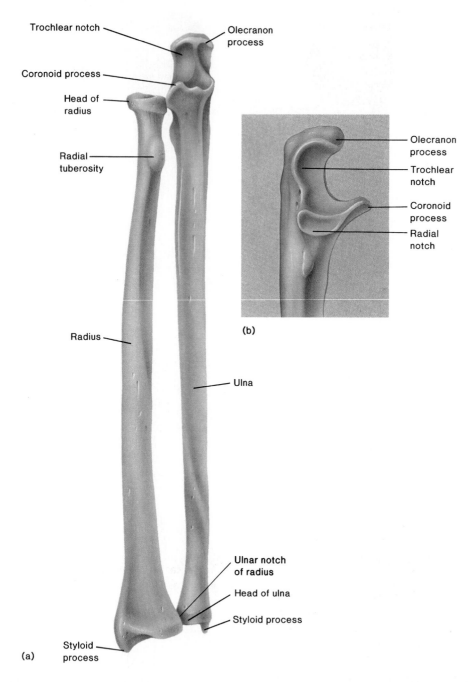

Ulna

The **ulna** (ul'nah) is longer than the radius and overlaps the end of the humerus posteriorly. At its upper end, the ulna has a wrenchlike opening, the *trochlear notch* (semilunar notch), which articulates with the trochlea of the humerus. There is a process on either side of this notch. The *olecranon process,* located above the trochlear notch, provides an attachment for the muscle (triceps brachii) that straightens the arm at the elbow. During this movement,

the olecranon process of the ulna fits into the olecranon fossa of the humerus. Similarly, the coronoid process, just below the trochlear notch, fits into the coronoid fossa of the humerus when the elbow is bent.

At the lower end of the ulna, its knoblike *head* articulates with a notch of the radius (ulnar notch) laterally and with a disk of fibrocartilage inferiorly (figure 6.52). This disk, in turn, joins a wrist bone (triangular). A medial *styloid process* at the distal end of the ulna provides attachments for the ligaments of the wrist.

FIGURE 6.53
The right hand viewed from the back.

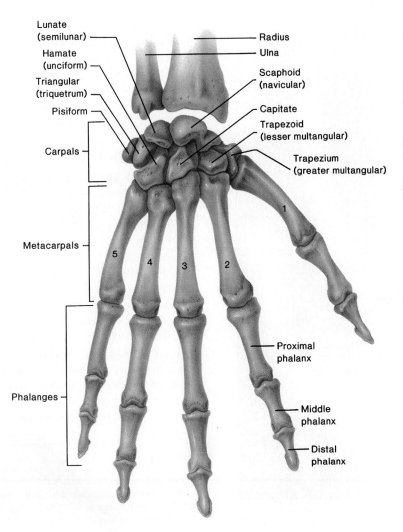

Lunate (semilunar)
Hamate (unciform)
Triangular (triquetrum)
Pisiform
Carpals
Metacarpals
Phalanges

Radius
Ulna
Scaphoid (navicular)
Capitate
Trapezoid (lesser multangular)
Trapezium (greater multangular)

Proximal phalanx
Middle phalanx
Distal phalanx

Hand

The hand is composed of a wrist, a palm, and five fingers (figures 6.53 and 6.54). The skeleton of the wrist consists of eight small **carpal** (kar′pel) **bones,** which are firmly bound in two rows of four bones each. The resulting compact mass is called a *carpus* (kar′pus).

The carpus is rounded on its proximal surface, where it articulates with the radius and with the fibrocartilaginous disk on the ulnar side. The carpus is concave anteriorly, forming a canal through which tendons and nerves extend to the palm. Its distal surface articulates with the metacarpal bones. The individual bones of the carpus are named in figure 6.53.

Five **metacarpal** (met″ah-kar′pal) **bones,** one in line with each finger, form the framework of the palm. These bones are cylindrical, with rounded distal ends that form the knuckles on a clenched fist. The metacarpals articulate proximally with the carpals and distally with the phalanges.

The metacarpal on the lateral side is the most freely movable; it permits the thumb to oppose the fingers when something is grasped in the hand. These bones are numbered one to five, beginning with the metacarpal of the thumb.

The **phalanges** (fah-lan′jēz) are the bones of the fingers. There are three in each finger—a proximal, a middle, and a distal phalanx—and two in the thumb (it lacks a middle phalanx). Thus, there are fourteen finger bones in each hand.

Chart 6.11 summarizes the bones of the pectoral girdle and upper limbs.

---

1. Locate and name each bone of the upper limb.
2. Explain how the bones of the upper limb articulate with one another.

FIGURE 6.54

X-ray film of the left hand. Note the small sesamoid bone associated with the joint at the base of the thumb (arrow).

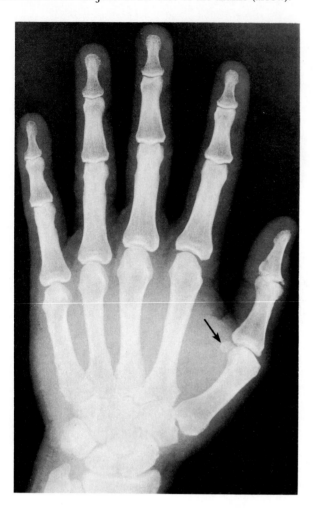

Pelvic Girdle

The **pelvic girdle** consists of the two coxal bones (hip bones), which articulate with each other anteriorly and with the sacrum posteriorly (figure 6.55). The sacrum and coccyx, and pelvic girdle together form the ringlike *pelvis,* which provides support for the trunk of the body and attachments for the legs. Weight of the body is transmitted through the pelvis to the legs and then onto the ground. The pelvis also protects the urinary bladder, the distal end of the large intestine, and internal reproductive organs.

Coxal Bones

Each **coxal** (kok′sal) **bone** (os coxa) develops from three parts—an ilium, an ischium, and a pubis. These parts fuse in the region of a cup-shaped cavity called the *acetabulum* (as″ĕ-tab′u-lum). This depression is on the lateral surface of the hip bone, and it receives the rounded head of the femur or thigh bone (figure 6.56).

The **ilium** (il′e-um) is the largest and uppermost portion of the coxal bone and it flares outward to form the prominence of the hip. The margin of this prominence is called the *iliac crest.*

Posteriorly, the ilium joins the sacrum at the *sacroiliac* (sa″kro-il′e-ak) *joint.* Anteriorly, a projection of the ilium, the *anterior superior iliac spine,* can be felt lateral to the groin and is an important surgical landmark. Below the anterior superior spine is the *anterior inferior iliac spine.* Both spines provide attachments for ligaments and muscles.

A common injury that occurs in contact sports such as football involves bruising the soft tissues and bone associated with the anterior superior iliac spine. This painful injury is called a *hip pointer* and may be prevented by wearing protective padding.

Chart 6.11 Bones of the pectoral girdle and upper limbs			
Name and number	**Location**	**Special features**	**Figure**
Clavicle (2)	Base of neck, between sternum and scapula	Sternal end, acromial end	6.46
Scapula (2)	Upper back, forming part of the shoulder	Body, spine, head, acromion process, coracoid process, glenoid cavity	6.48
Humerus (2)	Upper arm, between scapula and elbow	Head, greater tubercle, lesser tubercle, intertubercular groove, surgical neck, deltoid tuberosity, capitulum, trochlea, medial epicondyle, lateral epicondyle, coronoid fossa, olecranon fossa	6.51
Radius (2)	Lateral side of lower arm, between elbow and wrist	Head, radial tuberosity, styloid process	6.52
Ulna (2)	Medial side of lower arm, between elbow and wrist	Trochlear notch, olecranon process, head, styloid process	6.52
Carpal (16)	Wrist	Arranged in two rows of four bones each	6.53
Metacarpal (10)	Palm	One in line with each finger	6.53
Phalanx (28)	Finger	Three in each finger, two in each thumb	6.53

166   Chapter 6

FIGURE 6.55

(a) Anterior view and (b) posterior view of the pelvic girdle. This girdle provides an attachment for the legs, and together with the sacrum and coccyx forms the pelvis.

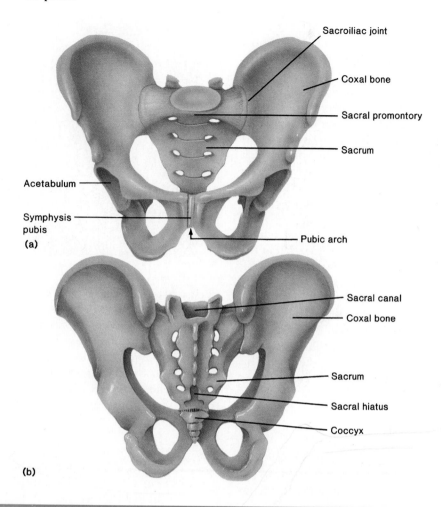

FIGURE 6.56

(a) Medial surface of the right coxal bone; (b) lateral view.

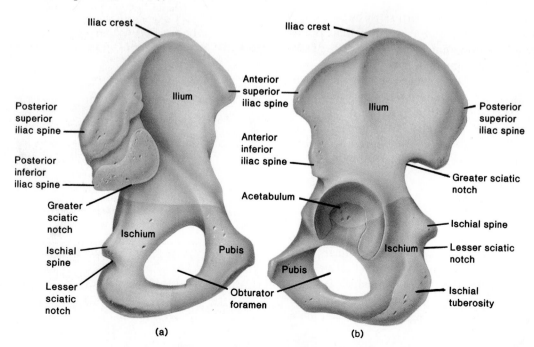

Located on the posterior border of the ilium, is the *posterior superior iliac spine* and the *posterior inferior iliac spine*. Below these spines is a deep indentation, the *greater sciatic notch*, through which a number of nerves and blood vessels pass.

The **ischium** (is′ke-um), which forms the lowest portion of the coxal bone, is L-shaped with its angle, the *ischial tuberosity*, pointing posteriorly and downward. This tuberosity has a rough surface that provides attachments for ligaments and leg muscles. It also supports the weight of the body when a person is sitting. Above the ischial tuberosity, near the junction of the ilium and ischium, is a sharp projection called the *ischial spine*. This spine, which can be felt during a vaginal examination, is used as a guide for determining the size of the pelvis. The distance between ischial spines represents the shortest diameter of the pelvic outlet.

The **pubis** (pu′bis) constitutes the anterior portion of the coxal bone. The two pubic bones come together at the midline to create a joint called the *symphysis pubis* (sim′fi-sis pubis). The angle formed by these bones below the symphysis is the *pubic arch*.

A portion of each pubis passes posteriorly and downward to join an ischium. Between the bodies of these bones on either side there is a large opening, the *obturator foramen*, which is the largest foramen in the skeleton. This foramen is covered and nearly closed by an obturator membrane. (See figure 6.57.)

Greater and Lesser Pelves

If a line is drawn along each side of the pelvis from the sacral promontory downward and anteriorly to the upper margin of the symphysis pubis, it marks the *pelvic brim* (linea terminalis). This margin separates the lower, or lesser (true), pelvis from the upper, or greater (false), pelvis. (See figure 6.58.)

The *greater pelvis* is bounded posteriorly by the lumbar vertebrae, laterally by the flared parts of the iliac bones, and anteriorly by the abdominal wall. The greater pelvis helps to support the abdominal organs.

The *lesser pelvis* is bounded posteriorly by the sacrum and coccyx, and laterally and anteriorly by the lower ilium, ischium, and pubis bones. This portion of the pelvis surrounds a short, canal-like cavity that has an upper inlet and a lower outlet. This cavity is of special interest because an infant passes through it during childbirth.

Sexual Differences in Pelves

Some structural differences exist between the male and female pelves, even though it may be difficult to find all of the "typical" characteristics in any one individual. These differences are related to the function of the female pelvis as a birth canal. Usually, the female iliac bones are more flared than those of the male, and consequently the female hips are usually broader. The angle of the female pubic

FIGURE 6.57
What features can you identify in this X-ray film of the pelvic girdle?

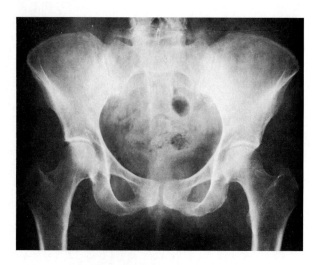

arch may be greater; there may be more distance between the ischial spines and the ischial tuberosities; and the sacral curvature may be shorter and flatter. Thus, the female pelvic cavity is usually wider in all diameters than that of the male. Also, the bones of the female pelvis are usually lighter, more delicate, and show less evidence of muscle attachments (figure 6.58). Chart 6.12 summarizes some of the sexual differences between the male and female skeleton.

Chart 6.12 Some sexual differences between the male and female skeletons	
Part	**Sexual Differences**
Skull	Female skull is relatively smaller and lighter, and its muscular attachments are less conspicuous. The female forehead is longer vertically, the facial area is rounder, the jaw is smaller, and the mastoid process is less prominent than those of a male.
Pelvis	Female pelvic bones are lighter, thinner, and have less obvious muscular attachments. The obturator foramina and the acetabula are smaller and farther apart than those of a male.
Pelvic cavity	Female pelvic cavity is wider in all diameters and is shorter and less funnel-shaped. The distances between the ischial spines and between the ischial tuberosities are greater than in a male.
Sacrum	Female sacrum is relatively wider, the sacral promontory projects forward to a lesser degree, and sacral curvature is bent more sharply posteriorly than in a male.
Coccyx	Female coccyx is more movable than that of a male.

1. Locate and name each pelvic bone.
2. Explain what is meant by the greater pelvis and the lesser pelvis.
3. How can a male and female pelvis be distinguished?

FIGURE 6.58
The female pelvis is usually wider in all diameters and roomier than that of the male. (*a*) Female pelvis; (*b*) male pelvis. Photographs of (*c*) male pelvis, and (*d*) female pelvis.

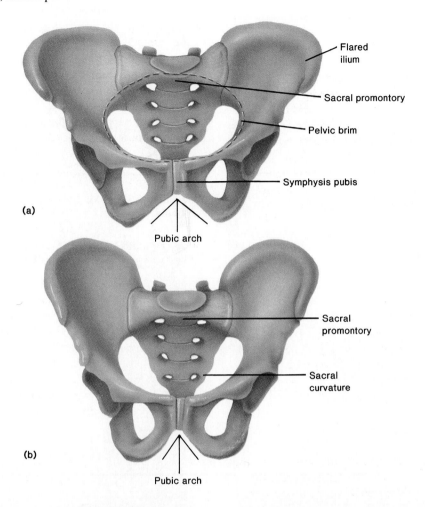

(a)

Flared ilium

Sacral promontory

Pelvic brim

Symphysis pubis

Pubic arch

(b)

Sacral promontory

Sacral curvature

Pubic arch

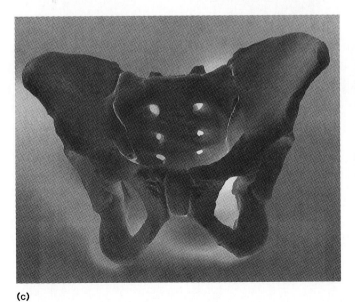

(c)

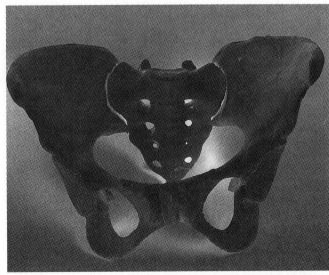

(d)

Lower Limb

Bones of the lower limb form the frameworks of the leg, ankle, instep, and toes. They include a femur, a tibia, a fibula, and several tarsals, metatarsals, and phalanges (figures 6.59 and 6.60).

Femur

The **femur** (fe'mur), or thigh bone, is the longest bone in the body and extends from the hip to the knee. A large, rounded head at its upper end projects medially into the acetabulum of the coxal bone. On the head, a pit called the *fovea capitis* marks the attachment of a ligament. Just below the head, are a constriction, or *neck,* and two large processes—an upper, lateral *greater trochanter* and a lower, medial *lesser trochanter.* These processes provide attachments for muscles of the legs and buttocks. On the posterior surface in the middle third of the shaft is a longitudinal crest called the *linea aspera.* This rough strip serves as an attachment for several muscles (figure 6.61).

At the lower end of the femur, two rounded processes, the *lateral* and *medial condyles,* articulate with the tibia of the lower leg. A patella also articulates with the femur on its distal anterior surface.

FIGURE 6.59

(*a*) The right leg viewed from the front; (*b*) lateral view and (*c*) posterior view of the knee.

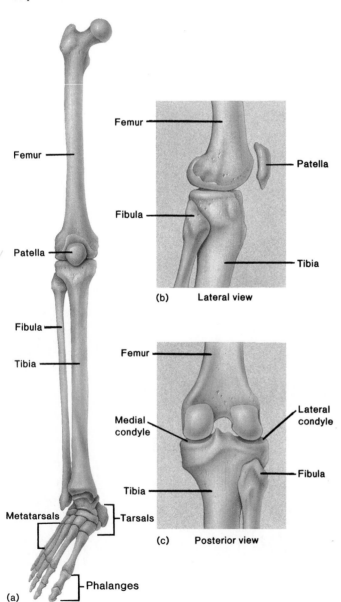

(b)　　Lateral view

(c)　　Posterior view

(a)

FIGURE 6.60

X-ray film of the left knee showing the ends of the femur, tibia, and fibula.

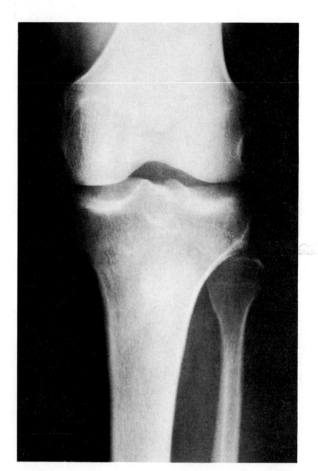

FIGURE 6.61

(a) Anterior surface and (b) posterior surface of the right femur. (c) Note the variation in shape of the proximal ends of these femurs.

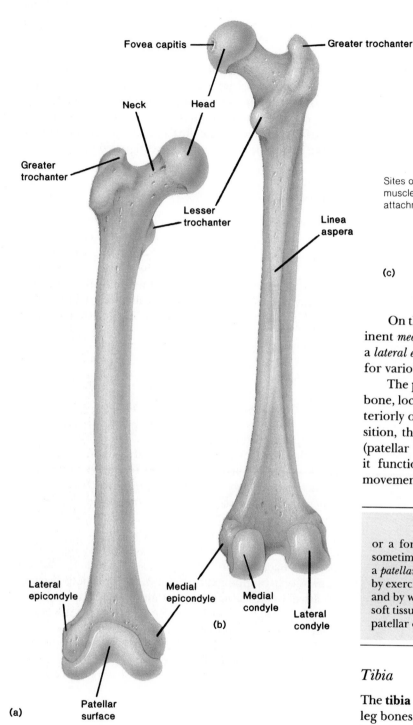

(a)

(b)

(c)

Fovea capitis

Greater trochanter

Neck

Head

Greater trochanter

Lesser trochanter

Linea aspera

Lateral epicondyle

Medial epicondyle

Medial condyle

Lateral condyle

Patellar surface

Sites of muscle attachments

On the medial surface at its distal end, there is a prominent *medial epicondyle,* and on the lateral surface there is a *lateral epicondyle.* These projections provide attachments for various muscles and ligaments.

The **patella** (pah-tel'ah), or kneecap, is a flat sesamoid bone, located in a tendon (patellar tendon), that passes anteriorly over the knee (see figure 6.59). Because of its position, the patella controls the angle at which a ligament (patellar ligament) continues toward the tibia, and thus it functions in lever actions associated with lower leg movements.

As a result of a blow to the knee or a forceful unnatural movement of the leg, the patella sometimes slips to one side. This painful condition is called a *patellar dislocation.* Such a displacement may be prevented by exercises that strengthen muscles associated with the knee and by wearing protective padding. Unfortunately, once the soft tissues that hold the patella in place have been stretched, patellar dislocation tends to recur.

Tibia

The **tibia** (tib'e-ah) (shinbone) is the larger of the two lower leg bones and is located on the medial side. Its upper end is expanded into *medial* and *lateral condyles,* which have

FIGURE 6.62
Bones of the right lower leg, viewed from the front.

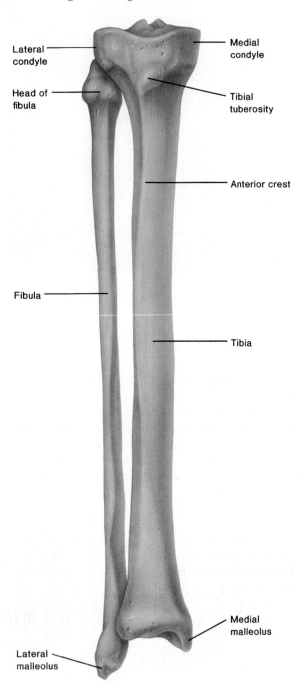

Lateral condyle

Head of fibula

Fibula

Lateral malleolus

Medial condyle

Tibial tuberosity

Anterior crest

Tibia

Medial malleolus

concave surfaces and articulate with the condyles of the femur. Below the condyles, on the anterior surface, is a process called the *tibial tuberosity,* which provides an attachment for the *patellar ligament*—a continuation of the patella-bearing tendon. A prominent *anterior crest* extends downward from the tuberosity and serves as an attachment for connective tissues in the lower leg.

At its lower end, the tibia expands to form a prominence on the inner ankle called the *medial malleolus* (male'o-lus), which serves as an attachment for ligaments. On its lateral side is a depression that articulates with the fibula. The inferior surface of the tibia's distal end articulates with a large bone (the talus) in the foot (figure 6.62).

Fibula

The **fibula** (fib'u-lah) is a long, slender bone located on the lateral side of the tibia. Its ends are slightly enlarged into an upper *head* and a lower *lateral malleolus.* The head articulates with the tibia just below the lateral condyle; however, it does not enter into the knee joint and does not bear any body weight. The lateral malleolus articulates with the ankle and forms a prominence on the lateral side (figure 6.62).

Foot

The foot consists of an ankle, an instep, and five toes. The ankle is composed of seven **tarsal** (tahr'sal) **bones,** forming a group called the *tarsus* (tahr'sus). These bones are arranged so that one of them, the **talus** (ta'lus), can move freely where it joins the tibia and fibula. The remaining tarsal bones are bound firmly together, forming a mass on which the talus rests. Individual bones of the tarsus are named in figures 6.63 and 6.64.

The largest of the ankle bones, the **calcaneus** (kalka'ne-us), or heel bone, is located below the talus where it projects backward to form the base of the heel. The calcaneus helps support the weight of the body and provides an attachment for muscles that move the foot.

The instep consists of five, elongated **metatarsal** (met"ah-tar'sal) **bones,** which articulate with the tarsus. They are numbered 1 to 5 beginning on the medial side (figure 6.64). The heads at the distal ends of these bones

FIGURE 6.63
The talus moves freely where it articulates with the tibia and fibula.

Fibula

Tibia

Talus

Medial
cuneiform

Navicular

Metatarsals

Phalanges

Tarsus

FIGURE 6.64

The right foot, viewed from above.

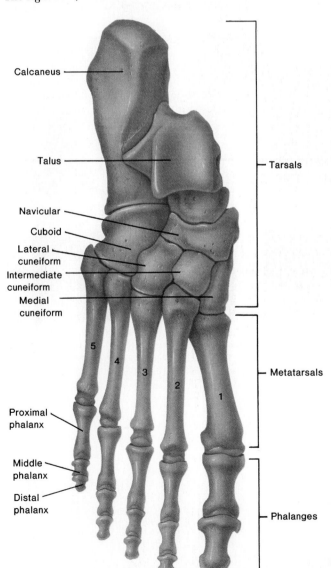

Calcaneus

Talus

Navicular

Cuboid

Lateral
cuneiform

Intermediate
cuneiform

Medial
cuneiform

Tarsals

5

4

3

2

1

Proximal
phalanx

Metatarsals

Middle
phalanx

Distal
phalanx

Phalanges

form the ball of the foot. The tarsals and metatarsals are arranged and bound by ligaments to form the arches of the foot. A longitudinal arch extends from the heel to the toe, and a transverse arch stretches across the foot. These arches provide a stable, springy base for the body. Sometimes, however, tissues that bind the metatarsals become weakened, producing fallen arches, or flat feet.

The **phalanges** of the toes are similar to those of the fingers. They are in line with the metatarsals and articulate with them. Each toe has three phalanges—a proximal, a middle, and a distal phalanx—except the great toe, which has only two and lacks the middle phalanx. Chart 6.13 summarizes the bones of the pelvic girdle and lower limbs. (See figure 6.65.)

1. Locate and name each bone of the lower limb.
2. Explain how the bones of the lower limb articulate with one another.
3. Describe how the foot is specialized to support the body.

Chart 6.13 Bones of the pelvic girdle and lower limbs

Name and number	Location	Special features	Figure
Coxal bone (2)	Hip, articulating with each other anteriorly and with the sacrum posteriorly	Ilium, iliac crest, anterior superior iliac spine, ischium, ischial tuberosity, ischial spine, obturator foramen, acetabulum, pubis	6.56
Femur (2)	Upper leg, between the hip and knee	Head, fovea capitis, neck, greater trochanter, lesser trochanter, linea aspera, lateral condyle, medial condyle	6.61
Patella (2)	Anterior surface of knee	A flat sesamoid bone located within a tendon	6.59
Tibia (2)	Medial side of lower leg, between knee and ankle	Medial condyle, lateral condyle, tibial tuberosity, anterior crest, medial malleolus	6.62
Fibula (2)	Lateral side of lower leg, between knee and ankle	Head, lateral malleolus	6.62
Tarsal (14)	Ankle	Freely movable talus that articulates with lower leg bones and six other bones bound firmly together	6.64
Metatarsal (10)	Instep	One in line with each toe, arranged and bound by ligaments to form arches	6.64
Phalanx (28)	Toe	Three in each toe, two in the great toe	6.64

FIGURE 6.65

(*a*) X-ray film of the left foot, viewed from the medial side; (*b*) from above. What features can you identify?

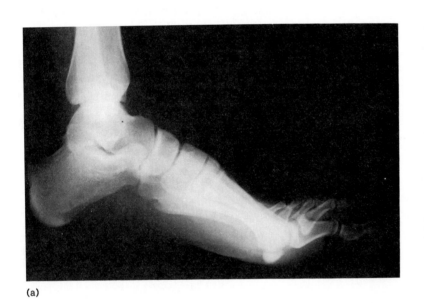

(a)

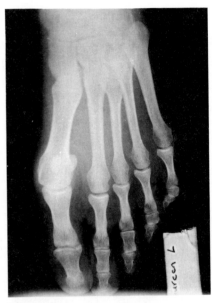

(b)

Appendicular Skeleton

Variations in arm and leg bones are primarily related to the size and muscle development of an individual. The lengths of these bones vary proportionally with overall height. The relationship between height and length of individual arm and leg bones is close enough to be used as a method of predicting height when only one of the arm or leg bones is present.

Other variations in these bones are due to differences in the amount of stress created by muscles pulling on the bones. Such stress stimulates bone growth and produces variations in the size of parts to which muscles are attached. (See figure 6.61.)

An inherited characteristic called *polydactyly* (pol″e-dak′ti-le) results in an individual having extra fingers or toes (figure 6.66).

FIGURE 6.66
X-ray film of the foot of a person with polydactyly.

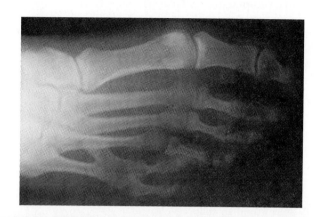

Clinical Terms Related to the Skeletal System

achondroplasia (a-kon″dro-pla′ze-ah)   an inherited condition in which formation of endochondral bone is retarded. The result is a type of dwarfism.

acromegaly (ak″ro-meg′ah-le)   a condition caused by an overproduction of growth hormone in adults and characterized by abnormal enlargement of facial features, hands, and feet.

Colles fracture (kol′ēz frak′tūre)   a fracture at the distal end of the radius in which the smaller fragment is displaced posteriorly.

epiphysiolysis (ep″ĭ-fiz″e-ol′ĭ-sis)   a separation or loosening of the epiphysis from the diaphysis of a bone.

laminectomy (lam″ĭ-nek′to-me)   surgical removal of a posterior vertebral arch usually to relieve the symptoms of a ruptured intervertebral disk.

lumbago (lum-ba′go)   a dull ache in the lumbar region of the back.

orthopedics (or″tho-pe′diks)   science of prevention, diagnosis, and treatment of diseases and abnormalities involving the skeletal and muscular systems.

ostalgia (os-tal′je-ah)   pain in a bone.

ostectomy (os-tek′to-me)   surgical removal of a bone.

osteitis (os″te-i′tis)   inflammation of bone tissue.

osteochondritis (os″te-o-kon-dri′tis)   inflammation of bone and cartilage tissues.

osteogenesis (os″te-o-jen′ĕ-sis)   development of bone.

osteogenesis imperfecta (os″te-o-jen′ĕ-sis im-per-fek′ta)   a congenital condition characterized by development of deformed and abnormally brittle bones.

osteoma (os″te-o′mah)   a tumor composed of bone tissue.

osteomalacia (os″te-o-mah-la′she-ah)   a softening of adult bone due to a disorder in calcium and phosphorus metabolism, usually caused by a dietary deficiency of vitamin D or by an inherited condition.

osteomyelitis (os″te-o-mi″ĕ-li′tis)   inflammation of bone caused by the action of bacteria or fungi.

osteonecrosis (os″te-o-ne-kro′sis)   death of bone tissue. This condition occurs most commonly in the head of the femur in elderly persons and may be due to obstructions in arteries that supply the bone.

osteopathology (os″te-o-pah-thol′o-je)   study of bone diseases.

osteotomy (os″te-ot′o-me)   cutting of a bone.

Chapter Summary

Introduction (page 122)
Individual bones are organs of the skeletal system. Bone contains very active tissues.

Bone Structure (page 122)
Bone structure reflects its function.

1.   Classification of bones: bones are grouped according to their shapes—long, short, flat, or irregular.
2.   Parts of a long bone
     a.   Epiphyses are covered with articular cartilage and articulate with other bones.
     b.   The shaft of a bone is called the diaphysis.
     c.   Except for the articular cartilage, a bone is covered by a periosteum.
     d.   Compact bone provides strength and resistance to bending.
     e.   Spongy bone provides strength where needed and reduces weight of bone.
     f.   The diaphysis contains a medullary cavity filled with marrow.

3. Microscopic structure
   a. Compact bone contains osteons cemented together.
   b. Osteonic canals contain blood vessels that nourish cells of osteons.
   c. Communicating canals connect osteonic canals transversely and communicate with the bone's surface and the medullary cavity.
   d. Cells of spongy bone are nourished by substances from the surface of the bony plates.

Bone Development and Growth (page 124)
1. Intramembranous bones
   a. Certain flat bones of the skull are intramembranous bones.
   b. They develop from layers of connective tissues.
   c. Bone tissue is formed by osteoblasts within the membranous layers.
   d. Mature bone cells are called osteocytes.
   e. Membranous tissues give rise to a periosteum.
2. Endochondral bones
   a. Most of the bones of the skeletal system are endochondral bones.
   b. They develop first as hyaline cartilage that is later replaced by bone tissue.
3. Growth of an endochondral bone
   a. Primary ossification center appears in the diaphysis, while secondary ossification centers appear in the epiphyses.
   b. An epiphyseal disk remains between the primary and secondary ossification centers.
   c. An epiphyseal disk consists of layers of cells: resting cells, young reproducing cells, older enlarging cells, and dying cells.
   d. The epiphyseal disk is responsible for growth in length.
   e. Long bones continue to grow in length until the epiphyseal disks are ossified.
   f. Growth in thickness is due to intramembranous ossification occurring beneath the periosteum.
   g. The medullary cavity is created by the action of osteoclasts.
4. Bone reorganization
   a. Bone is continually broken down and reformed.
   b. Osteoclasts resorb bone matrix and osteoblasts form new matrix.
   c. Physical stress stimulates bone development, while lack of exercise causes bone to become thinner and weaker.

Functions of Bones (page 131)
1. Support and protection
   a. Skeletal parts provide shape and form for body structures.
   b. Bones support and protect softer, underlying tissues.
2. Body movements
   a. Bones and muscles function together as levers.
   b. A lever consists of a rod, a pivot (fulcrum), the weight to be moved, and a force that supplies energy.
   c. Parts of a first-class lever are arranged weight-pivot-force; parts of a second-class lever are arranged pivot-weight-force; parts of a third-class lever are arranged pivot-force-weight.

3. Blood cell formation
   a. At different ages, hematopoiesis occurs in the yolk sac, liver, and spleen, and in red bone marrow.
   b. Red marrow functions in the production of blood cells and blood platelets.
4. Storage of minerals
   a. Intercellular material of bone tissue contains large quantities of calcium phosphate in the form of hydroxyapatite.
   b. When blood calcium concentrations are low, osteoclasts resorb bone, thus releasing calcium.
   c. When blood calcium concentrations are high, osteoblasts are stimulated to form bone matrix and store calcium.

Organization of the Skeleton (page 134)
1. Number of bones
   a. Usually there are 206 bones in the human skeleton, but the number may vary.
   b. Extra bones in sutures are called sutural bones.
2. Divisions of the skeleton
   a. The skeleton can be divided into axial and appendicular portions.
   b. The axial skeleton consists of the skull, hyoid bone, vertebral column, and thoracic cage.
   c. The appendicular skeleton consists of the pectoral girdle, upper limbs, pelvic girdle, and lower limbs.

The Skull (page 139)
The skull consists of twenty-two bones, which include eight cranial bones, thirteen immovable facial bones, and one mandible.

1. Cranium
   a. The cranium encloses and protects the brain, and provides attachments for muscles.
   b. Some cranial bones contain air-filled sinuses that help reduce the weight of the skull.
2. Facial skeleton
   Facial bones form the basic shape of the face and provide attachments for muscles.
3. Infantile skull
   a. Incompletely developed bones, separated by fontanels, enable the infantile skull to change shape slightly during birth.
   b. The proportions of the infantile skull are different from those of an adult skull, and its bones are less easily fractured.

Vertebral Column (page 150)
The vertebral column extends from the skull to the pelvis and protects the spinal cord. It is composed of vertebrae separated by intervertebral disks. It consists of thirty-three bones in an infant and twenty-six bones in an adult. It has four curvatures—cervical, thoracic, lumbar, and pelvic.

1. A typical vertebra
   a. A typical vertebra consists of a body, pedicles, laminae, a spinous process, transverse processes, and superior and inferior articulating processes.
   b. Notches on the lower surfaces of the pedicles form intervertebral foramina through which spinal nerves pass.

2. Cervical vertebrae
   a. Cervical vertebrae comprise the bones of the neck.
   b. Transverse processes bear transverse foramina.
   c. The atlas (first vertebra) supports and balances the head.
   d. The odontoid process of the axis (second vertebra) provides a pivot for the atlas when the head is turned from side to side.
3. Thoracic vertebrae
   a. Thoracic vertebrae are larger than cervical vertebrae.
   b. Their long, spinous processes slope downward, and facets on the sides of bodies articulate with the ribs.
4. Lumbar vertebrae
   a. Vertebral bodies of lumbar vertebrae are large and strong.
   b. Their transverse processes project back and spinous processes are directed horizontally.
5. Sacrum
   a. The sacrum is a triangular structure that bears rows of dorsal sacral foramina.
   b. It is united with the coxal bones at the sacroiliac joints.
   c. The sacral promontory provides a guide for determining the size of the pelvis.
6. Coccyx
   a. The coccyx forms the lowest part of the vertebral column.
   b. It acts as a shock absorber when a person sits.

Thoracic Cage (page 157)

The thoracic cage includes the ribs, thoracic vertebrae, sternum, and costal cartilages. It supports the shoulder girdle and arms, protects visceral organs, and functions in breathing.

1. Ribs
   a. Twelve pairs of ribs are attached to the thoracic vertebrae.
   b. Costal cartilages of vertebrosternal ribs join the sternum directly; those of vertebrochondral ribs join indirectly. The vertebral ribs lack cartilaginous attachments.
   c. A typical rib has a shaft, head, and tubercles that articulate with the vertebrae.
2. Sternum
   The sternum articulates with costal cartilages and clavicles.

Pectoral Girdle (page 159)

The pectoral girdle is composed of two clavicles and two scapulae. It forms an incomplete ring that supports the arms and provides attachments for muscles that move the arms.

1. Clavicles
   a. Clavicles are rodlike bones that run horizontally between the sternum and shoulder.
   b. They hold the shoulders in place and provide attachments for muscles.
2. Scapulae
   a. The scapulae are broad, triangular bones.
   b. They articulate with the humerus of each arm, and provide attachments for muscles of the arms and chest.

Upper Limb (page 160)

Bones of the limb provide frameworks and attachments for muscles, and function in levers that move the limb and its parts.

1. Humerus
   The humerus extends from the scapula to the elbow.
2. Radius
   The radius is located on the thumb side of the lower arm between the elbow and wrist.
3. Ulna
   The ulna is longer than the radius and overlaps the humerus posteriorly. It articulates with the radius laterally and with a disk of fibrocartilage inferiorly.
4. Hand
   a. The hand is composed of a wrist, palm, and five fingers.
   b. It includes eight carpals that form a carpus, five metacarpals, and fourteen phalanges.

Pelvic Girdle (page 166)

The pelvic girdle consists of two coxal bones that articulate with each other anteriorly and with the sacrum posteriorly. The sacrum, coccyx, and pelvic girdle form the pelvis. The girdle provides support for body weight and attachments for muscles, and protects visceral organs.

1. Coxal bones
   Each coxal bone consists of an ilium, ischium, and pubis, which are fused in the region of the acetabulum.
   a. The ilium, the largest portion of the coxal bone, joins the sacrum at the sacroiliac joint.
   b. The ischium is the lowest portion of the coxal bone.
   c. The pubis is the anterior portion of the coxal bone. Pubic bones are fused anteriorly at the symphysis pubis.
2. Greater and lesser pelves
   a. The lesser pelvis is below the pelvic brim; the greater pelvis is above it.
   b. The lesser pelvis functions as a birth canal; the greater pelvis helps to support abdominal organs.
3. Sexual differences in pelves
   a. Differences between male and female pelves are related to the function of the female pelvis as a birth canal.
   b. Usually, the female pelvis is more flared; pubic arch is broader; distance between the ischial spines and the ischial tuberosities is greater; and sacral curvature is shorter.

Lower Limb (page 170)

1. Femur
   a. The femur extends from the knee to the hip.
   b. Patella articulates with its anterior surface.
2. Tibia
   The tibia is located on the medial side of the lower leg and it articulates with the talus of the ankle.
3. Fibula
   The fibula is located on the lateral side of the tibia, and it bears a head and lateral malleolus that articulates with the ankle.
4. Foot
   a. The foot consists of an ankle, instep, and five toes.
   b. It includes seven tarsals that form the tarsus, five metatarsals, and fourteen phalanges.

Clinical Application of Knowledge

1. Why do you think incomplete, longitudinal fractures of bone shafts (greenstick fractures) are more common in children than in adults?
2. When a child's bone is fractured, growth may be stimulated at the epiphyseal disk of that bone. What problems might this extra growth create in an arm or leg before growth of the other limb compensates for the difference in length?
3. How would you explain the observation that elderly persons often develop bowed backs and appear shorter than they were in earlier years?
4. The walls of the maxillary sinuses are very thin. Which other structures might be affected by a tumor growing in a maxillary sinus and deforming its walls?
5. How is the repair of a fractured adult bone similar to endochondral bone formation?
6. How might the condition of an infant's fontanels be used to evaluate its development? How might these fontanels be used to estimate the intracranial pressure?

Review Activities

Part A

1. List four groups of bones based upon their shapes, and name an example from each group.
2. Sketch a typical long bone and label its epiphyses, diaphysis, medullary cavity, periosteum, and articular cartilages.
3. Distinguish between spongy and compact bone.
4. Explain how osteonic canals and communicating canals are related.
5. Explain how development of intramembranous bone differs from that of endochondral bone.
6. Distinguish between osteoblasts and osteocytes.
7. Explain the function of an epiphyseal disk.
8. Explain how a bone grows in thickness.
9. Define *osteoclast*.
10. Describe how bone is continually remodeled.
11. Explain the effects of exercise on bone structure.
12. Provide several examples to illustrate how bones support and protect body parts.
13. Describe a lever, and explain how its parts may be arranged to form first-, second-, and third-class levers.
14. Describe the functions of red and yellow bone marrow.
15. Distinguish between the axial and appendicular skeletons.
16. List the bones that form the pectoral and pelvic girdles.
17. Name the bones of the cranium and facial skeleton.
18. Explain the importance of fontanels.
19. Describe a typical vertebra.
20. Explain the differences between cervical, thoracic, and lumbar vertebrae.
21. Describe the locations of the sacroiliac joint, sacral promontory, and sacral hiatus.
22. Name the bones that comprise the thoracic cage.
23. Name the bones of the upper limb.
24. Name the bones that fuse to form a coxal bone.
25. List the major differences that may occur between the male and female pelves.
26. List the bones of the lower limb.

Part B
Match the parts listed in column I with the bones listed in column II.

I	II
1. Coronoid process	A. Ethmoid bone
2. Cribriform plate	B. Frontal bone
3. Foramen magnum	C. Mandible
4. Mastoid process	D. Maxillary bone
5. Palatine process	E. Occipital bone
6. Sella turcica	F. Temporal bone
7. Supraorbital foramen	G. Sphenoid bone
8. Temporal process	H. Zygomatic bone
9. Acromion process	I. Femur
10. Deltoid tuberosity	J. Fibula
11. Greater trochanter	K. Humerus
12. Lateral malleolus	L. Radius
13. Medial malleolus	M. Scapula
14. Olecranon process	N. Sternum
15. Radial tuberosity	O. Tibia
16. Xiphoid process	P. Ulna

REFERENCE PLATES

Human Skull

The following set of reference plates is presented to help you locate some of the more prominent features of the human skull. As you study these photographs, it is important to remember that human skulls vary in every characteristic. Also, the photographs included in this set depict bones from several different skulls.

PLATE 8
The skull, frontal view.

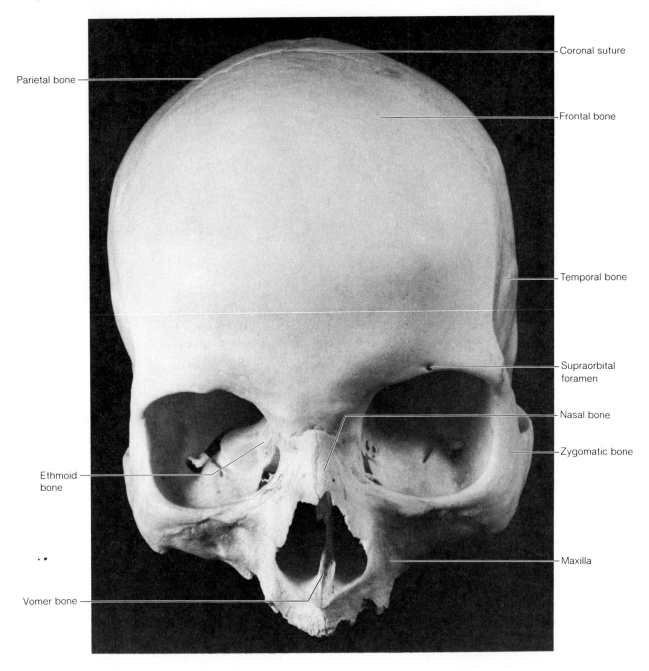

Parietal bone

Coronal suture

Frontal bone

Temporal bone

Supraorbital foramen

Nasal bone

Zygomatic bone

Ethmoid bone

Maxilla

Vomer bone

PLATE 9
The skull, left lateral view.

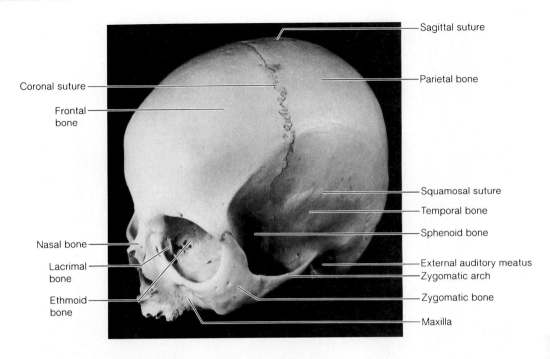

Sagittal suture

Parietal bone

Coronal suture

Frontal bone

Squamosal suture

Temporal bone

Sphenoid bone

Nasal bone

Lacrimal bone

External auditory meatus

Zygomatic arch

Zygomatic bone

Ethmoid bone

Maxilla

PLATE 10
The skull, left posterior view.

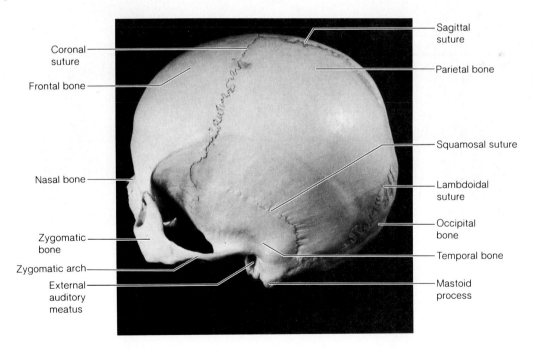

Sagittal suture

Coronal suture

Parietal bone

Frontal bone

Squamosal suture

Nasal bone

Lambdoidal suture

Occipital bone

Zygomatic bone

Temporal bone

Zygomatic arch

Mastoid process

External auditory meatus

PLATE 11
The skull, inferior view.

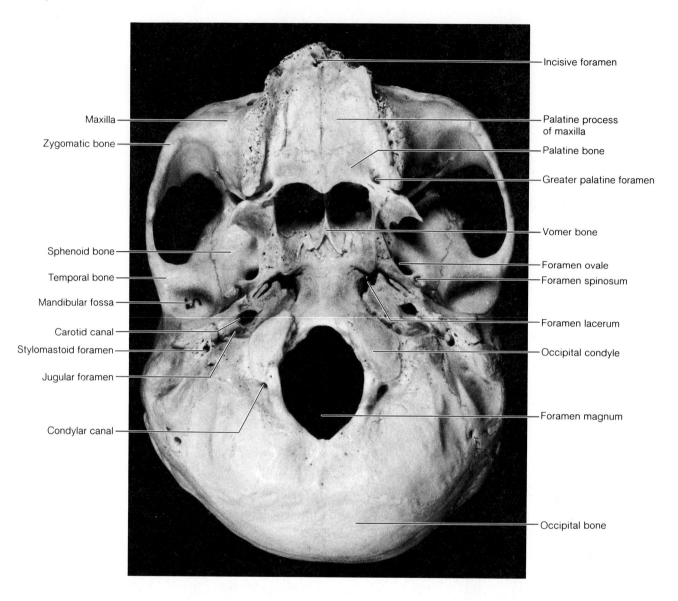

Incisive foramen

Maxilla

Zygomatic bone

Palatine process
of maxilla

Palatine bone

Greater palatine foramen

Sphenoid bone

Temporal bone

Mandibular fossa

Carotid canal

Stylomastoid foramen

Jugular foramen

Condylar canal

Vomer bone

Foramen ovale

Foramen spinosum

Foramen lacerum

Occipital condyle

Foramen magnum

Occipital bone

PLATE 12

Base of the skull, sphenoidal region.

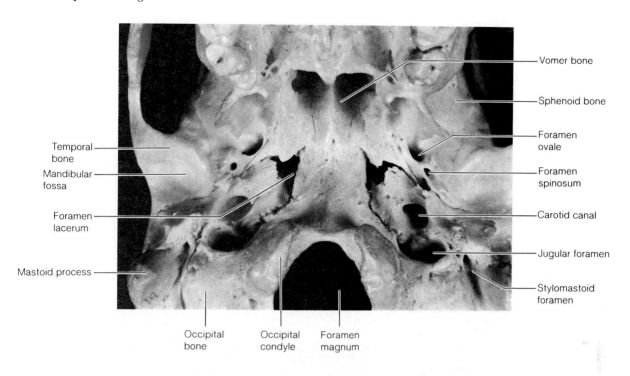

Temporal bone

Mandibular fossa

Foramen lacerum

Mastoid process

Vomer bone

Sphenoid bone

Foramen ovale

Foramen spinosum

Carotid canal

Jugular foramen

Stylomastoid foramen

Occipital bone

Occipital condyle

Foramen magnum

PLATE 13

Mandible, lateral view.

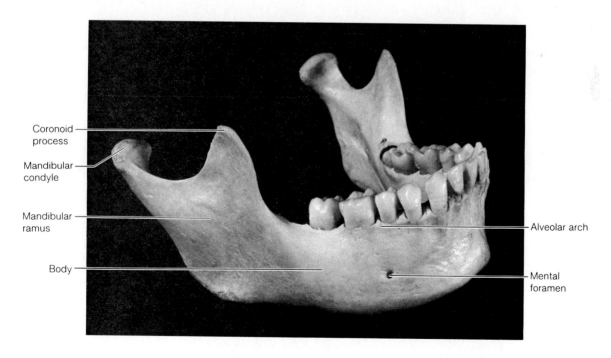

Coronoid process

Mandibular condyle

Mandibular ramus

Body

Alveolar arch

Mental foramen

PLATE 14
Temporal bone, left lateral view.

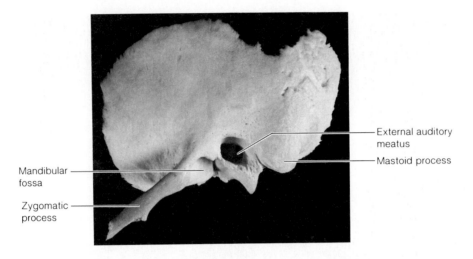

Mandibular fossa

Zygomatic process

External auditory meatus

Mastoid process

PLATE 15
Ethmoid bone, right lateral view.

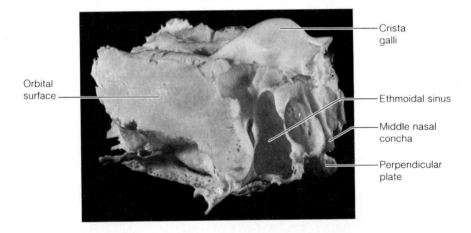

Orbital surface

Crista galli

Ethmoidal sinus

Middle nasal concha

Perpendicular plate

PLATE 16
Sphenoid bone, posterior view.

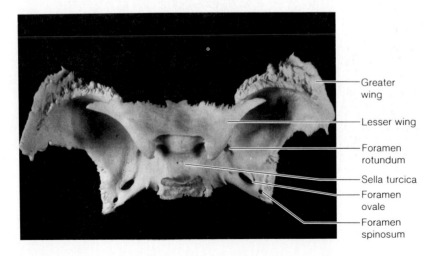

Greater wing

Lesser wing

Foramen rotundum

Sella turcica

Foramen ovale

Foramen spinosum

PLATE 17

The skull, median section.

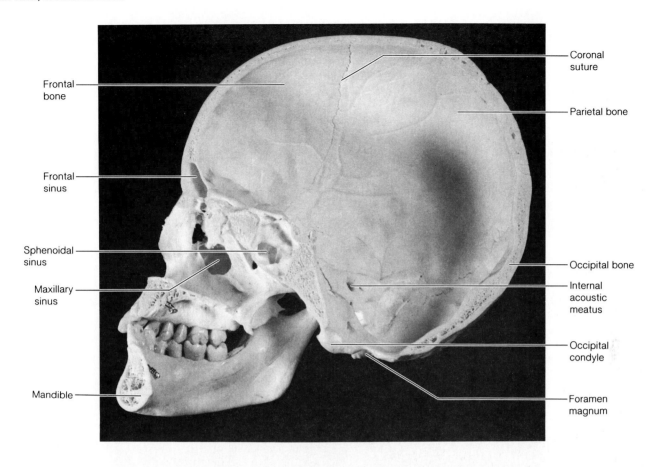

Frontal bone

Frontal sinus

Sphenoidal sinus

Maxillary sinus

Mandible

Coronal suture

Parietal bone

Occipital bone

Internal acoustic meatus

Occipital condyle

Foramen magnum

PLATE 18

Sphenoidal region, median section.

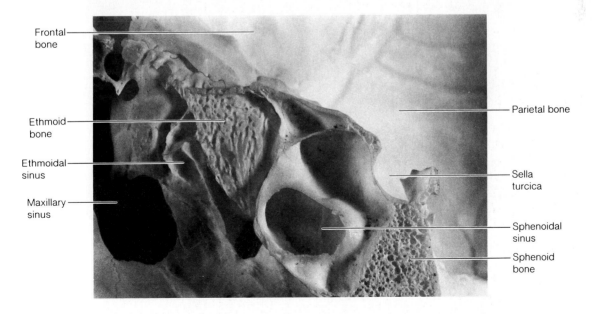

Frontal bone

Ethmoid bone

Ethmoidal sinus

Maxillary sinus

Parietal bone

Sella turcica

Sphenoidal sinus

Sphenoid bone

Human Skull   185

PLATE 19
The skull, floor of the cranial cavity.

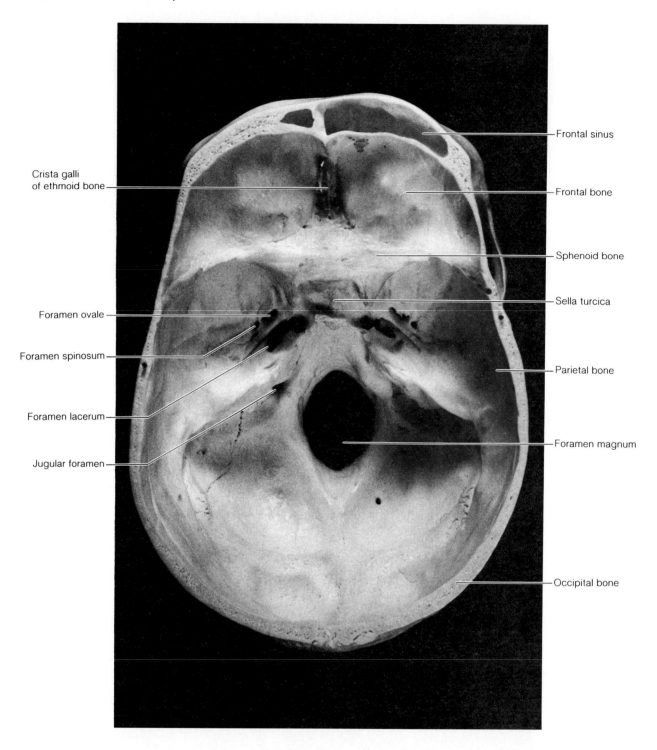

Crista galli
of ethmoid bone

Foramen ovale

Foramen spinosum

Foramen lacerum

Jugular foramen

Frontal sinus

Frontal bone

Sphenoid bone

Sella turcica

Parietal bone

Foramen magnum

Occipital bone

PLATE 20
Sphenoidal region, floor of the cranial cavity.

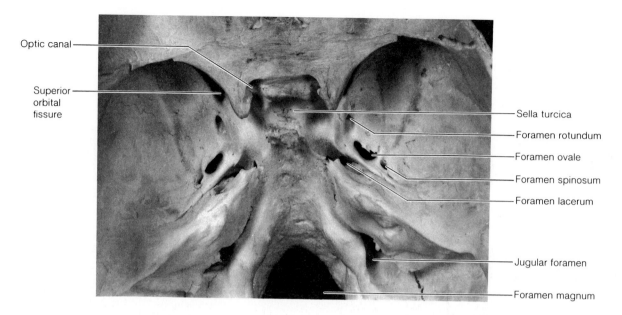

Optic canal

Superior
orbital
fissure

Sella turcica

Foramen rotundum

Foramen ovale

Foramen spinosum

Foramen lacerum

Jugular foramen

Foramen magnum

C H A P T E R 7

Joints of the Skeletal System

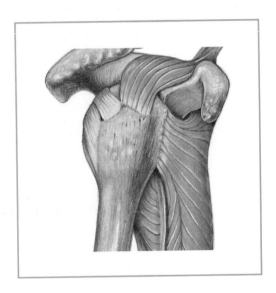

Joints are the junctions between the bones (or between bone and cartilage) of the skeletal system. That is, a joint occurs wherever two or more bones come together. Most joints function in lever systems that make movements possible by bending or straightening. Others, however, are relatively rigid structures that help hold bones in place or enable bones to grow.

This chapter describes how various types of joints are classified, how they differ in structure, and how they permit different movements. It also describes in detail the structures of several large, freely movable joints.

Chapter Objectives

After you have studied this chapter, you should be able to

1. Explain how joints can be classified according to structure and to the amount of movement they permit.

2. Describe how bones of fibrous joints are held together.

3. Describe how bones of cartilaginous joints are held together.

4. Describe the general structure of a synovial joint.

5. List six types of synovial joints and name an example of each type.

6. Explain how skeletal muscles produce movements at joints and identify several types of joint movements.

7. Describe the intervertebral joints and name the ligaments associated with these joints.

8. Describe the shoulder, elbow, hip, and knee joints, and explain how their articulating parts are held together.

9. Complete the review activities at the end of this chapter. Note that they are worded in the form of specific learning objectives. You may want to refer to them before reading the chapter.

Aids to Understanding Words

acetabul-, vinegar cup: *acetabulum*—cuplike depression of the coxal bone that articulates with the head of the femur.

annul-, a ring: *annul*ar ligament—a ring-shaped band of connective tissue within the elbow that encircles the head of the radius.

burs-, a pouch: prepatellar *burs*a—a fluid-filled sac between the skin and the patella.

condyl-, a knob: medial *condyle*—a rounded bony process at the distal end of the femur.

fov-, a pit: *fov*ea capitis—a pit in the head of the femur to which a ligament is attached.

glen-, joint socket: *glen*oid cavity—a depression in the scapula that articulates with the head of the humerus.

labr-, a lip: glenoidal *labr*um—a rim of fibrocartilage attached to the margin of the glenoid cavity.

menisc-, crescent: *menisc*us—a crescent-shaped, fibrocartilage structure found in certain joints.

ov-, egglike: syn*ov*ial fluid—thick fluid within a joint cavity that resembles egg white.

sutur-, a sewing: *sutur*e—a type of joint in which flat bones are interlocked by a set of tiny bony processes.

syndesm-, binding together: *syndesm*osis—a type of joint in which the bones are held together by long fibers of connective tissue.

Introduction

Wherever two or more bones (or cartilage and bone) meet, a **joint** is formed. Such joints, or **articulations,** represent the functional junctions between bones. They bind various parts of the skeletal system together, allow bone growth to occur, permit certain parts of the skeleton to change shape during childbirth, and enable body parts to move in response to skeletal muscle contractions.

Classification of Joints

Although joints vary considerably in structure and function, they can be classified according to the joint's structure or according to the amount of movement that can occur at each bony junction. On the basis of structure, joints are identified as fibrous, cartilaginous, and synovial. On the basis of movement, joints are classified as synarthroses (immovable), amphiarthroses (slightly movable), and diarthroses (freely movable).

Fibrous Joints

Fibrous joints are found between bones that come into close contact with one another. The bones at such joints are fastened tightly together by a thin layer of fibrous connective tissue. As a rule, no appreciable movement occurs between these bones; sometimes, however, a very small degree of motion is possible. The three types of fibrous joints are:

1. **Syndesmosis** (sin"des-mo′sis). In this type of joint, the bones are bound together by relatively long fibers of connective tissue that form an *interosseous ligament.* Because this ligament is flexible and may be twisted, the joint may permit some slight movement, and thus is amphiarthrotic (am"fe-ar-thro′tik). An example of a syndesmosis is found at the distal ends of the tibia and fibula, where they join to form the tibiofibular articulation. (See figure 7.1.)
2. **Suture** (su′chur). Sutures occur only between flat bones of the skull, where the relatively broad margins of adjacent bones grow together and become united by a thin layer of fibrous connective tissue called a *sutural ligament.* In the infantile skull, described in chapter 6, the skull is incompletely developed and many of the bones are separated by membranous areas called *fontanels.* (See figure 6.34.) These areas allow the skull to change shape slightly during childbirth, but as the bones continue to grow, the fontanels close and are replaced by sutures. With time, some of the bones at sutures become interlocked by a set of tiny bony processes, and the sutural ligament itself may be changed to bone. An example of such a suture can be found in the adult human skull where the parietal and occipital bones meet to

FIGURE 7.1
The articulation at the distal ends of the tibia and fibula provide an example of a syndesmosis.

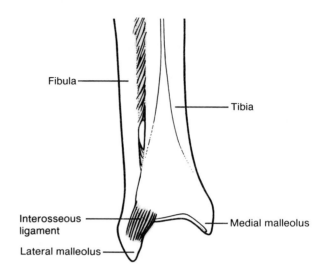

form the lambdoidal suture. Because they are immovable, sutures are synarthrotic (sin"ar-thro′tik) joints. (See figure 7.2.)

The obliteration of the sutures begins in early adulthood, usually before the age of 30. The process occurs first in the deeper parts of the sutures and extends slowly to the external surface. Since the obliteration is usually not complete until advanced age, the condition of the sutures may be used to judge the age of a human skull.

3. **Gomphosis** (gom-fo′sis). A gomphosis is a joint created by the union of a cone-shaped bony process and a bony socket. Such an articulation is formed by the peglike root of a tooth fastened to a jawbone by a *periodontal ligament* (membrane). This ligament surrounds the root and attaches it firmly to the jaw with bundles of thick collagenous fibers. A gomphosis is an example of a synarthrotic joint. (See figure 7.3.)

1. What is a joint?
2. How are joints classified?
3. Describe three types of fibrous joints.
4. What is the function of the fontanels?

Cartilaginous Joints

The bones of **cartilaginous joints** are connected by hyaline cartilage or fibrocartilage. The two types are:

1. **Synchondrosis** (sin"kon-dro′sis). In a synchondrosis, the bones are united by bands of hyaline cartilage. Many of these joints are temporary structures that disappear during the

FIGURE 7.2

(a) The fibrous joints between the bones of the cranium are immovable and are called *sutures*; (b) the bones at a suture are separated by a sutural ligament. (c) Medial view of the interlocking processes of a parietal bone. (Note that the grooves on the inside of this parietal bone mark the paths of blood vessels located near the surface of the brain.)

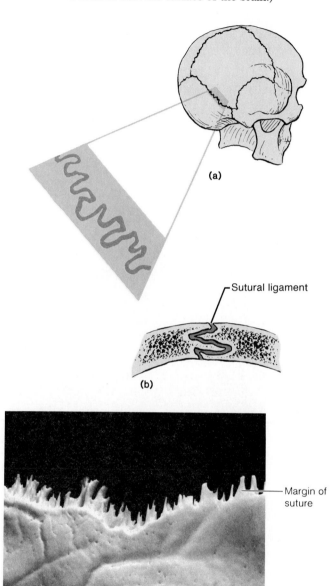

(a)

Sutural ligament

(b)

Margin of suture

Parietal bone

(c)

FIGURE 7.3

The articulation between the root of a tooth and the jawbone is a gomphosis.

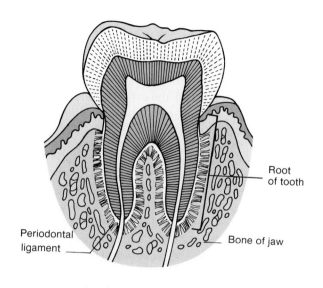

Root of tooth

Periodontal ligament

Bone of jaw

FIGURE 7.4

The articulation between the first rib and the sternum is an example of a synchondrosis.

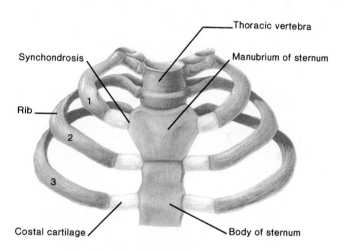

Thoracic vertebra

Synchondrosis

Manubrium of sternum

Rib

Costal cartilage

Body of sternum

growth process. An example is found in an immature long bone where an epiphysis is connected to a diaphysis by a band of hyaline cartilage (the epiphyseal disk—see figure 6.8). As described in chapter 6, this band functions in the growth of the bone and in time is converted from cartilage into bone. When this ossification is complete, usually before the age of twenty-five, movement no longer occurs at the joint. Thus, the joint is synarthrotic.

Another example of a synchondrosis occurs between the sternum and the first rib, which are united by costal cartilage. In this instance, the joint is permanent. It also allows some movement, since the costal cartilage can bend and twist. (See figure 7.4.)

Joints of the Skeletal System   191

Although the joint between the sternum and first rib is a synchondrosis, synovial joints are found between the sternum and ribs two through seven.

2. **Symphysis** (sim'fi-sis). The articular surfaces of the bones at a symphysis are covered by a thin layer of hyaline cartilage, and the cartilage, in turn, is attached to a pad of resilient fibrocartilage. A limited amount of movement occurs at such a joint whenever forces cause the cartilaginous pad to become compressed or deformed. The joint formed by the bodies of two adjacent vertebrae separated by an intervertebral disk is an example of a symphysis. (See figure 7.5.)

Each intervertebral disk is composed of a band of fibrocartilage (anulus fibrosus) that surrounds a gelatinous core (nucleus pulposus). The disk acts as a shock absorber and helps to equalize pressures between the vertebrae when the body moves. Since each disk is slightly flexible, limited motion occurs when the back is bent forward or to the side, or is twisted. These movements are limited since the bodies of the vertebrae are joined by an *anterior* and a *posterior longitudinal ligament*. (See figure 7.13.) Two other examples of this type of joint are the symphysis pubis and sacroiliac joints in the pelvic girdle. These joints normally allow only slight movements and thus are amphiarthrotic (am"fe-ar-thro'tik).

During pregnancy, hormonal changes cause relaxation of the symphysis pubis and sacroiliac joints and associated ligaments. As a result, greater movement occurs to allow an infant to pass through the birth canal during childbirth.

Synovial Joints

Most joints of the skeletal system are **synovial,** and they have much more complex structures than the fibrous or cartilaginous types. For example, these joints contain articular cartilage, a joint capsule, and synovial fluid. Because they are freely movable, synovial joints are diarthrotic (di"ar-thro-tik).

General Structure of a Synovial Joint

The articular ends of bones in a synovial joint are covered with a thin layer of hyaline cartilage. (See figure 7.6.) This layer, which is called the **articular cartilage,** is attached to the bone. The cartilage is resistant to wear and produces a minimum of friction when it is compressed as the joint is moved. It also transmits the weight load to the underlying bone.

FIGURE 7.5

(*a*) The symphysis pubis that separates the pubic bones of the pelvic girdle and (*b*) the intervertebral disks that separate the bodies of adjacent vertebrae are composed of fibrocartilage.

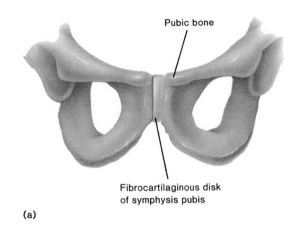

Pubic bone

Fibrocartilaginous disk of symphysis pubis

(a)

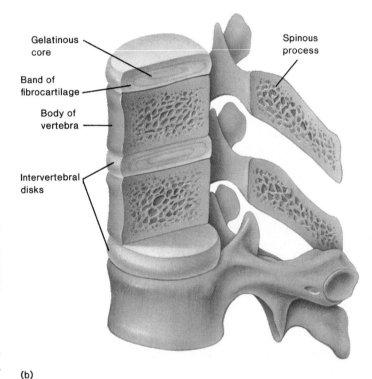

Gelatinous core

Spinous process

Band of fibrocartilage

Body of vertebra

Intervertebral disks

(b)

Typically, the articular cartilage lies on a layer of somewhat elastic spongy bone called the *subchondral plate*. This plate acts as a shock absorber, which helps protect the joint from stresses created by the load of body weight and by forces produced by contracting muscles.

Excessive mechanical stress may cause tiny fractures to appear in a subchondral plate. Although such fractures usually heal, the bone that regenerates may be less elastic than the original, and its protective function may be reduced.

FIGURE 7.6

The generalized structure of a synovial joint. What is the function of the synovial fluid within this type of joint?

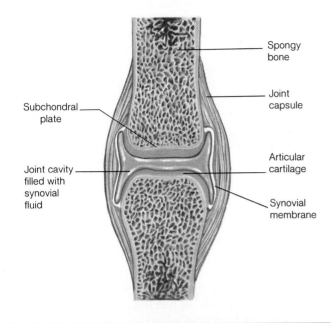

FIGURE 7.7

The articulating surfaces of the femur and tibia are separated by menisci; also there are several bursae associated with the knee joint.

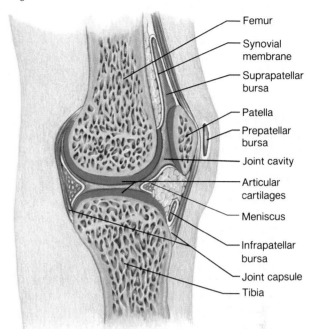

In addition to causing fractures in the subchondral plate, excessive mechanical stress due to obesity or certain athletic activities may damage the articular cartilage of various joints and cause it to deteriorate. Joints that are subjected to repeated overloading—such as the elbow of a baseball pitcher or the knee of a basketball player—are likely to develop the degenerative joint disease osteoarthritis.

The bones are held together by a tubular **joint capsule** that has two distinct layers. The outer layer consists largely of dense, white, fibrous connective tissue. It is attached to the periosteum of each bone around its articular end. Thus, the outer fibrous layer of the capsule completely encloses the other parts of the joint. It is, however, flexible enough to permit movement and strong enough to help prevent the articular surfaces from being pulled apart.

Bundles of strong, tough collagenous fibers called **ligaments** reinforce the joint capsule and help to bind the articular ends of the bones together. Some ligaments appear as thickenings in the fibrous layer of the capsule, while others are located outside the capsule. In either case, these ligaments also prevent excessive movement at the joint. That is, the ligament is relatively inelastic, and it becomes tightly drawn whenever a normal limit of movement has been achieved in the joint.

The inner layer of the joint capsule consists of a shiny, vascular lining of loose connective tissue called the **synovial membrane,** which is only a few cells thick. This membrane covers all of the surfaces within the joint capsule, except the areas covered by cartilage. The synovial membrane forms a closed sac called the *synovial cavity,* and into this joint cavity the membrane secretes a clear, viscous fluid

called **synovial fluid.** In some regions, the surface of the synovial membrane possesses villi as well as larger folds and projections that extend into the cavity. Besides filling spaces and irregularities of the joint cavity, these extensions increase the surface area of the synovial membrane. In addition, the membrane may include adipose tissue and form movable fatty pads within the joint. The synovial membrane also functions to reabsorb fluid. Thus, it may help remove substances from a joint cavity that is injured or infected.

Synovial fluid has a consistency similar to egg white, and it moistens and lubricates the smooth cartilaginous surfaces within the joint. It also helps supply articular cartilage with nutrients that are obtained from blood in vessels of the synovial membrane. The volume of synovial fluid present in a joint cavity is relatively small. Usually there is just enough to cover the articulating surfaces with a thin film of fluid—for example, the amount in the cavity of the knee is 0.5 ml or less.

Some synovial joints are partially or completely divided into two compartments by disks of fibrocartilage called **menisci** (sing. **meniscus**) located between the articular surfaces. Each meniscus is attached to the fibrous layer of the joint capsule peripherally, and its free surface projects into the joint cavity. In the case of the knee joint, crescent-shaped menisci cushion the articulating surfaces and help distribute the body weight onto these surfaces. (See figure 7.7.)

Certain synovial joints also have closed, fluid-filled sacs called **bursae** associated with them. Each bursa has an inner lining of synovial membrane, which may be continuous with the synovial membrane of a nearby joint cavity. These sacs contain synovial fluid and are commonly located between the skin and underlying bony prominences, as in the case of the patella of the knee or the olecranon process of the elbow. Bursae act as cushions and aid the movement of tendons that glide over bony parts or over other tendons. The names of bursae indicate their locations. Thus, there is a *suprapatellar bursa,* a *prepatellar bursa,* and an *infrapatellar bursa,* shown in figure 7.7.

Articular cartilage, along with other cartilaginous structures, lacks a direct blood supply (see chapter 4). Instead, it depends upon the surrounding synovial fluid for its supply of oxygen, nutrients, and other vital substances. Normal body movements create a forceful action within a joint that facilitates the passage of these substances into the cartilage. When a joint is immobilized or is not used for a prolonged time, lack of such action may result in degeneration of the articular cartilage.

Although degeneration of the cartilage may be reversed when joint movements are resumed, it is important to avoid exercises that cause excessive compression of the tissue during the period of regeneration. Otherwise, chondrocytes in the thinned cartilage may be injured, and the repair process may be halted.

---

1. Describe two types of cartilaginous joints.
2. What is the function of an intervertebral disk?
3. Describe the structure of a synovial joint.

Types of Synovial Joints

The articulating bones of synovial joints have a variety of shapes that allow different kinds of movement. Based upon the shapes of their parts and the movements they permit, these joints can be classified into six major types—ball-and-socket joints, condyloid joints, gliding joints, hinge joints, pivot joints, and saddle joints.

1. *Ball-and-socket joints.* A **ball-and-socket joint** (spheroidal joint) consists of a bone with a globular or slightly egg-shaped head that articulates with a cup-shaped cavity of another bone. Such a joint allows for a wider range of motion than does any other kind. Movements in all planes, as well as rotational movement around a central axis, are possible. The hip and shoulder contain joints of this type. (See figures 7.8*a* and 7.19.)

2. *Condyloid joints.* In a **condyloid joint** (ellipsoidal joint), an ovoid condyle of one bone fits into an elliptical cavity of another bone, as in the joints between the metacarpals and phalanges, and between the radius and the carpal bones. This type of joint permits a variety of movements in different planes; rotational movement, however, is not possible. (See figure 7.8*b*.)

3. *Gliding joints.* The articulating surfaces of **gliding joints** (arthrodial joint) are nearly flat or only slightly curved. These joints allow only sliding or back-and-forth motion. Most of the joints within the wrist and ankle as well as those between the articular processes of adjacent vertebrae belong to this group. (See figure 7.8*c*.)

4. *Hinge joints.* In a **hinge joint** (ginglymoidal joint), the convex surface of one bone fits into the concave surface of another, as in the elbow and the joints of the phalanges. Such a joint resembles the hinge of a door in that it permits movement in one plane only. (See figure 7.8*d*.)

5. *Pivot joints.* In a **pivot joint** (trochoidal joint), a cylindrical surface of one bone rotates within a ring formed of bone and a ligament. The movement at such a joint is limited to rotation about a central axis. The joint between the proximal ends of the radius and the ulna, where the head of the radius rotates in a ring formed by the radial notch of the ulna and a ligament (annular ligament), is of this type. Similarly, a pivot joint functions in the neck as the head is turned from side to side. In this case, the ring formed by a ligament (transverse ligament) and the anterior arch of the atlas rotates around the odontoid process (dens) of the axis. (See figure 7.8*e*.)

6. *Saddle joints.* A **saddle joint** (sellar joint) is formed between bones whose articulating surfaces have both concave and convex regions. The surface of one bone fits the complementary surface of the other. This arrangement permits a variety of movements, as in the case of the joint between the carpal (trapezium) and the metacarpal of the thumb. (See figure 7.8*f*.)

Chart 7.1 summarizes the types of joints.

FIGURE 7.8

(*a–f*) Types and examples of synovial joints.

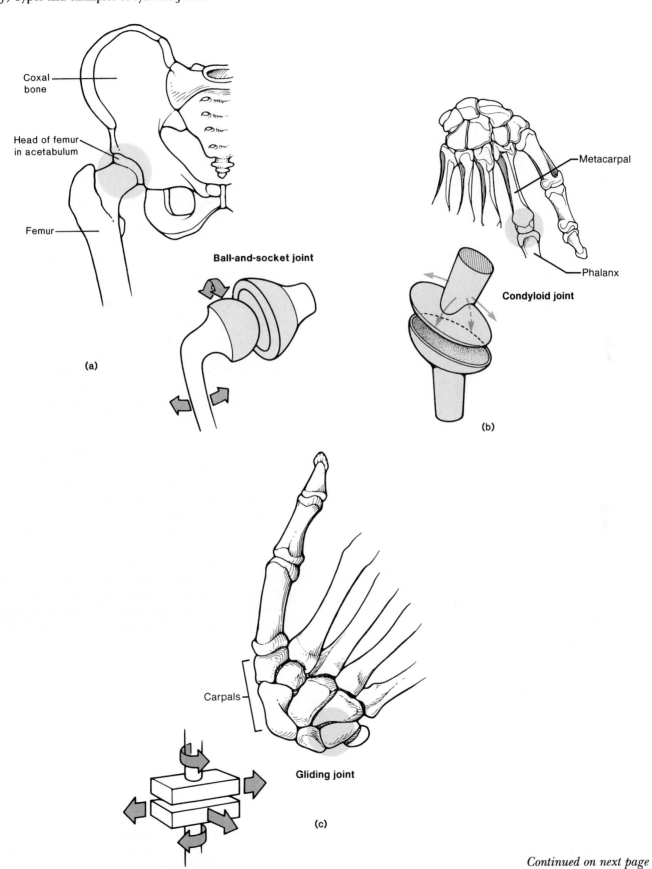

Coxal bone

Head of femur in acetabulum

Femur

Ball-and-socket joint

(a)

Metacarpal

Phalanx

Condyloid joint

(b)

Carpals

Gliding joint

(c)

Continued on next page

FIGURE 7.8—*Continued*

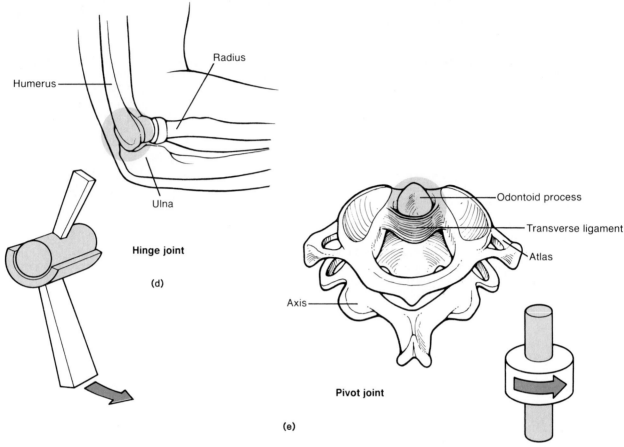

Hinge joint

(d)

Odontoid process

Transverse ligament

Atlas

Axis

Pivot joint

(e)

Humerus

Radius

Ulna

First metacarpal

Trapezium

Saddle joint

(f)

Types of Joint Movements

Movements at synovial joints are produced by actions of skeletal muscles. Typically, one end of a muscle is attached to a relatively immovable or fixed part on one side of a joint, and the other end of the muscle is fastened to a movable part on the other side. When the muscle contracts, its fibers pull its movable end (insertion) toward its fixed end (origin), and a movement occurs at the joint.

The following terms are used to describe movements at joints that occur in different directions and in different planes (figures 7.9, 7.10, and 7.11):

Abduction (ab-duk′shun) moving a part away from the midline (lifting the arm horizontally to form a right angle with the side of the body).

Adduction (ah-duk′shun) moving a part toward the midline (returning the arm from the horizontal position to the side of the body).

Flexion (flek′shun) bending parts at a joint so that the angle between them is decreased and the parts come closer together (bending the leg at the knee).

Extension (ek-sten′shun) straightening parts at a joint so that the angle between them is increased and the parts move further apart (straightening the leg at the knee).

Hyperextension (hi″per-ek-sten′shun) excessive extension of the parts at a joint, beyond the anatomical position (bending the head back beyond the upright position).

Chart 7.1 Types of joints

Type of joint	Description	Possible movements	Example
Fibrous	Articulating bones fastened together by thin layer of fibrous connective tissue		
1. *Syndesmosis*	Bones bound by interosseous ligament	Joint flexible and may be twisted (amphiarthrosis)	Tibiofibular articulation
2. *Suture*	Flat bones united by sutural ligament	None (synarthrosis)	Parietal bones articulate at sagittal suture of skull
3. *Gomphosis*	Cone-shaped process fastened in bony socket by periodontal ligament	None (synarthrosis)	Root of tooth united with jawbone
Cartilaginous	Articulating bones connected by hyaline cartilage or fibrocartilage		
1. *Synchondrosis*	Bones united by bands of hyaline cartilage	Movement occurs during growth process until ossification occurs (synarthrosis)	Joint between epiphysis and diaphysis of a long bone
2. *Symphysis*	Articular surfaces separated by thin layers of hyaline cartilage attached to band of fibrocartilage	Limited movement as when back is bent or twisted (amphiarthrosis)	Joints between bodies of adjacent vertebrae
Synovial	Articulating bones surrounded by joint capsule of ligaments and synovial membranes; ends of articulating bones covered by hyaline cartilage and separated by synovial fluid	Freely movable (diarthrosis)	
1. *Ball-and-socket*	Ball-shaped head of one bone articulates with cup-shaped socket of another	Movements in all planes and rotation	Shoulder, hip
2. *Condyloid*	Oval-shaped condyle of one bone articulates with elliptical cavity of another	Variety of movements in different planes, but no rotation	Joints between metacarpals and phalanges
3. *Gliding*	Articulating surfaces are nearly flat or slightly curved	Sliding or twisting	Joints between various bones of wrist and ankle
4. *Hinge*	Convex surface of one bone articulates with concave surface of another	Flexion and extension	Elbow and joints of phalanges
5. *Pivot*	Cylindrical surface of one bone articulates with ring of bone and fibrous tissue	Rotation	Joint between proximal ends of radius and ulna
6. *Saddle*	Articulating surfaces have both concave and convex regions; surface of one bone fits complementary surface of another	Variety of movements	Joint between carpal and metacarpal of thumb

Dorsiflexion (dor″si-flek′shun) flexing the foot at the ankle (bending the foot upward).

Plantar flexion (plan′tar flek′shun) extending the foot at the ankle (bending the foot downward).

Rotation (ro-ta′shun) moving a part around an axis (twisting the head from side to side).

Circumduction (ser″kum-duk′shun) moving a part so that its end follows a circular path (moving the finger in a circular motion without moving the hand).

Supination (soo″pi-na′shun) turning the hand so the palm is upward.

Pronation (pro-na′shun) turning the hand so the palm is downward.

Eversion (e-ver′zhun) turning the foot so the sole is outward.

Inversion (in-ver′zhun) turning the foot so the sole is inward.

Protraction (pro-trak′shun) moving a part forward (thrusting the chin forward).

Retraction (re-trak′shun) moving a part backward (pulling the chin backward).

Elevation (el″ĕ-va′shun) raising a part (shrugging the shoulders).

Depression (de-presh′un) lowering a part (drooping the shoulders).

FIGURE 7.9

Joint movements illustrating flexion, extension, hyperextension, dorsiflexion, plantar flexion, abduction, and adduction.

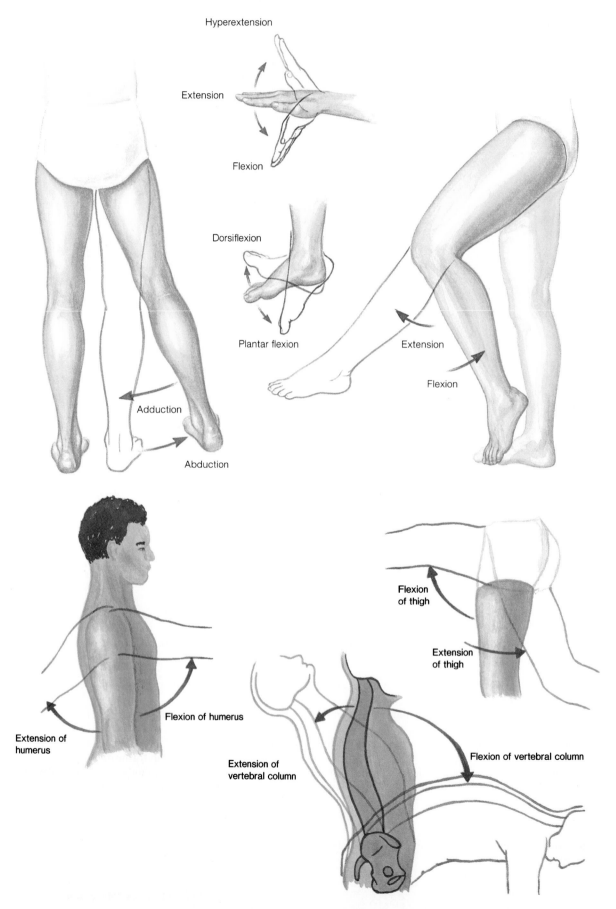

FIGURE 7.10

Joint movements illustrating rotation, circumduction, supination, and pronation.

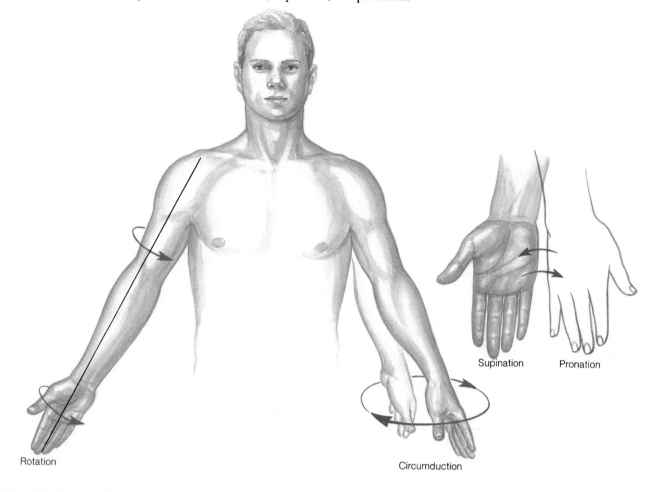

Rotation

Supination   Pronation

Circumduction

FIGURE 7.11

Joint movements illustrating eversion, inversion, protraction, retraction, elevation, and depression.

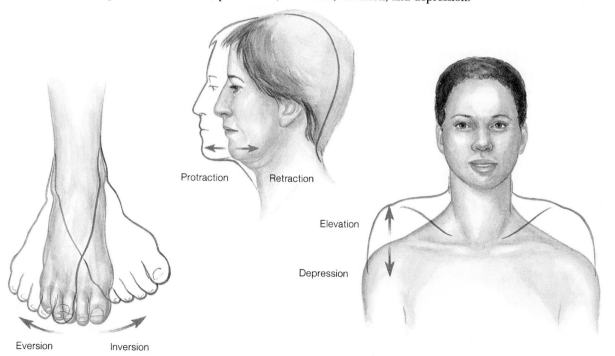

Protraction   Retraction

Elevation

Depression

Eversion   Inversion

Examples of Synovial Joints

The intervertebral joints are examples of relatively small synovial joints. They allow much of the movement possible in the vertebral column. The shoulder, elbow, hip, and knee are large synovial joints. Although these joints have much in common, each has a unique structure that is related to its specific function.

Intervertebral Joints

The joints between the vertebrae, from the second cervical to the sacrum, are of two types. In one type, the vertebral bodies are joined by cartilaginous joints (described previously). In the second type, synovial joints that occur between the nearly flat articular processes are of the gliding type (figure 7.12).

A joint capsule surrounds each intervertebral synovial joint (figure 7.13). The ligaments between the vertebral arches include the following:

1. **Ligamenta** (sing. *ligamentum*) **flavum** (fla′vum). These ligaments extend between adjacent laminae and contain some elastic tissue. They are thinnest and longest in the cervical area and are thickest in the lumbar region. They help limit flexion of the vertebral column.
2. **Supraspinous** (su″pra-spi′nus) **ligament.** This ligament connects the spines of the vertebrae from the seventh cervical to the sacrum. In the cervical area, it becomes the more elastic *ligamentum nuchae* (nu′ka).
3. **Interspinous** (in″ter-spi′nus) **ligaments.** The interspinous ligaments are thin and connect the spines of adjacent vertebrae. Their fibers blend with the ligamenta flavum and supraspinous ligaments.

Although movements between any two vertebrae are limited, the vertebral column as a whole is capable of a wide range of motion. These motions include flexion, extension, lateral flexion (bending to one side), rotation, and circumduction. The intervertebral joints of the cervical and lumbar areas demonstrate greater flexibility than those in the thoracic area.

FIGURE 7.12

The articulating processes of adjacent vertebrae form gliding joints.

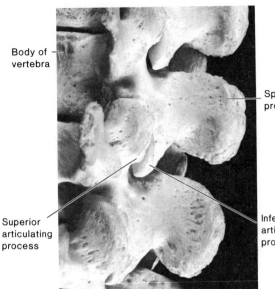

Body of vertebra

Spinous process

Superior articulating process

Inferior articulating process

Lifting heavy objects by bending from the waist (flexing the vertebral column) may cause tears in the ligaments between the lumbar vertebrae. The result may be increased movement at the intervertebral joints, leading to the rupture of an intervertebral disk. For this reason, it is suggested that when lifting heavy objects, the back be kept straight and the knees bent. This allows the lifting to be done by the strong leg muscles.

The Shoulder Joint

The **shoulder joint** is a ball-and-socket joint that consists of the rounded head of the humerus and the shallow glenoid cavity of the scapula. These parts are protected above by the coracoid and acromion processes of the scapula, and they are held together by various fibrous connective tissues and muscles.

The *joint capsule* of the shoulder is attached along the circumference of the glenoid cavity and the anatomical neck of the humerus. Although it completely envelopes the joint, the capsule is very loose and by itself is unable to keep the bones of the joint in close contact. However, the capsule is surrounded and reinforced by muscles and tendons, and these structures are largely responsible for keeping the articulating parts together. (See figure 7.14.)

FIGURE 7.13

Ligaments associated with intervertebral joints. (*a*) Sagittal view of the cervical area; (*b*) left lateral view of the lumbar area.

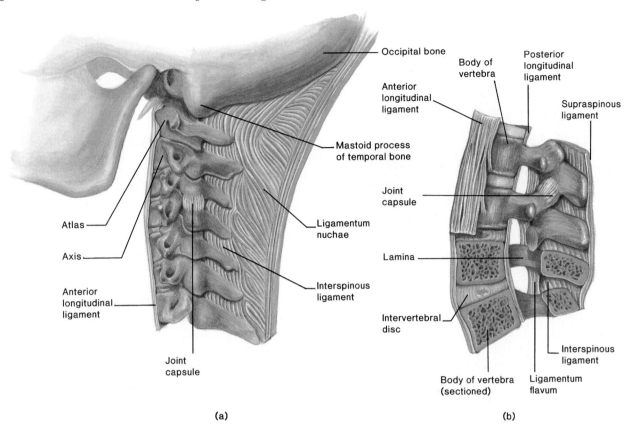

(a)

(b)

FIGURE 7.14

(*a*) The shoulder joint allows movements in all directions. (Note the bursa associated with this joint.) (*b*) Photograph of the shoulder joint with the articular surfaces exposed.

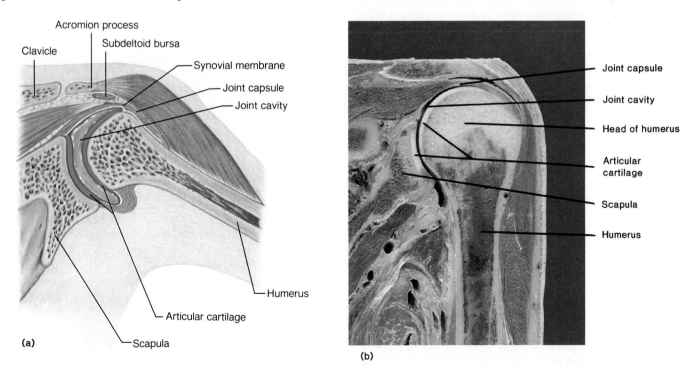

(a)

(b)

FIGURE 7.15

The tendons of four muscles form the rotator cuff and reinforce the shoulder joint.

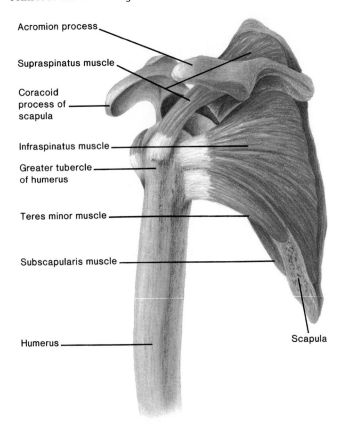

Acromion process

Supraspinatus muscle

Coracoid process of scapula

Infraspinatus muscle

Greater tubercle of humerus

Teres minor muscle

Subscapularis muscle

Humerus

Scapula

The tendons of four muscles (subscapularis, supraspinatus, infraspinatus, and teres minor muscles) blend with the fibrous layer of the shoulder joint capsule, forming the *rotator cuff*, which reinforces and supports the shoulder joint (figure 7.15). The rotator cuff is sometimes injured as a result of the centrifugal forces created when the shoulder joint is used for throwing.

The ligaments that help to prevent displacement of the articulating surfaces of the shoulder joint include the following:

1. **Coracohumeral** (kor″ah-ko-hu′mer-al) **ligament.** This ligament is composed of a broad band of connective tissue that connects the coracoid process of the scapula to the greater tubercle of the humerus. It strengthens the superior portion of the joint capsule.
2. **Glenohumeral** (gle″no-hu′mer-al) **ligaments.** These include three bands of fibers that appear as thickenings in the ventral wall of the joint capsule. They extend from the edge of the glenoid cavity to the lesser tubercle and the anatomical neck of the humerus.
3. **Transverse humeral ligament.** This ligament consists of a narrow sheet of connective tissue

fibers that run between the lesser and the greater tubercles of the humerus. Together with the intertubercular groove of the humerus, the ligament creates a canal (retinaculum) through which the long head of the biceps brachii muscle passes.

The shallow glenoid cavity is deepened by the **glenoidal labrum** (gle′noid-al la′brum). The glenoidal labrum is a rim of fibrocartilage that is attached along the margin of the glenoid cavity. (See figure 7.16.)

There are several bursae associated with the shoulder joint. The major ones include the *subscapular bursa,* located between the joint capsule and the tendon of the subscapularis muscle; the *subdeltoid bursa,* between the joint capsule and the deep surface of the deltoid muscle; the *subacromial bursa,* between the joint capsule and the under surface of the acromion process of the scapula; and the *subcoracoid bursa,* between the joint capsule and the coracoid process of the scapula. Of these, the subscapular bursa is usually continuous with the synovial cavity of the joint cavity, and although the others do not communicate with the joint cavity, they may be connected to each other. (See figures 7.14 and 7.16.)

Due to the looseness of its attachments and the relatively large articular surface of the humerus compared to the shallow depth of the glenoid cavity, the shoulder joint is capable of a very wide range of movement. These include flexion, extension, abduction, adduction, rotation, and circumduction. Such movements may also be aided by motion occurring simultaneously in the joint formed between the scapula and the clavicle.

Because the bones of the shoulder joint are held together mainly by supporting muscles rather than by bony structures and strong ligaments, the joint is somewhat weak. Consequently, the articulating surfaces may become displaced or dislocated rather easily. Such a *dislocation* most commonly occurs during forceful abduction, as when a person falls on an outstretched arm. This movement may cause the head of the humerus to press against the lower part of the joint capsule, where its wall is relatively thin and poorly supported by ligaments.

The Elbow Joint

The **elbow joint** is a complex structure that includes two articulations—a hinge joint between the trochlea of the humerus and the trochlear notch of the ulna, and a gliding joint between the capitulum of the humerus and a shallow depression (fovea) on the head of the radius. These unions are completely enclosed and held together by a joint capsule, whose sides are thickened by ulnar and radial collateral ligaments and whose anterior surface is reinforced by fibers from a muscle (brachialis) in the upper arm. (See figure 7.17.)

FIGURE 7.16

(a) The articulating surfaces of the shoulder are held together by ligaments; (b) the glenoidal labrum is a ligament composed of fibrocartilage.

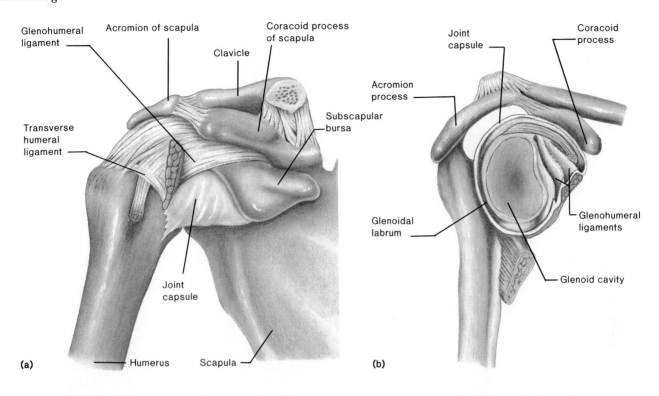

(a)

Glenohumeral ligament
Acromion of scapula
Coracoid process of scapula
Clavicle
Transverse humeral ligament
Subscapular bursa
Joint capsule
Humerus
Scapula

(b)

Joint capsule
Coracoid process
Acromion process
Glenoidal labrum
Glenohumeral ligaments
Glenoid cavity

FIGURE 7.17

(a) The elbow joint allows hinge movements as well as pronation and supination of the hand; (b) photograph of the elbow joint with the articular surfaces exposed.

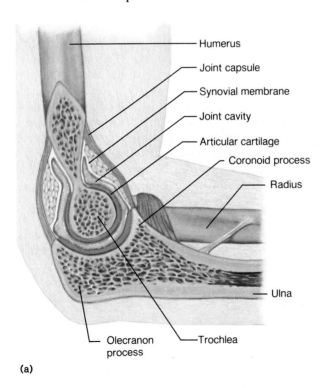

(a)

Humerus
Joint capsule
Synovial membrane
Joint cavity
Articular cartilage
Coronoid process
Radius
Ulna
Olecranon process
Trochlea

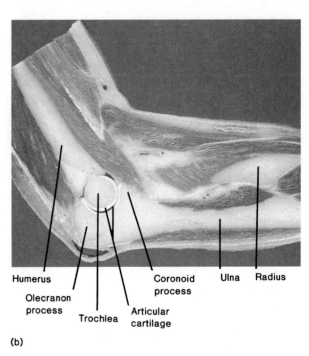

(b)

Humerus
Olecranon process
Trochlea
Articular cartilage
Coronoid process
Ulna
Radius

FIGURE 7.18
(a) The ulnar collateral ligament and (b) the radial collateral ligament strengthen the capsular wall of the elbow joint.

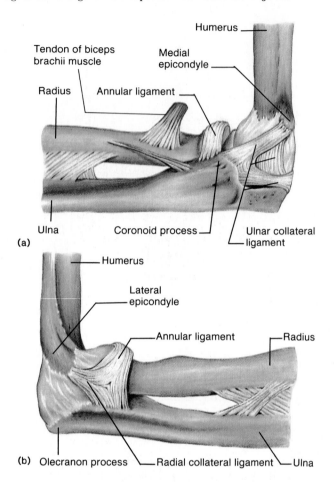

(a)

(b)

The **ulnar collateral ligament,** which consists of a thick band of fibrous connective tissue, is located in the medial wall of the capsule. The anterior portion of this ligament connects the medial epicondyle of the humerus to the medial margin of the coronoid process of the ulna. Its posterior part is attached to the medial epicondyle of the humerus and to the olecranon process of the ulna.

The **radial collateral ligament,** which strengthens the lateral wall of the joint capsule, is composed of a fibrous band extending between the lateral epicondyle of the humerus and the annular ligament of the radius. The *annular ligament,* in turn, is attached to the margin of the trochlear notch of the ulna. It encircles the head of the radius and functions to keep the head in contact with the radial notch of the ulna. The resulting radioulnar joint is also enclosed by the elbow joint capsule, so that its function is closely associated with the elbow. (See figure 7.18.)

The *synovial membrane* that forms the inner lining of the elbow capsule projects into the joint cavity between the radius and ulna, and partially divides the joint into humerus-ulnar and humerus-radial portions. Also, varying amounts of adipose tissue form fatty pads between the sy-

novial membrane and the fibrous layer of the joint capsule. These pads help protect nonarticular bony areas during joint movements.

The only movements that can occur at the elbow between the humerus and ulna are hinge-type movements—flexion and extension. The head of the radius, however, is free to rotate in the annular ligament, and this movement is responsible for pronation and supination of the hand.

Injuries to the elbow, shoulder, and knee are commonly diagnosed and treated using a procedure called *arthroscopy.* This procedure makes use of a thin, tubular instrument about 25 cm long, called an *arthroscope.* The instrument, which contains optical fibers, can be inserted through a small incision in the joint capsule. A surgeon can then view the interior of the joint directly or observe an image of the joint on a television screen. In either case, the surgeon can use the arthroscope to explore the joint cavity and to guide other instruments inserted through the capsule to repair or remove injured parts.

1. What parts help keep the articulating surfaces of the shoulder joint together?
2. What factors allow an especially wide range of motion in the shoulder?
3. What parts make up the hinge joint of the elbow?
4. What parts of the elbow permit pronation and supination of the hand?

The Hip Joint

The **hip joint** is a ball-and-socket joint that consists of the head of the femur and the cup-shaped acetabulum of the coxal bone (figure 7.19). A ligament (ligamentum capitis) is attached to a pit (fovea capitis) on the head of the femur and to connective tissue within the acetabulum. This attachment, however, seems to have little importance in holding the articulating bones together. Instead, it serves to carry blood vessels to the head of the femur.

A horseshoe-shaped ring of fibrocartilage (acetabular labrum) at the rim of the acetabulum deepens the cavity of the acetabulum. It encloses the head of the femur and helps hold it securely in place. In addition, a heavy, cylindrical joint capsule, which is reinforced with still other ligaments, surrounds the articulating structures and connects the neck of the femur to the margin of the acetabulum. (See figure 7.20.)

The major ligaments of the hip joint include the following:

1. **Iliofemoral** (il″e-o-fem′o-ral) **ligament.** This ligament consists of a Y-shaped band of very strong fibers that connect the anterior inferior iliac spine of the coxal bone to a bony line (intertrochanteric line) extending between the greater and lesser

FIGURE 7.19

(a) The acetabulum provides the socket for the head of the femur in the hip joint; (b) the pit in the head of the femur marks the attachment of a ligament that carries blood vessels to the head.

FIGURE 7.20

(a) The hip joint is held together by a ring of cartilage in the acetabulum and a joint capsule that is reinforced by ligaments; (b) photograph of the hip joint with the articular surfaces exposed.

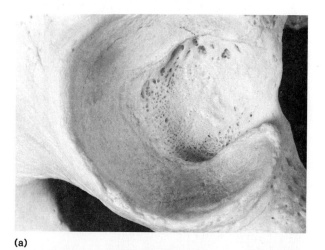

(a)

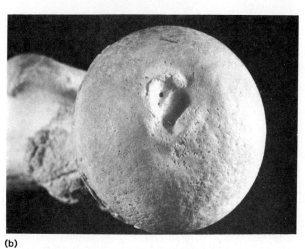

(b)

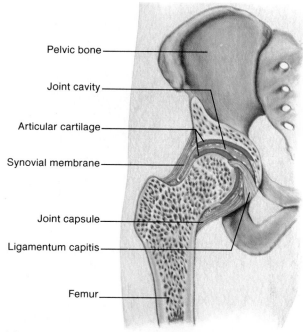

Pelvic bone

Joint cavity

Articular cartilage

Synovial membrane

Joint capsule

Ligamentum capitis

Femur

(a)

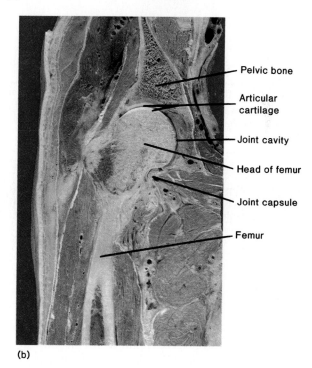

Pelvic bone

Articular cartilage

Joint cavity

Head of femur

Joint capsule

Femur

(b)

trochanters of the femur. The iliofemoral ligament is the strongest ligament in the body, and it helps to prevent extension of the femur when the body is standing erect.

2. **Pubofemoral** (pu″bo-fem′o-ral) **ligament.** The pubofemoral ligament extends between the superior portion of the pubis and the iliofemoral ligament. Its fibers also blend with the fibers of the joint capsule.

3. **Ischiofemoral** (is″ke-o-fem′o-ral) **ligament.** This ligament consists of a band of strong fibers that originate on the ischium just posterior to the acetabulum and blend with the fibers of the joint capsule. (See figure 7.21.)

As in the case of the shoulder, the joint capsule of the hip is surrounded by muscles. However, the articulating parts of the hip are held more closely together than those of the shoulder. Thus, there is considerably less freedom

FIGURE 7.21
The major ligaments of the hip joint. (*a*) Anterior view; (*b*) posterior view.

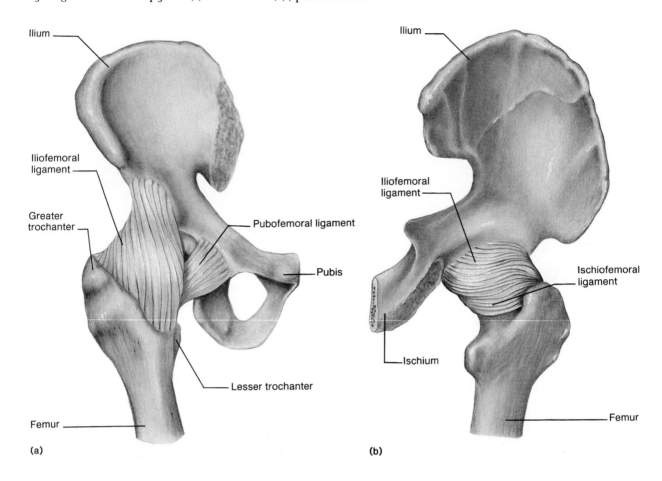

Ilium

Iliofemoral ligament

Greater trochanter

Pubofemoral ligament

Pubis

Lesser trochanter

Femur

(a)

Ilium

Iliofemoral ligament

Ischiofemoral ligament

Ischium

Femur

(b)

of movement at the hip joint, but its structure does permit a wide variety of movements, including extension, flexion, abduction, adduction, rotation, and circumduction.

To correct problems created by joint injury or disease, it is sometimes desirable to replace the articulating parts with artificial (prosthetic) devices. The hip joint, for example, can be totally replaced. In this procedure, called *total hip arthroplasty,* the acetabulum is replaced by a low-friction polyethylene socket that is fastened into the coxal bone with surgical bone cement. The head of the femur is replaced by a metallic, ball-shaped part.

The Knee Joint

The **knee joint** is the largest and most complex of the synovial joints. It consists of the medial and lateral condyles at the distal end of the femur, and the medial and lateral condyles at the proximal end of the tibia. In addition, the femur articulates anteriorly with the patella. Although the knee is sometimes considered a modified hinge joint, the articulations between the femur and tibia are of the condyloid type, and the joint between the femur and patella is a gliding joint.

The *joint capsule* of the knee is relatively thin, but it is greatly strengthened by ligaments and tendons of several muscles. Anteriorly, for example, the capsule is covered by the fused tendons of several muscles in the thigh. Fibers from these tendons descend to the patella, partially enclose it, and continue downward to the tibia. The capsule is attached to the margins of the femoral and tibial condyles as well as to the areas between these condyles. (See figure 7.22.)

The ligaments associated with the joint capsule, which help keep the articulating surfaces of the knee joint in contact, include the following:

1. **Patellar** (pah-tel′ar) **ligament.** This ligament represents a continuation of a tendon from a large muscle group in the thigh (quadriceps femoris). It consists of a strong, flat band that extends from the margin of the patella to the tibial tuberosity.

FIGURE 7.22

(*a*) The knee joint is the most complex of the synovial joints; (*b*) photograph of the knee joint with the articular surfaces exposed.

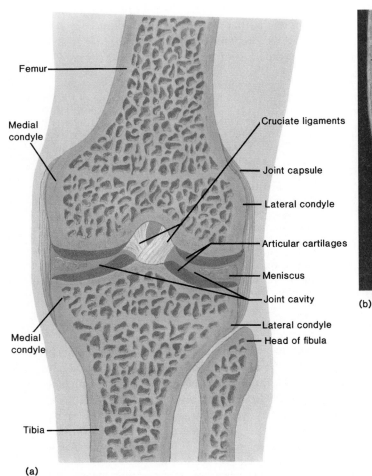

Femur
Medial condyle
Cruciate ligaments
Joint capsule
Lateral condyle
Articular cartilages
Meniscus
Joint cavity
Lateral condyle
Head of fibula
Medial condyle
Tibia

(a)

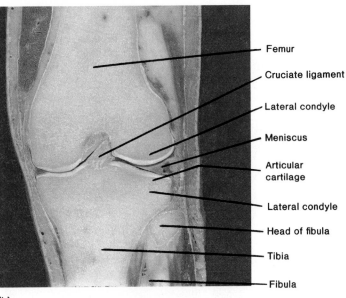

Femur
Cruciate ligament
Lateral condyle
Meniscus
Articular cartilage
Lateral condyle
Head of fibula
Tibia
Fibula

(b)

2. **Oblique popliteal** (ŏ-blēk pop-lit′e-al) **ligament.**
    This ligament connects the lateral condyle of the
    femur to the margin of the medial condyle of the
    tibia.

3. **Arcuate** (ar′ku-āt) **popliteal ligament.** This
    ligament appears as a Y-shaped system of fibers
    that extends from the lateral epicondyle of the
    femur and posterior intercondylar area of the tibia
    to the head of the fibula.

4. **Tibial collateral** (tib′e-al kŏ-lat′er-al) **ligament**
    (medial collateral ligament). This ligament is a
    broad, flat band of tissue that connects the medial
    condyle of the femur to the medial condyle of the
    tibia.

5. **Fibular** (fib′u-lar) **collateral ligament** (lateral
    collateral ligament). This ligament consists of a
    strong, round cord located between the lateral
    condyle of the femur and the head of the fibula.
    Both the tibial and fibular collateral ligaments help
    prevent lateral displacement of the knee.

In addition to the ligaments that strengthen the joint
capsule, there are two **cruciate** (kroo′she-āt) **ligaments**
within the joint, which help prevent displacement of the
articulating surfaces. These strong bands of fibrous tissue
stretch upward between the tibia and the femur, crossing
each other on the way. They are named according to their
positions of attachment to the tibia. Thus, the *anterior cruciate ligament* originates from the anterior intercondylar
area of the tibia and extends to the lateral condyle of the
femur. The *posterior cruciate ligament* connects the posterior intercondylar area of the tibia to the medial condyle
of the femur. These ligaments prevent the anterior and
posterior displacement of the knee. (See figure 7.23.)

One of the more common se-
rious knee injuries involves tearing the anterior cruciate ligament. Such a tear usually occurs when an athlete pivots
quickly on one leg in order to change direction. At the
moment of injury, the person often hears a pop from the knee,
and within about two hours the knee typically becomes severely swollen due to bleeding within the joint.

The surgical procedure to repair a torn ligament may
involve reattaching the injured part. However, if the ligament has been extensively damaged, it may be replaced by
substituting a ligament from a cadaver, an artificial ligament,
or a piece of ligament from another location. For example,
to repair a torn anterior cruciate ligament of the knee, a piece
of the individual's patellar ligament may be removed and attached in place of the damaged ligament.

FIGURE 7.23

Ligaments within the knee joint help to strengthen it.
(a) Anterior view; (b) posterior view.

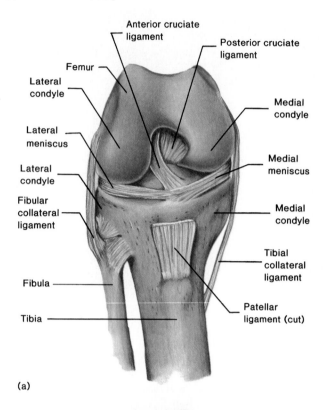

(a)

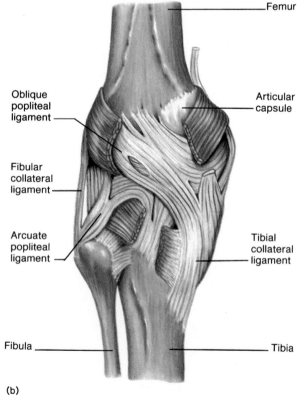

(b)

Between the articulating surfaces of the femur and tibia are two fibrocartilaginous *menisci.* Each meniscus is roughly C-shaped, with a thick rim and thin center, and is attached to the head of the tibia. The medial and lateral menisci form depressions that fit the corresponding condyles of the femur, thus compensating for the differences in shapes between the surfaces of the femur and tibia (figure 7.22).

Another common type of injury to the knee involves tearing or displacing a meniscus. Usually this occurs as a result of forcefully twisting the knee when the leg is flexed. Since the meniscus is composed of fibrocartilage, such an injury is likely to heal very slowly. Also, if a torn and displaced portion of cartilage becomes jammed between the articulating surfaces, movement of the joint may be impeded (ankylosis).

Magnetic resonance imaging has become an important technique for visualizing the menisci and assessing damage to them. (See figure 1.20)

Following such a knee injury, the synovial membrane may become inflamed (acute synovitis) and secrete fluid excessively. As a result, the joint cavity becomes distended. In this condition, the knee usually appears enlarged above and on the sides of the patella.

Several bursae are associated with the knee joint. These include a large extension of the knee joint cavity called the *suprapatellar bursa,* located between the anterior surface of the lower part of the femur and the muscle group (quadriceps femoris) above it; a large *prepatellar bursa,* between the patella and the skin; and a smaller *infrapatellar bursa,* between the upper part of the tibia and the patellar ligament. (See figure 7.22.)

As with a hinge joint, the basic structure of the knee joint permits flexion and extension. However, when the knee is flexed, rotation is also possible.

A patient with severe pain and loss of knee joint function as a result of rheumatoid arthritis or osteoarthritis may receive a knee replacement. During this surgical procedure called *total knee arthroplasty,* the damaged surfaces of the distal femur are removed and replaced with a smooth-surfaced metallic device. Similarly, the proximal surface of the tibia is removed and replaced by a device consisting of low-friction polyethelene attached to a metal plate. The metallic parts of these devices are connected to the bones by means of pegs, screws, or bone cement.

1. What ligaments help keep the articulating surfaces of the hip together?
2. What types of movement does the structure of the hip permit?
3. What types of joints are included within the knee?
4. What ligaments help hold the articulating surfaces of the knee together?

Disorders of Joints

Joints are subjected to considerable stress because they are used so frequently. They must provide for a great variety of body movements and some of them must support body weight. Injuries such as dislocations and sprains occur commonly during strenuous physical activity. In addition, joints may be affected by inflammation as well as by a number of degenerative diseases such as arthritis.

Dislocation

A *dislocation* (luxation) involves the displacement of the articulating bones of a joint. This condition usually occurs as the result of a fall or some other unusual body movement. The joints of the shoulders, knees, elbows, fingers, and jaw are common sites for such an injury. A dislocation is characterized by an obvious deformity of the joint, some loss of ability to move the parts involved, localized pain, and swelling. It presents a severe physical problem and requires medical attention (figure 7.24).

Sprains

Sprains are the result of overstretching or tearing the connective tissues, ligaments, and tendons associated with a joint, but without dislocating the articular bones. Usually sprains are caused by forceful wrenching or twisting movements involving joints of the wrists or ankles. For example, the ankle may be sprained if it is inverted excessively when running or jumping, causing the ligaments on its lateral surface to be stretched. In severe injuries, these tissues may be pulled loose from their attachments. A sprained joint is likely to be painful, swollen, and movement at the joint may be restricted. The immediate treatment for a sprain is rest; more serious cases require medical attention. However, immobilization of a joint, for even a short period, results in resorption of bone tissue and weakening of ligaments. Consequently, following such treatment, exercises may be needed to strengthen the joint.

Bursitis

Bursitis is an inflammation of a bursa, which may be caused by excessive use of a joint or by stress on a bursa. For example, the bursa between the heel bone (calcaneus) and the calcaneal (Achilles) tendon, may become inflamed as a result of a sudden increase in physical activity involving use of the feet. Similarly, a form of bursitis called "tennis elbow" involves the bursa between the olecranon process and the skin. Generally, bursitis is treated with rest, although severe cases may require medication prescribed by a physician.

Arthritis

Arthritis is a disease condition that causes inflamed, swollen, and painful joints. Although there are several types of arthritis, the most prevalent forms are rheumatoid arthritis and osteoarthritis.

Rheumatoid arthritis (RA) is the most painful and potentially crippling of the arthritic diseases. In this type, the syno-

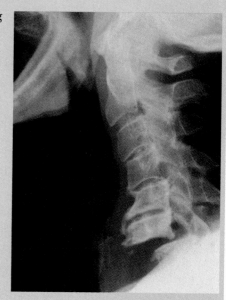

FIGURE 7.24
X-ray film showing a dislocated joint of a cervical vertebra.

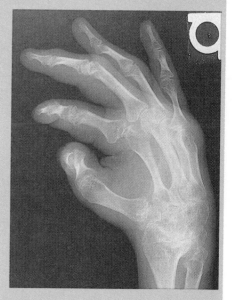

FIGURE 7.25
An X-ray film of a hand, showing changes caused by arthritis.

vial membrane of a freely movable joint becomes inflamed and grows thicker, forming a mass called a *pannus*. This change is usually followed by damage to the articular cartilages of the joint and by an invasion of the joint by fibrous tissues. These tissues interfere increasingly with joint movements, and, in time, they may become ossified so that the articulating bones become fused together (bony ankylosis). (See figure 7.25.)

Continued on next page

Rheumatoid arthritis may affect only a few joints or many joints. It may be accompanied by the development of other disorders, including anemia, osteoporosis, and muscular atrophy, as well as abnormal changes in the skin, eyes, lungs, blood vessels, and heart.

Osteoarthritis (degenerative joint disease) is the most common type of arthritis. It occurs as a result of aging and affects a large proportion of the population over sixty years of age. In this condition, the articular cartilages soften and disintegrate gradually so that the articular surfaces become roughened. Consequently, the joints involved are painful, and

their movement is somewhat restricted. Osteoarthritis is most likely to affect joints that have received the greatest use over a person's lifetime, such as those of the fingers, hips, knees, and the lower regions of the vertebral column. Other factors that seem to increase the chance of developing osteoarthritis include joint injuries and excess body weight.

As a rule, osteoarthritis develops relatively slowly, and its symptoms may be controlled by medications. In more severe cases, joint functions are disrupted and parts of joints may need to be replaced surgically.

Clinical Terms Related to Joints

ankylosis (ang″ki-lo′sis) loss of mobility of a joint.

arthralgia (ar-thral′je-ah) pain in a joint.

arthrocentesis (ar″thro-sen-te′sis) puncture and removal of fluid from a joint cavity.

arthrodesis (ar″thro-de′sis) surgery performed to fuse the bones at a joint.

arthrogram (ar′thro-gram) X-ray film of a joint after an injection of radiopaque fluid into the joint cavity.

arthrology (ar-throl′o-je) study of joints and the diseases involving them.

arthropathy (ar-throp′ah-the) any joint disease.

arthroplasty (ar′thro-plas″te) surgery performed to make a joint more movable.

arthroscopy (ar-thros′ko-pe) examination of the interior of a joint using a tubular instrument called an arthroscope.

arthrostomy (ar-thros′to-me) surgical opening of a joint to allow fluid drainage.

arthrotomy (ar-throt′o-me) surgical incision of a joint.

gout (gowt) metabolic disease in which excessive uric acid in the blood is deposited in joints, causing them to become inflamed, swollen, and painful.

hemarthrosis (hem″ar-thro′sis) blood in a joint cavity.

hydrarthrosis (hi″drar-thro′sis) accumulation of fluid within a joint cavity.

luxation (luk-sa′shun) dislocation of a joint.

subluxation (sub″luk-sa′shun) partial dislocation of a joint.

synovectomy (sin″o-vek′to-me) the surgical removal of the synovial membrane of a joint.

Chapter Summary

Introduction (page 190)

1. A joint is formed wherever two or more bones meet.
2. Joints are the functional junctions between bones.

Classification of Joints (page 190)

Joints can be classified according to structure and to the amount of movement they permit.

1. Fibrous joints
   a. Bones at fibrous joints are fastened tightly together by a layer of fibrous connective tissue.
   b. Little or no movement occurs at a fibrous joint.
   c. There are three types of fibrous joints.
      (1) A syndesmosis is characterized by bones bound by relatively long fibers of connective tissue.
      (2) A suture occurs where flat bones are united by a thin layer of connective tissue and become interlocked by a set of bony processes.
      (3) A gomphosis is created by the union of a cone-shaped bony process in a bony socket.
2. Cartilaginous joints
   a. Bones of cartilaginous joints are held together by a layer of cartilage.
   b. There are two types of cartilaginous joints.
      (1) A synchondrosis is characterized by bones united by hyaline cartilage that disappears as a result of growth.
      (2) A symphysis is a joint whose articular surfaces are covered by hyaline cartilage and attached to a pad of fibrocartilage.
3. Synovial joints
   a. Synovial joints have a more complex structure than other types of joints.
   b. These joints include articular cartilage, a joint capsule, and a synovial membrane.

General Structure of a Synovial Joint (page 192)

1. The articular ends of bones are covered by a layer of cartilage called articular cartilage.
2. The articular cartilage lies on a layer of spongy bone called a subchondral plate.
3. The bones are held together by a joint capsule that is strengthened by ligaments.
4. The inner layer of the joint capsule is lined by a synovial membrane that secretes synovial fluid.
5. Synovial fluid moistens and lubricates the articular surfaces.

6. Some synovial joints are divided into compartments by menisci.
7. Some synovial joints have fluid-filled bursae.
   a. Bursae are usually located between the skin and underlying bony prominences.
   b. Bursae act as cushions and aid the movement of tendons over bony parts.
   c. Bursae are named according to their locations.

Types of Synovial Joints (page 194)

1. Ball-and-socket joints
   a. In this type of joint, a globular head of a bone fits into a cup-shaped cavity of another.
   b. These joints permit a wide variety of movements.
   c. The hip and shoulder joints are ball-and-socket joints.
2. Condyloid joints
   a. A condyloid joint consists of an ovoid condyle of one bone that fits into an elliptical cavity of another.
   b. This joint permits a variety of movements.
   c. The joints between the metacarpals and phalanges are condyloid.
3. Gliding joints
   a. Articular surfaces of gliding joints are nearly flat.
   b. These joints permit the articular surfaces to slide back and forth.
   c. Most of the joints of the wrist and ankle are gliding joints.
4. Hinge joints
   a. In a hinge joint, a convex surface of one bone fits into a concave surface of another.
   b. This joint permits movement in one plane only.
   c. The elbow and the joints of the phalanges are of the hinge type.
5. Pivot joints
   a. In a pivot joint, a cylindrical surface of one bone rotates within a ring of bone or fibrous tissue.
   b. This joint permits rotational movement.
   c. The articulation between the proximal ends of the radius and ulna is a pivot joint.
6. Saddle joints
   a. A saddle joint is formed between bones that have complementary surfaces with both concave and convex regions.
   b. This joint permits a variety of movements.
   c. The articulation between the carpal and metacarpal of the thumb is a saddle joint.

Types of Joint Movements (page 196)

1. Muscles acting at synovial joints produce movements in different directions and in different planes.
2. Joint movements include: flexion, extension, hyperextension, dorsiflexion, plantar flexion, abduction, adduction, rotation, circumduction, supination, pronation, eversion, inversion, elevation, depression, protraction, and retraction.

Examples of Synovial Joints (page 200)

1. Intervertebral joints
   a. The synovial joints between articular processes are gliding joints.
   b. An articular capsule surrounds each intervertebral synovial joint.
   c. Several ligaments connect the parts of adjacent vertebrae.
   d. Movement between any two vertebrae is limited, but the whole vertebral column demonstrates great flexibility.
2. The shoulder joint
   a. The shoulder joint is a ball-and-socket joint that consists of the head of the humerus and the glenoid cavity of the scapula.
   b. A cylindrical joint capsule envelopes the joint.
      (1) The capsule is loose and by itself cannot keep the articular surfaces together.
      (2) It is reinforced by surrounding muscles and tendons.
   c. Several ligaments help to prevent displacement of bones.
   d. There are several bursae associated with the shoulder joint.
   e. Because its parts are loosely attached, the shoulder joint permits a wide range of movements.
3. The elbow joint
   a. The elbow includes a hinge joint between the humerus and the ulna, and a gliding joint between the humerus and radius.
   b. The joint capsule is reinforced by collateral ligaments.
   c. A synovial membrane partially divides the joint cavity into two portions.
   d. The joint between the humerus and ulna permits flexion and extension only.
4. The hip joint
   a. The hip joint is a ball-and-socket joint between the femur and the coxal bone.
   b. A ring of fibrocartilage deepens the cavity of the acetabulum.
   c. The articular surfaces are held together by a heavy joint capsule that is reinforced by ligaments.
   d. The hip joint permits a wide variety of movements.
5. The knee joint
   a. The knee joint includes two condyloid joints between the femur and tibia, and a gliding joint between the femur and patella.
   b. The joint capsule is relatively thin, but is strengthened by ligaments and tendons.
   c. Several ligaments, some of which are within the joint capsule, help keep the articular surfaces together.
   d. Two menisci separate the articulating surfaces of the femur and tibia, and help compensate for differences in the shapes of these surfaces.
   e. Several bursae are associated with the knee joint.
   f. The knee joint permits flexion and extension; when the leg is flexed at the knee, some rotation is possible.

Clinical Application of Knowledge

1. How would you explain to an athlete why damaged joint ligaments and cartilages are so slow to heal following an injury?
2. Compared to the shoulder and hip joints, in what way is the knee joint poorly protected and thus especially vulnerable to injuries?
3. Based on your knowledge of joint structures, which do you think could be most satisfactorily replaced by a prosthetic device—a hip joint or a knee joint? Why?
4. If a patient's lower arm and elbow were immobilized by a cast for several weeks, what changes would you expect to occur in the bones and joints of the arm?
5. Why is it important to encourage an inactive patient to keep all joints mobile, even if it is necessary to have another person move the joints (passive movement)?
6. How would you explain to a person with a dislocated shoulder that the shoulder is likely to become dislocated more easily in the future?

Review Activities

Part A

1. Define *joint.*
2. Explain how joints are classified.
3. Compare the structure of a fibrous joint with that of a cartilaginous joint.
4. Distinguish between a syndesmosis and a suture.
5. Describe a gomphosis and name an example.
6. Compare the structures of a synchondrosis and a symphysis.
7. Explain how the joints between adjacent vertebrae permit movement.
8. Describe the general structure of a synovial joint.
9. Describe how a joint capsule may be reinforced.
10. Explain the function of the synovial membrane.
11. Explain the function of synovial fluid.
12. Define *meniscus.*
13. Describe the general locations of bursae.
14. List six types of synovial joints and name an example of each type.
15. Describe the movements permitted by each type of synovial joint.
16. Identify the ligaments associated with the intervertebral joints.
17. What types of movements are permitted by the vertebral column?
18. Name the parts that comprise the shoulder joint.
19. Name the major ligaments associated with the shoulder joint.
20. Explain why the shoulder joint permits a wide range of movements.
21. Name the parts that comprise the elbow joint.
22. Describe the locations of the major ligaments associated with the elbow joint.
23. Name the movements permitted by the elbow joint.
24. Name the parts that comprise the hip joint.
25. Describe how the articular surfaces of the hip joint are held together.
26. Explain why there is less freedom of movement in the hip joint than in the shoulder joint.
27. Name the parts that comprise the knee joint.
28. Describe the major ligaments associated with the knee joint.
29. Explain the function of the menisci of the knee.
30. Describe the locations of the bursae associated with the knee joint.

Part B
Match the movements in column I with the descriptions in column II.

	I		II
1.	Rotation	A.	Turning the palm upward
2.	Supination	B.	Bending the leg at the knee
3.	Extension	C.	Bending the foot upward
4.	Eversion	D.	Turning the head to one side
5.	Dorsiflexion	E.	Turning the sole of the foot outward
6.	Flexion	F.	Straightening the arm at the elbow
7.	Pronation	G.	Lowering the shoulders
8.	Abduction	H.	Turning the palm downward
9.	Depression	I.	Moving the arm away from

CHAPTER 8

The Muscular System

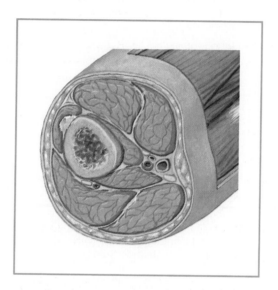

Muscles, the organs of the *muscular system*, consist largely of cells that are specialized to undergo contractions. When skeletal muscle cells contract, they pull on the body parts to which they are attached. This action usually causes movement, as when joints of the legs are flexed and extended during walking. But at other times, muscular contractions resist motion, as when they help to hold body parts in postural positions.

Chapter Outline

Chapter Objectives

After you have studied this chapter, you should be able to

1. Describe how connective tissue is included in the structure of a skeletal muscle.

2. Explain the anatomical relationship between motor nerve fibers and muscle fibers.

3. Explain how the locations of skeletal muscles are related to the movements they produce and how muscles interact to produce such movements.

4. Identify and describe the locations of the major skeletal muscles of each body region and describe the action of each muscle.

5. Complete the review activities at the end of this chapter. Note that the items are worded in the form of specific learning objectives. You may want to refer to them before reading the chapter.

Aids to Understanding Words

erg-, work: syn*erg*ist—muscle that works together with a prime mover to produce a movement.

fasc-, a bundle: *fasc*iculus—a bundle of muscle fibers.

fasci-, band: *fasci*a—layer or band of connective tissue that surrounds a skeletal muscle.

myo-, muscle: *myo*logy—the study of muscles.

syn-, together: *syn*ergist—muscle that works together with a prime mover to produce a movement.

voluntar-, of one's free will: *voluntary* muscle—muscle that can be controlled by conscious effort.

Introduction

There are three types of muscle tissues: skeletal muscle, smooth muscle, and cardiac muscle, as described in chapter 4. This chapter, however, is concerned with skeletal muscle, the type found in muscles that usually are attached to bones and are under conscious control (voluntary muscles).

Structure of a Skeletal Muscle

A skeletal muscle is an organ of the muscular system and is composed of several kinds of tissue. These include skeletal muscle tissue, nerve tissue, blood, and various connective tissues.

Connective Tissue Coverings

An individual skeletal muscle is separated from adjacent muscles and held in position by layers of fibrous connective tissue called **fascia.** This connective tissue surrounds each muscle and may project beyond the end of its muscle fibers to form a cordlike **tendon.** Fibers in a tendon intertwine with those in the periosteum of a bone, thus attaching the muscle to the bone. In other cases, the connective tissues associated with a muscle form broad, fibrous sheets called **aponeuroses,** which may be attached to the coverings of adjacent muscles (figure 8.1).

A tendon or the connective tissue sheath of a tendon (tenosynovium) may become painfully inflamed and swollen following an injury or the repeated stress of athletic activity. These conditions are called *tendinitis* and *tenosynovitis*, respectively. The tendons most commonly affected by tendinitis are those associated with the joint capsules of the shoulder, elbow, and hip, and those involved with moving the wrist, hand, thigh, and foot.

The layer of connective tissue that closely surrounds a skeletal muscle is called the *epimysium.* Other layers of connective tissue, called the *perimysium,* extend inward from the epimysium and separate the muscle tissue into small sections. These sections contain bundles of skeletal muscle fibers called *fascicles* (fasciculi). Each muscle fiber within a fascicle (fasciculus) is surrounded by a layer of connective tissue in the form of a thin, delicate covering called the *endomysium* (figure 8.2).

Thus, all parts of a skeletal muscle are enclosed in layers of connective tissue. This arrangement allows the parts to move independently. Also, numerous blood vessels and nerves pass through these layers (figure 8.3).

The fascia associated with the individual organs of the muscular system is part of a complex network of fasciae that extends throughout the body. The portion of the network that surrounds and penetrates the muscles is called *deep fascia.* Additional layers surround groups of muscles

FIGURE 8.1

Various connective tissues attach skeletal muscles to bones or to other muscles.

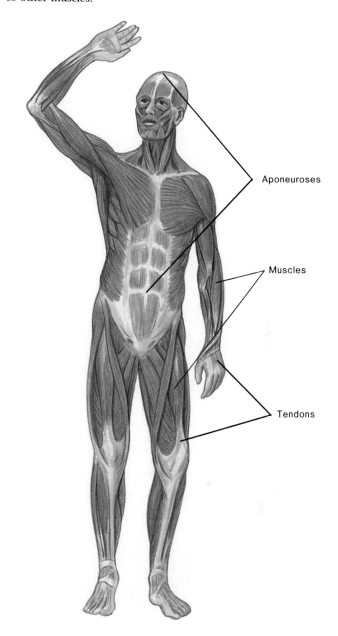

Aponeuroses

Muscles

Tendons

forming units called *compartments.* The deep fascia also includes bands of connective tissue that help hold tendons close to bones. At various places, the deep fascia is attached to the *superficial fascia,* which is also called the subcutaneous layer—a layer of adipose and loose connective tissue just beneath the skin. The network is also continuous with the *subserous fascia* that forms the connective tissue layer of the serous membranes covering organs in various body cavities and lining those cavities (see chapter 5).

FIGURE 8.2

(a) A skeletal muscle is composed of a variety of tissues, including layers of connective tissue. (b) Fascia covers the surface of the muscle, epimysium lies beneath the fascia, and perimysium extends into the structure of the muscle and separates muscle cells into fascicles. (c) Individual muscle fibers are separated by endomysium.

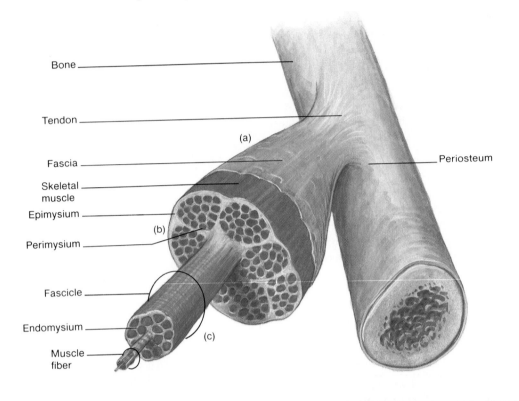

FIGURE 8.3

Scanning electron micrograph of a rat's eye muscle surrounded by its connective tissue sheath, the epimysium (×215).
R. G. Kessel and R. H. Kardon, *Tissues and Organs: A Text Atlas of Scanning Electron Microscopy,* © 1979, W. H. Freeman & Co.

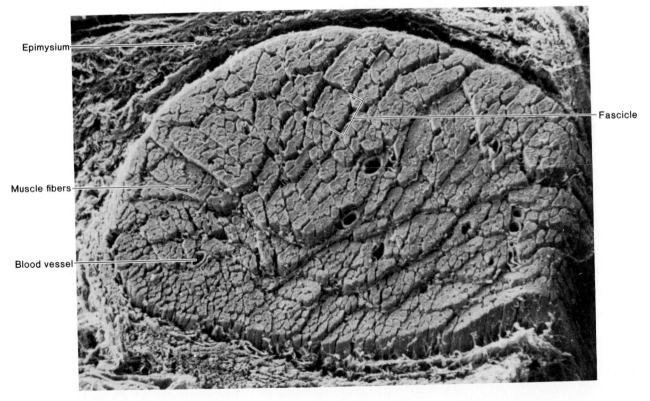

FIGURE 8.4

(*a*) A neuromuscular junction includes the end of a motor neuron and the motor end plate of a muscle fiber; (*b*) micrograph of a neuromuscular junction.

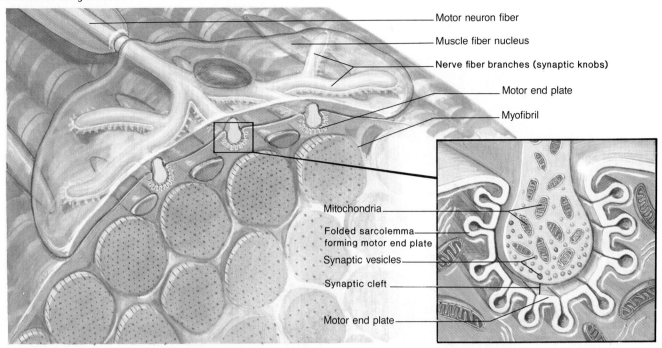

(a)

The space occupied by a particular group of muscles, blood vessels, and nerves and tightly enclosed by relatively inelastic fascia constitutes a *compartment.* There are many such spaces in the arms and legs. If an injury causes fluid, such as blood from an internal hemorrhage, to accumulate within a compartment, the pressure inside will rise. The increased pressure, in turn, may interfere with blood flow into the region, thus reducing the supply of oxygen and nutrients to the affected tissues. This condition, called *compartment syndrome,* often produces severe, unrelenting pain, and if the compartmental pressure remains elevated, the enclosed muscles and nerves may be irreversibly damaged.

Treatment for compartment syndrome may involve making a surgical incision through the fascia (fasciotomy) to relieve the excessive pressure and restore the circulation of blood.

1. What types of tissues make up a skeletal muscle?
2. Describe how connective tissue is associated with a skeletal muscle.

The Neuromuscular Junction

Each skeletal muscle fiber is a single cell of a skeletal muscle. A muscle fiber responds to a stimulus from a nerve cell (neuron) by contracting and then relaxing. Long extensions of nerve cells called *nerve fibers* reach to every muscle fiber. These nerve fibers are extensions of **motor neurons** that pass outward from the brain or spinal cord. Usually, a skeletal muscle fiber will contract only when it is stimulated by the action of a motor neuron.

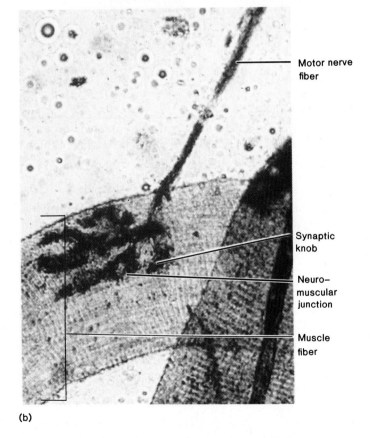

(b)

The site where a nerve fiber and muscle fiber meet is called a **neuromuscular junction** (myoneural junction). At this junction, the muscle fiber membrane is specialized to form a **motor end plate.** In this region of a muscle fiber, nuclei and mitochondria are abundant and the sarcolemma is extensively folded (figure 8.4).

FIGURE 8.5

A motor unit consists of one motor neuron and all the muscle fibers with which it communicates.

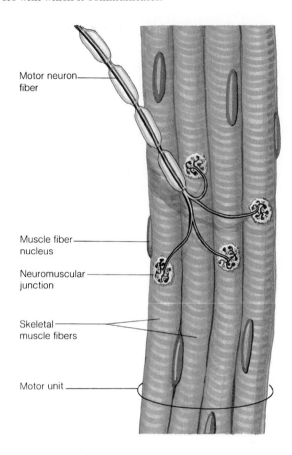

Motor neuron fiber

Muscle fiber nucleus

Neuromuscular junction

Skeletal muscle fibers

Motor unit

The distal portion of a motor nerve fiber divides into many short branches, which have tiny enlargements called *synaptic knobs* at their terminal ends. Each of these projects into a depression, called the *synaptic cleft,* formed by the motor end plate. The knobs come very close to the motor end plate but do not make direct contact with it. The cytoplasm at the end of a synaptic knob contains many mitochondria and tiny *synaptic vesicles.* These vesicles store chemicals called *neurotransmitters* (such as acetylcholine).

When a nerve impulse traveling from the brain or spinal cord reaches the terminal end of a motor nerve fiber, some of the synaptic vesicles release a neurotransmitter into the synaptic cleft. This action stimulates the muscle fiber to contract.

Motor Units

Motor nerve fibers are densely branched. By means of these branches, one motor nerve fiber may be connected to many muscle fibers. Furthermore, when a motor nerve fiber transmits an impulse, all of the muscle fibers connected to it are stimulated to contract simultaneously. Together, a motor neuron and the muscle fibers it controls constitute a **motor unit** (figure 8.5).

The number of muscle fibers in a motor unit varies considerably. The fewer muscle fibers in the motor units, however, the finer the movements that can be produced in a particular muscle. For example, the motor units of the muscles that move the eyes may contain fewer than ten muscle fibers per motor unit and can produce very slight movements. Conversely, the motor units of the large muscles in the back may include a hundred or more muscle fibers. When these motor units are stimulated, the movements produced are coarse in comparison with those of the eye muscles.

If some of the motor nerve fibers innervating a muscle are lost due to injury or disease, their motor units become paralyzed. However, branches from remaining uninjured nerve fibers may grow to join the paralyzed muscle fibers, creating new motor units that have several times the usual number of muscle fibers. As a result, some muscular functions may be restored, although the degree of control over the muscle fibers is diminished.

1. Describe a neuromuscular junction.
2. Define a motor unit.

Skeletal Muscle Actions

Skeletal muscles are responsible for a great variety of body movements. The action of each muscle—that is, the movement it causes—depends largely upon the kind of joint it is associated with and the way it is attached on either side of that joint.

Origin and Insertion

One end of a skeletal muscle is usually fastened to a relatively immovable or fixed part, and the other end is connected to a movable part on the other side of a joint. The immovable end is called the **origin** of the muscle, and the movable one is its **insertion.** When a muscle contracts, its insertion is pulled toward its origin (figure 8.6).

Some muscles have more than one origin or insertion. The *biceps brachii* in the upper arm, for example, has two origins. This is reflected in its name, *biceps,* which means *two heads.* (Note: The head of a muscle is the part nearest the origin.) As figure 8.6 shows, one head is attached to the coracoid process of the scapula, and the other arises from a tubercle above the glenoid cavity of the scapula. The muscle extends along the anterior surface of the humerus and is inserted by means of a tendon on the radial tuberosity of the radius. When the biceps brachii contracts, its insertion is pulled toward its origin, and the arm bends at the elbow.

Use and Disuse of Skeletal Muscles

Skeletal muscles are very responsive to use and disuse. For example, those that are forcefully exercised tend to enlarge. This phenomenon is called *muscular hypertrophy*. Conversely, a muscle that is not used undergoes *atrophy*—that is, it decreases in size and strength.

The way a muscle responds to use also depends on the type of exercise involved. For instance, when a muscle contracts relatively weakly as occurs during swimming and running exercises, its fatigue-resistant red fibers are most likely to be activated. As a result, these fibers develop more mitochondria, and more extensive capillary networks develop around the fibers. Such changes increase the fibers' abilities to resist fatigue during prolonged periods of exercise, although their sizes and strengths may remain unchanged.

Forceful exercise, such as weightlifting, in which a muscle exerts more than 75% of its maximum tension involves the muscle's fatigable white fibers. In response, existing muscle fibers develop new filaments, and as their diameters increase, the whole muscle enlarges. However, no new muscle fibers are produced during hypertrophy.

Since the strength of a contraction is directly related to the diameter of the muscle fibers, an enlarged muscle is capable of producing stronger contractions than before. However, such a change does not increase the muscle's ability to resist fatigue during activities such as running or swimming.

If exercise is discontinued, there is a reduction in the capillary networks and in the number of mitochondria within the muscle fibers. Also the number of filaments decreases and the entire muscle atrophies. Such atrophy commonly occurs when limbs are immobilized by casts, or when accidents or diseases interfere with motor nerve impulses. A muscle that cannot be exercised may decrease to less than one-half its usual size within a few months.

The fibers of muscles whose motor neurons are severed not only decrease in size, but may also become fragmented and, in time, may be replaced by fat or fibrous connective tissue. However, if such a muscle is reinnervated within the first few months following an injury, its function may be restored. Meanwhile, atrophy may be delayed by treatments in which electrical stimulation is used to cause muscular contractions against loads.

FIGURE 8.6

The biceps brachii has two heads that originate on the scapula. This muscle is inserted on the radius by means of a tendon. What movement results as this muscle contracts?

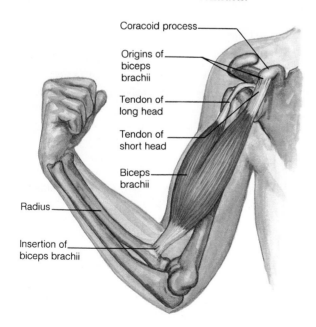

Coracoid process

Origins of biceps brachii

Tendon of long head

Tendon of short head

Biceps brachii

Radius

Insertion of biceps brachii

Sometimes the end of a muscle changes its function in different body movements; that is, the origin may become the insertion or vice versa. For instance, a large muscle in the chest, the *pectoralis major*, connects the humerus to bones of the thorax. If the arm moves across the chest, the end of the muscle attached to the humerus acts as the insertion. When a person hangs from a bar to do chinning exercises, however, the arm becomes fixed and the body is pulled up. In this movement, the end attached to the humerus acts as the origin.

Similarly, the *latissimus dorsi* muscle in the back has its origin on the pelvic girdle and vertebral column and its insertion on the proximal end of the humerus. Usually it functions to pull the arm toward the back, as when rowing a boat or swimming. During chinning exercises, however, the end attached to the humerus becomes the origin of the muscle, and the end attached to the pelvis and vertebral column moves.

Interaction of Skeletal Muscles

Skeletal muscles almost always function in groups rather than singly. Consequently, when a particular body movement occurs, a person must do more than cause a single muscle to contract; instead, that person decides which movement will occur, and the appropriate group of muscles responds to the decision.

By carefully observing body movements, it is possible to determine the particular roles of various muscles. For instance, when the arm is lifted horizontally away from the side, a *deltoid* muscle is responsible for most of the movement and so is said to be the **prime mover.** However, while the prime mover is acting, certain nearby muscles are also contracting. They help hold the shoulder steady and in this way make the action of the prime mover more effective. Muscles that assist the prime mover are called **synergists.**

Still other muscles act as **antagonists** to prime movers. These muscles are capable of resisting a prime mover's action and are responsible for movement in the opposite direction—the antagonist of the prime mover that raises the arm can lower the arm, or the antagonist of the prime mover that bends the arm can straighten it. If both a prime mover and its antagonist contract simultaneously, the part they act upon remains rigid. Consequently, smooth body movements depend upon the antagonists relaxing when the prime movers are contracting. These complex actions are controlled by the nervous system.

Sometimes a skeletal muscle contracts but the parts to which it is attached do not move. This happens, for instance, when a person pushes against the wall of a building. Tension within the muscles increases, but the wall does not move, and the muscles remain the same length. Contractions of this type are called *isometric.* Isometric contractions occur continuously in postural muscles that function to stabilize skeletal parts and hold the body upright.

At other times, muscles shorten when they contract. For example, if a person lifts an object, the tautness in the muscles remains unchanged, their attached ends pull closer together, and the object is moved. This type of contraction is termed *isotonic.* Figure 8.7 illustrates these two types of contraction.

Skeletal muscles can contract either isometrically or isotonically, and most body actions involve both types of contraction. In walking, for instance, certain leg muscles contract isometrically and keep the limb stiff as it touches the ground, while other muscles contract isotonically, causing the leg to bend and lift upward.

FIGURE 8.7

(*a*) Isotonic contractions occur when a muscle contracts and shortens; (*b*) isometric contractions occur when a muscle contracts, but does not shorten.

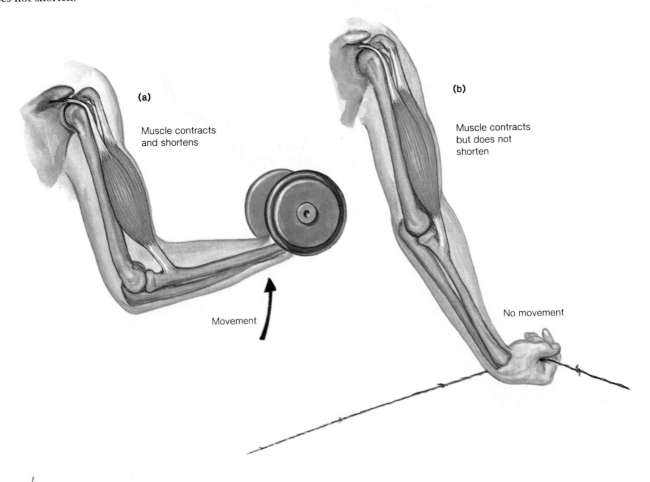

(a)

Muscle contracts and shortens

Movement

(b)

Muscle contracts but does not shorten

No movement

Major Skeletal Muscles

The following section concerns the locations, actions, and attachments of some of the major skeletal muscles of the body. (Figures 8.8 and 8.9 show the locations of superficial skeletal muscles—that is, those near the surface.) Notice that the names of these muscles often describe them in some way. A name may indicate a muscle's size, shape, lo-

cation, action, number of attachments, or the direction of its fibers, as in the following examples:

Pectoralis major a muscle of large size (*major*) located in the pectoral region or chest.

Deltoid shaped like a delta or triangle.

Extensor digitorum acts to extend the digits (fingers or toes).

Biceps brachii a muscle with two heads (*biceps*), or points of origin, and located in the brachium or arm.

Sternocleidomastoid attached to the sternum, clavicle, and mastoid process.

External oblique located near the outside, with fibers that run obliquely or in a slanting direction.

FIGURE 8.8
Anterior view of superficial skeletal muscles.

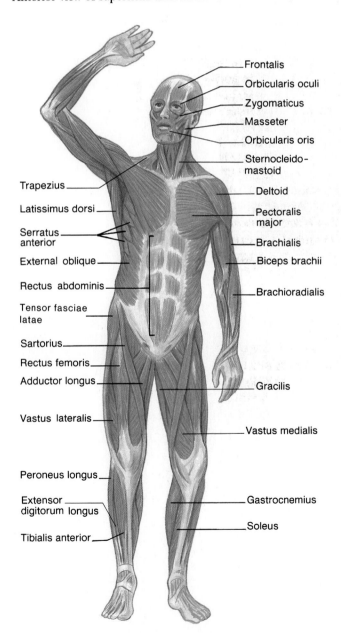

Frontalis
Orbicularis oculi
Zygomaticus
Masseter
Orbicularis oris
Sternocleido-mastoid
Deltoid
Pectoralis major
Brachialis
Biceps brachii
Brachioradialis
Gracilis
Vastus medialis
Gastrocnemius
Soleus

Trapezius
Latissimus dorsi
Serratus anterior
External oblique
Rectus abdominis
Tensor fasciae latae
Sartorius
Rectus femoris
Adductor longus
Vastus lateralis
Peroneus longus
Extensor digitorum longus
Tibialis anterior

FIGURE 8.9
Posterior view of superficial skeletal muscles.

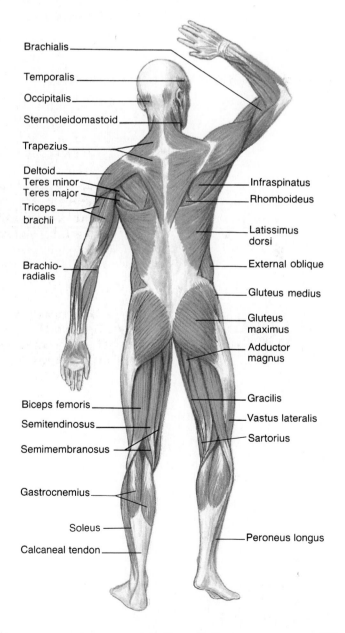

Brachialis
Temporalis
Occipitalis
Sternocleidomastoid
Trapezius
Deltoid
Teres minor
Teres major
Triceps brachii
Brachio-radialis
Biceps femoris
Semitendinosus
Semimembranosus
Gastrocnemius
Soleus
Calcaneal tendon

Infraspinatus
Rhomboideus
Latissimus dorsi
External oblique
Gluteus medius
Gluteus maximus
Adductor magnus
Gracilis
Vastus lateralis
Sartorius
Peroneus longus

Muscles of Facial Expression

A number of small muscles that lie beneath the skin of the face and scalp enable us to communicate feelings through facial expression. Many of these muscles are located around the eyes and mouth, and they are responsible for expressions such as surprise, sadness, anger, fear, disgust, and pain. As a group, the muscles of facial expression connect the bones of the skull to connective tissue in various regions of the overlying skin. They include the following (figure 8.10 and chart 8.1):

Epicranius
Orbicularis oculi
Orbicularis oris
Buccinator
Zygomaticus
Platysma

FIGURE 8.10

(*a*) Muscles of expression and mastication; isolated views of (*b*) the temporalis and buccinator, and (*c*) the lateral and medial pterygoid muscles.

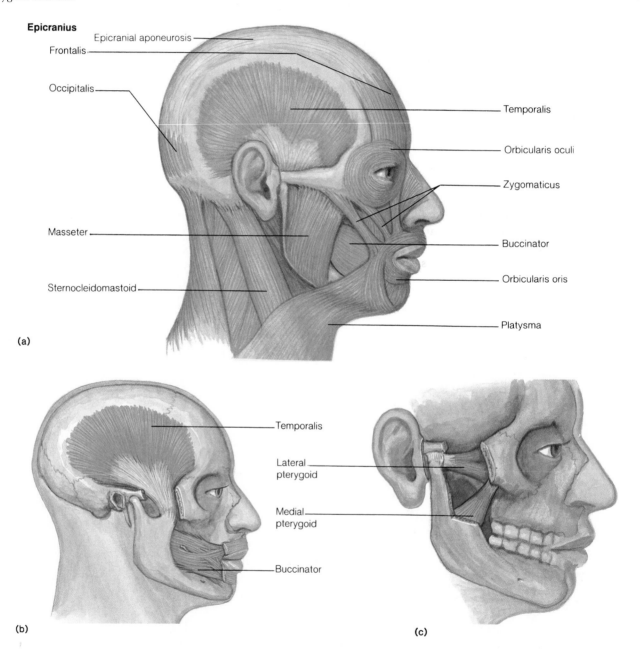

Chart 8.1 Muscles of facial expression

Muscle	Origin	Insertion	Action	Innervation*
Epicranius	Occipital bone	Skin and muscles around eye	Raises eyebrow, as when surprised	Facial n.
Orbicularis oculi	Maxillary and frontal bones	Skin around eye	Closes eye, as in blinking	Facial n.
Orbicularis oris	Muscles near the mouth	Skin of central lip	Closes lips, protrudes lips, as in kissing	Facial n.
Buccinator	Outer surfaces of maxilla and mandible	Orbicularis oris	Compresses cheeks inward, as in blowing air	Facial n.
Zygomaticus	Zygomatic bone	Orbicularis oris	Raises corner of mouth, as in smiling	Facial n.
Platysma	Fascia in upper chest	Lower border of mandible	Draws angle of mouth downward, as in pouting	Facial n.

*The term *innervation* refers to the nerve supply to a body part (n. stands for nerve).
Note: The nerves listed in the charts in chapter 8 are discussed in greater detail in chapter 9.

The **epicranius** (ep″ĭ-kra′ne-us) covers the upper part of the cranium and consists of two muscular parts: the *frontalis* (frun-ta′lis), which lies over the frontal bone, and the *occipitalis* (ok-sip″ĭ-ta′lis), which lies over the occipital bone. These parts are united by a broad, tendinous membrane called the *epicranial aponeurosis* (galea aponeurotica), which covers the cranium like a cap. Contraction of the epicranius raises the eyebrows and causes the skin of the forehead to wrinkle horizontally, as when a person expresses surprise. Headaches often result from sustained contraction of this muscle.

The **orbicularis oculi** (or-bik′u-la-rus ok′u-li) is a ring-like band of muscle, called a *sphincter muscle*, that surrounds the eye. It lies in the subcutaneous tissue of the eyelid and causes the eye to close or blink. At the same time, it compresses the nearby tear gland, or *lacrimal gland*, aiding the flow of tears over the surface of the eye. Contraction of the orbicularis oculi also creates the folds, or crow's feet, that radiate laterally from the corner of the eye.

The **orbicularis oris** (or-bik′u-la-rus o′ris) is a sphincter muscle that encircles the mouth. It lies between the skin and the mucous membranes of the lips, extending upward to the nose and downward to the region between the lower lip and chin. The orbicularis oris is sometimes called the kissing muscle because it causes the lips to close and pucker.

The **buccinator** (buk′sĭ-na″tor) is located in the wall of the cheek. Its fibers are directed forward from the bones of the jaws to the angle of the mouth, and when they contract the cheek is compressed inward. This action helps hold food in contact with the teeth when a person is chewing. The buccinator also aids in blowing air out of the mouth, and for this reason, it is sometimes called the trumpeter muscle.

The **zygomaticus** (zi″go-mat′ik-us) extends from the zygomatic arch downward to the corner of the mouth. When it contracts, the corner of the mouth is drawn up, as in smiling or laughing.

The **platysma** (plah-tiz′mah) is a thin, sheetlike muscle whose fibers extend from the chest upward over the neck to the face. It functions to pull the angle of the mouth downward, as in pouting. The platysma also helps lower the mandible.

The muscles that move the eye are described in chapter 10 and shown in figure 10.27.

Muscles of Mastication and Swallowing

Chewing movements are produced by four pairs of muscles that are attached to the mandible. Three pairs of these muscles act to close the lower jaw, as in biting; the fourth pair can lower the jaw, cause side-to-side grinding motions of the mandible, and pull the mandible forward, causing it to protrude. The muscles of mastication are shown in figure 8.10 and listed in chart 8.2. They include the following:

Masseter
Temporalis
Medial pterygoid
Lateral pterygoid

The **masseter** (mas-se′ter) is a thick, flattened muscle that can be felt just in front of the ear when the teeth are clenched. Its fibers extend downward from the zygomatic arch to the mandible. The masseter functions primarily to raise the jaw, but it can also control the rate at which the jaw falls open in response to gravity.

The **temporalis** (tem-po-ra′lis) is a fan-shaped muscle located on the side of the skull above and in front of the ear. Its fibers, which also raise the jaw, pass downward beneath the zygomatic arch to the mandible.

The **medial pterygoid** (ter′-ĭ-goid) extends back and downward from the sphenoid, palatine, and maxillary bones to the ramus of the mandible. It closes the jaw.

The fibers of the **lateral pterygoid** are directed forward from the region just below the mandibular condyle

FIGURE 8.11
Anterior and lateral neck muscles.

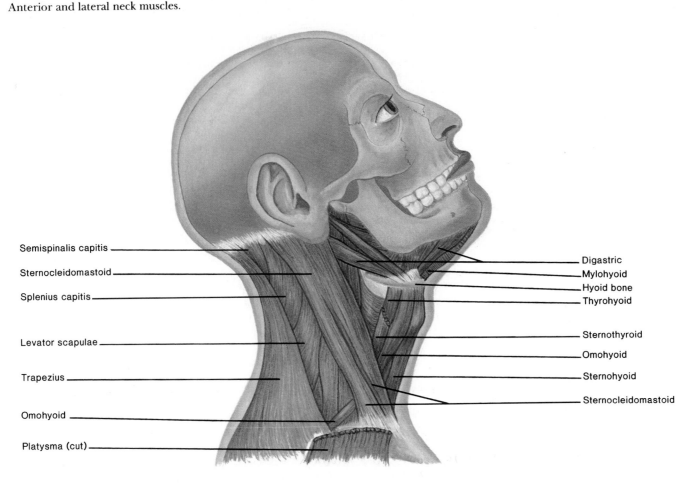

Semispinalis capitis

Sternocleidomastoid

Splenius capitis

Levator scapulae

Trapezius

Omohyoid

Platysma (cut)

Digastric
Mylohyoid
Hyoid bone
Thyrohyoid

Sternothyroid

Omohyoid

Sternohyoid

Sternocleidomastoid

to the sphenoid bone. This muscle can open the mouth, pull the mandible forward making it protrude, and move the mandible from side to side.

Sometimes an individual who is emotionally tense or has a poor bite (malocclusion) uses his or her jaw muscles to grind or clench the teeth excessively. This action may create stress on the temporomandibular joint—the articulation between the mandibular condyle of the mandible and the mandibular fossa of the temporal bone. As a result, the person may experience a variety of unpleasant symptoms, including headache, earache, and pain in the jaw, neck, or shoulder. This condition is called *temporomandibular joint syndrome* (TMJ syndrome).

The following muscles assist in the actions of swallowing. Most of these muscles are attached to the hyoid bone, which is raised during swallowing. These muscles are shown in figure 8.11 and are listed in chart 8.2. They are:

Digastric
Mylohyoid
Sternohyoid
Sternothyroid
Thyrohyoid
Omohyoid

The **digastric** (di-gas'trik) has two muscular parts that are joined by a tendon. These parts are attached to the mandible and the mastoid process of the temporal bone. A loop of connective tissue holds the tendon to the hyoid bone. This muscle depresses the mandible and elevates the hyoid bone—actions that occur during swallowing.

The **mylohyoid** (mi"lo-hi-oyd') is also attached to the mandible and the hyoid bone and forms the floor of the oral cavity. It raises the floor of the mouth and the hyoid bone during swallowing.

The **sternohyoid** (ster"no-hi-oyd') is a thin, straplike muscle that extends from the clavicle and sternum to the hyoid bone. The sternohyoid muscle lowers the hyoid bone after swallowing.

Chart 8.2 Muscles of mastication and swallowing

Muscle	Origin	Insertion	Action	Innervation	Figure
Masseter	Lower border of zygomatic arch	Lateral surface of mandible	Elevates mandible	Trigeminal n.	8.10
Temporalis	Temporal bone	Coronoid process and anterior ramus of mandible	Elevates mandible	Trigeminal n.	8.10
Medial pterygoid	Sphenoid, palatine, and maxillary bones	Medial surface of mandible	Elevates mandible	Trigeminal n.	8.10
Lateral pterygoid	Sphenoid bone	Anterior surface of mandibular condyle	Depresses and protracts mandible, and moves it from side to side	Trigeminal n.	8.10
Digastric	Mastoid process of temporal bone	Hyoid bone	Depresses mandible, and raises hyoid	Inferior alveolar and facial nerves	8.11
Mylohyoid	Mandible	Hyoid bone	Elevates floor of mouth, raises hyoid	Inferior alveolar n.	8.11
Sternohyoid	Medial end of clavicle, manubrium of sternum	Hyoid bone	Lowers hyoid	C1, 2, 3 nerves	8.11
Sternothyroid	Manubrium of sternum and costal cartilage of first rib	Thyroid gland	Pulls larynx down	C1, 2, 3 nerves	8.11
Thyrohyoid	Larynx	Hyoid bone	Lowers hyoid bone, raises larynx	Hypoglossal and C1 nerves	8.11
Omohyoid	Upper border of scapula	Hyoid bone	Lowers hyoid bone	C1, 2, 3 nerves	8.11

The **sternothyroid** (ster″no-thi-royd′) extends from the sternum and first rib to the thyroid gland and lowers the larynx after swallowing.

The **thyrohyoid** (thi-ro-hi-oyd′) is a small muscle that passes from the larynx to the hyoid bone. It lowers the hyoid bone and raises the larynx.

The **omohyoid** (o″mo-hi-oyd′) consists of two parts joined by a tendon. It extends from the scapula to the hyoid bone. A loop of fascia attached to the clavicle holds the tendon, so that the muscle forms an angle at the tendon. The omohyoid lowers the hyoid bone.

Muscles That Move the Head

Head movements result from the actions of paired muscles in the neck and upper back. These muscles are responsible for flexing, extending, and rotating the head. They are shown in figures 8.12, 8.15, and listed on chart 8.3. Muscles that move the head include the following:

Sternocleidomastoid
Splenius capitis
Semispinalis capitis
Longissimus capitis

The **sternocleidomastoid** (ster″no-kli″do-mas′toid) is a long muscle in the side of the neck that extends upward from the thorax to the base of the skull behind the ear. When the sternocleidomastoid on one side contracts, the face is turned to the opposite side. When both muscles contract, the head is bent toward the chest. If the head is fixed in position by other muscles, the sternocleidomastoids can raise the sternum—an action that aids forceful inhalation.

The **splenius capitis** (sple′ne-us kap′ĭ-tis) is a broad, straplike muscle located in the back of the neck. It connects the base of the skull to the vertebrae in the neck and upper thorax. A splenius capitis acting singly causes the head to rotate and bend toward one side. Acting together, these muscles bring the head into an upright position.

The **semispinalis capitis** (sem″e-spi-na′lis kap′ĭ-tis) is a broad, sheetlike muscle extending upward from the vertebrae in the neck and thorax to the occipital bone. It functions to extend the head, bend it to one side, or rotate it.

The **longissimus capitis** (lon-jis′ĭ-mus kap′ĭ-tis) is a narrow band of muscle that ascends from the vertebrae of the neck and thorax to the temporal bone. It also functions to extend the head, bend it to one side, or rotate it.

FIGURE 8.12
Deep muscles of the posterior neck help to move the head. (The splenius capitis is removed on the left to show the underlying muscles.)

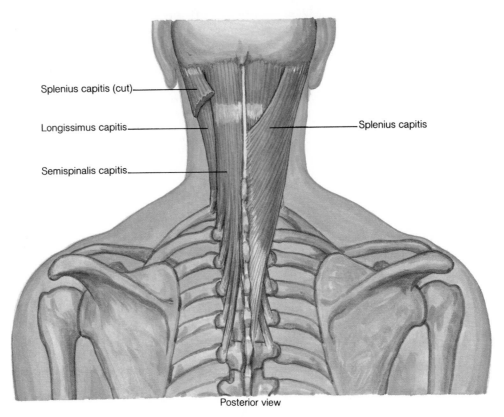

Splenius capitis (cut)

Longissimus capitis

Semispinalis capitis

Splenius capitis

Posterior view

Chart 8.3 Muscles that move the head

Muscle	Origin	Insertion	Action	Innervation	Figure
Sternocleido-mastoid	Anterior surface of sternum and upper surface of clavicle	Mastoid process of temporal bone	Pulls head to one side, flexes neck, or raises sternum	Accessory, C2, C3 nerves	8.15
Splenius capitis	Spinous processes of lower cervical and upper thoracic vertebrae	Mastoid process of temporal bone	Rotates head, bends head to one side, or extends neck	Cervical spinal nerves	8.12
Semispinalis capitis	Processes of lower cervical and upper thoracic vertebrae	Occipital bone	Extends head, bends head to one side, or rotates head	Cervical and thoracic spinal nerves	8.12
Longissimus capitis	Processes of lower cervical and upper thoracic vertebrae	Mastoid process of temporal bone	Extends head, bends head to one side, or rotates head	Lower cervical, thoracic, lumbar spinal nerves	8.12

FIGURE 8.13

(a) Deep back muscles; (b) anterior view of iliacus and quadratus lumborum.

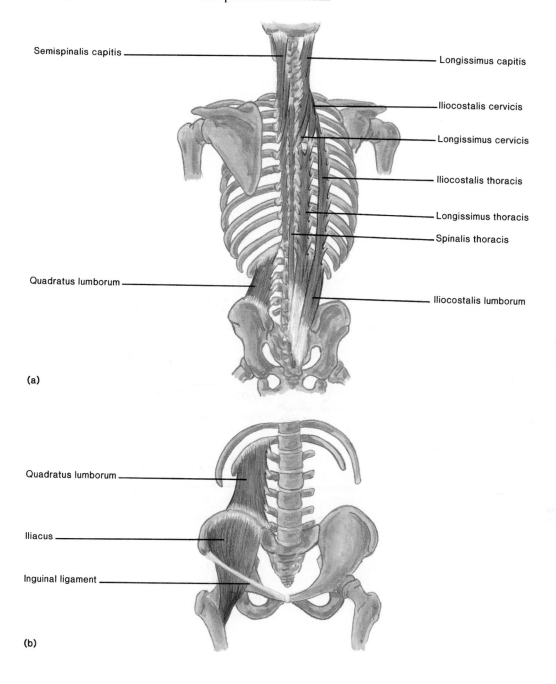

Semispinalis capitis

Longissimus capitis

Iliocostalis cervicis

Longissimus cervicis

Iliocostalis thoracis

Longissimus thoracis

Spinalis thoracis

Quadratus lumborum

Iliocostalis lumborum

(a)

Quadratus lumborum

Iliacus

Inguinal ligament

(b)

Muscles That Move the Vertebral Column

Movements of the vertebral column result from the actions of muscles that are attached to the pelvic girdle, vertebrae, ribs, and skull. These muscles are shown in figure 8.13 and listed in chart 8.4. They include the following:

Erector spinae
   Iliocostalis
   Longissimus
   Spinalis
Quadratus lumborum

The **erector spinae** (e-rek′tor spi′ne) is a muscle group that is located along the posterior vertebral column from the sacrum to the cranium. It includes, from lateral to medial, the *iliocostalis* (il″ĭ-o-kos-ta′lis), *longissimus* (lon-jis′i-mus), and *spinalis* (spi-na′lis) muscle groups. These muscles, together with the **quadratus lumborum** (kwad-ra′tus lumbo′rum) are the primary extensors of the vertebral column.

Chart 8.4 Muscles that move the vertebral column

Muscle	Origin	Insertion	Action	Innervation
Iliocostalis (lumborum, thoracis, and cervicis parts)	Iliac crest, sacrum, lumbar vertebrae, last 2 thoracic vertebrae, ribs 3–12	Ribs, transverse process of lower 4 cervical vertebrae	Extends vertebral column, bends column to one side	Lower cervical, thoracic, and lumbar spinal nerves
Longissimus (thoracis and cervicis parts)	Transverse processes of lumbar and first 5 thoracic vertebrae	Transverse processes of thoracic and cervical vertebrae 2–6 and lower 8 ribs	Extends vertebral column, bends column to one side	Lower cervical, thoracic, and lumbar spinal nerves
Spinalis thoracis	Spinous processes of last 2 thoracic and first 2 lumbar vertebrae	Spinous processes of first 4 thoracic vertebrae	Extends vertebral column	Thoracic spinal nerves
Quadratus lumborum	Iliac crest	Last rib and transverse processes of first 4 lumbar vertebrae	Bends vertebral column to side, extends vertebral column	T12; L1, 2, 3 spinal nerves

(handwritten above chart 8.5: Attach to Scapula)

Chart 8.5 Muscles that move the pectoral girdle

Muscle	Origin	Insertion	Action	Innervation	Figure
Trapezius	Occipital bone and spines of cervical and thoracic vertebrae	Clavicle, spine, and acromion process of scapula	Rotates scapula; various fibers raise scapula, pull scapula medially, or pull scapula and shoulder downward	Accessory n.	8.14
Rhomboideus major and minor	Spines of upper thoracic vertebrae	Medial border of scapula	Raises and adducts scapula	Dorsal scapular n.	8.14
Levator scapulae	Transverse processes of cervical vertebrae	Medial margin of scapula	Elevates scapula	Dorsal scapular, C3–C5 nerves	8.16
Serratus anterior	Outer surfaces of upper ribs	Ventral surface of scapula	Pulls scapula anteriorly and downward	Long thoracic n.	8.15
Pectoralis minor	Sternal ends of upper ribs	Coracoid process of scapula	Pulls scapula forward and downward or raises ribs	Pectoral n.	8.15

(handwritten annotations around chart: "when got R & L get trapazoid"; "Moves interior angles in of Scap"; "Lateral Upward Rotation of Inferior angle / elevates"; "turns Scapula (downward) Rotation"; "Superior Angle"; "downw. Rot of Scapula"; "Abd: Protract Terminal Rotation (up)"; "Rotation of Shoulder")

Muscles That Move the Pectoral Girdle

The muscles that move the pectoral girdle are closely associated with those that move the upper arm. A number of these chest and shoulder muscles connect the scapula to nearby bones and act to move the scapula upward, downward, forward, and backward. These muscles are shown in figures 8.14, 8.15, and listed on chart 8.5. They include:

Trapezius
Rhomboideus major
Levator scapulae
Serratus anterior
Pectoralis minor

The **trapezius** (trah-pe′ze-us) is a large, triangular muscle in the upper back that extends horizontally from the base of the skull and the cervical and thoracic vertebrae to the shoulder. Its fibers are arranged in three groups—upper, middle, and lower. Together these fibers rotate the scapula. The upper fibers acting alone raise the scapula and shoulder, as when the shoulders are shrugged to express a feeling of indifference. The middle fibers pull the scapula toward the vertebral column, and the lower fibers draw the scapula and shoulder downward. When the shoulder is fixed in position by other muscles, the trapezius can pull the head backward or to one side.

FIGURE 8.14

(*a*) Muscles of the posterior shoulder. (The trapezius is removed on the right to show underlying muscles.) Isolated views of (*b*) trapezius, (*c*) deltoid, and (*d*) rhomboideus and latissimus dorsi muscles.

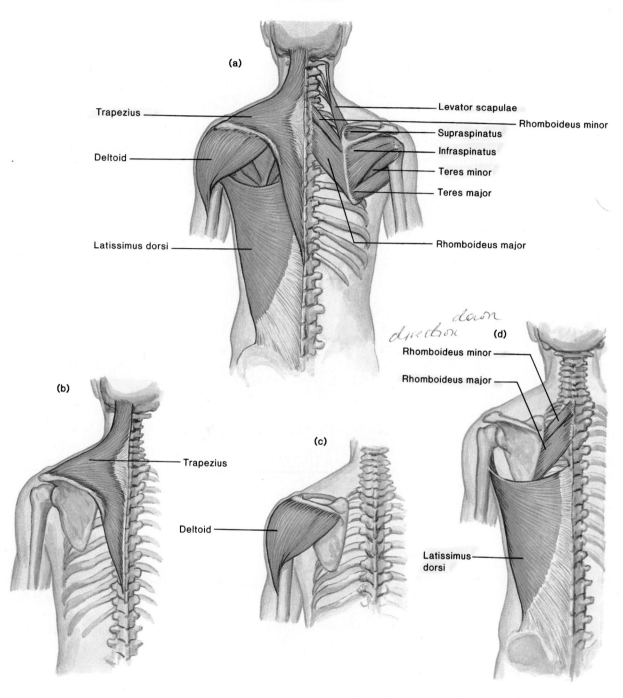

(a)

Trapezius

Deltoid

Latissimus dorsi

Levator scapulae

Rhomboideus minor

Supraspinatus

Infraspinatus

Teres minor

Teres major

Rhomboideus major

(b)

Trapezius

(c)

Deltoid

direction *down*

(d)

Rhomboideus minor

Rhomboideus major

Latissimus dorsi

FIGURE 8.15

(a) Muscles of the anterior chest and abdominal wall. (The left pectoralis major is removed to show the pectoralis minor.)
(b) Isolated view of the internal and external intercostal muscles.

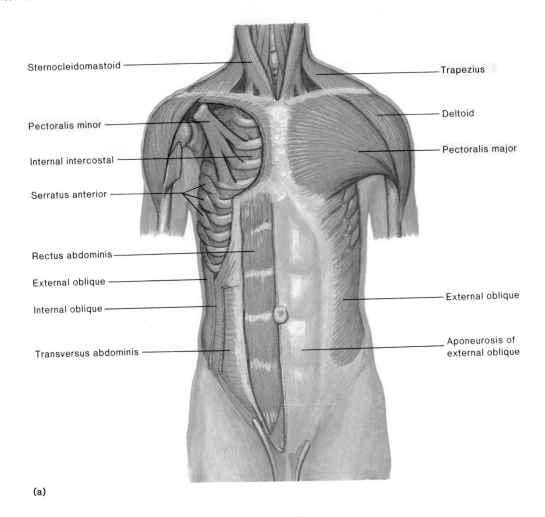

Sternocleidomastoid

Pectoralis minor

Internal intercostal

Serratus anterior

Rectus abdominis

External oblique

Internal oblique

Transversus abdominis

Trapezius

Deltoid

Pectoralis major

External oblique

Aponeurosis of
external oblique

(a)

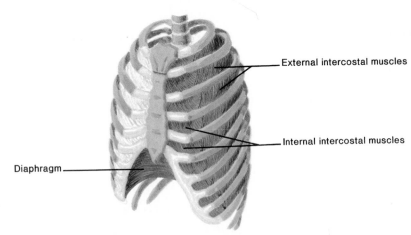

External intercostal muscles

Internal intercostal muscles

Diaphragm

(b)

The **rhomboideus** (rom-boid′e-us) **major** and **minor** connect the upper thoracic vertebrae to the scapula. These muscles act to raise the scapula and to adduct it.

The **levator scapulae** (le-va′tor scap′u-lē) is a straplike muscle that runs almost vertically through the neck, connecting the cervical vertebrae to the scapula. It functions to elevate the scapula.

The **serratus anterior** (ser-ra′tus an-te′re-or) is a broad, curved muscle located on the side of the chest. It arises as fleshy, narrow strips on the upper ribs and extends along the medial wall of the axilla to the anterior surface of the scapula. It functions to pull the scapula downward and anteriorly and is used to thrust the shoulder forward, as when pushing something.

The **pectoralis** (pek″to-ra′lis) **minor** is a thin, flat muscle that lies beneath the larger pectoralis major. It extends laterally and upward from the ribs to the scapula and serves to pull the scapula forward and downward. When other muscles fix the scapula in position, the pectoralis minor can raise the ribs and thus aid forceful inhalation.

The **intercostal muscles**, located between the ribs, and the **diaphragm** are described in chapter 13.

A small, triangular region in the back, where the trapezius overlaps the superior border of the latissimus dorsi and the underlying rhomboideus major, is called the *triangle of auscultation*. This area, which is near the medial border of the scapula, becomes enlarged when a person bends forward with the arms folded across the chest. By placing the bell of a stethoscope within the triangle of auscultation, a physician usually can hear the sounds of the respiratory organs clearly.

Muscles That Move the Upper Arm

The upper arm is one of the more freely movable parts of the body. Its many movements are made possible by muscles that connect the humerus to various regions of the pectoral girdle, ribs, and vertebral column (figures 8.14–8.18). These muscles can be grouped according to their primary actions—flexion, extension, abduction, and rotation—as follows (chart 8.6):

Flexors
  Coracobrachialis
  Pectoralis major
Extensors
  Teres major
  Latissimus dorsi

Abductors
  Supraspinatus
  Deltoid
Rotators
  Subscapularis
  Infraspinatus
  Teres minor

Flexors

The **coracobrachialis** (kor″ah-ko-bra′ke-al-is) extends from the scapula to the middle of the humerus along its medial surface. It acts to flex and adduct the upper arm.

The **pectoralis major** is a thick, fan-shaped muscle located in the upper chest. Its fibers extend from the center of the thorax through the armpit to the humerus. This muscle functions primarily to pull the upper arm forward and across the chest. It can also rotate the humerus medially and adduct the arm from a raised position.

Extensors

The **teres** (te′rēz) **major** connects the scapula to the humerus. It extends the humerus and can also adduct and rotate the upper arm medially.

Muscle	Origin	Insertion	Action	Innervation	Figure
Coracobrachialis	Coracoid process of scapula	Shaft of humerus	Flexes and adducts the upper arm	Musculocutaneous n.	8.18
Pectoralis major	Clavicle, sternum, and costal cartilages of upper ribs	Intertubercular groove of humerus	Flexes and adducts humerus, rotates humerus, or adducts arm	Pectoral n.	8.15
Teres major	Lateral border of scapula	Intertubercular groove of humerus	Extends humerus, or adducts and rotates arm medially	Lower subscapular n.	8.16
Latissimus dorsi	Spines of sacral, lumbar, and lower thoracic vertebrae, iliac crest, and lower ribs	Intertubercular groove of humerus	Extends and adducts the arm and rotates humerus inwardly, or pulls the shoulder downward and back	Thoracodorsal n.	8.14
Supraspinatus	Posterior surface of scapula	Greater tubercle of humerus	Abducts the upper arm	Suprascapular n.	8.16
Deltoid	Acromion process, spine of the scapula, and the clavicle	Deltoid tuberosity of humerus	Abducts upper arm, extends humerus, or flexes humerus	Axillary n.	8.14
Subscapularis	Anterior surface of scapula	Lesser tubercle of humerus	Rotates arm medially	Subscapular n.	8.18
Infraspinatus	Posterior surface of scapula	Greater tubercle of humerus	Rotates arm laterally	Suprascapular n.	8.16
Teres minor	Lateral border of scapula	Greater tubercle of humerus	Rotates arm laterally	Axillary n.	8.16

Chart 8.6 Muscles that move the upper arm

FIGURE 8.16

(a) Muscles of the posterior surface of the scapula and the upper arm; (b) and (c) muscles associated with the scapula. (d) Isolated view of the triceps brachii.

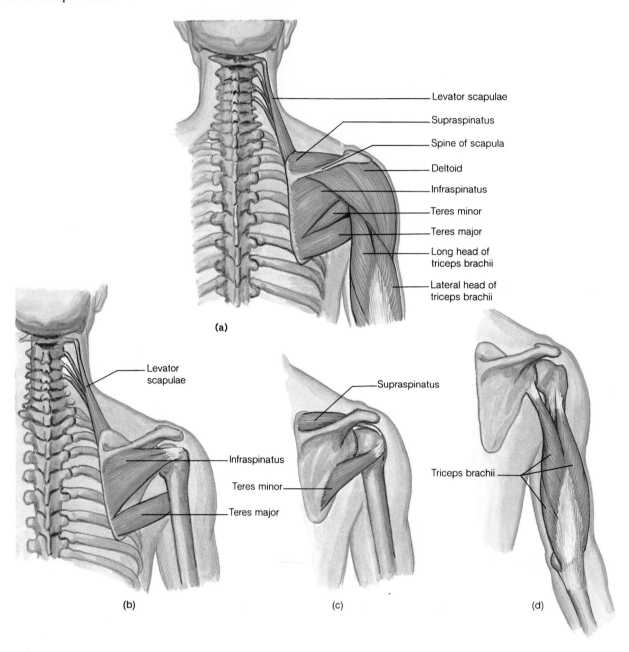

Levator scapulae
Supraspinatus
Spine of scapula
Deltoid
Infraspinatus
Teres minor
Teres major
Long head of triceps brachii
Lateral head of triceps brachii

(a)

Levator scapulae
Infraspinatus
Teres minor
Teres major

(b)

Supraspinatus
Teres minor

(c)

Triceps brachii

(d)

The **latissimus dorsi** (lah-tis′ĭ-mus dor′si) is a wide, triangular muscle that curves upward from the lower back, around the side, and to the armpit. It can extend and adduct the arm, and rotate the humerus inwardly. It also acts to pull the shoulder downward and back. This muscle is used to pull the arm back in swimming, climbing, and rowing movements.

Abductors

The **supraspinatus** (su″prah-spi′na-tus) is located in the depression above the spine of the scapula on its posterior surface. It connects the scapula to the greater tubercle of the humerus and acts to abduct the upper arm.

The **deltoid** (del′toid) is a thick, triangular muscle that covers the shoulder joint. It connects the clavicle and scapula to the lateral side of the humerus and acts to abduct the upper arm. The deltoid's posterior fibers can extend the humerus, and its anterior fibers can flex the humerus.

> If the humerus is fractured at its surgical neck, the nerve that supplies the deltoid muscle (axillary nerve) may be damaged. If this occurs, the muscle is likely to decrease in size and become weakened. In order to test the deltoid for such weakness, a physician may ask a patient to abduct the arm against some resistance and maintain that posture for a time.

Rotators

The **subscapularis** (sub-scap'u-lar-is) is a large, triangular muscle that covers the anterior surface of the scapula. It connects the scapula to the humerus and functions to rotate the upper arm medially.

The **infraspinatus** (in"frah-spi'na-tus) occupies the depression below the spine of the scapula on its posterior surface. The fibers of this muscle attach the scapula to the humerus and act to rotate the upper arm laterally.

The **teres minor** is a small muscle connecting the scapula to the humerus. It acts to rotate the upper arm laterally.

Muscles That Move the Forearm

Most forearm movements are produced by muscles that connect the radius or ulna to the humerus or pectoral girdle. A group of muscles located along the anterior surface of the humerus acts to flex the elbow, while a single posterior muscle serves to extend this joint. Other muscles cause movements at the radioulnar joint and are responsible for rotating the forearm.

The muscles that move the forearm are shown in figures 8.16–8.19 and listed on chart 8.7. They include the following:

Flexors	Rotators
Biceps brachii	*Supinator*
Brachialis	*Pronator teres*
Brachioradialis	*Pronator quadratus*
Extensor	
Triceps brachii	

FIGURE 8.17

Cross section of the upper arm.

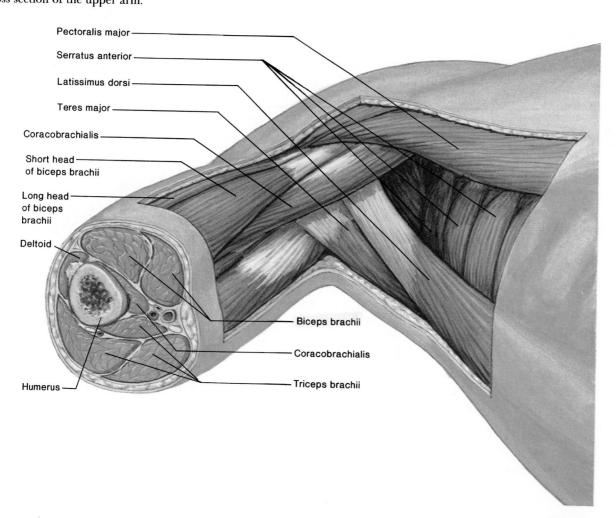

Pectoralis major
Serratus anterior
Latissimus dorsi
Teres major
Coracobrachialis
Short head of biceps brachii
Long head of biceps brachii
Deltoid
Humerus
Biceps brachii
Coracobrachialis
Triceps brachii

FIGURE 8.18

(*a*) Muscles of the anterior shoulder and the upper arm, with the rib cage removed. (*b–d*) Isolated views of muscles associated with the upper arm.

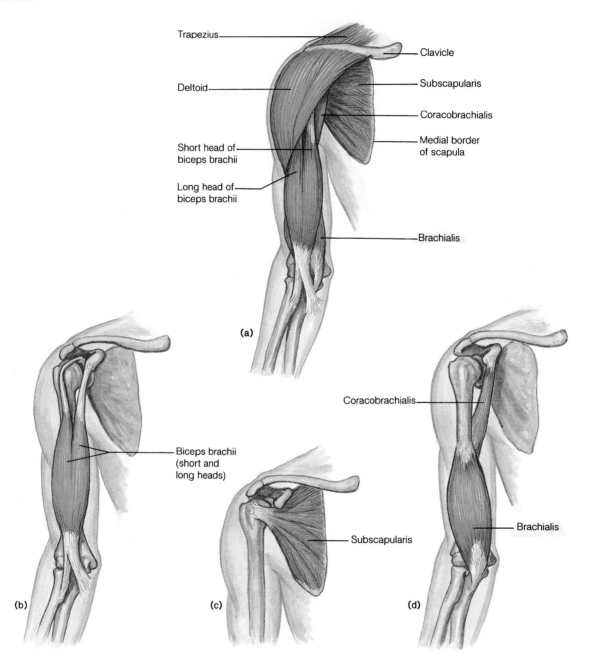

Flexors

The **biceps brachii** (bi′seps bra′ke-i) is a fleshy muscle that forms a long, rounded mass on the anterior side of the upper arm. It connects the scapula to the radius, and functions to flex the arm at the elbow and to rotate the hand laterally (supination), as when a person turns a doorknob or screwdriver.

The **brachialis** (bra′ke-al-is) is a large muscle beneath the biceps brachii. It connects the shaft of the humerus to the ulna and is the strongest flexor of the elbow.

The **brachioradialis** (bra″ke-o-ra″de-a′lis) connects the humerus to the radius and aids in flexing the elbow.

Extensor

The **triceps brachii** (tri′seps bra′ke-i) has three heads and is the only muscle on the back of the upper arm. It connects the humerus and scapula to the ulna, and is the primary extensor of the elbow.

FIGURE 8.19

(*a*) Muscles of the anterior forearm. (*b–e*) Isolated views of muscles associated with the anterior forearm.

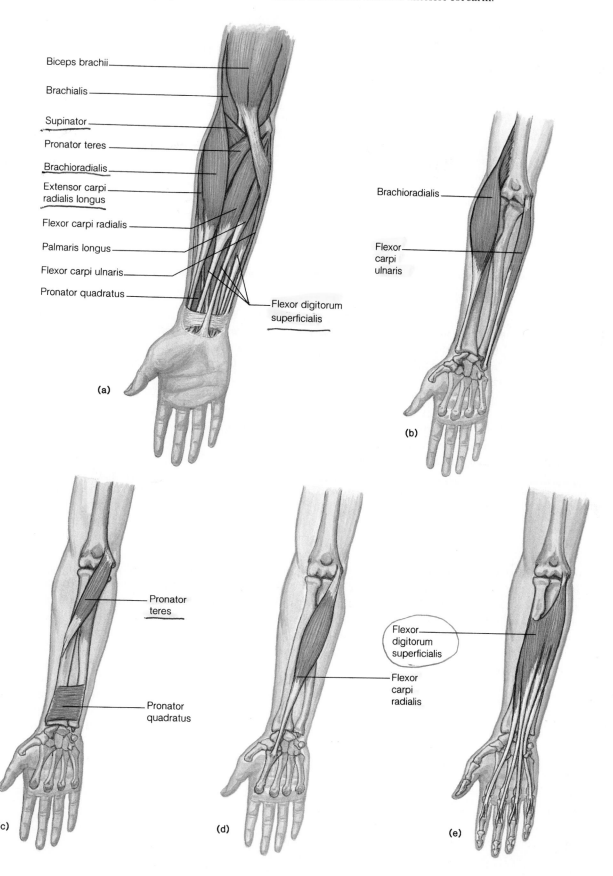

Biceps brachii

Brachialis

Supinator

Pronator teres

Brachioradialis

Extensor carpi radialis longus

Flexor carpi radialis

Palmaris longus

Flexor carpi ulnaris

Pronator quadratus

Flexor digitorum superficialis

(a)

Brachioradialis

Flexor carpi ulnaris

(b)

Pronator teres

Pronator quadratus

(c)

Flexor digitorum superficialis

Flexor carpi radialis

(d)

(e)

Chart 8.7 Muscles that move the forearm

Muscle	Origin	Insertion	Action	Innervation
Biceps brachii	Coracoid process and tubercle above glenoid cavity of scapula	Radial tuberosity of radius	Flexes arm at elbow and rotates hand laterally *flexes shoulder*	Musculocutaneous n.
Brachialis	Anterior shaft of humerus	Coronoid process of ulna	Flexes arm at elbow	Musculocutaneous, median, and radial nerves
Brachioradialis	Distal lateral end of humerus	Lateral surface of radius above styloid process	Flexes arm at elbow	Radial n.
Triceps brachii	Tubercle below glenoid cavity, and lateral and medial surfaces of humerus	Olecranon process of ulna *elbow*	Extends arm at elbow *shoulder extensor*	Radial n.
Supinator	Lateral epicondyle of humerus and crest of ulna	Lateral surface of radius	Rotates forearm laterally	Radial n.
Pronator teres	Medial epicondyle of humerus and coronoid process of ulna	Lateral surface of radius	Rotates arm medially	Median n.
Pronator quadratus	Anterior distal end of ulna	Anterior distal end of radius	Rotates arm medially	Median n.

Rotators

The **supinator** (su'pĭ-na-tor) is a short muscle whose fibers run from the ulna and the lateral end of the humerus to the radius. It assists the biceps brachii in rotating the forearm laterally (supination).

The **pronator teres** (pro-na'tor te'rēz) is a short muscle connecting the ends of the humerus and ulna to the radius. It functions to rotate the arm medially, as when the hand is turned so the palm is facing downward (pronation).

The **pronator quadratus** (pro-na'tor kwod-ra'tus) runs from the distal end of the ulna to the distal end of the radius. It assists the pronator teres in rotating the arm medially.

Muscles That Move the Wrist, Hand, and Fingers

Many muscles are responsible for wrist, hand, and finger movements. They originate from the distal end of the humerus, and from the radius and ulna. The two major groups of these muscles are flexors on the anterior side of the forearm and extensors on the posterior side. These muscles are shown in figures 8.19–8.21 and listed on chart 8.8. They include the following:

Flexors

Flexor carpi radialis
Flexor carpi ulnaris
Palmaris longus
Flexor digitorum profundus
Flexor digitorum superficialis
Flexor pollicis longus

Extensors

Extensor carpi radialis longus
Extensor carpi radialis brevis
Extensor carpi ulnaris
Extensor digitorum
Extensor pollicis brevis
Extensor pollicis longus
Abductor pollicis longus

Flexors

The **flexor carpi radialis** (flek'sor kar-pi' ra"de-a'lis) is a fleshy muscle that runs medially on the anterior side of the forearm. It extends from the distal end of the humerus into the hand, where it is attached to metacarpal bones. The flexor carpi radialis functions to flex and abduct the wrist.

The **flexor carpi ulnaris** (flek'sor kar-pi' ul-na'ris) is located along the medial border of the forearm. It connects the distal end of the humerus and the proximal end of the ulna to carpal and metacarpal bones. It serves to flex and adduct the wrist.

The **palmaris longus** (pal-ma'ris long'gus) is a slender muscle located on the medial side of the forearm between the flexor carpi radialis and the flexor carpi ulnaris. It connects the distal end of the humerus to fascia of the palm and functions to flex the wrist.

The **flexor digitorum profundus** (flek'sor dij"ĭ-to'rum pro-fun'dus) is a large muscle that connects the ulna to the distal phalanges. It acts to flex the distal joints of the fingers, as when a fist is made.

FIGURE 8.20

(a) Muscles of the posterior forearm. (b) and (c) Isolated views of muscles associated with the posterior forearm.

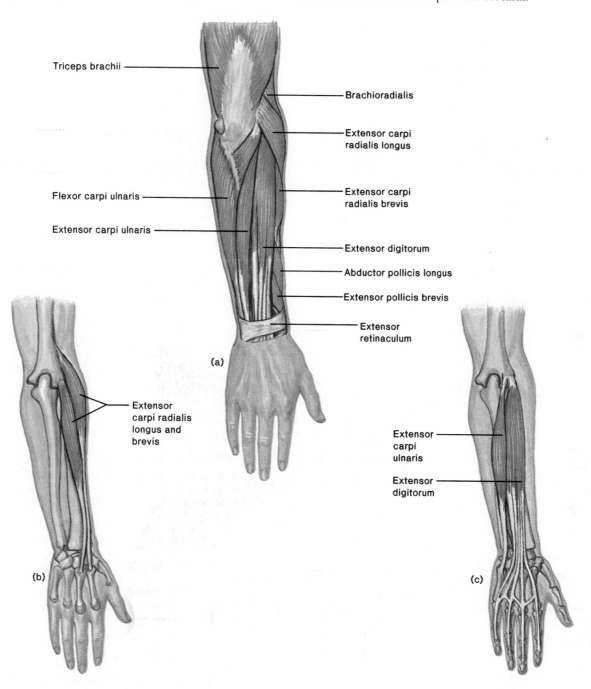

Triceps brachii

Brachioradialis

Extensor carpi radialis longus

Flexor carpi ulnaris

Extensor carpi ulnaris

Extensor carpi radialis brevis

Extensor digitorum

Abductor pollicis longus

Extensor pollicis brevis

Extensor retinaculum

(a)

Extensor carpi radialis longus and brevis

(b)

Extensor carpi ulnaris

Extensor digitorum

(c)

The **flexor digitorum superficialis** (flek'sor dij''ĭ-to'rum su''per-fish''e-a'lis) is a large muscle located beneath the flexor carpi ulnaris. It arises by three heads—one from the medial epicondyle of the humerus, one from the medial side of the ulna, and one from the radius. It is inserted in the tendons of the fingers and acts to flex the fingers and, by a combined action, to flex the hand.

The **flexor pollicis longus** (flek'sor pol'ĭ-sis long'us) is a deep muscle that is located along the anterior surface of the radius and extends from the radial tuberosity to the base of the distal phalanx of the thumb. This muscle flexes the thumb.

FIGURE 8.21

A cross section of the forearm.

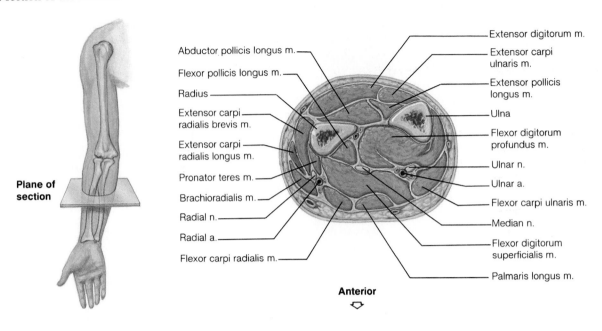

Plane of section

Abductor pollicis longus m.

Flexor pollicis longus m.

Radius

Extensor carpi radialis brevis m.

Extensor carpi radialis longus m.

Pronator teres m.

Brachioradialis m.

Radial n.

Radial a.

Flexor carpi radialis m.

Extensor digitorum m.

Extensor carpi ulnaris m.

Extensor pollicis longus m.

Ulna

Flexor digitorum profundus m.

Ulnar n.

Ulnar a.

Flexor carpi ulnaris m.

Median n.

Flexor digitorum superficialis m.

Palmaris longus m.

Anterior

Chart 8.8 Muscles that move the wrist, hand, and fingers

Muscle	Origin	Insertion	Action	Innervation	Figure
Flexor carpi radialis	Medial epicondyle of humerus	Base of second and third metacarpals	Flexes and abducts wrist	Median n.	8.19
Flexor carpi ulnaris	Medial epicondyle of humerus and olecranon process	Carpal and metacarpal bones	Flexes and adducts wrist	Ulnar n.	8.19
Palmaris longus	Medial epicondyle of humerus	Fascia of palm	Flexes wrist	Median n.	8.19
Flexor digitorum profundus	Anterior surface of ulna	Bases of distal phalanges in fingers two through five	Flexes distal joints of fingers	Median, ulnar nerves	8.21
Flexor digitorum superficialis	Medial epicondyle of humerus, coronoid process of ulna, and radius	Tendons of fingers	Flexes fingers and hand	Median n.	8.19
Flexor pollicis longus	Radial tuberosity	Base of distal phalanx of thumb	Flexes thumb	Branch of median n.	8.21
Extensor carpi radialis longus	Distal end of humerus	Base of second metacarpal	Extends wrist and abducts hand	Radial n.	8.20
Extensor carpi radialis brevis	Lateral epicondyle of humerus	Base of second and third metacarpals	Extends wrist and abducts hand	Radial n.	8.20
Extensor carpi ulnaris	Lateral epicondyle of humerus	Base of fifth metacarpal	Extends and adducts wrist	Radial n.	8.20
Extensor digitorum	Lateral epicondyle of humerus	Posterior surface of phalanges in fingers two through five	Extends fingers	Radial n.	8.20
Extensor pollicis brevis	Radius	Base of proximal phalanx of thumb	Extends thumb	Posterior interosseous n.	8.20
Extensor pollicis longus	Ulna	Base of distal phalanx of thumb	Extends thumb	Posterior interosseous n.	8.21
Abductor pollicis longus	Shafts of radius and ulna	Base of first metacarpal	Abducts and extends thumb	Posterior interosseous n.	8.20

Extensors

The **extensor carpi radialis longus** (eks-ten′sor kar-pi′ ra″de-a′lis long′gus) runs along the lateral side of the forearm, connecting the humerus to the hand. It functions to extend the wrist and assists in abducting the hand.

The **extensor carpi radialis brevis** (eks-ten′sor kar-pi′ ra″de-a′lis bre′vis) is a companion of the extensor carpi radialis longus and is located medially to it. This muscle runs from the humerus to metacarpal bones and functions to extend the wrist. It also assists in abducting the hand.

The **extensor carpi ulnaris** (eks-ten′sor kar-pi′ ulna′ris) is located along the posterior surface of the ulna and connects the humerus to the hand. It acts to extend the wrist and assists in adducting it.

The **extensor digitorum** (eks-ten′sor dij″i-to′rum) runs medially along the back of the forearm. It connects the humerus to the posterior surface of the phalanges and functions to extend the fingers.

The **extensor pollicis brevis** (eks-ten′sor pol′i-sis bre′vis) and the **extensor pollicis longus** both act to extend the thumb. The extensor pollicis brevis extends from the radius to the base of the proximal phalanx; the extensor pollicis longus passes from the ulna to the base of the distal phalanx of the thumb.

The **abductor pollicis longus** (ab-duk′tor pol′i-sis long′us) runs deep along the posterior surface of the radius, becoming superficial near the wrist. It connects the shafts of the radius and ulna to the base of the first metacarpal. This muscle acts to abduct the thumb, and together with the extensor pollicis brevis and longus, extends the thumb.

A structure called the *extensor retinaculum* consists of a group of heavy connective tissue fibers in the posterior fascia of the wrist. It connects the lateral margin of the radius with the medial border of the styloid process of the ulna and certain bones of the wrist. The retinaculum gives off branches of connective tissue to the underlying wrist bones, creating a series of sheathlike compartments through which the tendons of the extensor muscles pass to the wrist and fingers (figure 8.20). These compartments are lined with a synovial membrane that also covers the tendons passing through them. The synovial membrane produces a small amount of synovial fluid that allows a tendon to move freely within a compartment.

The anterior fascia of the wrist forms the *flexor retinaculum*. This fascia creates the *carpal tunnel*, between the carpal bones and the retinaculum, through which the flexor muscle tendons pass (figure 8.19). The carpal tunnel is also lined with synovial membrane.

> The median nerve also passes through the carpal tunnel. If the compartment's synovial membranes or the joints between the carpal bones become inflamed, the result may be increased pressure on the median nerve. This condition is called *carpal tunnel syndrome*, and it causes pain, a burning sensation, and muscular weakness in the hand and fingers. These symptoms may be treated by surgically cutting the flexor retinaculum to relieve the pressure.

Muscles of the Abdominal Wall

Although the walls of the chest and pelvic regions are supported directly by bone, those of the abdomen are not. Instead, the anterior and lateral walls of the abdomen are composed of broad, flattened muscles arranged in layers. These muscles connect the rib cage and vertebral column to the pelvic girdle. A band of tough connective tissue, called the **linea alba,** (figure 8.22) extends from the xiphoid process of the sternum to the symphysis pubis. It serves as an attachment for some of the abdominal wall muscles.

Contraction of these muscles decreases the size of the abdominal cavity and increases the pressure inside. This action helps to press air out of the lungs during forceful exhalation, and also aids in defecation, urination, vomiting, and childbirth.

The abdominal wall muscles (figures 8.15, 8.22, and chart 8.9) include the following:

External oblique
Internal oblique
Transversus abdominis
Rectus abdominis

Chart 8.9 Muscles of the abdominal wall

Muscle	Origin	Insertion	Action	Innervation
External oblique	Outer surfaces of lower ribs	Outer lip of iliac crest and linea alba	Tenses abdominal wall and compresses abdominal contents	Intercostal 7–12 nerves
Internal oblique	Crest of ilium and inguinal ligament	Cartilages of lower ribs, linea alba, and crest of pubis	Same as above	Intercostal 7–12 nerves
Transversus abdominis	Costal cartilages of lower ribs, processes of lumbar vertebrae, lip of iliac crest, and inguinal ligament	Linea alba and crest of pubis	Same as above	Intercostal 7–12 nerves
Rectus abdominis	Crest of pubis and symphysis pubis	Xiphoid process of sternum and costal cartilages	Same as above, also flexes vertebral column	Intercostal 7–12 nerves

FIGURE 8.22
(*a–d*) Isolated muscles of the abdominal wall; (*e*) transverse section through the abdominal wall.

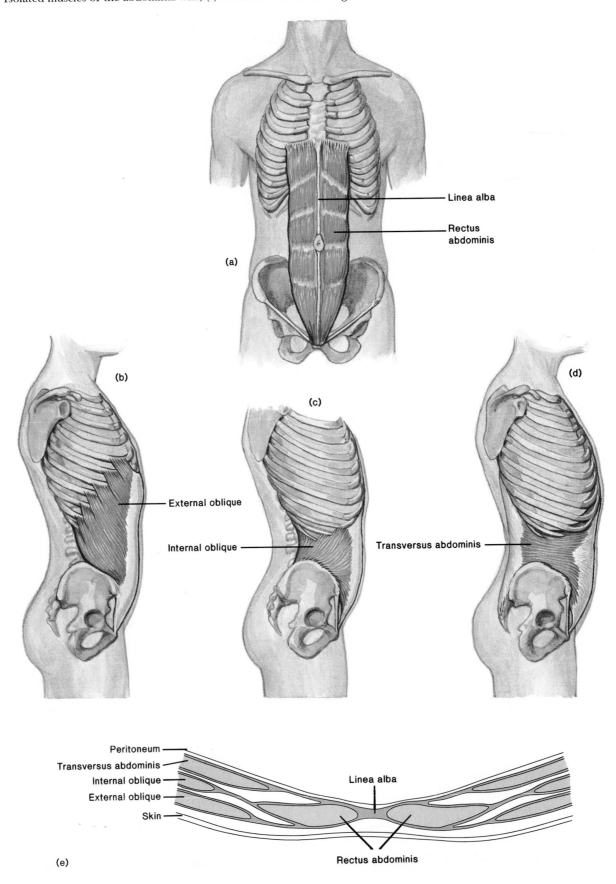

Linea alba

Rectus abdominis

(a)

(b)

(c)

(d)

External oblique

Internal oblique

Transversus abdominis

Peritoneum
Transversus abdominis
Internal oblique
External oblique
Skin

Linea alba

Rectus abdominis

(e)

The **external oblique** (eks-ter'nal ŏ-blēk) is a broad, thin sheet of muscle whose fibers slant downward from the lower ribs to the pelvic girdle and the linea alba. When this muscle contracts, it tenses the abdominal wall and compresses the contents of the abdominal cavity.

Similarly, the **internal oblique** (in-ter'nal ŏ-blēk) is a broad, thin sheet of muscle located beneath the external oblique. Its fibers run up and forward from the pelvic girdle to the lower ribs. Its function is similar to that of the external oblique.

The **transversus abdominis** (trans-ver'sus ab-dom'ĭ-nis) forms a third layer of muscle beneath the external and internal obliques. Its fibers run horizontally from the lower ribs, lumbar vertebrae, and ilium to the linea alba and pubic bones. It functions in the same manner as the external and internal obliques.

The **rectus abdominis** (rek'tus ab-dom'ĭ-nis) is a long, straplike muscle that connects the pubic bones to the ribs and sternum. It is crossed transversely by three or more fibrous bands that give it a segmented appearance. The muscle functions with other abdominal wall muscles to compress the contents of the abdominal cavity, and it also helps to flex the vertebral column.

Muscles of the Pelvic Outlet

The outlet of the pelvis is spanned by two muscular sheets—a deeper **pelvic diaphragm** and a more superficial **urogenital diaphragm.** The pelvic diaphragm forms the floor of the pelvic cavity, and the urogenital diaphragm fills the space within the pubic arch. The muscles of the male and female pelvic outlets include the following (figure 8.23 and chart 8.10):

Pelvic diaphragm
Levator ani
Coccygeus

Urogenital diaphragm
Superficial transversus perinei
Bulbospongiosus
Ischiocavernosus
Sphincter urethrae

Pelvic Diaphragm

The **levator ani** (le-va'tor ah-ni') muscles form a thin sheet across the pelvic outlet. They are connected at the midline posteriorly by a ligament that extends from the tip of the coccyx to the anal canal. Anteriorly, they are separated in the male by the urethra and the anal canal; and in the female by the urethra, vagina, and anal canal. These muscles help to support the pelvic viscera and provide sphincterlike action in the anal canal and vagina.

An *external anal sphincter,* which is under voluntary control, and an *internal anal sphincter,* which is formed of involuntary muscle fibers of the intestine, encircle the anal canal and keep it closed.

The **coccygeus** (kok-sij'e-us) is a fan-shaped muscle that extends from the ischial spine to the coccyx and sacrum. It aids the levator ani in its functions.

Urogenital Diaphragm

The **superficial transversus perinei** (su''per-fish'al trans-ver'sus per''ĭ-ne'i) consists of a small bundle of muscle fibers that passes medially from the ischial tuberosity along the posterior border of the urogenital diaphragm. It assists other muscles in supporting the pelvic viscera.

In males, the **bulbospongiosus** (bul''bo-spon''je-o'sus) muscles are united surrounding the base of the penis. They assist in emptying the urethra. In females, these muscles are separated medially by the vagina and act to constrict the vaginal opening. They can also retard the flow of blood in veins, which helps maintain an erection in the penis of the male and the clitoris of the female.

Chart 8.10 Muscles of the pelvic outlet				
Muscle	**Origin**	**Insertion**	**Action**	**Innervation**
Levator ani	Pubic bone and ischial spine	Coccyx	Supports pelvic viscera, and provides sphincterlike action in anal canal and vagina	Pudendal n.
Coccygeus	Ischial spine	Sacrum and coccyx	Same as above	S4, S5 nerves
Superficial transversus perinei	Ischial tuberosity	Central tendon	Supports pelvic viscera	Pudendal n.
Bulbospongiosus	Central tendon	Males: urogenital diaphragm and fascia of penis Females: pubic arch and root of clitoris	Males: assists emptying urethra Females: constricts vagina	Pudendal n. Pudendal n.
Ischiocavernosus	Ischial tuberosity	Pubic arch	Assists the function of the bulbospongiosus	Pudendal n.
Sphincter urethrae	Margins of pubis and ischium	Fibers of each unite with those from other side	Opens and closes urethra	Pudendal n.

FIGURE 8.23
(a) External view of muscles of the male pelvic outlet, and (b) female pelvic outlet; (c) internal view of pelvic and urogenital diaphragms.

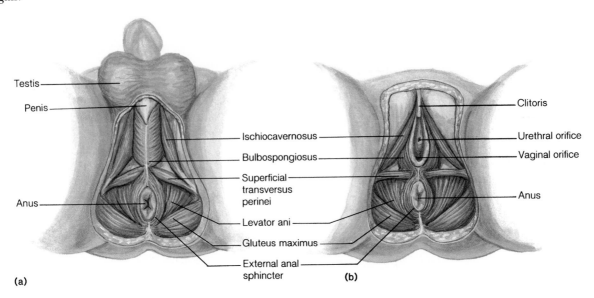

(a)

Testis

Penis

Ischiocavernosus

Bulbospongiosus

Superficial transversus perinei

Anus

Levator ani

Gluteus maximus

External anal sphincter

(b)

Clitoris

Urethral orifice

Vaginal orifice

Anus

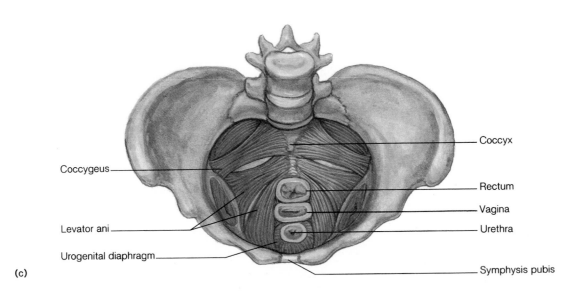

(c)

Coccygeus

Levator ani

Urogenital diaphragm

Coccyx

Rectum

Vagina

Urethra

Symphysis pubis

The **ischiocavernosus** (is″ke-o-kav″er-no′sus) **muscle** is a tendinous structure that extends from the ischial tuberosity to the margin of the pubic arch. It assists the function of the bulbospongiosus muscle.

The **sphincter urethrae** (sfingk′ter u-re′thrē) are muscles that arise from the margins of the pubic and ischial bones. Each arches around the urethra and unites with the one on the other side. Together they act as a sphincter that closes the urethra by compression and opens it by relaxation, thus helping to control the flow of urine.

Muscles That Move the Thigh

The muscles that move the thigh are attached to the femur and to some part of the pelvic girdle. They can be separated into anterior and posterior groups. The muscles of the anterior group act primarily to flex the thigh; those of the posterior group extend, abduct, or rotate it. The muscles in these groups are shown in figures 8.24–8.26 and listed on chart 8.11. They include the following:

Anterior group	Posterior group
Psoas major	*Gluteus maximus*
Iliacus	*Gluteus medius*
	Gluteus minimus
	Tensor fasciae latae

FIGURE 8.24

(a) Muscles of the anterior right thigh. Isolated views of (b) vastus intermedius; (c–e) adductors of the thigh; (f–g) flexors of the thigh.

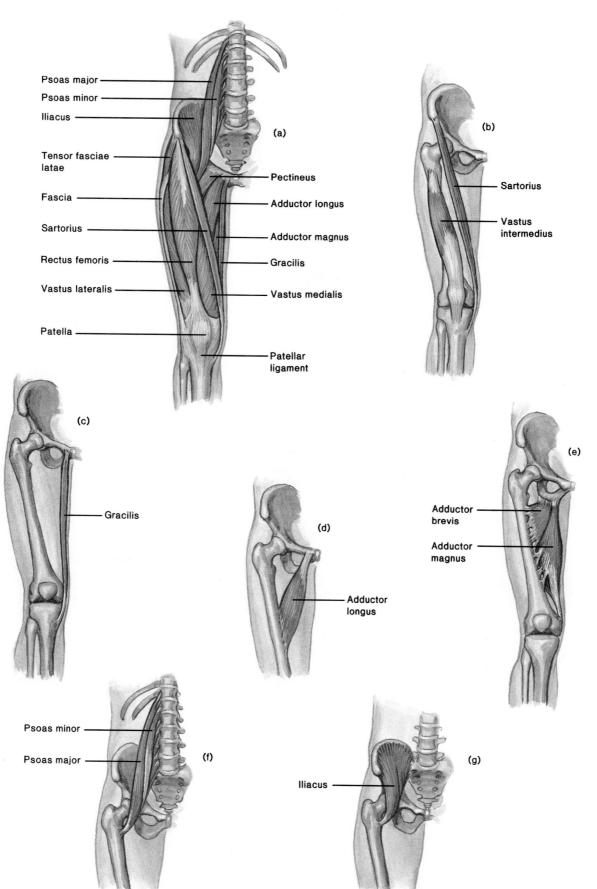

FIGURE 8.25

(*a*) Muscles of the lateral right thigh. (*b–d*) Isolated views of the gluteal muscles.

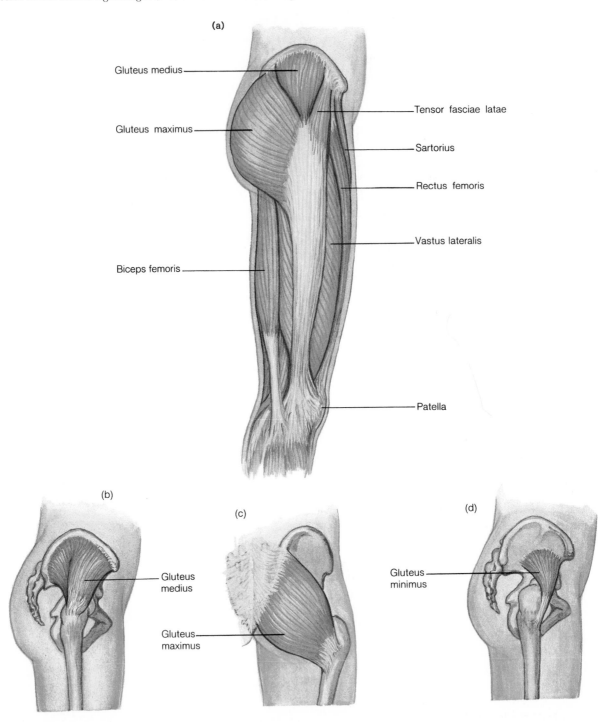

Still another group of muscles attached to the femur and pelvic girdle functions to adduct the thigh. This group includes:

Pectineus
Adductor longus
Adductor magnus
Adductor brevis
Gracilis

Anterior Group

The **psoas** (so'as) **major** is a long, thick muscle that connects the lumbar vertebrae to the femur. It functions to flex the thigh. The **psoas minor** is located anterior to the psoas major and is a much smaller muscle. It runs from the last thoracic and first lumbar vertebrae to the ilium and pubis of a coxal bone. Since it extends only to the pelvic girdle, it acts as a weak flexor of the vertebral column.

FIGURE 8.26

(a) Muscles of the posterior right thigh. (b) and (c) Isolated views of muscles that flex the leg at the knee.

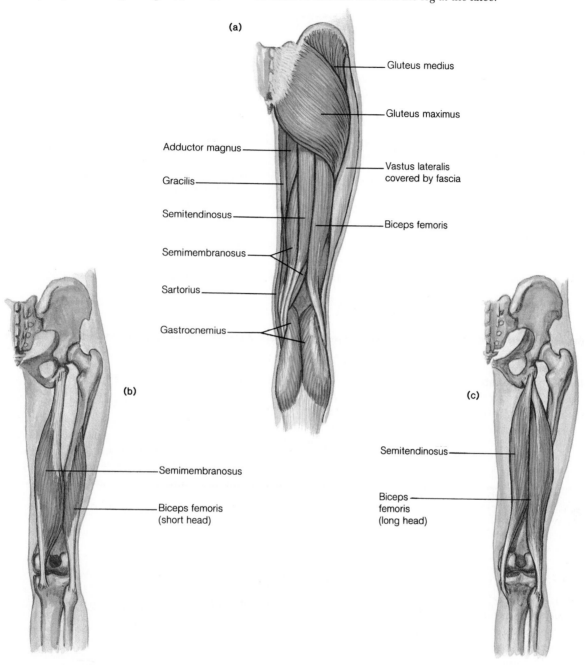

(a)

Gluteus medius

Gluteus maximus

Adductor magnus

Vastus lateralis
covered by fascia

Gracilis

Semitendinosus

Biceps femoris

Semimembranosus

Sartorius

Gastrocnemius

(b)

(c)

Semimembranosus

Semitendinosus

Biceps femoris
(short head)

Biceps
femoris
(long head)

The **iliacus** (il′e-ak-us), a large, fan-shaped muscle, lies along the lateral side of the psoas major. The iliacus and the psoas major are the primary flexors of the thigh, and they serve to advance the leg in walking movements.

Because of their common insertion and action, the iliacus and psoas major are sometimes described as the iliopsoas muscle.

Posterior Group

The **gluteus maximus** (gloo′te-us mak′si-mus) is the largest muscle in the body and covers a large part of each buttock.

It connects the ilium, sacrum, and coccyx to the femur by fascia of the thigh and acts to extend the thigh. The gluteus maximus causes the leg to straighten at the hip when a person walks, runs, or climbs. It is also used to raise the body from a sitting position.

The **gluteus medius** (gloo′te-us me′de-us) is partly covered by the gluteus maximus. Its fibers extend from the ilium to the femur, and they function to abduct the thigh and rotate it medially.

The **gluteus minimus** (gloo′te-us min′i-mus) lies beneath the gluteus medius and is its companion in attachments and functions.

Chart 8.11 Muscles that move the thigh

Muscle	Origin	Insertion	Action	Innervation	Figure
Psoas major	Lumbar intervertebral disks, bodies and transverse processes of lumbar vertebrae	Lesser trochanter of femur	Flexes thigh	Branches of L1–3 nerves	8.24
Iliacus	Iliac fossa of ilium	Lesser trochanter of femur	Flexes thigh	Femoral n.	8.24
Gluteus maximus	Sacrum, coccyx, and posterior surface of ilium	Posterior surface of femur and fascia of thigh	Extends leg at hip	Inferior gluteal n.	8.25
Gluteus medius	Lateral surface of ilium	Greater trochanter of femur	Abducts and rotates thigh medially	Superior gluteal n.	8.25
Gluteus minimus	Lateral surface of ilium	Greater trochanter of femur	Same as gluteus medius	Superior gluteal n.	8.25
Tensor fasciae latae	Anterior iliac crest	Fascia of thigh	Abducts, flexes, and rotates thigh medially	Superior gluteal n.	8.25
Pectineus	Pubic bone	Posterior surface of femur	Adducts and flexes thigh	Femoral n.	8.24
Adductor longus	Pubic bone near symphysis pubis	Posterior surface of femur	Adducts, flexes, and rotates thigh laterally	Obturator n.	8.24
Adductor magnus	Ischial tuberosity	Posterior surface of femur	Adducts, extends, and rotates thigh laterally	Obturator, branch of sciatic n.	8.24
Adductor brevis	Pubic bone	Posterior surface of femur	Adducts, flexes, and rotates thigh laterally	Obturator n.	8.24
Gracilis	Lower edge of symphysis pubis	Medial surface of tibia	Adducts thigh, flexes leg at knee	Obturator n.	8.24

The **tensor fasciae latae** (ten'sor fash'ē-e lah-tē) connects the ilium to the fascia of the thigh, which continues downward to the tibia. This muscle functions to abduct and flex the thigh, and to rotate it medially.

The gluteus medius and gluteus minimus help support and maintain the normal position of the pelvis. If these muscles are paralyzed as a result of injury or disease, the pelvis tends to drop to one side whenever the foot on that side is raised. Consequently, the person walks with a waddling limp, called the *gluteal gait*.

Thigh Adductors

The **pectineus** (pek-tin'e-us) extends from the pubic bone to the femur, and acts to adduct and flex the thigh.

The **adductor longus** (ah-duk'tor long'gus) is a long, triangular muscle that runs from the pubic bone to the femur. It adducts the thigh, and assists in flexing and rotating it laterally.

The **adductor magnus** (ah-duk'tor mag'nus) is the largest adductor of the thigh. It is a triangular muscle that connects the ischium to the femur. It adducts the thigh, and assists in extending and rotating it laterally.

The **adductor brevis** (ah-duk'tor brev'is) is found beneath the pectineus and adductor longus muscles. It connects the pubic bone and the femur, and adducts the thigh.

The **gracilis** (gras'il-is) is a long, straplike muscle that passes from the pubic bone to the tibia. It functions to adduct the thigh and to flex the leg at the knee.

Muscles That Move the Lower Leg

The muscles that move the lower leg connect the tibia or fibula to the femur or the pelvic girdle (figures 8.24–8.27, and chart 8.12). They can be separated into two major groups—those that cause flexion at the knee and those that cause extension at the knee. The muscles of these groups include the following:

Flexors
Biceps femoris
Semitendinosus
Semimembranosus
Sartorius
Extensor
Quadriceps femoris group

When skeletal muscles are contracted very forcefully, they may generate up to 50 pounds of pull for each square inch of muscle cross section. Consequently, large muscles such as those in the thigh can pull with several hundred pounds of force. Occasionally, this force is so great that the tendons of muscles are torn away from their attachments on bones.

Flexors

As its name implies, the **biceps femoris** (bi'seps fem'or-is) has two heads, one attached to the ischium and the other attached to the femur. This muscle passes along the back of the thigh on the lateral side and connects to the proximal ends of the fibula and tibia. The biceps femoris is one

FIGURE 8.27
A cross section of the thigh.

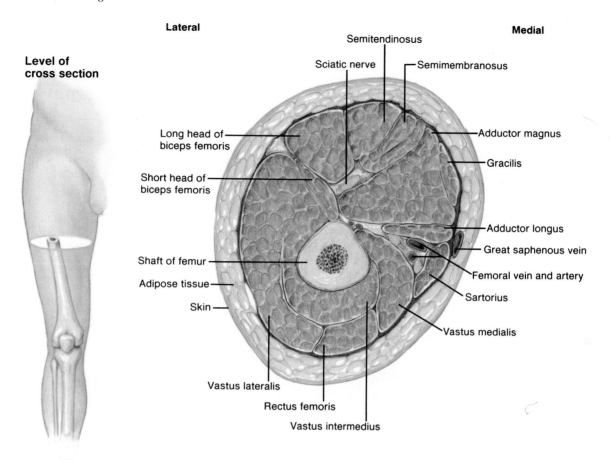

Chart 8.12 Muscles that move the lower leg					
Muscle	**Origin**	**Insertion**	**Action**	**Innervation**	**Figure**
Hamstring group Biceps femoris	Ischial tuberosity and linea aspera of femur	Head of fibula and lateral condyle of tibia	Flexes and rotates leg laterally and extends thigh	Tibial n.	8.26
Semitendinosus	Ischial tuberosity	Medial surface of tibia	Flexes and rotates leg medially and extends thigh	Tibial n.	8.26
Semimembranosus	Ischial tuberosity	Medial condyle of tibia	Flexes and rotates leg medially and extends thigh	Tibial n.	8.26
Sartorius	Anterior superior iliac spine	Medial surface of tibia	Flexes leg and thigh, abducts thigh, rotates thigh laterally, and rotates leg medially	Femoral n.	8.24
Quadriceps femoris group Rectus femoris	Spine of ilium and margin of acetabulum			Femoral n.	8.24
Vastus lateralis	Greater trochanter and posterior surface of femur	Patella by common tendon, which continues as patellar ligament to tibial tuberosity	Extends leg at knee	Femoral n.	8.24
Vastus medialis	Medial surface of femur			Femoral n.	8.24
Vastus intermedius	Anterior and lateral surfaces of femur			Femoral n.	8.24

FIGURE 8.28
(a) Muscles of the anterior right lower leg. (b–d) Isolated views of muscles associated with the anterior lower leg.

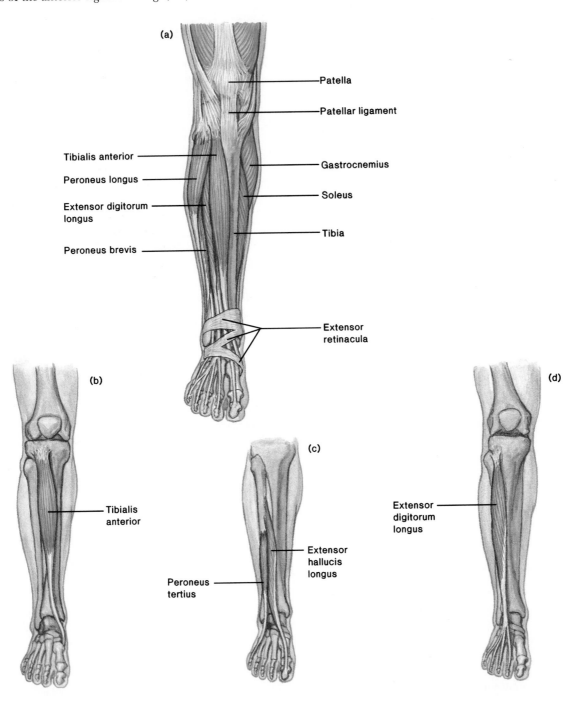

(a)

Patella

Patellar ligament

Tibialis anterior

Peroneus longus

Extensor digitorum longus

Peroneus brevis

Gastrocnemius

Soleus

Tibia

Extensor retinacula

(b)

Tibialis anterior

(c)

Peroneus tertius

Extensor hallucis longus

(d)

Extensor digitorum longus

of the hamstring muscles, and its tendon (hamstring) can be felt as a lateral ridge behind the knee. This muscle functions to flex and rotate the leg laterally and to extend the thigh.

The **semitendinosus** (sem″e-ten′di-no-sus) is another of the hamstring muscles. It is a long, bandlike muscle on the back of the thigh toward the medial side, connecting the ischium to the proximal end of the tibia. The semitendinosus is so named because it becomes tendinous in the middle of the thigh, continuing to its insertion as a long, cordlike tendon. It functions to flex and rotate the leg medially, and to extend the thigh.

The **semimembranosus** (sem″e-mem′brah-no-sus) is the third hamstring muscle and is the most medially located muscle in the back of the thigh. It connects the ischium to the tibia, and functions to flex and rotate the leg medially and to extend the thigh.

The **sartorius** (sar-to're-us), the longest muscle in the body, is an elongated, straplike muscle that passes obliquely across the front of the thigh and then descends over the medial side of the knee. It connects the ilium to the tibia and functions to flex the leg and the thigh. It can also abduct the thigh and rotate it laterally.

Extensor

The large, fleshy muscle group called **quadriceps femoris** (kwod'ri-seps fem'or-is) occupies the front and sides of the thigh, and is the primary extensor of the knee. It is composed of four muscles—*rectus femoris, vastus lateralis, vastus medialis,* and *vastus intermedius.* These parts connect the ilium and femur to a common *patellar tendon,* which passes over the front of the knee and attaches to the patella. This tendon then continues as the *patellar ligament* to the tibia.

Muscles That Move the Ankle, Foot, and Toes

A number of muscles that function to move the ankle, foot, and toes are located in the lower leg (figures 8.28–8.31, and chart 8.13). They attach the femur, tibia, and fibula to various bones of the foot, and are responsible for a variety of movements—moving the foot upward (dorsiflexion) or downward (plantar flexion), and turning the sole of the foot inward (inversion) or outward (eversion). These muscles include the following:

Dorsal flexors
Tibialis anterior
Peroneus tertius
Extensor digitorum longus
Extensor hallucis longus

Chart 8.13 Muscles that move the ankle, foot, and toes

Muscle	Origin	Insertion	Action	Innervation	Figure
Tibialis anterior	Lateral condyle and lateral surface of tibia	Tarsal bone (cuneiform) and first metatarsal	Dorsiflexion and inversion of foot	Deep peroneal n.	8.28
Peroneus tertius	Anterior surface of fibula	Dorsal surface of fifth metatarsal	Dorsiflexion and eversion of foot	Deep peroneal n.	8.28
Extensor digitorum longus	Lateral condyle of tibia and anterior surface of fibula	Dorsal surfaces of second and third phalanges of four lateral toes	Dorsiflexion and eversion of foot and extension of toes	Deep peroneal n.	8.28
Extensor hallucis longus	Anterior fibula and interosseus ligament	Distal phalanx of great toe	Dorsiflexion and eversion of foot and extension of great toe	Deep peroneal n.	8.28
Gastrocnemius	Lateral and medial condyles of femur	Posterior surface of calcaneus	Plantar flexion of foot and flexion of leg at knee	Tibial n.	8.30
Soleus	Head and shaft of fibula and posterior surface of tibia	Posterior surface of calcaneus	Plantar flexion of foot	Tibial n.	8.30
Plantaris	Above lateral condyle of femur	Posterior surface of calcaneus	Plantar flexion of foot and flexion of leg at knee	Tibial n.	8.30
Flexor digitorum longus	Posterior surface of tibia	Distal phalanges of four lateral toes	Plantar flexion and inversion of foot and flexion of four lateral toes	Tibial n.	8.30
Tibialis posterior	Lateral condyle and posterior surface of tibia and posterior surface of fibula	Tarsal and metatarsal bones	Plantar flexion and inversion of foot	Tibial n.	8.30
Peroneus longus	Lateral condyle of tibia and head and shaft of fibula	Tarsal and metatarsal bones	Plantar flexion and eversion of foot; also supports arch	Superficial peroneal n.	8.29
Peroneus brevis	Shaft of fibula	Fifth metatarsal	Plantar flexion and eversion of foot	Superficial peroneal n.	8.29

FIGURE 8.29

(a) Muscles of the lateral right lower leg. Isolated views of (b) peroneus longus and (c) peroneus brevis.

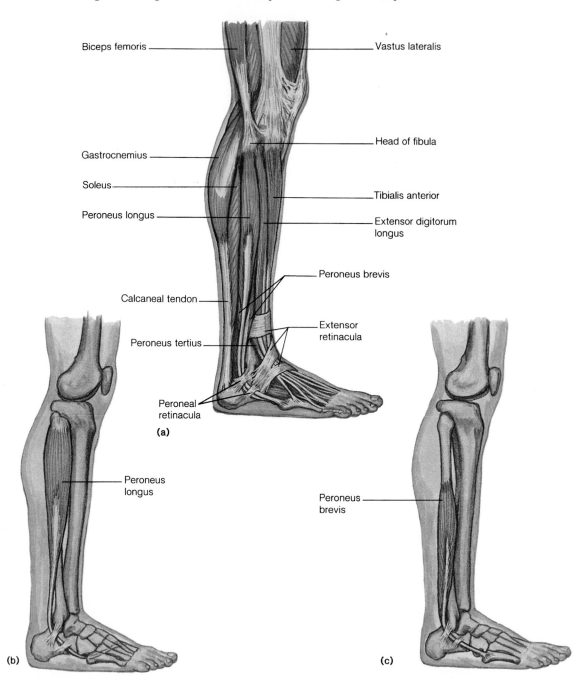

Biceps femoris

Gastrocnemius

Soleus

Peroneus longus

Calcaneal tendon

Peroneus tertius

Peroneal retinacula

Vastus lateralis

Head of fibula

Tibialis anterior

Extensor digitorum longus

Peroneus brevis

Extensor retinacula

(a)

Peroneus longus

(b)

Peroneus brevis

(c)

Plantar flexors
  Gastrocnemius
  Soleus
  Plantaris
  Flexor digitorum longus
Invertor
  Tibialis posterior
Evertors
  Peroneus longus
  Peroneus brevis

Dorsal Flexors

The **tibialis anterior** (tib″e-a′lis an-te′re-or) is an elongated, spindle-shaped muscle located on the front of the lower leg. It arises from the surface of the tibia, passes medially over the distal end of the tibia, and attaches to bones of the ankle and foot. Contraction of the tibialis anterior causes dorsiflexion and inversion of the foot.

The **peroneus tertius** (per″o-ne′us ter′shus) is a muscle of variable size that connects the fibula to the lateral side of the foot. It functions in dorsiflexion and eversion of the foot.

FIGURE 8.30

(a) Muscles of the posterior right lower leg. (b–e) Isolated views of muscles associated with the posterior right lower leg.

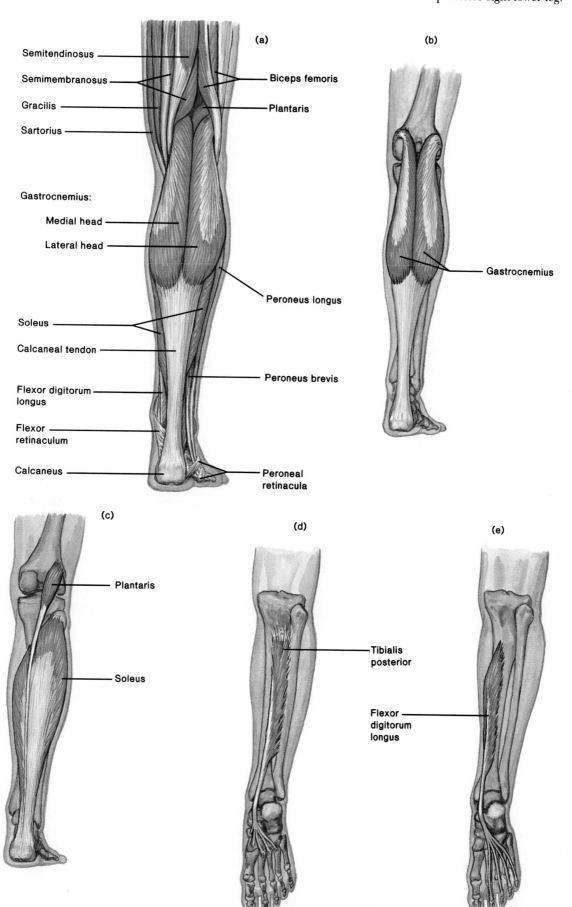

Semitendinosus

Semimembranosus

Gracilis

Sartorius

Biceps femoris

Plantaris

Gastrocnemius:

Medial head

Lateral head

Peroneus longus

Soleus

Calcaneal tendon

Peroneus brevis

Flexor digitorum longus

Flexor retinaculum

Calcaneus

Peroneal retinacula

(a)

(b)

Gastrocnemius

(c)

Plantaris

Soleus

(d)

Tibialis posterior

(e)

Flexor digitorum longus

FIGURE 8.31
A cross section of the lower leg.

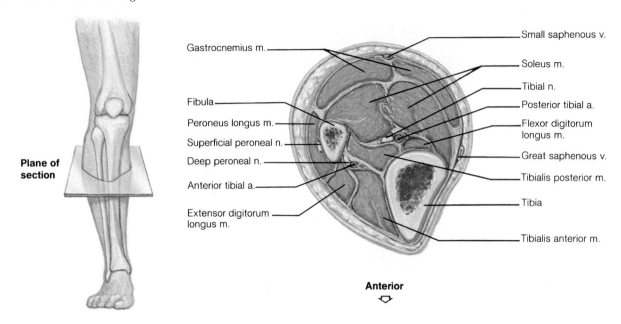

The **extensor digitorum longus** (eks-ten′sor dij″ĭ-to′rum long′gus) is situated along the lateral side of the lower leg just behind the tibialis anterior. It arises from the proximal end of the tibia and the shaft of the fibula. Its tendon divides into four parts as it passes over the front of the ankle. These parts continue over the surface of the foot and attach to the four lateral toes. The actions of the extensor digitorum longus include dorsiflexion of the foot, eversion of the foot, and extension of the toes.

The **extensor hallucis longus** (eks-ten′sor hal-u′sis long′us) connects the fibula and interosseus ligament to the great toe. It acts in dorsiflexion and eversion of the foot and extension of the great toe.

Although muscle fibers and the connective tissues associated with them are flexible and somewhat elastic, they can be torn if they are overstretched. This type of injury is common in athletes and is called a *muscle strain*, or *muscle pull*. The seriousness of the injury depends on the degree of damage sustained by the tissues. In a mild strain, for example, only a few muscle fibers may be injured, the fascia remains intact, and there is little loss of function. In a severe strain, many muscle fibers as well as fascia are torn, and muscle function may be lost completely. A severe strain is very painful and is accompanied by discoloration and swelling of tissues due to the rupture of blood vessels. Such an injury may require surgery to reconnect the separated tissues.

Plantar Flexors

The **gastrocnemius** (gas″trok-ne′me-us), at the back of the lower leg, forms part of the calf. It arises by two heads from the femur. The distal end of this muscle joins the strong calcaneal tendon (*Achilles tendon*), which descends to the heel and attaches to the calcaneus. The gastrocnemius is a powerful plantar flexor of the foot, which aids in pushing the body forward when a person walks or runs. It also functions to flex the leg at the knee.

Although it is the thickest and strongest human tendon, the calcaneal tendon may be partially or completely torn as a result of strenuous athletic activity. This injury occurs most frequently in middle-aged athletes, who run or play games that involve quick movements and directional changes. A torn calcaneal tendon usually requires surgical treatment.

The **soleus** (so′le-us) is a thick, flat muscle located beneath the gastrocnemius, and together, these two muscles make up the calf of the leg. The soleus arises from the tibia and fibula, and it extends to the heel by way of the calcaneal tendon. It acts with the gastrocnemius to cause plantar flexion of the foot.

The **plantaris** (plan-tah′ris) is a small muscle located behind the knee. It has a long, thin tendon that extends between the gastrocnemius and soleus, and becomes part of the calcaneal tendon. While the plantaris plays only a minor role in plantar flexion, its tendon may be ruptured by sudden dorsiflexion of the foot. This can occur while running or jumping, and such a rupture may cause severe pain.

The **flexor digitorum longus** (flek′sor dij″ĭ-to′rum long′gus) extends from the posterior surface of the tibia to the foot. Its tendon passes along the plantar surface of the foot, where it divides into four parts that attach to the terminal bones of the four lateral toes. This muscle assists in plantar flexion of the foot, flexion of the four lateral toes, and inversion of the foot.

Invertor

The **tibialis posterior** (tib″e-a′lis pos-tēr′e-or) is the deepest of the muscles on the back of the lower leg. It connects the fibula and tibia to ankle bones by means of a tendon that curves under the medial malleolus. This muscle assists in inversion and plantar flexion of the foot.

Evertor

The **peroneus longus** (per″o-ne′us long′gus) is a long, straplike muscle located on the lateral side of the lower leg. The **peroneus brevis** lies beneath the peroneus longus. These muscles connect the tibia and the fibula to the foot by means of stout tendons that pass behind the lateral malleolus. They function in eversion of the foot, assist in plantar flexion, and help support the arch of the foot.

As in the wrist, fascia in various regions of the ankle is thickened to form retinacula. Anteriorly, for example, *extensor retinacula* connect the tibia and fibula as well as the calcaneus and fascia of the sole. These retinacula form sheaths for tendons crossing the front of the ankle.

Posteriorly, on the inside, a *flexor retinaculum* runs between the medial malleolus and the calcaneus, and forms sheaths for tendons passing beneath the foot. *Peroneal retinacula* connect the lateral malleolus and the calcaneus, providing sheaths for tendons on the lateral side of the ankle (figures 8.29 and 8.30).

Muscles

Although the descriptions of muscles given in the text are the most common forms, many variations also are found. Muscles may vary in presence, attachments, and form.

Muscles such as the peroneus tertius, palmaris longus, flexor carpi radialis, psoas minor, semimembranosus, plantaris, and gastrocnemius may be missing on one or both sides in some individuals.

In other individuals, muscles may vary in the origins and insertions. For example, the latissimus dorsi may have fewer attachments to the ribs and vertebrae, the trapezius may lack an attachment to the occipital bone, and the flexor digitorum superficialis may lack a tendon to the fifth digit.

In other cases, a muscle may have extra parts called muscle slips. The slips may provide additional attachments to bones.

Muscles also show variations in shape and size. The biceps brachii and gastrocnemius may have a third head, the flexor digitorum superficialis may lack the portion attached to the radius, and the deltoid may be separated into three parts. The hamstring muscles may vary in length. If they are short, an individual will have difficulty bending over from the waist.

Clinical Terms Related to the Muscular System

contracture (kon-trak′chur)   a condition in which there is great resistance to the stretching of a muscle.

convulsion (kun-vul′shun)   an involuntary contraction of muscles.

fibrosis (fi-bro′sis)   a degenerative disease in which skeletal muscle tissue is replaced by fibrous connective tissue.

fibrositis (fi″bro-si′tis)   an inflammatory condition of fibrous connective tissues, especially in the muscle fascia. This disease is also called muscular rheumatism.

muscular dystrophy (mus′ku-lar dis′tro-fe)   a progressively crippling disease of unknown cause in which the muscles gradually weaken and atrophy.

myalgia (mi-al′je-ah)   pain resulting from any muscular disease or disorder.

myasthenia gravis (mi″as-the′ne-ah grav′is)   chronic disease characterized by muscles that are weak and easily fatigued. It results from a disorder at some of the neuromuscular junctions so that a stimulus is not transmitted from the motor neuron to the muscle fiber.

myology (mi-ol′o-je)   the study of muscles.

myoma (mi-o′mah)   a tumor composed of muscle tissue.

myopathy (mi-op′ah-the)   any muscular disease.

myositis (mi″o-si′tis)   an inflammation of skeletal muscle tissue.

myotomy (mi-ot′o-me)   the cutting of muscle tissue.

paralysis (pah-ral′i-sis)   the loss of ability to move a body part.

paresis (pah-re′sis)   a partial or slight paralysis of muscles.

shin splints   a soreness on the front of the lower leg due to slight fractures of the tibia or fibula, torn fascia of the leg muscles, or damage to the periosteum of the tibia. This often occurs as a result of running long distances or running on hard surfaces.

torticollis (tor″ti-kol′is)   a condition in which the neck muscles, such as the sternocleidomastoids, contract involuntarily. It is more commonly called wryneck.

Chapter Summary

Introduction (page 215)
Skeletal muscles usually are attached to bones and under conscious control.

Structure of a Skeletal Muscle (page 215)
Skeletal muscles are composed of nerve, vascular, and various connective tissues, as well as skeletal muscle tissue.

1. Connective tissue coverings
   a. Skeletal muscles are covered with fascia.
   b. Other connective tissues surround cells and groups of cells within the muscle's structure.
   c. Fascia is part of a complex network of connective tissue that extends throughout the body.
2. The neuromuscular junction
   a. Muscle fibers are stimulated to contract by motor neurons.
   b. The motor end plate of a muscle fiber lies on one side of a neuromuscular junction.
   c. The motor nerve fiber secretes a neurotransmitter, which stimulates the muscle fiber.
3. Motor units
   a. One motor neuron and the muscle fibers associated with it constitute a motor unit.
   b. Finer movements can be produced in muscles whose motor units contain small numbers of muscle fibers.

Skeletal Muscle Actions (page 218)
The type of movement produced by a muscle depends on the way it is attached on either side of a joint.

1. Origin and insertion
   a. The movable end of a muscle is its insertion, and the immovable end is its origin.
   b. Some muscles have more than one origin or insertion.
   c. Sometimes the end of a muscle changes its function in different body movements.
2. Interaction of skeletal muscles
   a. Skeletal muscles function in groups.
   b. A prime mover is responsible for most of a movement. Synergists aid prime movers. Antagonists can resist the movement of a prime mover.
   c. Smooth movements depend upon antagonists giving way to the actions of prime movers.

Major Skeletal Muscles (page 221)
Muscle names often describe sizes, shapes, locations, actions, number of attachments, or direction of fibers.

1. Muscles of facial expression lie beneath the skin of the face and scalp, and are used to communicate feelings through facial expression.
2. Muscles of mastication and swallowing
   a. These muscles are attached to the mandible and are used in chewing.
   b. Other muscles are attached to the hyoid and aid swallowing.
3. Muscles that move the head are in the neck and upper back.
4. Muscles that move the vertebral column are attached to the pelvic girdle, vertebrae, ribs, and skull.
5. Most muscles that move the pectoral girdle connect the scapula to nearby bones and are closely associated with muscles that move the upper arm.
6. Muscles that move the upper arm connect the humerus to various regions of the pectoral girdle, ribs, and vertebral column.
7. Muscles that move the forearm connect the radius and ulna to the humerus or pectoral girdle.
8. Muscles that move the wrist, hand, and fingers
   a. These muscles arise from the distal end of the humerus, and from the radius and ulna.
   b. Retinacula form sheaths for tendons of the extensor muscles.
9. Muscles of the abdominal wall connect the rib cage and vertebral column to the pelvic girdle.
10. Muscles of the pelvic outlet form the floor of the pelvic cavity and fill the space of the pubic arch.
11. Muscles that move the thigh are attached to the femur and to some part of the pelvic girdle.
12. Muscles that move the lower leg connect the tibia or fibula to the femur or pelvic girdle.
13. Muscles that move the ankle, foot, and toes
   a. These muscles attach the femur, tibia, and fibula to various bones of the foot.
   b. Retinacula form sheaths for tendons passing to the foot.

Clinical Application of Knowledge

1. Following childbirth, a woman may experience urinary incontinence when sneezing or coughing. What muscles of the pelvic floor should be strengthened by exercise to help control this problem?
2. Several important nerves and blood vessels course through the muscles of the gluteal region. In order to avoid the possibility of damaging such parts, intramuscular injections into this region usually are made into the lateral, superior portion of the gluteus medius. What landmarks would help you locate this muscle in a patient?
3. Following an injury to a nerve, the muscles it supplies with motor nerve fibers may become paralyzed. How would you explain to a patient the importance of having the disabled muscles moved passively or causing them to contract by using electrical stimulation?
4. After a knee joint injury, a patient is given exercises to strengthen the thigh muscles. Why must both the quadriceps femoris and hamstrings groups be included in the exercises? What kinds of exercises might strengthen these muscles without causing further injury to the knee joint?

Review Activities

Part A

1. Distinguish between a tendon and an aponeurosis.
2. Describe the connective tissue coverings of a skeletal muscle.
3. Distinguish between deep fascia, superficial fascia, and subserous fascia.
4. Describe a neuromuscular junction.
5. Define *motor unit* and explain how the number of fibers within a unit affects muscular contractions.
6. Distinguish between a muscle's origin and insertion.
7. Name two muscles that have more than one origin.
8. Define *prime mover, synergist,* and *antagonist.*
9. Describe the location, action, or size of the following muscles based on their names:
   a. gluteus maximus
   b. adductor longus
   c. levator scapulae
   d. temporalis
   e. tibialis anterior
   f. sternohyoid

Part B

Match the muscles in column I with the descriptions and functions in column II.

I	II
1. Buccinator	A. Inserted on the coronoid process of the mandible.
2. Epicranius	B. Draws the corner of the mouth upward.
3. Medial pterygoid	C. Can raise and adduct the scapula.
4. Platysma	D. Can pull the head into an upright position.
5. Rhomboideus major	
6. Splenius capitis	

7. Temporalis
8. Zygomaticus
9. Biceps brachii
10. Brachialis
11. Deltoid
12. Latissimus dorsi
13. Pectoralis major
14. Pronator teres
15. Teres minor
16. Triceps brachii
17. Biceps femoris
18. External oblique
19. Gastrocnemius
20. Gluteus maximus
21. Gluteus medius
22. Gracilis
23. Rectus femoris
24. Tibialis anterior
25. Digastric
26. Erector spinae

E. Consists of two parts—the frontalis and the occipitalis.
F. Raises the hyoid.
G. Extends over the neck from the chest to the face.
H. Pulls the jaw to the side in grinding movements.
I. Primary extensor of the elbow.
J. Pulls the shoulder back and downward.
K. Abducts the arm.
L. Rotates the arm laterally.
M. Pulls the arm forward and across the chest.
N. Rotates the arm medially.
O. Strongest flexor of the elbow.
P. Strongest supinator of the forearm.
Q. Extends the vertebral column.
R. A member of the quadriceps femoris group.
S. A plantar flexor of the foot.
T. Compresses the contents of the abdominal cavity.
U. Largest muscle in the body.
V. A hamstring muscle.
W. Adducts the thigh.
X. Abducts the thigh.
Y. Inverts the foot.
Z. Compresses the cheeks.

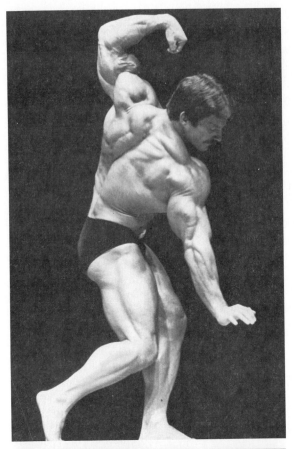

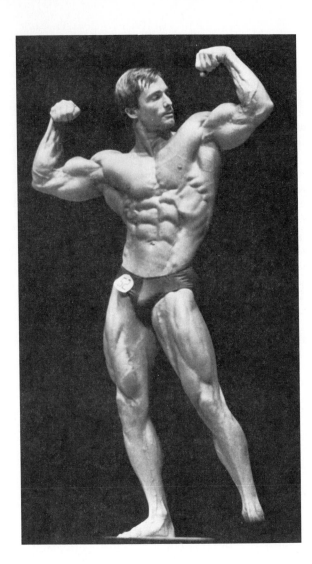

Part C
What muscles can you identify in the bodies of these models?

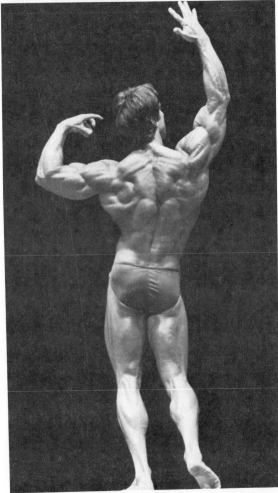

REFERENCE PLATES

Surface Anatomy

The following set of reference plates is presented to help you locate some of the more prominent surface features in various regions of the body. For the most part, the labeled structures are easily seen or palpated through the skin. Locate as many of these features as possible on your body as a review.

PLATE 21
Surface anatomy of head and neck, lateral view.

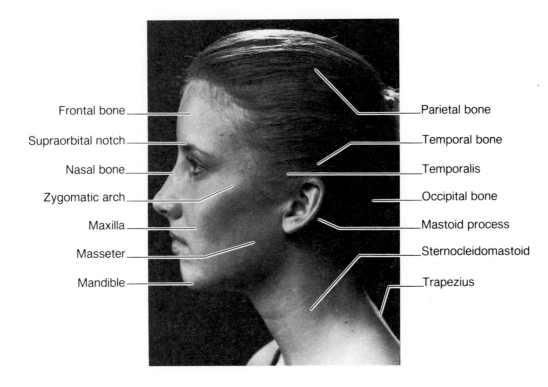

Frontal bone
Supraorbital notch
Nasal bone
Zygomatic arch
Maxilla
Masseter
Mandible

Parietal bone
Temporal bone
Temporalis
Occipital bone
Mastoid process
Sternocleidomastoid
Trapezius

PLATE 22
Surface anatomy of arm and thorax, lateral view.

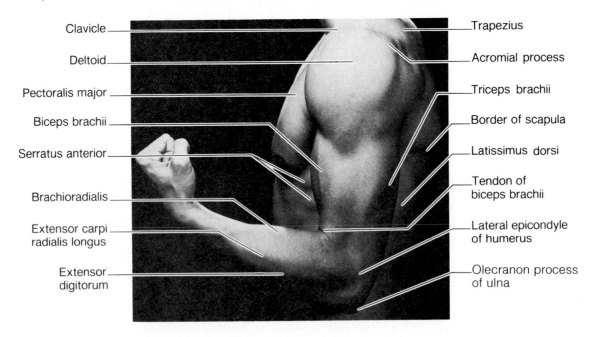

Clavicle
Deltoid
Pectoralis major
Biceps brachii
Serratus anterior
Brachioradialis
Extensor carpi radialis longus
Extensor digitorum

Trapezius
Acromial process
Triceps brachii
Border of scapula
Latissimus dorsi
Tendon of biceps brachii
Lateral epicondyle of humerus
Olecranon process of ulna

PLATE 23
Surface anatomy of back and arms, posterior view.

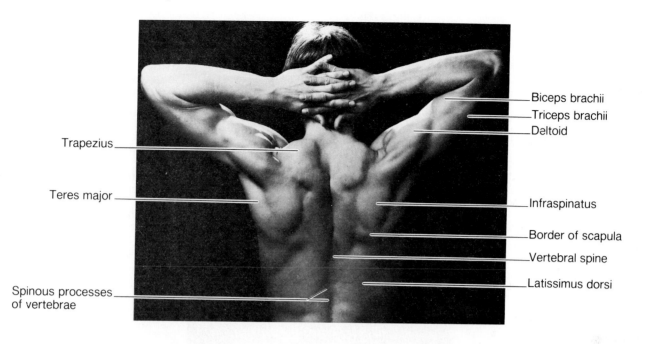

Trapezius

Teres major

Spinous processes
of vertebrae

Biceps brachii
Triceps brachii
Deltoid

Infraspinatus

Border of scapula

Vertebral spine

Latissimus dorsi

PLATE 24
Surface anatomy of torso and arms, anterior view.

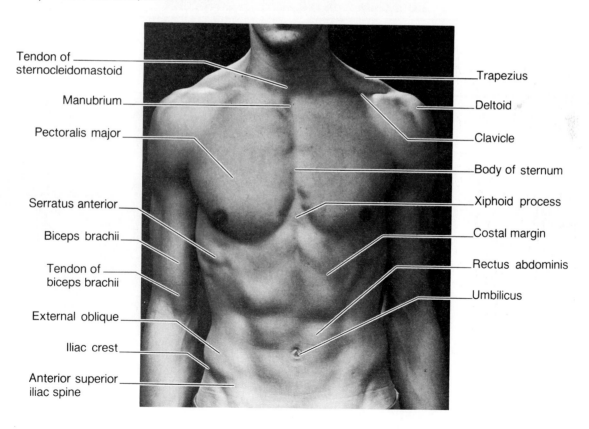

Tendon of
sternocleidomastoid

Manubrium

Pectoralis major

Serratus anterior

Biceps brachii

Tendon of
biceps brachii

External oblique

Iliac crest

Anterior superior
iliac spine

Trapezius

Deltoid

Clavicle

Body of sternum

Xiphoid process

Costal margin

Rectus abdominis

Umbilicus

PLATE 25
Surface anatomy of torso and upper legs, posterior view.

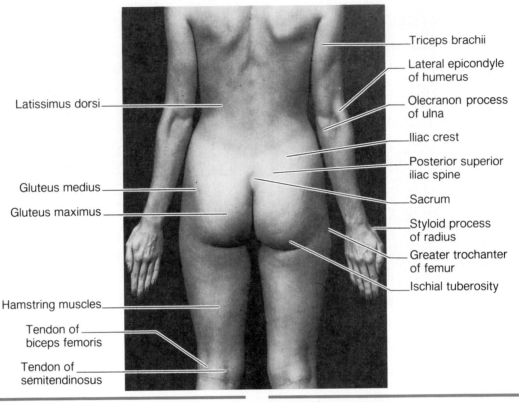

Triceps brachii

Lateral epicondyle
of humerus

Olecranon process
of ulna

Iliac crest

Latissimus dorsi

Posterior superior
iliac spine

Sacrum

Gluteus medius

Gluteus maximus

Styloid process
of radius

Greater trochanter
of femur

Ischial tuberosity

Hamstring muscles

Tendon of
biceps femoris

Tendon of
semitendinosus

PLATE 26
Surface anatomy of the arm, anterior view.

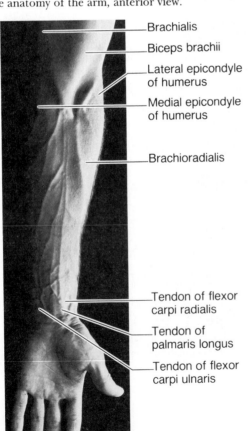

Brachialis

Biceps brachii

Lateral epicondyle
of humerus

Medial epicondyle
of humerus

Brachioradialis

Tendon of flexor
carpi radialis

Tendon of
palmaris longus

Tendon of flexor
carpi ulnaris

PLATE 27
Surface anatomy of the hand.

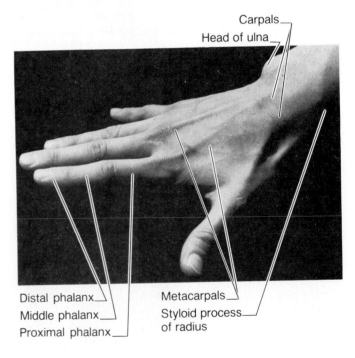

Carpals

Head of ulna

Distal phalanx

Middle phalanx

Proximal phalanx

Metacarpals

Styloid process
of radius

PLATE 28

Surface anatomy of knee and surrounding area, anterior view.

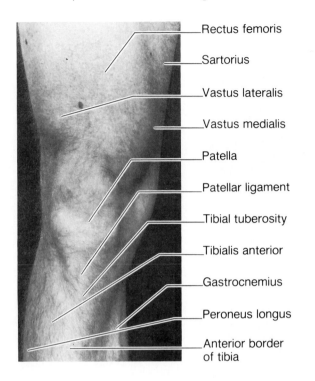

— Rectus femoris

— Sartorius

— Vastus lateralis

— Vastus medialis

— Patella

— Patellar ligament

— Tibial tuberosity

— Tibialis anterior

— Gastrocnemius

— Peroneus longus

— Anterior border of tibia

PLATE 29

Surface anatomy of knee and surrounding area, lateral view.

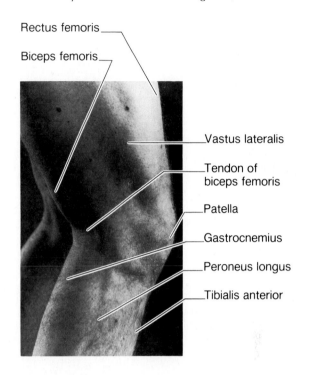

Rectus femoris

Biceps femoris

— Vastus lateralis

— Tendon of biceps femoris

— Patella

— Gastrocnemius

— Peroneus longus

— Tibialis anterior

PLATE 30

Surface anatomy of ankle and lower leg, medial view.

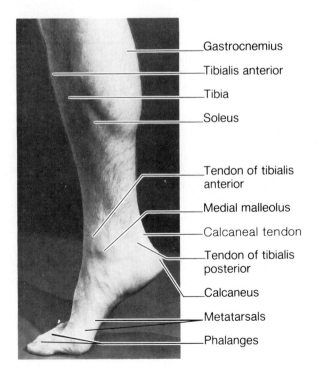

— Gastrocnemius

— Tibialis anterior

— Tibia

— Soleus

— Tendon of tibialis anterior

— Medial malleolus

— Calcaneal tendon

— Tendon of tibialis posterior

— Calcaneus

— Metatarsals

— Phalanges

PLATE 31

Surface anatomy of the ankle and foot.

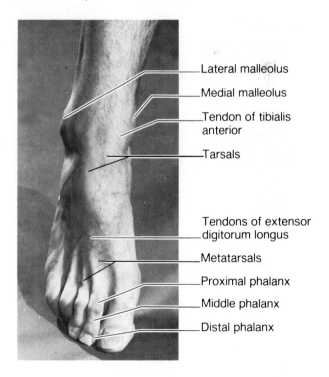

— Lateral malleolus

— Medial malleolus

— Tendon of tibialis anterior

— Tarsals

— Tendons of extensor digitorum longus

— Metatarsals

— Proximal phalanx

— Middle phalanx

— Distal phalanx

U N I T 3

Integration and Coordination

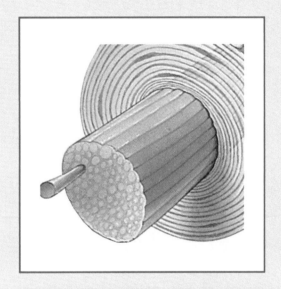

The chapters of unit 3 are concerned with the structures and functions of the nervous and endocrine systems. They describe how the organs of these systems keep the parts of the human body functioning together as a whole and how these organs help maintain a stable internal environment, which is vital to the survival of the organism.

CHAPTER 9

The Nervous System

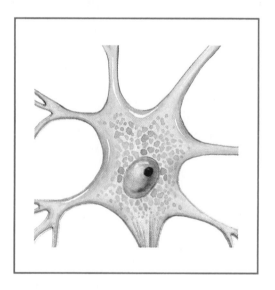

Neurons, the structural and functional units of the nervous system, communicate with one another by means of nerve impulses. Some are specialized to detect changes that occur inside and outside the body, and can transmit impulses to processing centers within the brain or spinal cord. Other neurons gather the incoming information, integrate it, and act on it in various ways. Still others can transmit signals to muscles and glands, causing them to respond.

These functions are essential in the control and coordination of the body, enabling its parts to work together to maintain a stable internal environment. The organs of the nervous system can be divided into two major groups. The brain and spinal cord comprise the central nervous system, while nerves that connect the brain and spinal cord to other body parts form the peripheral nervous system. The peripheral nervous system can be subdivided further into a somatic system, composed of the peripheral nerves that communicate with skin and skeletal muscles, and an autonomic system, composed of the peripheral nerves that communicate with visceral organs.

Chapter Outline

Chapter Objectives

After you have studied this chapter, you should be able to

1. Explain the general functions of the nervous system.

2. Describe the general structure of a neuron.

3. Name four types of neuroglial cells and describe the functions of each.

4. Describe two ways neurons are organized in neuronal pools.

5. Explain how neurons are classified.

6. Describe a reflex arc and explain what is meant by reflex behavior.

7. Describe the structure of the spinal cord and its major functions.

8. Name the major parts of the brain and describe the functions of each.

9. Distinguish between motor, sensory, and association areas of the cerebral cortex.

10. Describe the formation and function of cerebrospinal fluid.

11. List the major parts of the peripheral nervous system and describe the structure of a peripheral nerve.

12. Name the cranial nerves and list their major functions.

13. Explain how spinal nerves are named, and explain their functions.

14. Describe the general characteristics of the autonomic nervous system.

15. Distinguish between the sympathetic and the parasympathetic divisions of the autonomic nervous system.

16. Complete the review activities at the end of this chapter. Note that the items are worded in the form of specific learning objectives. You may want to refer to them before reading the chapter.

Aids to Understanding Words

astr-, starlike: *astr*ocyte—a star-shaped neuroglial cell.

chiasm-, a cross: optic *chiasm*a—an X-shaped structure produced by the crossing over of optic nerve fibers.

dendr-, tree: *dendr*ite—branched nerve fibers that serve as receptor surfaces of a neuron.

ependym-, tunic or covering: *ependym*a—neuroglial cells that line spaces within the brain and spinal cord.

funi-, small cord or fiber: *funi*culus—a major nerve tract or bundle of myelinated nerve fibers within the spinal cord.

gangli-, a swelling: *gangli*on—a mass of neuron cell bodies.

-lemm, rind or peel: neuri*lemm*a—a sheath that surrounds the myelin of a nerve fiber.

mening-, membrane: *mening*es—membranous coverings of the brain and spinal cord.

moto-, moving: *moto*r neuron—neuron that stimulates a muscle to contract or a gland to release a secretion.

oligo-, few: *oligo*dendrocyte—small neuroglial cell with few cellular processes.

peri-, all around: *peri*pheral nervous system—portion of the nervous system that consists of the nerves branching from the brain and spinal cord.

plex-, interweaving: *plex*us—a network of interweaving spinal nerves.

syn-, together: *syn*apse—junction between two neurons.

Introduction

Organs of the nervous system, like other organs, are composed of various kinds of tissues, including nerve tissue, connective tissues, and blood. These organs can be divided into two groups. One group, consisting of the brain and spinal cord, forms the **central nervous system (CNS),** and the other, which includes the nerves (peripheral nerves) that connect the central nervous system to other body parts, is called the **peripheral nervous system (PNS)** (figure 9.1). Together these parts have three general functions—a sensory function, an integrative function, and a motor function.

General Functions of the Nervous System

The sensory function of the nervous system involves sensory *receptors* at the ends of peripheral nerves. These receptors are specialized to gather information by detecting changes that occur inside and outside the body.

The information that is gathered is converted to signals in the form of *nerve impulses,* which are transmitted over peripheral nerves to the central nervous system. There the signals are integrated—that is, they are brought together. As a result of this integrative function, conscious or subconscious decisions are made and then acted upon by means of motor functions.

The motor functions of the nervous system employ peripheral nerves, which carry impulses from the central nervous system to responsive parts called *effectors.* These effectors are outside the nervous system and include muscles that contract when they are stimulated by nerve impulses, and glands that may produce a secretion when they are stimulated.

Thus, the nervous system can detect changes occurring in the body, make decisions on the basis of the information received, and cause muscles or glands to respond. Typically, these responses are directed toward counteracting the effects of the changes, and in this way the nervous system helps maintain stable internal conditions.

Nerve Tissue

The nerve tissue of the brain, spinal cord, and nerves consists of masses of nerve cells, or **neurons,** that are the structural and functional units of the nervous system. These cells are specialized to react to physical and chemical changes occurring in their surroundings. They also conduct nerve impulses to other neurons and to cells outside the nervous system. (See figure 9.2.)

As mentioned in chapter 4, **neuroglial cells** are accessory cells within nerve tissue. They greatly outnumber the neurons and function much like connective tissue cells in other body structures; that is, they fill spaces and surround or support various parts.

Neuron Structure

Although neurons vary considerably in size and shape, they have certain features in common. For example, every neuron has a cell body and tubular processes filled with cytoplasm that conduct nerve impulses to or from the cell body (figure 9.3).

FIGURE 9.1

The nervous system consists of the brain, spinal cord, and peripheral nerves.

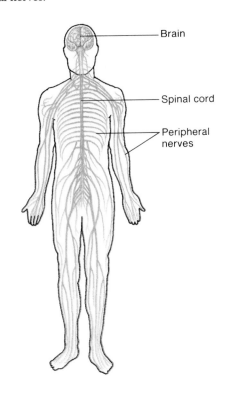

FIGURE 9.2

Neurons are the structural and functional units of the nervous system ($\times 50$).

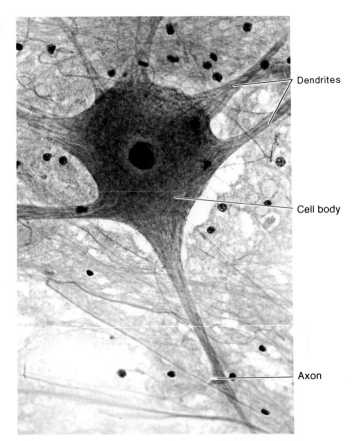

FIGURE 9.3

(*a*) Motor neuron and (*b*) sensory neuron.

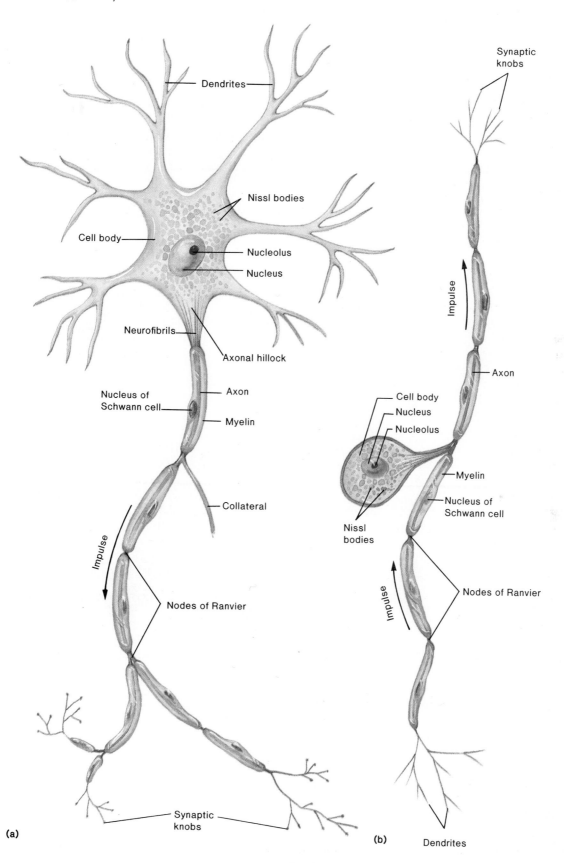

The **cell body** (perikaryon) contains a mass of cytoplasm, a cell membrane, and various other organelles. Inside the cell body are mitochondria, lysosomes, a Golgi apparatus, a centrosome, and numerous microtubules. There also is a network of fine threads called **neurofibrils,** which extend into the cell processes and provide support for these processes. Scattered throughout the cytoplasm are masses of rough endoplasmic reticulum called **Nissl bodies**. Ribosomes attached to the surfaces of these membranes manufacture vital protein molecules. Cytoplasmic inclusions are common.

Near the center of the cell body there is a large, spherical nucleus with a conspicuous nucleolus. This nucleus apparently does not undergo mitosis after the nervous system is developed, and consequently mature neurons seem to be incapable of reproduction.

Two kinds of nerve fibers, **dendrites** and **axons,** extend from the cell bodies of most neurons. Although a neuron usually has many dendrites, it has only one axon.

In most neurons, the dendrites are relatively short and highly branched. These branches, together with the membrane of the cell body, provide the main receptive surfaces

FIGURE 9.4

(*a*) The portion of a Schwann cell that is tightly wound around an axon forms the myelin sheath; the cytoplasm and nucleus of the Schwann cell form the neurilemmal sheath. (*b*) A small axon lying in a longitudinal groove of a Schwann cell lacks a myelin sheath.

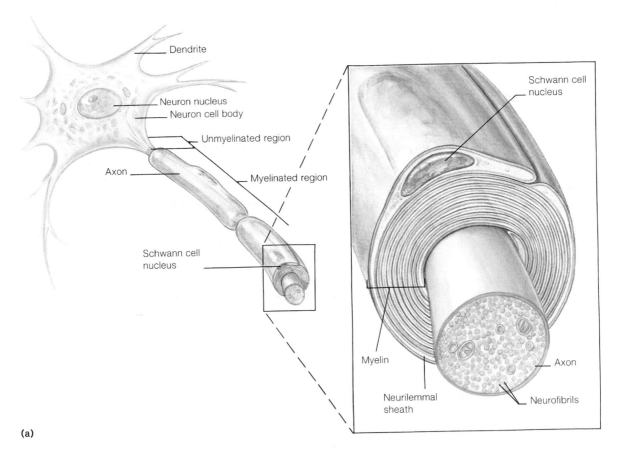

(a)

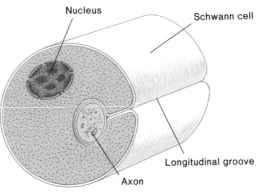

(b)

of the neuron with which fibers from other neurons communicate. Often the dendrites possess tiny, thornlike spines (dendritic spines) on their surfaces, which serve as contact points for parts of other neurons.

The axon (ak'son), which usually arises from a slight elevation of the cell body (axon hillock), is a slender, cylindrical process with a nearly smooth surface and uniform diameter. It is specialized to conduct nerve impulses away from the cell body. Many mitochondria, microtubules, and neurofibrils occur within the cytoplasm of the axon. Although it begins as a single fiber, an axon may give off branches called *collaterals*. Near its end, it may have many fine branches, each with a specialized ending called a *synaptic knob*, which contacts the receptive surface of another cell.

Larger axons of peripheral nerves are commonly enclosed in sheaths composed of peripheral neuroglial cells called **Schwann cells.** These cells are tightly wound around the axons, somewhat like a bandage wrapped around a finger. As a result, the axons are coated with many layers of cell membranes that have little or no cytoplasm between them. These membranes are composed largely of a substance called *myelin* (mi'e-lin), which forms a **myelin sheath** on the outside of an axon. In addition, the portions of the Schwann cells that contain cytoplasm and nuclei remain outside the myelin sheath and comprise a **neurilemma** (neurilemmal sheath), which surrounds the myelin sheath. This sheath is not continuous, but is interrupted by constrictions called *nodes of Ranvier,* which occur between adjacent Schwann cells (figures 9.4 and 9.5).

The smallest axons are also enclosed by Schwann cells, but the Schwann cells are not wound around these axons. Consequently such axons lack myelin sheaths.

Axons that possess myelin sheaths are called *myelinated* (medullated) nerve fibers, while those that lack these sheaths are *unmyelinated* (non-medullated) nerve fibers (figure 9.5). While Schwann cells form myelin sheaths around peripheral nerve fibers, other neuroglial cells (oligodendrocytes) form these sheaths within the brain and spinal cord. Groups of myelinated fibers appear white, and form the white matter in the brain and spinal cord. Unmyelinated nerve tissue appears gray. Thus, the gray matter within the brain and spinal cord contains many unmyelinated nerve fibers and cell bodies.

A myelin sheath functions in nerve impulse conduction. Myelinated fibers conduct impulses more rapidly than unmyelinated fibers.

The speed of nerve impulse conduction is also related to the diameter of the fiber—the greater the diameter, the faster the impulse. For example, an impulse on a thick myelinated fiber, such as a motor fiber associated with a skeletal muscle, might travel 120 meters per second, while an impulse on a thin unmyelinated fiber, such as a sensory fiber associated with the skin, might move only 0.5 meter per second.

FIGURE 9.5

(*a*) A transmission electron micrograph of myelinated and unmyelinated axons in cross section. (*b*) Light micrograph of a myelinated nerve fiber (longitudinal section), showing a node of Ranvier (×300).

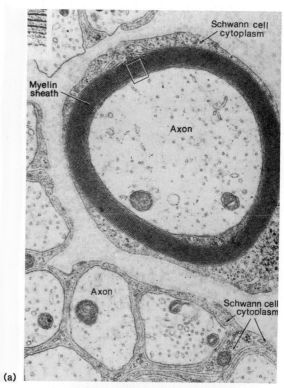

(a)

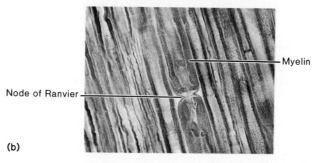

(b)

1. List the general functions of the nervous system.
2. Describe a neuron.
3. What is meant by the term *nerve fiber*?
4. Explain where myelin is found in the peripheral nervous system.

Neuroglial Cells

As mentioned earlier, neuroglial cells fill spaces, support neurons, and provide frameworks within the organs of the nervous system. They also enclose neurons in ways that prevent contact between nearby cells except at particular sites (figures 9.6 and 9.7).

FIGURE 9.6

Types of neuroglial cells found within the central nervous system include (*a*) microglial cell, (*b*) oligodendrocyte, (*c*) astrocyte, and (*d*) ependymal cell.

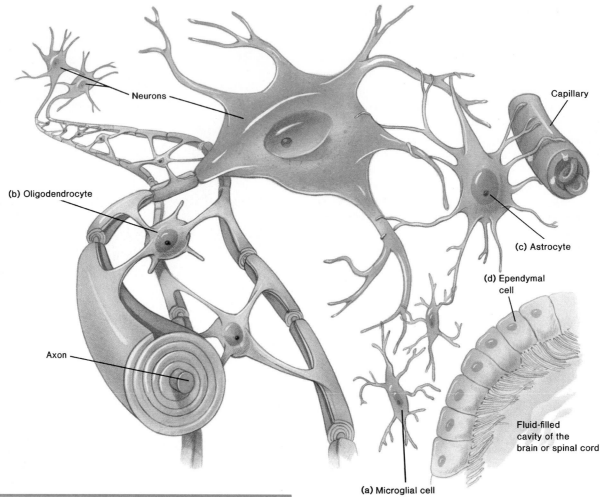

FIGURE 9.7

A scanning electron micrograph of a neuron cell body and some neuroglial cells associated with it (about ×10,000).
R. G. Kessel and R. H. Kardon, *Tissues and Organs: A Text Atlas of Scanning Electron Microscopy,* © 1979, W. H. Freeman & Co.

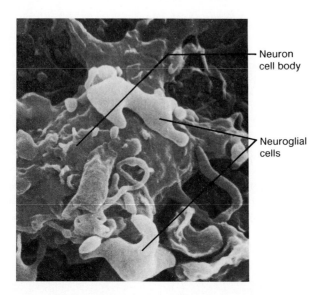

Within the peripheral nervous system, the neuroglial cells include the Schwann cells previously described. In the central nervous system, the neuroglial cells greatly outnumber the neurons. They include the following types:

1. **Astrocytes.** As their name implies, astrocytes are star-shaped cells. They are the most numerous neuroglial cells and are commonly found between neurons and blood vessels, where they seem to provide structural support and hold parts together by means of numerous cellular processes. They also respond to injury of brain tissue and are responsible for the formation of scar tissue that fills spaces and closes gaps following injuries. Astrocytes may have a nutritive function involving the transport of substances from blood vessels to neurons.

2. **Oligodendrocytes.** Oligodendrocytes resemble astrocytes, but are smaller and have fewer processes. They are commonly arranged in rows along nerve fibers, and they function in the formation of myelin within the brain and spinal cord.

Regeneration of a Nerve Fiber

Injury to a cell body is most likely to cause the death of the neuron; however, a damaged axon may be regenerated. For example, if an axon in a peripheral nerve is separated from its cell body by injury or disease, the distal portion of the axon and its myelin sheath deteriorates within a few weeks. Macrophages remove the fragments of myelin and other cellular debris. Although some Schwann cells may also degenerate, a thin basement membrane and a layer of connective tissue (endoneurium) surrounding the Schwann cells will remain. These parts form a tube that leads back to the original connection of the axon.

The proximal end of the injured axon develops sprouts shortly after the injury, and one of these sprouts may grow into the tube formed by the basement membrane and connective tissue. At the same time, remaining Schwann cells proliferate along the length of the degenerating fiber, and form new myelin around the growing axon.

The growth of such a regenerating fiber is slow (3 to 4 millimeters per day), but eventually the new fiber may reestablish the former connection (figure 9.8).

If an axon of a nerve fiber within the central nervous system is separated from its cell body, the distal portion of the axon degenerates, although the rate of degeneration is somewhat slower. However, the axons lack connective tissue sheaths, and the myelin-producing oligodendrocytes fail to proliferate following an injury. Consequently, if the proximal end of a damaged axon begins to grow, there is no tube of sheath cells to guide it, and a functionally significant regeneration is unlikely to take place.

If a peripheral nerve is severed, it is very important that the two cut ends be closely connected as soon as possible. The regenerating sprouts of the nerve fibers can then more easily reach the tubes formed by the basement membranes and connective tissues on the other side of the gap.

When the gap exceeds 3 millimeters, the regenerating fibers tend to form a tangled mass called a *neuroma*. A neuroma composed of sensory nerve fibers is likely to be painfully sensitive to pressure. The development of such growths sometimes complicates a patient's recovery following the amputation of a limb.

FIGURE 9.8

If a myelinated axon is injured (*a*) the proximal portion of the fiber may survive, but (*b*) the portion distal to the injury degenerates. (*c*) and (*d*) In time, the proximal portion may develop extensions that grow into the tube of basement membrane and connective tissue cells previously occupied by the fiber. Thus, (*e*) the former connection may be reestablished.

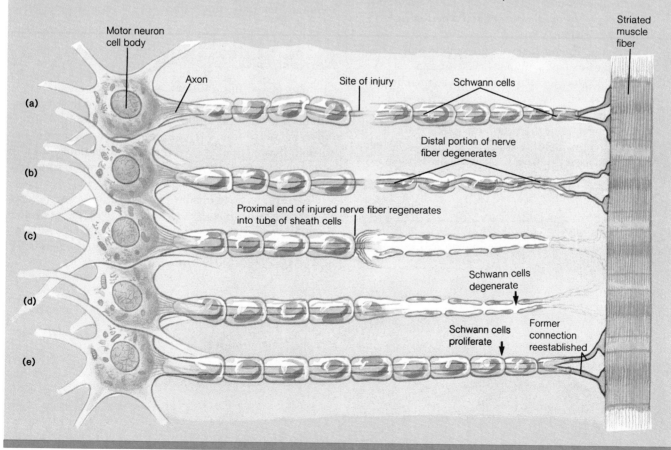

Unlike the Schwann cells of the peripheral nervous system, oligodendrocytes can send out a number of cellular processes, each of which wraps tightly around a nearby axon. In this way, a single oligodendrocyte may provide myelin for many axons. However, these cells do not form neurilemmal sheaths.

Although myelin begins to form on nerve fibers during the fourteenth week of development, many of the nerve fibers in a newborn infant are not completely myelinated. Consequently, the nervous system is unable to function as effectively as that of an older child or adult. An infant's responses to stimuli are therefore coarse and undifferentiated, and may involve its whole body. The great increase in brain size in an infant's first year is due mostly to the development of myelin sheaths around neurons in the brain. Essentially all myelinated fibers have begun to develop sheaths by the time a child starts to walk. Myelination continues into adolescence.

Any interference with the supply of essential nutrients during the developmental years may result in an insufficient amount of myelin formation. This, in turn, may cause impaired function of the nervous system.

---

3. **Microglia.** Microglial cells are relatively small and have fewer processes than other types of neuroglial cells. These cells are scattered throughout the central nervous system, where they help support neurons and break down bacterial cells and cellular debris. They usually increase in number whenever the brain or spinal cord is inflamed because of injury or disease.

4. **Ependyma.** Ependymal cells are cuboidal or columnar in shape and may have cilia and microvilli. They form an epithelial-like membrane that is one cell thick and covers the inside of spaces within the brain, called *ventricles*. They also form the inner lining of the *central canal* that extends downward through the spinal cord, and they cover the specialized capillaries called *choroid plexuses*, which are associated with the ventricles of the brain.

---

1. What is a neuroglial cell?
2. Name and describe four types of neuroglial cells.

The Synapse

Within the nervous system, nerve impulses travel from neuron to neuron along complex nerve pathways. The junction between the parts of two such neurons is called a **synapse.** Actually, these cells, called *presynaptic* and *postsynaptic neurons,* are not in direct contact at the synapse. There is a gap called a *synaptic cleft* between them, and an impulse must cross this gap to continue along a nerve pathway (figure 9.9).

Axons usually have several rounded synaptic knobs at their terminal ends. These knobs contain numerous membranous sacs, called *synaptic vesicles.* When a nerve impulse reaches a knob, some of the vesicles respond by releasing a substance called a **neurotransmitter** (figures 9.10 and 9.11).

Within the brain and spinal cord, the synaptic knobs of a thousand or more nerve fibers may communicate with the dendrites and cell body of each neuron (figure 9.12).

---

1. Describe a synapse.
2. Describe the structures found in a synaptic knob.

Organization of Neurons

The way the nervous system processes nerve impulses and acts upon them reflects, in part, the organization of neurons and their nerve fibers within the brain and spinal cord.

Neuronal Pools

The neurons within the central nervous system are organized into groups called *neuronal pools,* which have varying numbers of cells. Each pool receives impulses from input (afferent) nerve fibers. These impulses are processed according to the special characteristics of the pool, and any resulting impulses are conducted away on output (efferent) fibers.

Each input fiber divides many times as it enters, and its branches spread over a certain region of the neuronal pool. The branches give off smaller branches and their synaptic knobs form hundreds of synapses with the dendrites and cell bodies of the neurons in the pool.

FIGURE 9.9

For an impulse to continue from one neuron to another, it must cross the synaptic cleft at a synapse. A synapse may occur (*a*) between an axon and a dendrite, or (*b*) between an axon and a cell body.

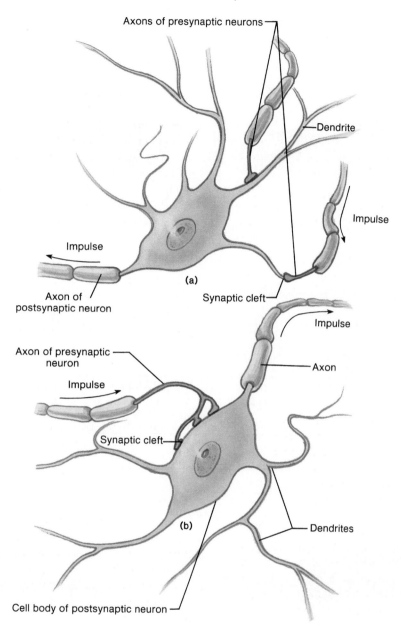

Convergence

Any single neuron in a neuronal pool may receive impulses from two or more incoming fibers. Furthermore, these fibers may originate from different parts of the nervous system, and are said to *converge* when they lead to the same neuron (figure 9.13).

Convergence allows the nervous system to bring together a variety of information, process it, and respond to it. An example of a converging pool is found in the rods and bipolar neurons of the eye. (See chapter 10.)

Divergence

Impulses leaving a neuron of a neuronal pool often *diverge* by passing into several other output fibers. For example, one neuron may synapse with two others; each of these, in turn, may synapse with several others; and so forth. Such an arrangement of diverging nerve fibers can cause an impulse to be *amplified*—that is, to be spread to increasing numbers of neurons within the pool (figure 9.13). Motor pathways from the brain and spinal cord form diverging pools.

FIGURE 9.10

(a) When a nerve impulse reaches the synaptic knob at the end of an axon, (b) synaptic vesicles release a neurotransmitter substance that moves across the synaptic cleft.

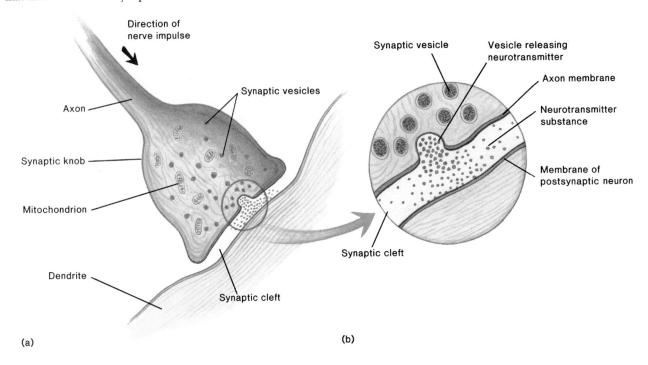

(a)

(b)

FIGURE 9.11

A transmission electron micrograph of a synaptic knob filled with synaptic vesicles.

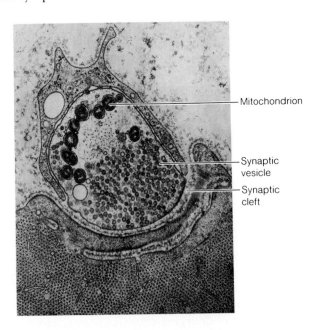

FIGURE 9.12

Within the brain and spinal cord, thousands of nerve fibers may synapse with a single neuron.

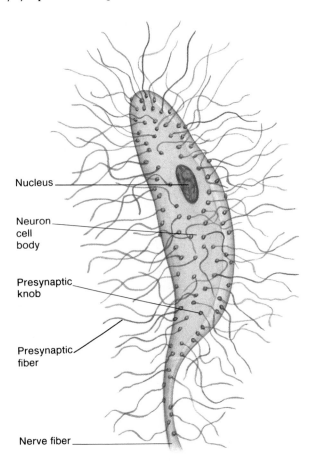

FIGURE 9.13
(*a*) Nerve fibers of neurons 1 and 2 converge to the cell body of neuron 3; (*b*) the nerve fiber of neuron 4 diverges to the cell bodies of neurons 5 and 6.

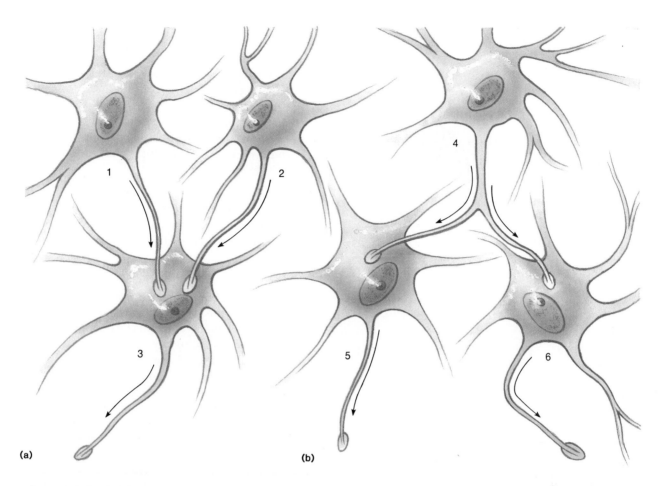

(a)   (b)

---

1. What is a neuronal pool?
2. What is meant by convergence?
3. What is the relationship between divergence and amplification?

Classification of Neurons and Nerves

Neurons differ in the structure, size, and shape of their cell bodies. They also vary in the length and size of their axons and dendrites, and in the number of synaptic knobs by which they communicate with other neurons.

Neurons also vary in function. Some carry impulses into the brain or spinal cord, others transmit impulses from the brain or spinal cord, and still others conduct impulses from neuron to neuron within the brain or spinal cord.

Classification of Neurons

On the basis of *structural* differences, neurons can be classified into three major groups, as shown in figure 9.14:

1. **Bipolar neurons.** The cell body of a bipolar neuron has only two nerve fibers, one arising from either end. Although these fibers have similar structural characteristics, one serves as an axon and the other as a dendrite. Such neurons are found within specialized parts of the eyes, nose, and ears.

2. **Unipolar neurons.** Each unipolar neuron has a single nerve fiber extending from its cell body. A short distance from the cell body, this fiber divides into two branches: One branch is connected to a peripheral body part and serves as a dendrite, and the other enters the brain or spinal cord and serves as an axon. Unipolar neuron cell bodies occur in groups called *ganglia,* which are located outside the brain and spinal cord. (Note: The sensory neuron illustrated in figure 9.3 is unipolar.)

3. **Multipolar neurons.** Multipolar neurons have many nerve fibers arising from their cell bodies. Only one fiber of each neuron is an axon; the rest are dendrites. Most neurons whose cell bodies lie within the brain or spinal cord are of this type.

FIGURE 9.14
Structural types of neurons include (*a*) the bipolar neuron, (*b*) the unipolar neuron, and (*c*) the multipolar neuron. Where can examples of each of these be found in the body?

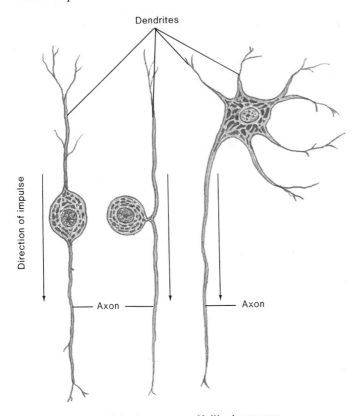

Dendrites

Direction of impulse

Axon — — Axon

Bipolar neuron   **Unipolar neuron**   **Multipolar neuron**

(a)   (b)   (c)

Neurons can also be classified on the basis of their *functional* differences into the following groups:

1. **Sensory neurons** (afferent neurons) are those that carry nerve impulses from peripheral body parts into the brain or spinal cord. These neurons have specialized *receptor ends* at the tips of their dendrites, or they have dendrites that are closely associated with receptor cells located in the skin or various sensory organs.

    Changes that occur inside or outside the body are likely to stimulate receptor ends or receptor cells, triggering sensory nerve impulses. The impulses travel along the sensory neuron fibers, which lead to the brain or spinal cord, and are processed in these parts by other neurons. Most sensory neurons are unipolar (figure 9.14).

2. **Interneurons** (also called association, intercalated, or internuncial neurons) lie within the brain or spinal cord. They are multipolar and form links

between other neurons. Interneurons transmit impulses from one part of the brain or spinal cord to another. That is, they may direct incoming sensory impulses to appropriate parts for processing and interpreting. Other incoming impulses are transferred to motor neurons.

3. **Motor neurons** (efferent neurons) are multipolar and carry nerve impulses out of the brain or spinal cord to **effectors**—parts of the body capable of responding, such as muscles or glands. When motor impulses reach muscles, for example, these effectors are stimulated to contract; when motor impulses reach glands, the glands are stimulated to release secretions.

Two specialized groups of motor neurons supply impulses to smooth and cardiac muscles. The *accelerator neurons* cause an increase in muscular activities, while the *inhibitory neurons* cause such actions to decrease.

Types of Nerves

Although a nerve fiber is an extension of a neuron, a **nerve** is a cordlike bundle (or group of bundles) of nerve fibers held together by layers of connective tissues (figure 9.15).

Like nerve fibers, nerves that conduct impulses into the brain or spinal cord are called **sensory nerves,** and those that carry impulses out to muscles or glands are termed **motor nerves.** Most nerves, however, include both sensory and motor fibers, and they are called **mixed nerves.**

Nerves originating from the spinal cord that communicate with other body parts are called *spinal nerves,* while those originating from the brain that communicate with other body parts are *cranial nerves.*

---

1. Explain how neurons are classified according to structure and function.
2. How is a neuron related to a nerve?
3. What is a mixed nerve?

Nerve Pathways

The routes followed by nerve impulses as they travel through the nervous system are called *nerve pathways.* The simplest of these pathways includes only a few neurons and is called a reflex arc.

Reflex Arcs

A **reflex arc** begins with a receptor at the end of a sensory nerve fiber. This fiber usually leads to several interneurons within the central nervous system, which serve as a processing or *reflex center.* Fibers from interneurons may

FIGURE 9.15
A nerve is composed of bundles of nerve fibers held together
by connective tissues.

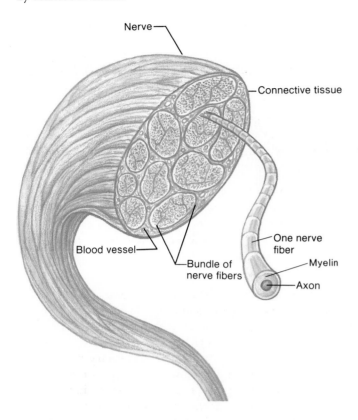

connect with interneurons in other parts of the nervous
system. They also communicate with motor neurons, whose
fibers pass outward to effectors. (See figure 9.16.)

Such a reflex arc represents the behavioral unit of the
nervous system. That is, it constitutes the structural and
functional basis for the simplest acts—the reflexes.

Reflex Behavior

Reflexes are automatic, unconscious responses to changes
occurring in or out of the body. They are mechanisms that
help control many of the body's involuntary processes such
as heart rate, breathing rate, blood pressure, and digestive
activities. Reflexes are also involved in the automatic actions of swallowing, sneezing, coughing, and vomiting. The
two reflex arcs described in the following paragraphs involve skeletal muscles. In other reflexes, the effectors may
be smooth muscle of a visceral organ or cardiac muscle of
the heart.

The *knee-jerk reflex* (patellar tendon reflex) is an example of a simple reflex that employs only two neurons—
a sensory neuron communicating directly with a motor
neuron. This reflex is initiated by striking the patellar ligament just below the patella. As a result, the quadriceps
femoris group of muscles, which is attached to the patella
by a tendon, is pulled slightly, and stretch receptors located within the muscles are stimulated. These receptors,
in turn, trigger impulses that pass along the fiber of a sensory neuron into the lumbar region of the spinal cord.

FIGURE 9.16
A reflex arc usually includes a receptor, sensory neuron, interneurons, motor neuron, and an effector.

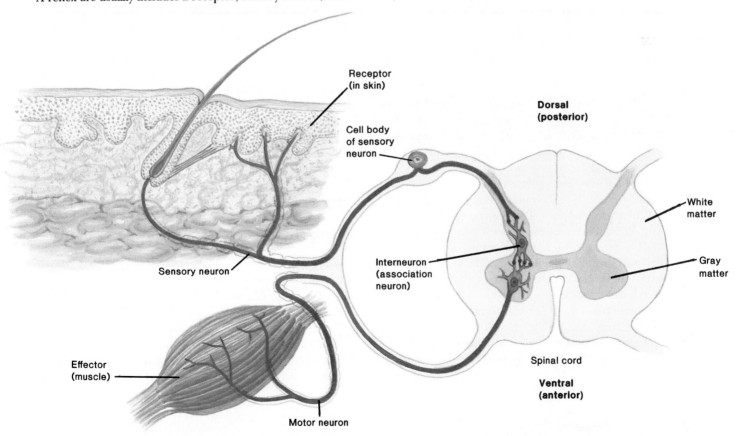

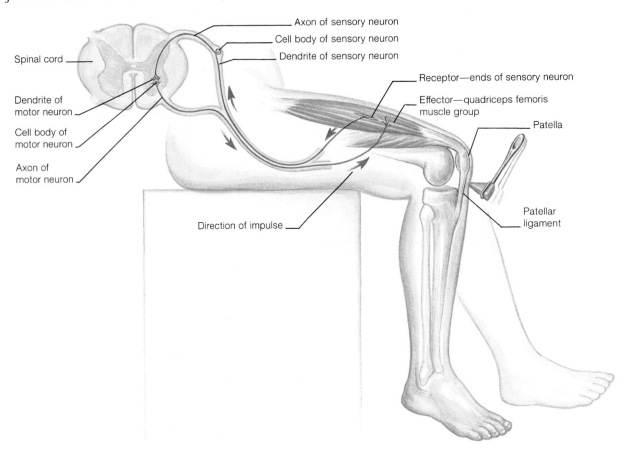

Within the cord, the sensory axon forms a synapse with a dendrite of a motor neuron. The impulse then continues along the axon of the motor neuron and travels back to the quadriceps femoris. The muscles respond by contracting, and the reflex is completed as the lower leg extends (figure 9.17).

This reflex is helpful in maintaining an upright posture. For example, if a person is standing still and the knee begins to bend as a result of gravity, the quadriceps femoris is stretched, the reflex is triggered, and the leg straightens again.

Another type of reflex, called a *withdrawal reflex*, occurs when a person unexpectedly touches a finger to something painful. When this happens, the skin receptors are activated, and impulses travel on sensory neurons to interneurons of a reflex center and to motor neurons. The motor neurons stimulate the flexor muscles in the arm, and the muscles contract, causing the part to be pulled away from the painful stimulus.

At the same time, some of the incoming impulses stimulate interneurons that inhibit the action of the antagonistic extensor muscles. This inhibition (reciprocal innervation) allows flexor muscles to effectively withdraw the hand.

Concurrent with the withdrawal reflex, other interneurons in the spinal cord carry sensory impulses to the brain, and the person becomes aware of the painful experience and may feel pain. A withdrawal reflex is, of course, protective because it prevents excessive tissue damage when a body part touches something potentially harmful. Chart 9.1 summarizes the parts of a reflex arc.

1. What is a nerve pathway?
2. Describe a reflex arc.
3. Describe the events that occur during a knee-jerk reflex.

The Meninges

The organs of the central nervous system (CNS) are surrounded by bones, membranes, and fluid. More specifically, the brain lies within the cranial cavity of the skull, while the spinal cord, which is continuous with the brain, occupies the vertebral canal within the vertebral column. Beneath these bony coverings, the brain and spinal cord are protected by membranes called meninges located between the bone and the soft tissues of the nervous system.

Chart 9.1 Parts of a reflex arc

Part	Description	Function
Receptor	The receptor end of a dendrite or a specialized receptor cell in a sensory organ	Sensitive to a specific type of internal or external change
Sensory neuron	Dendrite, cell body, and axon of a sensory neuron	Transmits nerve impulse from the receptor into the brain or spinal cord
Interneuron	Dendrite, cell body, and axon of a neuron within the brain or spinal cord	Serves as a processing center; conducts nerve impulse from the sensory neuron to a motor neuron
Motor neuron	Dendrite, cell body, and axon of a motor neuron	Transmits nerve impulse from the brain or spinal cord out to an effector
Effector	A muscle or gland outside the nervous system	Responds to stimulation by the motor neuron and produces the reflex or behavioral action.

FIGURE 9.18

(*a*) The brain and spinal cord are enclosed by bone and by membranes called meninges. (*b*) The meninges include three layers: dura mater, arachnoid mater, and pia mater.

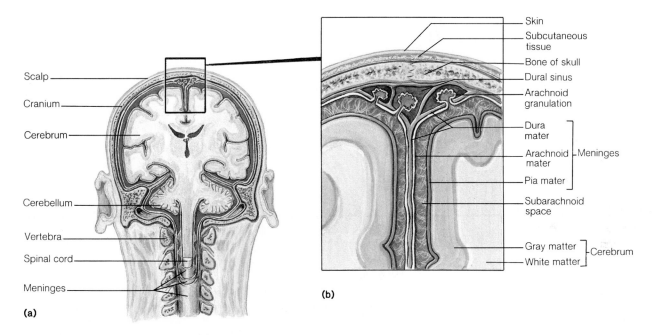

(a)

(b)

The **meninges** (me-nin′jēz) have three layers—dura mater, arachnoid mater, and pia mater (figure 9.18).

The **dura mater** is the outermost layer. It is composed primarily of tough, white fibrous connective tissue and contains many blood vessels and nerves. It is attached to the inside of the cranial cavity and forms the internal periosteum of the surrounding skull bones.

In some regions, the dura mater extends inward between lobes of the brain and forms partitions that support and protect these parts (chart 9.2). In other areas, the dura mater splits into two layers, forming channels called *dural sinuses,* shown in figure 9.18. Venous blood flows through these channels as it returns from the brain to vessels leading to the heart.

Chart 9.2 Partitions of the dura mater

Partition	Location
Falx cerebri	Extends downward into the longitudinal fissure, and separates the right and left cerebral hemispheres
Falx cerebelli	Separates the right and left cerebellar hemispheres
Tentorium cerebelli	Separates the occipital lobes of the cerebrum from the cerebellum

FIGURE 9.19

(*a*) The dura mater forms a tubular sheath around the spinal cord; (*b*) the epidural space between the dural sheath and the bone of the vertebra is filled with tissues that provide a protective pad around the cord.

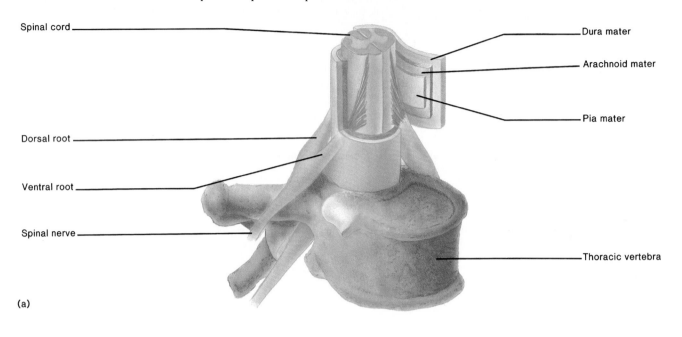

Spinal cord

Dorsal root

Ventral root

Spinal nerve

Dura mater

Arachnoid mater

Pia mater

Thoracic vertebra

(a)

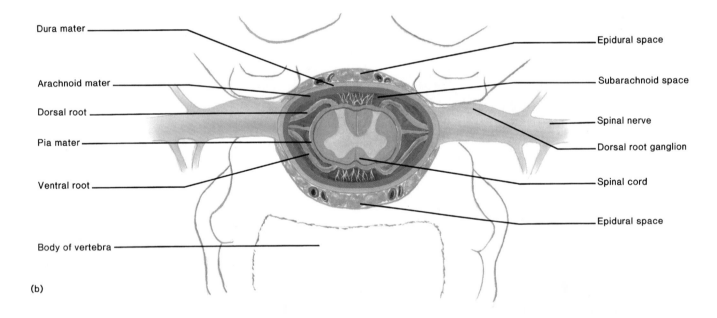

Dura mater

Arachnoid mater

Dorsal root

Pia mater

Ventral root

Body of vertebra

Epidural space

Subarachnoid space

Spinal nerve

Dorsal root ganglion

Spinal cord

Epidural space

(b)

The dura mater continues into the vertebral canal as a strong, tubular sheath that surrounds the spinal cord. It is attached to the cord at regular intervals by bands of pia mater, called *denticulate ligaments,* that extend the length of the spinal cord on either side. The dural sheath terminates as a blind sac at the level of the second sacral vertebra, below the end of the cord. The sheath around the spinal cord is not attached directly to the vertebrae, but is separated by the *epidural space,* which lies between the dural sheath and the bony walls (figure 9.19). This space contains blood vessels, loose connective tissue, and fat tissue, which provide a protective pad around the spinal cord.

A blow to the head may cause some blood vessels associated with the brain to rupture, and the escaping blood may collect in the space beneath the dura mater. This condition, called subdural hematoma, can create increasing pressure between the rigid bones of the skull and the soft tissues of the brain. Unless the accumulating blood is drained promptly, the resulting compression of the brain may lead to functional losses or even death.

The **arachnoid mater** is a thin, netlike membrane that lacks blood vessels and is located between the dura and pia maters. It spreads over the brain and spinal cord, but generally does not dip into the grooves and depressions on their surfaces. Many thin strands extend from its undersurface and are attached to the pia mater.

Between the arachnoid and pia maters is a *subarachnoid space* that contains clear, watery **cerebrospinal fluid.**

The **pia mater** is very thin and contains many nerves and blood vessels that aid in nourishing the underlying cells of the brain and spinal cord. The pia mater is attached to the surfaces of these organs and follows their irregular contours, passing over the high areas and dipping into the depressions.

An inflammation of the meninges is called *meningitis.* This condition is usually caused by certain bacteria or viruses that invade the cerebrospinal fluid. Although meningitis may involve the dura mater, it is more commonly limited to the arachnoid and pia maters.

Meningitis occurs most often in infants and children, and is considered one of the more serious childhood infections. Possible complications of this disease include loss of vision or hearing, paralysis, mental retardation, or death.

1. Describe the meninges.
2. Name the layers of the meninges.
3. Explain where cerebrospinal fluid occurs.

The Spinal Cord

The **spinal cord** is a slender nerve column that passes downward from the brain into the vertebral canal. Although it is continuous with the brain, the spinal cord is said to begin where nerve tissue leaves the cranial cavity at the level of the foramen magnum. The cord tapers to a point, called the *conus medullaris,* and terminates near the intervertebral disk that separates the first and second lumbar vertebrae. From this point the *filum terminale,* a thin cordlike extension of the pia mater, extends and attaches to the coccyx (figure 9.20).

FIGURE 9.20

(a) The spinal cord begins at the level of the foramen magnum. At what level does it terminate? (b) Dorsal view of the spinal cord with the spinal nerves removed.

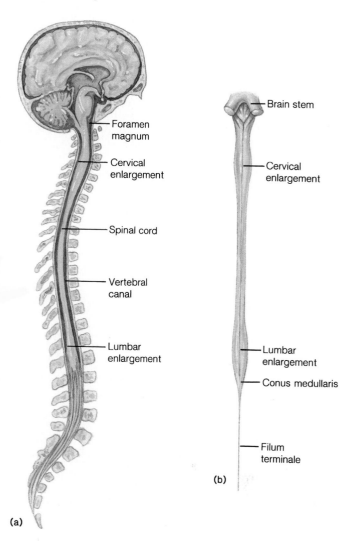

(a)

(b)

Structure of the Spinal Cord

The spinal cord consists of thirty-one segments, each of which gives rise to a pair of **spinal nerves.** These nerves branch out to various body parts and connect them with the central nervous system.

In the neck region, a bulge in the spinal cord called the *cervical enlargement,* gives off nerves to the arms. A similar thickening in the lower back, the *lumbar enlargement,* gives off nerves to the legs.

Two grooves, a deep *anterior median fissure* and a shallow *posterior median sulcus,* extend the length of the spinal cord, dividing it into right and left halves. A cross

FIGURE 9.21

(a) A cross section of the spinal cord. (b) Identify the parts of the spinal cord in this micrograph.

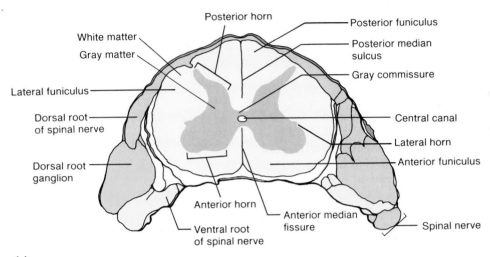

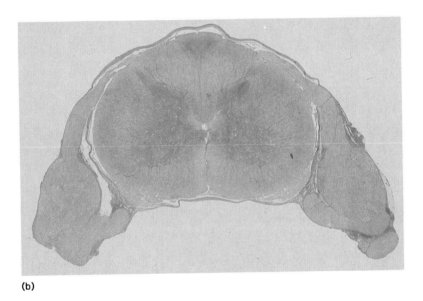

section of the cord (figure 9.21) reveals that it consists of a core of gray matter surrounded by white matter. The pattern produced by the gray matter roughly resembles a butterfly with its wings outspread. The upper and lower wings of gray matter are called the *posterior horns* and the *anterior horns*, respectively. Between them on either side there is a protrusion of gray matter called the *lateral horn*. Neurons with large cell bodies in the anterior horns (anterior horn cells) give rise to motor fibers that pass through spinal nerves to various skeletal muscles. However, the majority of neurons in the gray matter are interneurons.

A horizontal bar of gray matter in the middle of the spinal cord, the *gray commissure*, connects the wings of the gray matter on the right and left sides. This bar surrounds the **central canal,** which is continuous with the ventricles of the brain and contains cerebrospinal fluid. Although the

central canal is prominent during embryonic development, it usually disappears before adulthood.

The white matter of the spinal cord is divided by the gray matter into three regions on each side. These regions are known as the *anterior, lateral,* and *posterior funiculi.* Each funiculus consists of longitudinal bundles of myelinated nerve fibers that comprise major nerve pathways called **nerve tracts** (figure 9.21).

Functions of the Spinal Cord

The spinal cord has two major functions—to conduct nerve impulses and to serve as a center for spinal reflexes.

The nerve tracts of the spinal cord provide a two-way system of communication between the brain and parts outside the nervous system. Tracts that conduct impulses from

FIGURE 9.22

Major (*a*) ascending and (*b*) descending tracts within a cross section of the spinal cord.

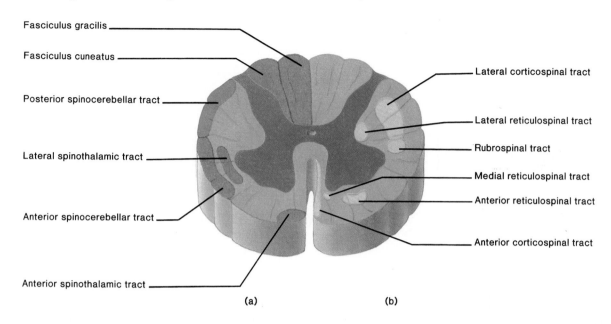

Fasciculus gracilis

Fasciculus cuneatus

Posterior spinocerebellar tract

Lateral spinothalamic tract

Anterior spinocerebellar tract

Anterior spinothalamic tract

Lateral corticospinal tract

Lateral reticulospinal tract

Rubrospinal tract

Medial reticulospinal tract

Anterior reticulospinal tract

Anterior corticospinal tract

(a)   (b)

body parts and carry sensory information to the brain are called **ascending tracts;** those that conduct motor impulses from the brain to muscles and glands are **descending tracts.**

The nerve fibers within these tracts are axons, and usually all the axons within a given tract originate from neuron cell bodies located in the same part of the nervous system and end together in some other part. The names that identify nerve tracts often reflect these common origins and terminations. For example, a *spinothalamic* tract begins in the spinal cord and carries sensory impulses associated with the sensations of pain and touch to the thalamus of the brain; a *corticospinal* tract originates in the cortex of the brain and carries motor impulses downward through the spinal cord and spinal nerves. These impulses function in the control of skeletal muscle movements.

Ascending Tracts

Among the major ascending tracts of the spinal cord are the following (figure 9.22):

1. **Fasciculus gracilis** (fah-sik′u-lus gras′il-is) and **fasciculus cuneatus** (ku′ne-at-us). These tracts are located in the posterior funiculi of the spinal cord. Their fibers conduct sensory impulses from the skin, muscles, tendons, and joints to the brain, where they are interpreted as sensations of touch, pressure, and body movement.

    In a part at the base of the brain called the medulla oblongata, most of these fibers cross over (decussate) from one side to the other—that is, those ascending on the left side of the spinal cord

pass across to the right side and vice versa. As a result, the impulses originating from sensory receptors on the left side of the body reach the right side of the brain, and those originating on the right side of the body reach the left side of the brain (figure 9.23).

2. **Spinothalamic** (spi″no-thah-lam′ik) **tracts.** The *lateral* and *anterior spinothalamic tracts* are located in the lateral and anterior funiculi, respectively. Impulses in these tracts cross over in the spinal cord. The lateral tracts conduct impulses originating in the skin to the brain and give rise to sensations of pain and temperature. Impulses carried on fibers of the anterior tracts are interpreted as touch.

Persons suffering from severe, unremitting pain are sometimes treated with a surgical operation called a *cordotomy*. This is done only as a last resort. In this procedure, fibers in the lateral spinothalamic tracts on the side opposite the affected area are severed above the level of the pain receptors that are being stimulated.

3. **Spinocerebellar** (spi″no-ser″ĕ-bel′ar) **tracts.** The *posterior* and *anterior spinocerebellar tracts* are found near the surface in the lateral funiculi of the spinal cord. Fibers in the posterior tracts remain uncrossed, while those in the anterior tracts cross over in the cord. Impulses conducted on their

FIGURE 9.23
Sensory impulses originating in skin receptors ascend in the fasciculus cuneatus tract and cross over in the medulla of the brain.

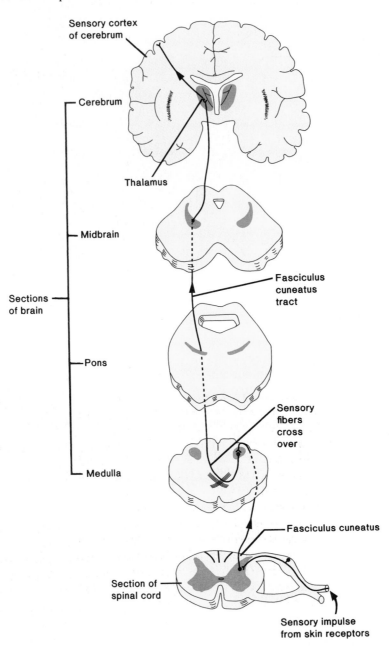

fibers originate in the muscles of the legs and trunk, and travel to the cerebellum of the brain. These impulses are necessary for the coordination of muscular movements.

Descending Tracts

The major descending tracts of the spinal cord include the following (figure 9.22):

1. **Corticospinal** (kor″ti-ko-spi′nal) **tracts.** The *lateral* and *anterior corticospinal tracts* occupy the lateral and anterior funiculi, respectively. Most of the

fibers of the lateral tracts cross over in the lower portion of the medulla oblongata. Those of the anterior tracts descend uncrossed. The corticospinal tracts conduct motor impulses from the brain to spinal nerves and outward to various skeletal muscles. Thus, they function in the control of voluntary movements (figure 9.24).

The corticospinal tracts also are called *pyramidal tracts* after the pyramid-shaped areas in the medulla oblongata through which they pass. Other descending tracts are called *extrapyramidal tracts,* and they include the reticulospinal and rubrospinal tracts.

FIGURE 9.24
Motor pathways of the corticospinal tract begin in the cerebral cortex, cross over in the medulla, and descend in the spinal cord. There, these fibers synapse with neurons that travel in spinal nerves supplying skeletal muscles.

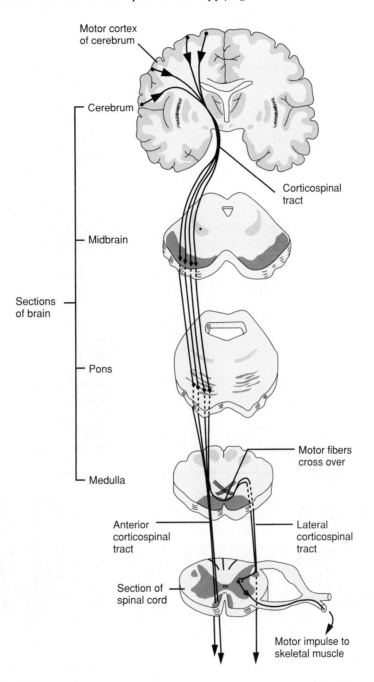

2. **Reticulospinal** (re-tik″u-lo-spi′nal) **tracts.** The *lateral reticulospinal tracts* are located in the lateral funiculi, while the *anterior* and *medial reticulospinal tracts* are in the anterior funiculi. Some fibers in the lateral tracts cross over, while others remain uncrossed. Those of the anterior and medial tracts remain uncrossed. Motor impulses transmitted on the reticulospinal tracts originate in the brain, and function in the control of muscular tone and in the activity of the sweat glands.

3. **Rubrospinal** (roo″bro-spi′nal) **tracts.** The fibers of the rubrospinal tracts cross over in the brain and pass through the lateral funiculi. They carry motor impulses from the brain to skeletal muscles, and are involved with muscular coordination and posture control.

The disease called *poliomyelitis* is caused by viruses that sometimes affect motor neurons, including those in the anterior horns of the spinal cord. When this happens, the person may develop paralysis in the muscles innervated by the affected neurons, but may not suffer any sensory losses in these parts.

Another condition involving motor neurons is called *amyotrophic lateral sclerosis* (ALS). In this disorder, motor neurons degenerate within the spinal cord, brain stem, and cerebral cortex. Later, these neurons are replaced by fibrous tissue. The early signs of ALS include loss of dexterity (particularly in fine finger movements), wasting of hand muscles, severe muscle cramps, difficulty in walking, and problems with swallowing. The cause of ALS, which is also called Lou Gehrig's disease, is unknown.

In addition to serving as a pathway for various nerve tracts, the spinal cord functions in many reflexes, such as the knee-jerk and withdrawal reflexes described earlier. Such reflexes are called **spinal reflexes,** because their reflex arcs pass through the spinal cord.

1. Describe the structure of the spinal cord.
2. What is meant by ascending and descending tracts?
3. What is the consequence of fibers crossing over?
4. Name the major tracts of the spinal cord and list the kinds of impulses each conducts.

A CLINICAL APPLICATION

Spinal Cord Injuries

Injuries to the spinal cord may be caused indirectly, as by a blow to the head or by a fall, or they may be caused by forces applied directly to the cord. The consequences will depend on the amount of damage sustained by the cord.

Normal spinal reflexes depend on two-way communication between the spinal cord and the brain. When nerve pathways are injured, the cord's reflex activities in sites below the injury are usually depressed. At the same time, there is a lessening of sensations and muscular tone in the parts innervated by the affected fibers. This condition is called *spinal shock,* and it may last for days or weeks; normal reflex activity may return eventually. However, if nerve fibers are severed, some of the cord's functions are likely to be permanently lost.

Less severe injuries to the spinal cord—as may be sustained from a blow to the head, whiplash in an automobile accident, or the rupture of an intervertebral disk, which cause the cord to be compressed or distorted—are often accompanied by pain, weakness, and muscular atrophy in the regions supplied by the damaged nerve fibers.

Among the more common causes of direct injury to the spinal cord are gunshot wounds, stabbings, and fractures or dislocations of vertebrae during a vehicular accident. Regardless of the cause, if nerve fibers in ascending tracts are cut, sensations arising from receptors below the level of the injury will be lost. If descending tracts are damaged, the result will be a loss of motor functions.

For example, if the right lateral corticospinal tract is severed in the neck near the first cervical vertebra, control of the voluntary muscles in the right arm and leg is lost, and the limbs become paralyzed (hemiplegia). Problems of this type, involving fibers of the descending tracts, are said to produce the *upper motor neuron syndrome.* There is usually uncoordinated reflex activity (hyperreflexia) during which the flexor and extensor muscles of affected limbs alternately undergo spasms.

If, on the other hand, motor neurons or their fibers in the horns of the spinal cord are injured, the resulting condition is called *lower motor neuron syndrome.* Reflex activity is lost.

The Brain

The **brain** is the largest and most complex part of the nervous system. It occupies the cranial cavity, and is composed of about one hundred billion (10^{11}) multipolar neurons and innumerable nerve fibers, by which these neurons communicate with one another and with neurons in other parts of the system.

The brain contains nerve centers associated with sensory functions, and is responsible for sensations and perceptions. It issues motor commands to skeletal muscles, and carries on higher mental functions, such as memory and reasoning. It also includes centers associated with the co-

ordination of muscular movements, and contains centers and nerve pathways involved in the regulation of visceral activities.

The basic structure of the brain reflects the way it forms during early development. It begins as a tubelike structure (neural tube) that gives rise to the central nervous system. The portion that becomes the brain forms cavities or vesicles at one end. These cavities persist in the mature brain as fluid-filled spaces called *ventricles* and the tubes that connect them. The tissue surrounding the spaces differentiates into the cerebrum, cerebellum, and brain stem (figure 9.25).

FIGURE 9.25
The major portions of the brain include the cerebrum, cerebellum, and brain stem.

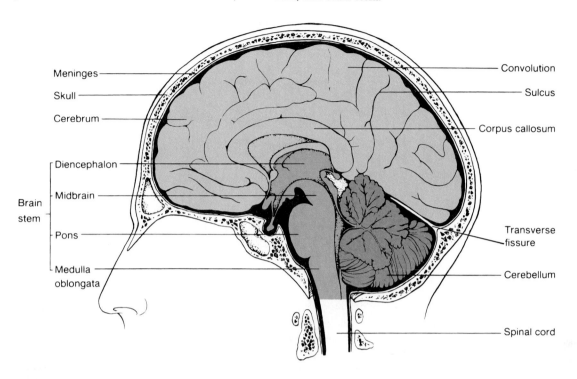

Occasionally during early development, the neural tube does not close completely. If this happens in the anterior end, the brain fails to develop or only a rudimentary one forms. This condition is called *anencephaly*, and it usually results in the death of the developing offspring.

When the neural tube defect occurs in the posterior portion, the vertebral column remains open and the spinal cord is exposed to some degree. This condition is called *spina bifida*. If the spinal cord is covered by the developing skin, the problem may be corrected surgically, and the child may have only minor problems. However, if the nerve tissue is protruding from the site of the defect at birth, the child is likely to suffer irreversible brain damage and some degree of paralysis, and will require extensive medical and surgical treatment.

Structure of the Cerebrum

The **cerebrum** (ser'e-brum) is the largest part of the mature brain. It consists of two large masses called **cerebral hemispheres,** which are essentially mirror images of each other (figure 9.26). These hemispheres are connected by a deep bridge of nerve fibers called the **corpus callosum** and are separated by a layer of dura mater called the *falx cerebri.*

The surface of the cerebrum is marked by numerous ridges, or **convolutions** (gyri), which are separated by grooves. A shallow groove is called a **sulcus,** and a very deep groove is a **fissure.** Although the arrangement of these elevations and depressions is complex, they form

fairly distinct patterns in all normal brains. For example, a *longitudinal fissure* separates the right and left cerebral hemispheres; a *transverse fissure* separates the cerebrum from the cerebellum; and various sulci divide each hemisphere into lobes (figures 9.25 and 9.26).

The lobes of the cerebral hemispheres (figure 9.26) are named after the skull bones that they underlie. They include the following:

1. **Frontal lobe.** The frontal lobe forms the anterior portion of each cerebral hemisphere. Its posterior border is formed by a *central sulcus* (fissure of Rolando) that passes out from the longitudinal fissure at a right angle. The *lateral sulcus* (fissure of Sylvius) that passes out from the under surface of the brain along its sides, forms the inferior border of the frontal lobe.

2. **Parietal lobe.** The parietal lobe is posterior to the frontal lobe and is separated from it by the central sulcus.

3. **Temporal lobe.** The temporal lobe lies below the frontal and parietal lobes, and is separated from them by the lateral sulcus.

4. **Occipital lobe.** The occipital lobe forms the posterior portion of each cerebral hemisphere and is separated from the cerebellum by a shelflike extension of dura mater called the tentorium cerebelli. There is no distinct boundary between the occipital lobe and the parietal and temporal lobes.

FIGURE 9.26
Lobes of the cerebral hemispheres are distinguished by color. (*a*) Lateral view of the right hemisphere; (*b*) hemispheres viewed from above; (*c*) lateral view of the left cerebral hemisphere with the insula exposed.

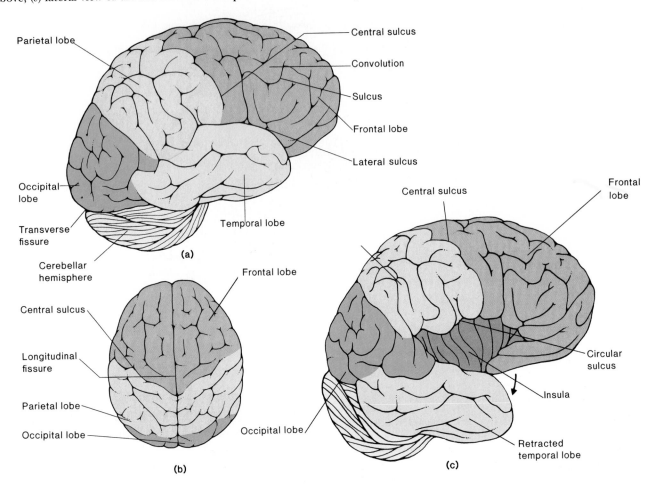

5. **Insula.** The insula (island of Reil) is located deep within the lateral sulcus and is covered by parts of the frontal, parietal, and temporal lobes. It is separated from them by a circular sulcus.

A thin layer of gray matter (2 to 5 millimeters thick) called the **cerebral cortex** constitutes the outermost portion of the cerebrum. This layer forms the convolutions and the sulci, and it extends into the fissures. (See reference plates 32, 33, and 35.) It is estimated to contain nearly 75% of all the neuron cell bodies in the nervous system.

Just beneath the cerebral cortex are masses of white matter, making up the bulk of the cerebrum. These masses contain bundles of myelinated nerve fibers that connect neuron cell bodies of the cortex with other parts of the nervous system. Some of these fibers pass from one cerebral hemisphere to the other by way of the corpus callosum, while others carry sensory or motor impulses from portions of the cortex to nerve centers in the brain or spinal cord.

Functions of the Cerebrum

The cerebrum is concerned with higher brain functions; that is, it contains centers for interpreting sensory impulses arriving from various sense organs as well as centers for initiating voluntary muscular movements. It stores the information of memory and utilizes this information in reasoning processes. It also functions in determining a person's intelligence and personality.

Functional Regions of the Cortex

The regions of the cerebral cortex that perform specific functions have been located by using a variety of techniques. For example, persons who have suffered brain injuries or have had portions of their brains removed surgically have been studied. Their impaired abilities provide clues about the functions of the specific parts that were injured or removed.

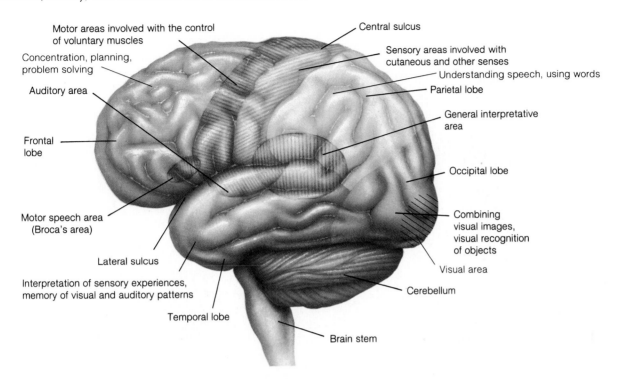

In other studies, areas of the cortex have been exposed surgically and stimulated mechanically or electrically. Then the responses in certain muscles or specific sensations that resulted were observed.

As a result of such investigations, it is possible to map the functional regions of the cerebral cortex. Although there is considerable overlap in these areas, the cortex can be divided into sections known as motor, sensory, and association areas.

Motor Areas

The *primary motor areas* of the cerebral cortex lie in the frontal lobes, just anterior to the central sulcus (precentral gyrus), and in the anterior wall of this sulcus (figure 9.27). As figure 9.28 shows, cells in these motor areas send impulses to various voluntary muscles. Cells in the upper portions of the motor areas send impulses to muscles in the legs and thighs; those in the middle portions control muscles in the shoulders and arms; and those in the lower portions activate muscles of the head, face, and tongue.

The nervous tissue in the motor areas contains numerous, large *pyramidal cells,* named because of their pyramid-shaped cell bodies. These cells form the beginnings of the motor pathways. Impulses from the pyramidal cells travel downward through the cerebrum and brain stem, and into the spinal cord along the *corticospinal tract* and other nerve tracts. Many of the nerve fibers in these tracts cross over from one side of the brain stem to the other and

descend as the spinal tracts. Within the spinal cord, the nerve fibers synapse with motor neurons in the gray matter of the anterior horns. Axons of the motor neurons lead outward through peripheral nerves to various skeletal muscles (figure 9.24).

In addition to the primary motor areas, certain other regions of the frontal lobe are involved with motor functions. For example, a region called *Broca's area* is just anterior to the primary motor cortex and above the lateral sulcus. This area usually occurs only in the left cerebral hemisphere. It coordinates the complex muscular actions of the mouth, tongue, and larynx, which make speech possible. A person with an injury to this area may be able to understand spoken words, but cannot speak.

Above Broca's area is a region called the *frontal eye field.* The motor cortex in this area controls the voluntary movements of the eyes and eyelids. Nearby is the cortex responsible for movements of the head that direct the eyes. Another region, just in front of the primary motor area, controls the muscular movements of the hands and fingers that make such skills as writing possible (figure 9.27).

Sensory Areas

Sensory areas, which occur in several lobes of the cerebrum, function in interpreting impulses that arrive from various sensory receptors. These interpretations give rise to feelings or sensations. For example, the sensations of temperature, touch, pressure, and pain involving the skin

FIGURE 9.28
(*a*) Motor areas involved with the control of voluntary muscles; (*b*) sensory areas involved with cutaneous and certain other senses.

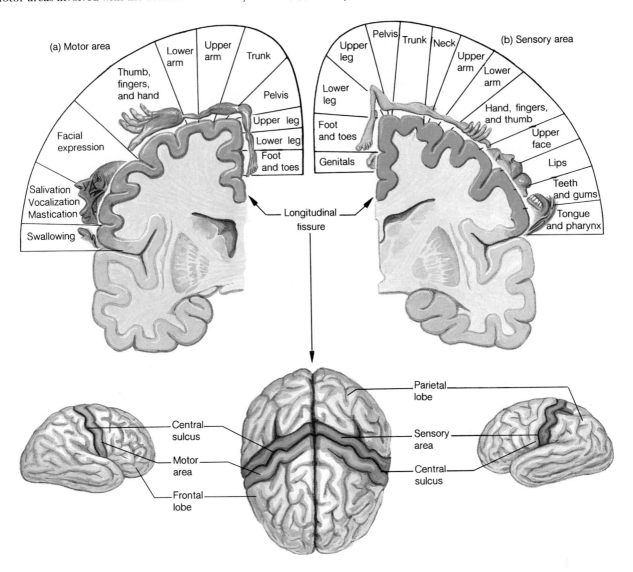

arise in the anterior portions of the parietal lobes along the central sulcus (postcentral gyrus) and in the posterior wall of this sulcus (figures 9.27 and 9.28). The posterior parts of the occipital lobes are concerned with vision, while the anterior portions of the temporal lobes near the lateral sulcus contain the centers for hearing. The sensory areas for taste are located near the bases of the central sulci along the lateral sulci, and the sense of smell arises from centers deep within the cerebrum.

Like motor fibers, sensory fibers (such as those in the fasciculus cuneatus tract) cross over. Thus, the centers in the right cerebral hemisphere interpret impulses originating from the left side of the body and vice versa (figure 9.23). However, the sensory areas concerned with vision receive impulses from both eyes, and those for hearing receive impulses from both ears.

Association Areas

Association areas occupy the anterior portions of the frontal lobes and are widespread in the lateral portions of the parietal, temporal, and occipital lobes. They analyze and interpret sensory experiences, and are involved with memory, reasoning, verbalizing, judgment, and emotional feelings (figure 9.27).

Association tracts are composed of bundles of myelinated nerve fibers that allow communication between neurons of one convolution and those of another. Longer bundles carry nerve impulses between the lobes of each hemisphere. The corpus callosum, mentioned earlier, contains similar nerve fiber tracts that transmit impulses from one hemisphere to the other.

Of particular importance is the region where the parietal, temporal, and occipital association areas come together near the posterior end of the lateral sulcus. This region is called the *general interpretative area,* and it plays the primary role in complex thought processing. Its function makes it possible for a person to recognize words and arrange them to express a thought, and to read and understand ideas presented in writing. Chart 9.3 summarizes the functions of the cerebral lobes.

Basal Nuclei

The **basal nuclei** (basal ganglia) are masses of gray matter located deep within the cerebral hemispheres. They are called the *caudate nucleus, putamen,* and *globus pallidus.* Although the precise function of these parts is not completely understood, the neuron cell bodies they contain are known to serve as relay stations for motor impulses originating in the cerebral cortex and passing into the brain stem and spinal cord. For example, some motor fibers from the cerebral cortex synapse in the basal nuclei, then extend through the brain stem and into the rubrospinal and reticulospinal tracts. Impulses from these parts normally aid in controlling various muscular activities (figure 9.29).

1. Describe the cerebrum.
2. Where in the brain are the primary motor and sensory regions located?
3. Explain the functions of association areas.
4. Describe the location and function of the basal nuclei.

Chart 9.3 Functions of the cerebral lobes	
Lobe	**Functions**
Frontal lobes	Motor areas control movements of voluntary skeletal muscles.
	Association areas carry on higher intellectual processes such as those required for concentrating, planning, complex problem-solving, and judging the consequences of behavior.
Parietal lobes	Sensory areas are responsible for the sensations of temperature, touch, pressure, and pain involving skin.
	Association areas function in understanding speech, and in using words to express thoughts and feelings.
Temporal lobes	Sensory areas are responsible for hearing.
	Association areas are used in interpreting sensory experiences and in remembering visual scenes, music, and other complex sensory patterns.
Occipital lobes	Sensory areas are responsible for vision.
	Association areas function in combining visual images with other sensory experiences.

FIGURE 9.29

A frontal section of the left cerebral hemisphere reveals the basal nuclei (basal ganglia).

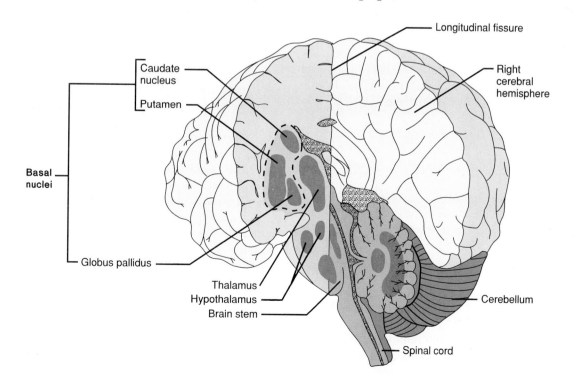

FIGURE 9.30
(a) Anterior view of the ventricles within the cerebral hemispheres and brain stem; (b) lateral view.

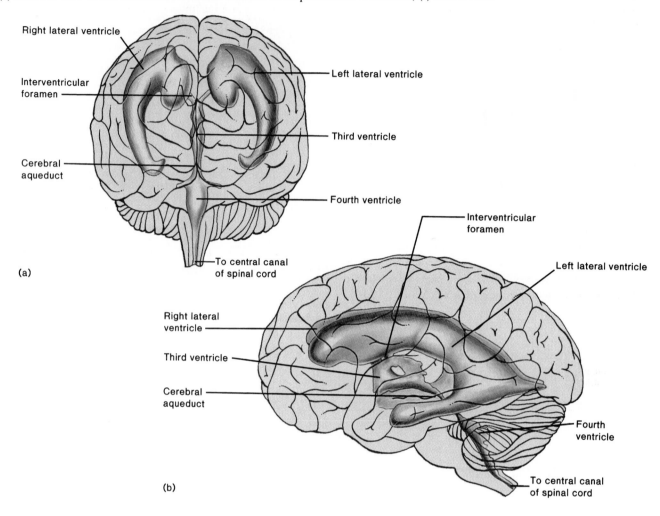

The Ventricles and Cerebrospinal Fluid

Within the cerebral hemispheres and brain stem is a series of interconnected cavities called **ventricles,** shown in figure 9.30. These spaces are continuous with the central canal of the spinal cord and, like it, they are filled with cerebrospinal fluid.

The largest ventricles are the *lateral ventricles* (first and second ventricles), which extend into the cerebral hemispheres and occupy portions of the frontal, temporal, and occipital lobes.

A narrow space that constitutes the *third ventricle* is located in the midline of the brain, beneath the corpus callosum. This ventricle communicates with the lateral ventricles through openings (*interventricular foramina*) in its anterior end.

The *fourth ventricle* is located in the brain stem just in front of the cerebellum. It is connected to the third ventricle by a narrow canal, the *cerebral aqueduct* (aqueduct of Sylvius), which passes lengthwise through the brain stem (midbrain). This ventricle is continuous with the central canal of the spinal cord and has openings in its roof that lead into the subarachnoid space of the meninges.

Cerebrospinal Fluid

The cerebrospinal fluid (CSF) is secreted by tiny cauliflower-like masses of specialized capillaries from the pia mater called **choroid plexuses** (ko'roid plek'sus-es). These structures project into the cavities of the ventricles. They are covered by epithelium-like *ependymal cells* of the neuroglia (figure 9.31).

Although choroid plexuses occur in the medial walls of the lateral ventricles and the roofs of the third and fourth ventricles, most of the cerebrospinal fluid seems to arise in the lateral ventricles. From there it circulates slowly into the third and fourth ventricles, and into the central canal of the spinal cord. It also enters the subarachnoid space of the meninges by passing through the wall of the fourth ventricle near the cerebellum.

The cerebrospinal fluid completes its circuit by being reabsorbed into the blood. This reabsorption occurs gradually through fingerlike structures called *arachnoid granulations* that project from the subarachnoid space into the blood-filled dural sinuses (figure 9.31).

Cerebrospinal fluid is a clear, somewhat viscid liquid. Its primary function seems to be protective. Since it occupies the subarachnoid space of the meninges,

FIGURE 9.31
Cerebrospinal fluid is secreted by choroid plexuses in the walls of the ventricles. The fluid circulates from the ventricles to the central canal. It enters the subarachnoid space near the fourth ventricle, and is reabsorbed into the blood of the dural sinuses through arachnoid granulations.

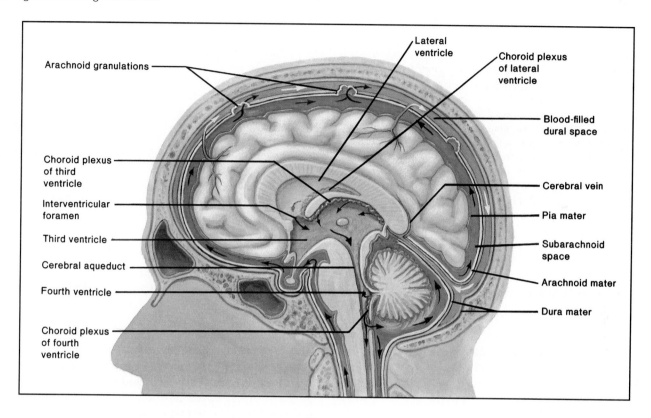

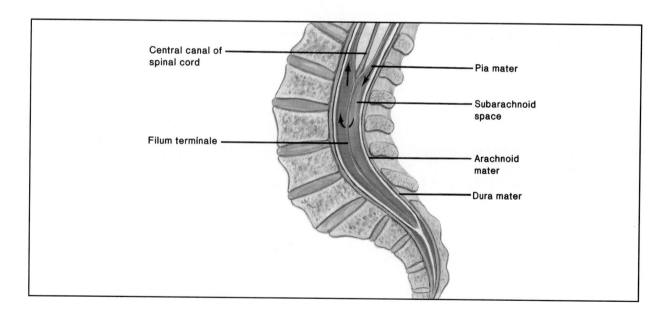

A CLINICAL APPLICATION

Cerebral Injuries

The effects of injuries to the cerebral cortex depend on which areas are damaged and to what extent. When particular portions of the cortex are injured, the special functions of these portions are likely to be lost or at least decreased.

It is often possible to deduce the location and extent of a brain injury by determining what abilities the patient is missing. For example, if the motor area of one frontal lobe has been damaged, the person is likely to be partially or completely paralyzed on the opposite side of the body. Similarly, if the visual cortex of one occipital lobe is injured, the person may suffer partial blindness in both eyes; if both visual cortices are damaged, the blindness may be total.

A person with damage to the association areas of the frontal lobes may have difficulty in concentrating on complex mental tasks. Such an individual usually appears disorganized and is easily distracted.

If the general interpretative area is injured, the person may be unable to interpret sounds as words or understand ideas presented in writing. However, if the general interpretative area is destroyed in a child, the corresponding region on the other side of the brain may be able to take over the functions, and the child's language abilities may develop normally. If such an injury occurs in an adult, the other hemisphere may develop only limited interpretative functions, and the person is likely to have a severe intellectual disability.

Brain damage may also interfere with memory. Generally, the amount of stored memory that is lost as a result of injury is roughly proportional to the amount of cerebral cortex damaged.

---

cerebrospinal fluid completely surrounds the brain and spinal cord. In effect, these organs float in the fluid that supports and protects them by absorbing forces that might otherwise jar and damage their delicate tissues. Cerebrospinal fluid also provides a pathway to the blood for waste substances.

> In an infant, an excess of cerebrospinal fluid may cause an enlargement of the ventricles and the cranium (figure 9.32). This condition is called *hydrocephalus*, or "water on the brain," and is often treated by inserting a shunt that drains fluid away from the cranial cavity.

1. Where are the ventricles of the brain located?
2. Which structures form cerebrospinal fluid?
3. Describe the pattern of cerebrospinal fluid circulation.

The Brain Stem

The region of the brain that connects the cerebrum to the spinal cord is called the brain stem. It consists of the diencephalon, midbrain, pons, and medulla oblongata. These parts include numerous tracts of nerve fibers and several masses of gray matter called *nuclei*, which are groups of neuron cell bodies and unmyelinated nerve fibers. (Note: nuclei are located within the central nervous system) (figures 9.25 and 9.33).

The Diencephalon

The *diencephalon* (di''en-sef'ah-lon) is located between the cerebral hemispheres and above the midbrain. It generally surrounds the third ventricle and is composed largely of gray matter organized into nuclei. Among these, a dense nucleus, called the *thalamus,* bulges into the third ventricle from each side. Another region of the diencephalon that includes many nuclei is called the *hypothalamus.* It lies below the thalamic nuclei, and forms the lower walls and floor of the third ventricle.

Other parts of the diencephalon include: (a) the **optic tracts** and **optic chiasma,** which is formed by the optic nerve fibers crossing over; (b) the **infundibulum,** a conical process behind the optic chiasma to which the pituitary gland is attached; (c) the **posterior pituitary gland,** which hangs from the floor of the hypothalamus; (d) the **mammillary** (mam'i-ler''e) **bodies,** which appear as two rounded structures behind the infundibulum; and (e) the **pineal gland,** which forms as a cone-shaped evagination from the roof of the diencephalon (see chapter 11).

The **thalamus** (thal'ah-mus) serves as a central relay station for sensory impulses ascending from other parts of the nervous system to the cerebral cortex. It receives all sensory impulses (except those associated with the sense of smell) and channels them to appropriate regions of the cortex for interpretation. In addition, all regions of the cerebral cortex can communicate with the thalamus by means of descending fibers.

The **hypothalamus** is interconnected by nerve fibers to the cerebral cortex, thalamus, and other parts of the

FIGURE 9.32

CT scans of the human brain. (a) Normal ventricles. (b) Ventricles enlarged due to excessive accumulation of fluid (hydrocephalism).

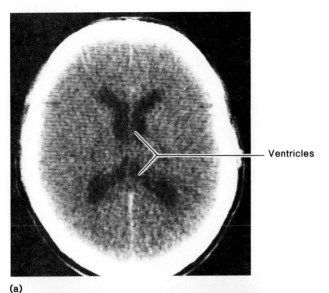

Ventricles

(a)

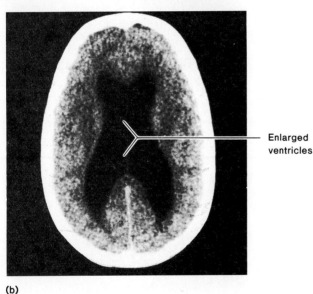

Enlarged ventricles

(b)

brain stem so that it can receive impulses from them and send impulses to them. The nuclei of the hypothalamus play key roles in regulating a variety of visceral activities and by serving as a link between the nervous and endocrine systems.

Among the many important functions of the nuclei in the hypothalamus are the following:

1. Regulation of heart rate and blood pressure.
2. Regulation of body temperature.
3. Regulation of water and electrolyte balance.
4. Control of hunger and regulation of body weight.
5. Control of movements and glandular secretions of the stomach and intestines.
6. Production of substances that stimulate the pituitary gland to release various hormones.
7. Regulation of sleep and wakefulness.

> In infants, the hypothalamus is less effective in regulating body temperature than it is in older children and adults. Consequently, changes in environmental temperatures may be reflected in corresponding changes in an infant's body temperature. In a cold environment, for example, an infant's body temperature may drop to a level that can threaten its life.

Structures in the general region of the diencephalon also play important roles in the control of emotional responses. Portions of the cerebral cortex in the medial parts of the frontal and temporal lobes (cingulate gyrus) are interconnected with the hypothalamus, thalamus, basal nuclei, olfactory nerve and cortex area, *hippocampus,* and *amygdala.* Together these structures comprise a complex called the **limbic system** (figure 9.34).

The limbic system is involved in emotional experience and expression, and can modify the way a person acts. It produces such feelings as fear, anger, pleasure, and sorrow.

The Midbrain

The **midbrain** (mesencephalon) is a short section of the brain stem located between the diencephalon and the pons. It contains bundles of myelinated nerve fibers that join lower parts of the brain stem and spinal cord with higher parts of the brain. The midbrain includes several masses of gray matter that serve as reflex centers, and the cerebral aqueduct that connects the third and fourth ventricles (figure 9.31).

Two prominent bundles of nerve fibers on the underside of the midbrain comprise the *cerebral peduncles.* These fibers include the corticospinal tracts and are the main motor pathways between the cerebrum and lower parts of the nervous system. Beneath the cerebral peduncles are large bundles of sensory fibers that carry impulses upward to the thalamus.

Two pairs of rounded knobs on the upper surface of the midbrain mark the location of four nuclei known collectively as *corpora quadrigemina.* The upper masses, the *superior colliculi,* contain the centers for certain visual reflexes, such as those responsible for moving the eyes to view something as the head is turned. The lower masses, the *inferior colliculi,* contain the auditory reflex centers that operate when it is necessary to move the head so that sounds can be heard more distinctly.

Near the center of the midbrain is a mass of gray matter called the *red nucleus.* This nucleus communicates with the cerebellum and with centers of the spinal cord, and it functions in reflexes concerned with maintaining posture.

FIGURE 9.33

(*a*) Anterior view of the brain stem; (*b*) posterior view of the brain stem with the cerebellum removed, exposing the fourth ventricle.

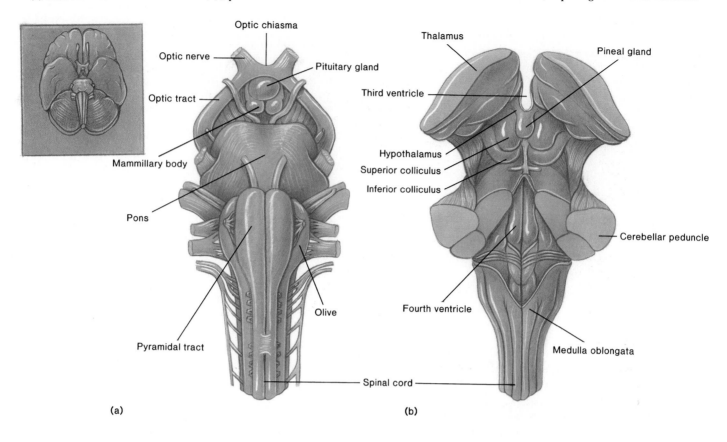

(a)   (b)

FIGURE 9.34

The structures of the limbic system.

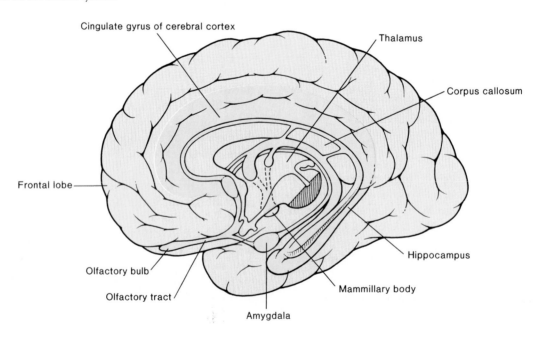

The Pons

The **pons** appears as a rounded bulge on the underside of the brain stem where it separates the midbrain from the medulla oblongata. The dorsal portion of the pons consists largely of longitudinal nerve fibers, which relay impulses to and from the medulla oblongata and the cerebrum. Its anterior portion contains large bundles of transverse nerve fibers, which transmit impulses from the cerebrum to centers within the cerebellum.

Several nuclei of the pons relay sensory impulses from peripheral nerves to higher brain centers. Other nuclei function with centers of the medulla oblongata in regulating the rate and depth of breathing (figure 9.33).

Medulla Oblongata

The **medulla oblongata** (me-dul'ah ob"long-ga'tah) is an enlarged continuation of the spinal cord extending from the level of the foramen magnum to the pons. Its posterior surface is flattened to form the floor of the fourth ventricle, and its anterior surface is marked by the corticospinal tracts, most of whose fibers cross over at this level. On each side of the medulla oblongata is an oval swelling called the *olive,* from which a large bundle of nerve fibers arises and passes to the cerebellum.

Because of its location, all ascending and descending nerve fibers connecting the brain and spinal cord must pass through the medulla oblongata. As in the spinal cord, the white matter of the medulla surrounds a central mass of gray matter. Here, however, the gray matter is broken up into nuclei that are separated by nerve fibers. Some of these nuclei relay ascending impulses to the other side of the brain stem and then onto higher brain centers. The *nucleus gracilis* and the *nucleus cuneatus,* for example, receive sensory impulses from fibers of the fasciculus gracilis and the fasciculus cuneatus and pass them on to the thalamus or the cerebellum.

Other nuclei within the medulla oblongata function as control centers for vital visceral activities. These centers include the following:

1. **Cardiac center.** Impulses originating in the cardiac center are transmitted to the heart on peripheral nerves. Impulses on these nerves can cause the heart rate to decrease or increase.
2. **Vasomotor center.** Certain cells of the vasomotor center initiate impulses that travel to smooth muscles in the walls of blood vessels and stimulate them to contract. This action causes constriction of the vessels (vasoconstriction). Other cells of the vasomotor center can produce the opposite effect—dilation of blood vessels.
3. **Respiratory center.** The respiratory center functions with centers in the pons to regulate the rate, rhythm, and depth of breathing. These cells send impulses on motor fibers to the diaphragm and intercostal muscles.

FIGURE 9.35

The reticular formation extends from the upper portion of the spinal cord into the diencephalon. What is the function of this complex network of nerve fibers?

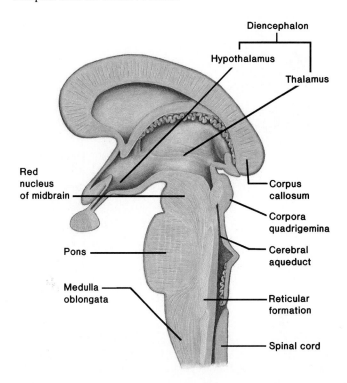

Still other nuclei within the medulla oblongata function as centers for certain nonvital reflexes, including those associated with coughing, sneezing, swallowing, and vomiting. Since the medulla contains vital reflex centers, injuries to this part of the brain stem are often fatal.

Reticular Formation

Scattered throughout the medulla oblongata, pons, and midbrain is a complex network of nerve fibers associated with tiny islands of gray matter. This network, the **reticular formation** (reticular activating system), extends from the upper portion of the spinal cord into the diencephalon (figure 9.35). Its intricate system of nerve fibers interconnects centers of the hypothalamus, basal nuclei, cerebellum, and cerebrum with fibers in all the major ascending and descending tracts.

When sensory impulses reach the reticular formation, it responds by activating the cerebral cortex into a state of wakefulness. Without this arousal, the cortex remains unaware of stimulation and cannot interpret sensory information or carry on thought processes. If the reticular formation ceases to function, as in certain injuries, the person remains unconscious (a comatose state) and cannot be aroused even with strong stimulation.

In addition, the reticular formation plays a role in regulating various motor activities so that coordinated muscular movements are smooth. It exerts an influence on spinal reflexes so that some are inhibited and others are enhanced.

FIGURE 9.36

The cerebellum, which is located below the occipital lobes of the cerebrum, communicates with other parts of the nervous system by means of the cerebellar peduncles.

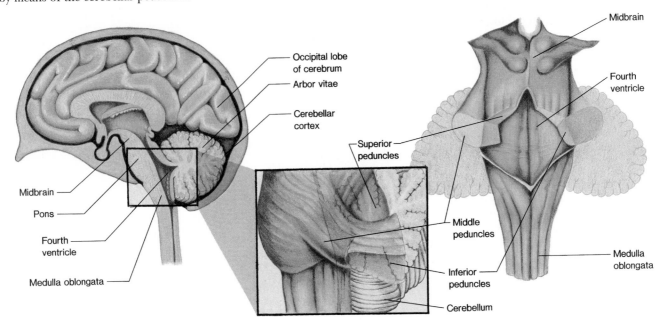

1. What are the major functions of the thalamus? The hypothalamus?
2. What parts of the brain are included in the limbic system?
3. What vital reflex centers are located in the brain stem?
4. What is the function of the reticular formation?

The Cerebellum

The **cerebellum** (ser″e-bel′um) is a large mass of tissue located below the occipital lobes of the cerebrum and posterior to the pons and medulla oblongata. It consists of two lateral hemispheres partially separated by a layer of dura mater called the *falx cerebelli*. These hemispheres are connected in the midline by a structure called the **vermis** (figures 9.36 and 9.37).

Like the cerebrum, the cerebellum is composed primarily of white matter with a thin layer of gray matter, the **cerebellar cortex,** on its surface. This cortex is doubled over on itself in a series of complex folds with myelinated nerve fibers branching into them. A cut into the cerebellum reveals a treelike pattern of white matter, called the *arbor vitae*, surrounded by gray matter. A number of nuclei lie deep within each cerebellar hemisphere, the largest and most important of which is the *dentate nucleus.*

The cerebellum communicates with other parts of the central nervous system by means of three pairs of nerve tracts called **cerebellar peduncles** (ser″ĕ-bel′ar pedung′k′ls). One pair, the *inferior peduncles*, bring sensory information concerning the actual position of body parts such as limbs and joints to the cerebellum via the spinal cord and medulla oblongata. The *middle peduncles* transmit

FIGURE 9.37

What structures can you identify in this sagittal section of the brain?

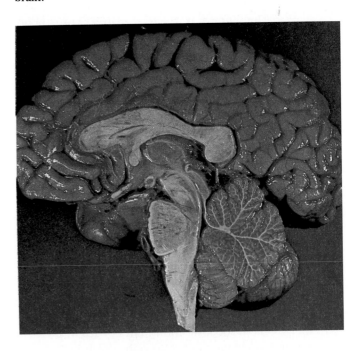

information from the cerebral cortex about the desired position of these body parts. After integrating and analyzing the information from these two sources, the cerebellum sends impulses from the dentate nucleus via the *superior peduncles* to the red nucleus of the midbrain (figure 9.36). In response, motor impulses travel downward through the pons, medulla oblongata, and spinal cord to cause movements of body parts into the desired positions. This activity of the cerebellum makes rapid and complex muscular movements possible.

Thus, the cerebellum is the center for controlling and coordinating of skeletal muscles and maintaining posture. The sensory impulses it receives come from receptors in muscles, tendons, and joints (proprioceptors), and from special sense organs, such as the eyes and ears (see chapter 10). Damage to the cerebellum is likely to result in tremors, inaccurate movements of voluntary muscles, reeling walk, and loss of equilibrium.

1. Where is the cerebellum located?
2. What are the major structures and functions of the cerebellum?
3. What kinds of receptors provide information to the cerebellum?

The Peripheral Nervous System

The **peripheral nervous system (PNS)** consists of the nerves that branch out from the central nervous system (CNS) and connect it to other body parts. The PNS includes the *cranial nerves* that arise from the brain and the *spinal nerves* that arise from the spinal cord.

The peripheral nervous system can also be subdivided into somatic and autonomic nervous systems. Generally, the **somatic system** consists of the cranial and spinal nerve fibers that connect the CNS to the skin and skeletal mus-

cles, and it is involved with conscious activities. The **autonomic nervous system** includes those fibers that connect the CNS to visceral organs such as the heart, stomach, intestines, and various glands (figure 9.38). It is concerned with unconscious activities. Chart 9.4 outlines the subdivisions of the nervous system.

Structure of Peripheral Nerves

As described earlier, a peripheral nerve consists of bundles of nerve fibers surrounded by connective tissue. The outermost layer of the connective tissue, called the *epineurium,* is dense and includes many collagenous fibers. Each bundle of nerve fibers (fascicle) is, in turn, enclosed in a sleeve of less dense connective tissue called the *perineurium.* The individual nerve fibers are surrounded by a small amount of loose connective tissue called *endoneurium* (figures 9.39 and 9.40).

Chart 9.4 Subdivisions of the nervous system

1. Central nervous system (CNS)
   a. Brain
   b. Spinal cord
2. Peripheral nervous system (PNS)
   a. Cranial nerves arising from the brain
      (1) Somatic fibers connecting to the skin and skeletal muscles
      (2) Autonomic fibers connecting to visceral organs
   b. Spinal nerves arising from the spinal cord
      (1) Somatic fibers connecting to the skin and skeletal muscles
      (2) Autonomic fibers connecting to visceral organs

FIGURE 9.38

The peripheral nervous system (PNS) includes motor and sensory neurons that branch from the central nervous system (CNS) and connect with other body parts.

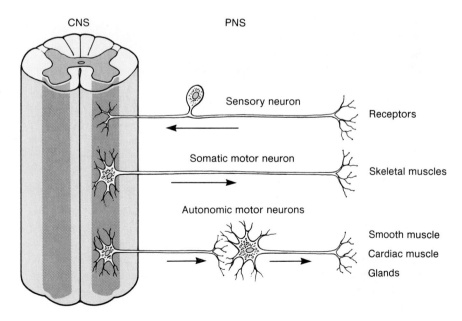

FIGURE 9.39

The structure of a peripheral nerve.

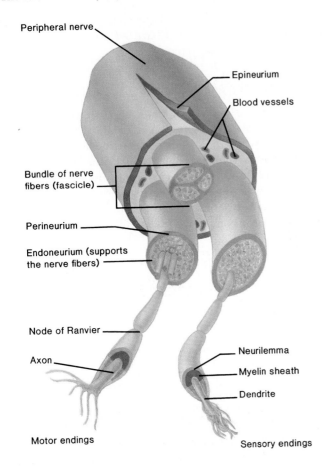

- Peripheral nerve
- Epineurium
- Blood vessels
- Bundle of nerve fibers (fascicle)
- Perineurium
- Endoneurium (supports the nerve fibers)
- Node of Ranvier
- Axon
- Neurilemma
- Myelin sheath
- Dendrite
- Motor endings
- Sensory endings

Blood vessels are usually found in the epineurium and perineurium, and they give rise to a network of capillaries in the endoneurium.

The Cranial Nerves

Twelve pairs of cranial nerves arise from various locations on the underside of the brain. With the exception of the first pair, which begins within the cerebrum, these nerves originate from the brain stem. They pass from their sites of origin through various foramina of the skull and lead to parts of the head, neck, and trunk.

Although most cranial nerves are mixed nerves, some of those associated with special senses, such as smell and vision, contain only sensory fibers. Others that are closely involved with the activities of muscles and glands are composed primarily of motor fibers and have only limited sensory functions.

When sensory fibers are present in cranial nerves, the neuron cell bodies to which the fibers are attached are located outside the brain and are usually in groups called *ganglia* (sing., *ganglion*). On the other hand, motor neuron cell bodies are typically located within the gray matter of the brain.

Cranial nerves are designated either by a number or a name. The numbers indicate the order in which the nerves arise from the brain, going from anterior to posterior. The names describe their primary functions or the general distribution of their fibers (figure 9.41).

The first pair of cranial nerves, the **olfactory nerves (I),** are associated with the sense of smell and contain only sensory neurons. These neurons are located in the lining

FIGURE 9.40

Scanning electron micrograph of the cross section of a nerve (about ×1,000). Note the bundles or fascicles of nerve fibers.
R. G. Kessel and R. H. Kardon, *Tissues and Organs: A Text Atlas of Scanning Electron Microscopy,* © 1979, W. H. Freeman & Co.

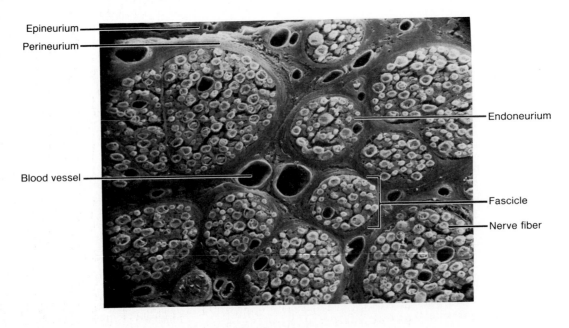

- Epineurium
- Perineurium
- Endoneurium
- Blood vessel
- Fascicle
- Nerve fiber

FIGURE 9.41

Except for the first pair, the cranial nerves arise from the brain stem. They are identified either by numbers indicating their order, or by names describing their function or the general distribution of their fibers.

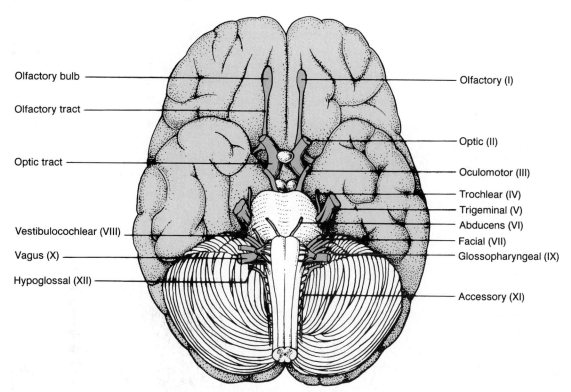

Olfactory bulb

Olfactory tract

Optic tract

Vestibulocochlear (VIII)

Vagus (X)

Hypoglossal (XII)

Olfactory (I)

Optic (II)

Oculomotor (III)

Trochlear (IV)

Trigeminal (V)

Abducens (VI)

Facial (VII)

Glossopharyngeal (IX)

Accessory (XI)

of the upper nasal cavity where they serve as *olfactory receptor cells*. Axons from these receptors pass upward through the cribriform plates of the ethmoid bone and into *olfactory bulbs* that lie just beneath the frontal lobes of the cerebrum. Sensory impulses travel from these bulbs along *olfactory tracts* to cerebral centers where they are interpreted. The result is the sensation of smell.

The second pair of cranial nerves, the **optic nerves (II)**, lead from the eyes to the brain and are associated with the sense of vision. The sensory cell bodies of the nerve fibers occur in ganglion cell layers within the eyes, and their axons pass through the *optic canals* of the orbits and continue into the brain.

Some of the fibers in each optic nerve cross over to the other side of the brain. Specifically, the fibers arising from the medial half of each eye cross over, while those arising from the lateral sides do not. This crossing produces the X-shaped *optic chiasma* in the hypothalamus.

Sensory impulses transmitted on the optic nerves continue along *optic tracts* to centers in the thalamus and then travel to the visual cortices of the occipital lobes.

The third pair of cranial nerves, the **oculomotor** (ok″u-lo-mo′tor) **nerves (III)**, arise from the midbrain and pass into the orbits of the eyes through the superior orbital fissures. One component of each nerve connects to a number of voluntary muscles. These include the *levator palpebrae superioris muscles*, which function to raise the eyelids, as well as most of the muscles attached to the eye surfaces that cause them to move—the *superior rectus, medial rectus, inferior rectus,* and *inferior oblique* muscles (figure 9.42).

A second portion of each oculomotor nerve is part of the autonomic nervous system, supplying involuntary muscles inside the eyes. These muscles help in adjusting the amount of light that enters the eyes and help focus the lenses of the eyes.

Although the fibers of the oculomotor nerves are primarily motor, some sensory fibers are present. These transmit sensory information to the brain concerning the condition of various muscles.

The fourth pair, the **trochlear** (trok′le-ar) **nerves (IV)**, are the smallest cranial nerves. They arise from the midbrain and carry motor impulses through the superior orbital fissures to a pair of external eye muscles, the *superior oblique muscles,* which are not supplied by the oculomotor nerves. The trochlear nerves also contain some sensory fibers that transmit information about the condition of certain muscles (figure 9.42).

The fifth pair, the **trigeminal** (tri-jem′i-nal) **nerves (V)**, are the largest of the cranial nerves and arise from the pons. They are mixed nerves, but their sensory portions are more extensive than their motor portions. Each sensory component includes three large branches: the ophthalmic, maxillary, and mandibular divisions (figure 9.43).

The *ophthalmic division* consists of sensory fibers that bring impulses to the brain from the surface of the eye, the tear gland, and the skin of the anterior scalp, forehead, and upper eyelid. The fibers of the *maxillary division* carry sensory impulses from the upper teeth, upper gum, and upper lip, as well as from the mucous lining of the palate and the skin of the face. The *mandibular division* includes

The Nervous System   301

FIGURE 9.42
The oculomotor, trochlear, and abducens nerves control the muscles that move the eyes.

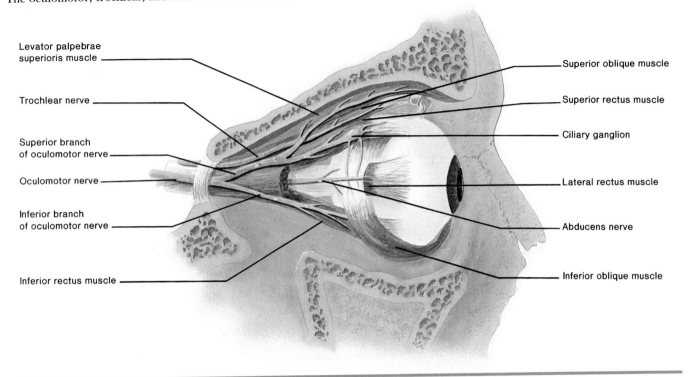

Levator palpebrae superioris muscle

Trochlear nerve

Superior branch of oculomotor nerve

Oculomotor nerve

Inferior branch of oculomotor nerve

Inferior rectus muscle

Superior oblique muscle

Superior rectus muscle

Ciliary ganglion

Lateral rectus muscle

Abducens nerve

Inferior oblique muscle

FIGURE 9.43
The trigeminal nerve has three large branches that supply various parts of the head and face.

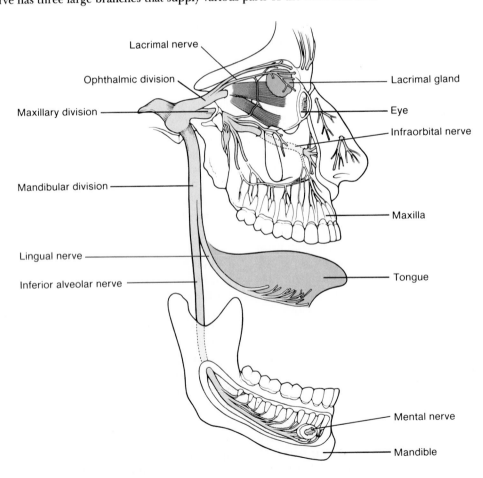

Lacrimal nerve

Ophthalmic division

Maxillary division

Mandibular division

Lingual nerve

Inferior alveolar nerve

Lacrimal gland

Eye

Infraorbital nerve

Maxilla

Tongue

Mental nerve

Mandible

both motor and sensory fibers. The sensory branches transmit impulses from the scalp behind the ear, the skin of the jaw, the lower teeth, the lower gum, and the lower lip. The motor branches supply the muscles of mastication and certain muscles in the floor of the mouth.

The nerve fibers of the three divisions of the trigeminal nerve pass through different openings in the skull to reach these parts. Those of the ophthalmic division pass through the superior orbital fissure, those of the maxillary division pass through the foramen rotundum, and those of the mandibular division pass downward through the foramen ovale.

A disorder of the trigeminal nerve called *trigeminal neuralgia* (tic douloureux) is characterized by severe recurring pain in the face and forehead on the affected side. If the pain cannot be controlled with drugs, the sensory portion of the nerve is sometimes severed surgically. Although this procedure may relieve the pain, the patient loses other sensations in the parts supplied by the sensory branch. Consequently, persons who have had such surgery must be cautious when eating or drinking hot foods or liquids, because they may not sense burning. They should also inspect their mouths daily for the presence of food particles or damage to their cheeks from biting, which they may not feel.

The sixth pair of cranial nerves, the **abducens** (ab-du'senz) **nerves (VI)**, are quite small and originate from the pons near the medulla oblongata. They enter the orbits of the eyes through the superior orbital fissures and supply motor impulses to a pair of external eye muscles, the *lateral rectus muscles*. The sensory fibers of the nerves provide the brain with information concerning the condition of certain muscles (figure 9.42).

The seventh pair of cranial nerves, the **facial** (fa'shal) **nerves (VII)**, arise from the lower part of the pons, pass through the internal acoustic meatuses, and emerge on the sides of the face. Their sensory branches are associated with taste receptors on the anterior two-thirds of the tongue, and some of their motor fibers transmit impulses to muscles of facial expression. Still other motor fibers of these nerves function in the autonomic nervous system by stimulating secretions from tear glands and certain salivary glands (submandibular and sublingual glands). (See figure 9.44.)

The eighth pair of cranial nerves, the **vestibulocochlear** (ves-tib″u-lo-kok'le-ar) **nerves (VIII**, or acoustic nerves), are sensory nerves that arise from the medulla oblongata and pass through the internal acoustic meatuses. Each of these nerves has two distinct parts—a vestibular branch and a cochlear branch.

The neuron cell bodies of the *vestibular branch* fibers are located in ganglia near the vestibule and semicircular canals of the inner ear. These structures contain receptors that are sensitive to changes in the position of the head. The impulses they initiate pass into the cerebellum, where they are used in reflexes associated with maintaining equilibrium.

The neuron cell bodies of the *cochlear branch* fibers are located in a ganglion of the cochlea, a part of the inner ear that houses the hearing receptors. Impulses from this branch pass through the pons and medulla oblongata on their way to the temporal lobe where they are interpreted. (See chapter 10.)

FIGURE 9.44
The facial nerve is associated with the taste receptors on the tongue and with the muscles of facial expression.

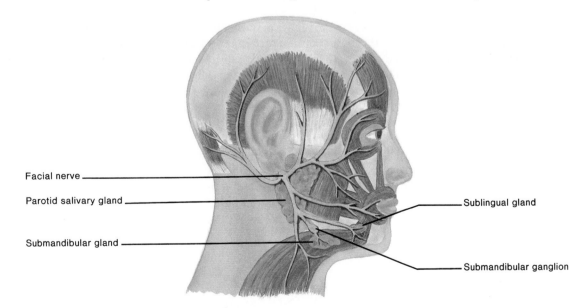

Facial nerve

Parotid salivary gland

Submandibular gland

Sublingual gland

Submandibular ganglion

FIGURE 9.45

The glossopharyngeal nerve is associated with the pharynx, posterior tongue, and carotid arteries.

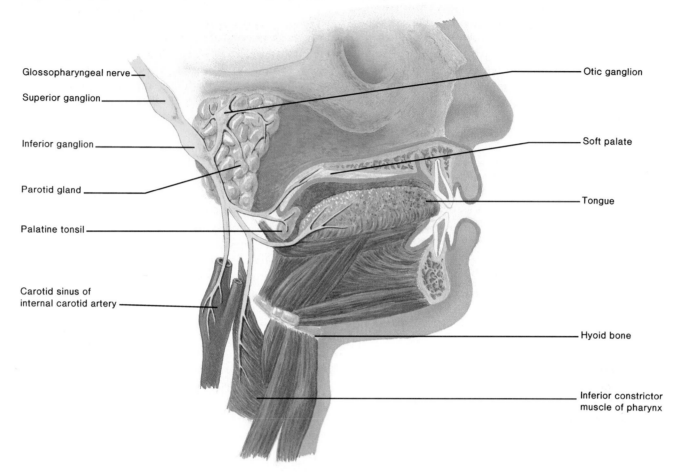

Glossopharyngeal nerve

Superior ganglion

Inferior ganglion

Parotid gland

Palatine tonsil

Carotid sinus of internal carotid artery

Otic ganglion

Soft palate

Tongue

Hyoid bone

Inferior constrictor muscle of pharynx

The ninth pair of cranial nerves, the **glossopharyngeal** (glos″o-fah-rin′je-al) **nerves (IX),** are associated with the tongue and pharynx, as the name implies. These nerves arise from the medulla oblongata and pass through the jugular foramina. Although they are mixed nerves, their predominant fibers are sensory. These fibers carry impulses from the lining of the pharynx, tonsils, and posterior third of the tongue to the brain. Fibers in the motor component of the glossopharyngeal nerves innervate constrictor muscles in the wall of the pharynx that function in swallowing.

Other branches of the glossopharyngeal nerves function in the autonomic nervous system. Some sensory fibers, for example, conduct impulses from special receptors in the wall of an artery in the neck (carotid artery) to the vasomotor center in the medulla oblongata. This information is used to regulate blood pressure. Certain autonomic motor fibers within the glossopharyngeal nerves lead to the parotid salivary gland in front of the ear, and can stimulate it to secrete saliva (figure 9.45).

The tenth pair of cranial nerves, the **vagus** (va′gus) **nerves (X),** originate in the medulla oblongata and extend downward through the jugular foramina to the neck into the chest and abdomen. These nerves are mixed, and although they contain both somatic and autonomic branches, the autonomic fibers are the predominant ones.

Among the somatic components are motor fibers that carry impulses to muscles of the larynx. These fibers are associated with speech and with swallowing reflexes that employ muscles in the soft palate and pharynx. Vagal sensory fibers carry impulses from the linings of the pharynx, larynx, and esophagus, and from the viscera of the thorax and abdomen to the brain.

One way to test the functioning of a person's vagus nerves is to gently touch an object, such as a tongue depressor, to the lateral wall of the pharynx. This stimulates the pharyngeal sensory receptors and triggers nerve impulses to travel on sensory neurons to the reflex center in the medulla oblongata. Motor fibers of the vagus nerve then conduct impulses to the muscles of the pharynx, causing them to contract (gag reflex). Failure of the gag reflex may indicate injury to the reflex pathway.

Autonomic motor fibers of the vagus nerves supply the heart and a variety of smooth muscles and glands in the visceral organs of the thorax and abdomen. (See figure 9.46.)

The eleventh pair of cranial nerves, the **accessory** (ak-ses′o-re) **nerves (XI,** or spinal accessory nerves), originate in the medulla oblongata and the spinal cord; thus, they have both cranial and spinal branches.

Each *cranial branch* of an accessory nerve originates in the medulla oblongata and passes through the jugular foramen where it joins a vagus nerve. It carries impulses to muscles of the soft palate, pharynx, and larynx. The *spinal branch* originates in the cervical region of the spinal cord, passes upward through the foramen magnum, then out through the jugular foramen and into the neck. It descends into the neck and supplies motor fibers to the trapezius and sternocleidomastoid muscles (figure 9.47).

The twelfth pair of cranial nerves, the **hypoglossal** (hi″po-glos′al) **nerves (XII),** arise from the medulla oblongata and pass through the hypoglossal canals and into the tongue. They consist primarily of motor fibers that carry impulses to muscles that move the tongue in speaking, chewing, and swallowing (figure 9.47).

The functions of the cranial nerves are summarized in chart 9.5.

The consequences of cranial nerve injuries depend on the location and extent of the injuries. For example, if only one member of a nerve pair is damaged, loss of function is limited to the affected side, but if both nerves are injured, losses occur on both sides. Also, if a nerve is severed completely, the functional loss is total; if the cut is incomplete, the loss may be partial.

FIGURE 9.46

The vagus nerve extends from the medulla oblongata downward into the chest and abdomen to supply many visceral organs.

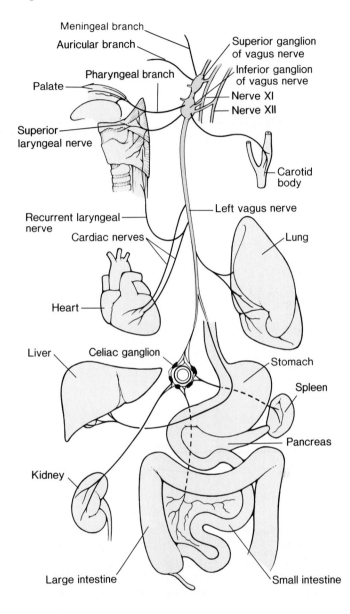

1. Define peripheral nervous system.
2. Distinguish between somatic and autonomic nerve fibers.
3. Describe the structure of a peripheral nerve.
4. Name the cranial nerves and list the major functions of each.

Chart 9.5 Functions of cranial nerves

Nerve	Type	Function	Figure
I Olfactory	Sensory	Sensory fibers transmit impulses associated with the sense of smell.	9.41
II Optic	Sensory	Sensory fibers transmit impulses associated with the sense of vision.	9.41
III Oculomotor	Primarily motor	Motor fibers transmit impulses to muscles that raise the eyelids, move the eyes, adjust the amount of light entering the eyes, and focus the lenses. Some sensory fibers transmit impulses associated with the condition of muscles.	9.42
IV Trochlear	Primarily motor	Motor fibers transmit impulses to muscles that move the eyes. Some sensory fibers transmit impulses associated with the condition of muscles.	9.42
V Trigeminal	Mixed		9.43
Ophthalmic division		Sensory fibers transmit impulses from the surface of the eyes, tear glands, scalp, forehead, and upper eyelids.	
Maxillary division		Sensory fibers transmit impulses from the upper teeth, upper gum, upper lip, lining of the palate, and skin of the face.	
Mandibular division		Sensory fibers transmit impulses from the scalp, skin of the jaw, lower teeth, lower gum, and lower lip. Motor fibers transmit impulses to muscles of mastication and to muscles in the floor of the mouth.	
VI Abducens	Primarily motor	Motor fibers transmit impulses to muscles that move the eyes. Some sensory fibers transmit impulses associated with the condition of muscles.	9.42
VII Facial	Mixed	Sensory fibers transmit impulses associated with taste receptors of the anterior tongue. Motor fibers transmit impulses to muscles of facial expression, tear glands, and salivary glands.	9.44
VIII Vestibulocochlear	Sensory		
Vestibular branch		Sensory fibers transmit impulses associated with the sense of equilibrium.	10.14
Cochlear branch		Sensory fibers transmit impulses associated with the sense of hearing.	
IX Glossopharyngeal	Mixed	Sensory fibers transmit impulses from the pharynx, tonsils, posterior tongue, and carotid arteries. Motor fibers transmit impulses to muscles of the pharynx used in swallowing and to salivary glands.	9.45
X Vagus	Mixed	Somatic motor fibers transmit impulses to muscles associated with speech and swallowing; autonomic motor fibers transmit impulses to the heart and to smooth muscles and glands of visceral organs in the thorax and abdomen. Sensory fibers transmit impulses from the pharynx, larynx, esophagus, and visceral organs of the thorax and abdomen.	9.46
XI Accessory	Motor		
Cranial branch		Motor fibers transmit impulses to muscles of the soft palate, pharynx, and larynx.	9.47
Spinal branch		Motor fibers transmit impulses to muscles of the neck and back.	
XII Hypoglossal	Motor	Motor fibers transmit impulses to muscles that move the tongue.	9.47

FIGURE 9.47

The accessory nerves supply the muscles of the soft palate, pharynx, and larynx, and some neck muscles. The hypoglossal nerves supply the muscles of the tongue.

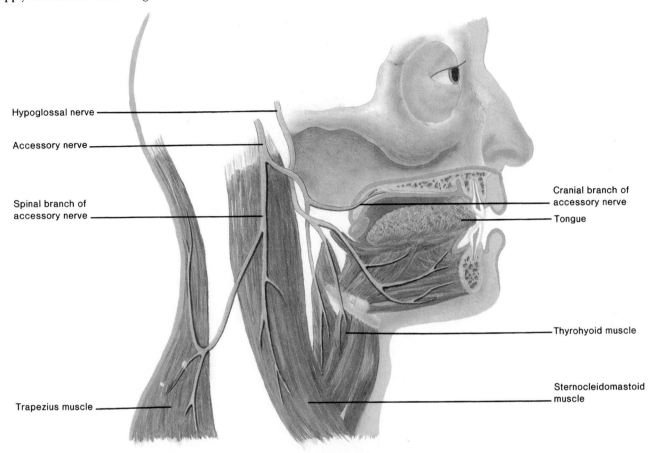

The Spinal Nerves

Thirty-one pairs of **spinal nerves** originate from the spinal cord. They are mixed nerves and provide a two-way communication system between the spinal cord and parts in the arms, legs, neck, and trunk.

Although spinal nerves are not named individually, they are grouped according to the vertebral level from which they arise, and each nerve is numbered in sequence (figure 9.48). Thus, there are eight pairs of *cervical nerves* (numbered C1 to C8), twelve pairs of *thoracic nerves* (numbered T1 to T12), five pairs of *lumbar nerves* (numbered L1 to L5), five pairs of *sacral nerves* (numbered S1 to S5), and one pair of *coccygeal nerves* (Co).

The nerves arising from the upper part of the spinal cord pass outward almost horizontally, while those from the lower portions of the spinal cord descend at sharp angles. This arrangement is a consequence of growth. In early life, the spinal cord extends the entire length of the vertebral column, but with age the column grows more rapidly than the cord. Thus, the adult spinal cord ends at the level between the first and second lumbar vertebrae, so the lumbar, sacral, and coccygeal nerves descend to their exits beyond the end of the cord. These descending nerves form a structure called the *cauda equina* (horse's tail) (figure 9.48).

Each spinal nerve emerges from the cord by two short branches, or *roots*, which lie within the vertebral canal. The **dorsal root** (sensory root) can be identified by an enlargement called the *dorsal root ganglion*. This ganglion contains the cell bodies of the sensory neurons whose dendrites conduct impulses inward from peripheral body parts. The axons of these neurons extend through the dorsal root and into the spinal cord, where they form synapses with dendrites of other neurons.

FIGURE 9.48

There are thirty-one pairs of spinal nerves.

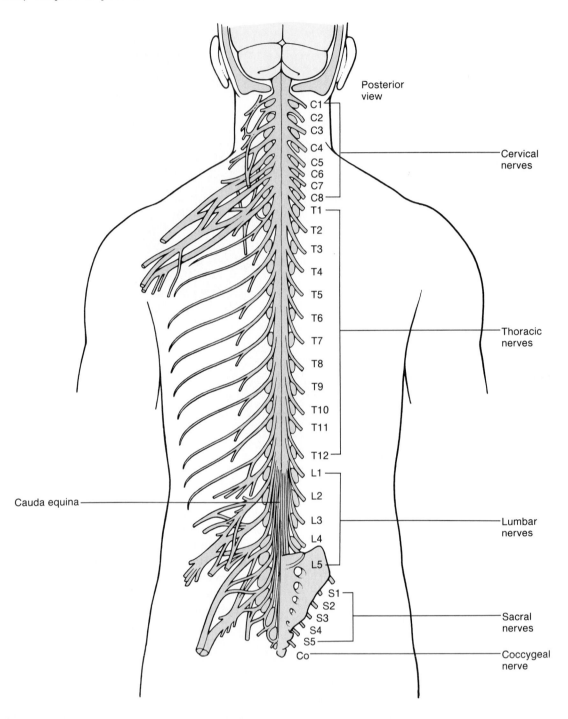

Posterior view

Cervical nerves

Thoracic nerves

Cauda equina

Lumbar nerves

Sacral nerves

Coccygeal nerve

An area of skin where a group of sensory nerve fibers lead to a particular dorsal root is called a *dermatome*. Dermatomes are highly organized, but they vary considerably in size and shape, as indicated in figure 9.49. A map of the dermatomes is often useful in localizing the sites of injuries to dorsal roots or the spinal cord.

The **ventral root** (motor root) of each spinal nerve consists of axons from motor neurons whose cell bodies are located within the gray matter of the cord.

A ventral root and a dorsal root unite to form a spinal nerve, which passes outward from the vertebral canal through an *intervertebral foramen*. Just beyond its foramen, each spinal nerve divides into several parts. One of these

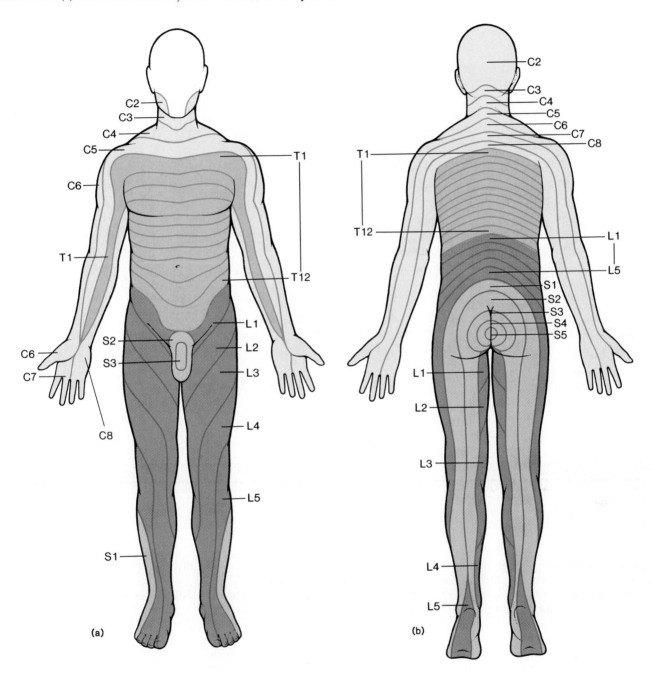

(a)

(b)

parts, the small *meningeal branch,* reenters the vertebral canal through the intervertebral foramen and supplies the meninges and blood vessels of the cord, as well as the intervertebral ligaments and the vertebrae.

As figure 9.50 shows, a *posterior branch* (posterior ramus) of each spinal nerve turns posteriorly and innervates the muscles and skin of the back. The main portion of the nerve, the *anterior branch* (anterior ramus), con-

tinues forward to supply muscles and skin on the front and sides of the trunk and limbs.

The spinal nerves in the thoracic and lumbar regions have a fourth branch, the *visceral branch,* which is part of the autonomic nervous system.

Except in the thoracic region, anterior branches of the spinal nerves combine to form complex networks called **plexuses** instead of continuing directly to the peripheral

FIGURE 9.50
Each spinal nerve has a posterior and an anterior branch; the thoracic and lumbar spinal nerves also have a visceral branch.

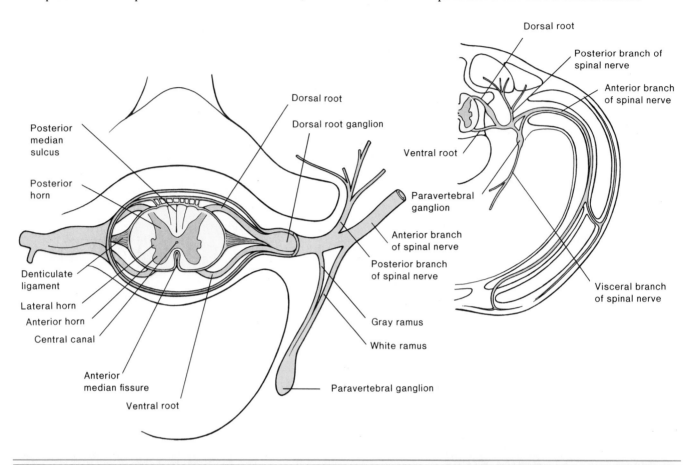

Spinal Nerve Injuries

Spinal nerves may be injured in a variety of ways including birth injuries, dislocations and fractures of vertebrae, stabs, gunshot wounds, and pressure from tumors in surrounding tissues.

The nerves of the cervical plexuses are sometimes compressed by the sudden bending of the neck, called *whiplash,* which may occur during rear end automobile collisions. A victim of such an injury may suffer continuing headaches and pain in the neck and skin, which are supplied by the cervical nerves.

If the phrenic nerves associated with the cervical plexuses are severed or damaged by a broken or dislocated vertebra, partial or complete paralysis of the diaphragm may result.

Sometimes people whose occupations require prolonged abduction of the arm, as in painting or typing, develop intermittent or constant pain in the neck, shoulder, or region of the arm due to excessive pressure on the brachial plexus. This condition, called *thoracic outlet syndrome,* may also be caused by congenital malformations of skeletal parts that compress the plexus during arm and shoulder movements.

Nerves of a newborn's brachial plexuses may be stretched or injured during childbirth when the shoulders are in a fixed position and excessive pull is applied to the head. In such cases, the newborn may suffer losses of sensory and motor functions in the arms on the injured sides, and the arms may wither as muscles atrophy.

As a result of degenerative changes, an intervertebral disk in the lumbar region may rupture and press against the sciatic nerve or its roots. This may produce a condition called *sciatica,* which is characterized by pain in the lower back and gluteal region that sometimes radiates into the thigh, calf, ankle, and foot. Sciatica is most common in persons forty to fifty years of age. It usually involves compression of spinal nerve roots between L2 and S1, some of which contain fibers of the sciatic nerve.

Although most persons with sciatica recover spontaneously after a period of rest, others require treatment with drugs or surgery. In some cases, a surgical procedure called a *laminectomy* may be performed. In this procedure, the bony lamina of a vertebra is removed so that the surgeon can reach the displaced portion of the intervertebral disk and relieve the pressure on the spinal nerve.

FIGURE 9.51

The anterior branches of the spinal nerves in the thoracic region give rise to intercostal nerves. Those in other regions combine to form complex networks called *plexuses*.

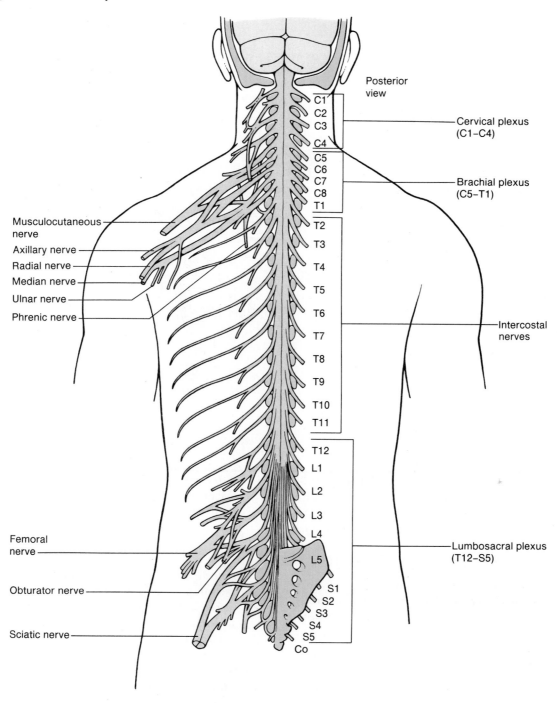

body parts. In a plexus, the fibers of various spinal nerves are sorted and recombined, so that fibers associated with a particular peripheral part reach it in the same nerve, even though the fibers originate from different spinal nerves (figure 9.51).

Cervical Plexuses

The **cervical plexuses** lie deep in the neck on either side. They are formed by the anterior branches of the first four cervical nerves. Fibers from these plexuses supply the muscles and skin of the neck. In addition, fibers from the third, fourth, and fifth cervical nerves form the right and left **phrenic** (fren'ik) **nerves,** which conduct motor impulses to the muscle fibers of the diaphragm.

Brachial Plexuses

The anterior branches of the lower four cervical nerves and the first thoracic nerve give rise to **brachial plexuses.** These nets of nerve fibers are located deep within the shoulders between the neck and the axillae (armpits). The

FIGURE 9.52
Nerves of the brachial plexus.

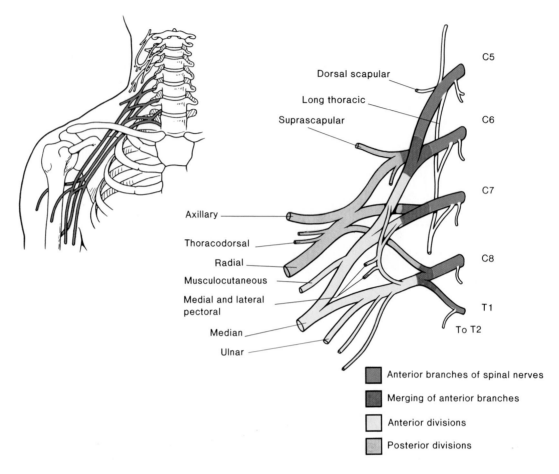

anterior branches merge at three points and then split into anterior and posterior divisions. The nerves of the anterior division primarily supply the flexor muscles of the arm, while those of the posterior division nerves supply the extensor muscles of the arm (figure 9.52). The major branches emerging from the brachial plexuses include the following:

1. *Musculocutaneous nerves* supply muscles of the arms on the anterior sides, and the skin of the forearms.
2. *Ulnar nerves* supply muscles of the forearms and hands, and the skin of the hands.
3. *Median nerves* supply muscles of the forearms, and the muscles and skin of the hands.
4. *Radial nerves* supply muscles of the arms on the posterior sides, and skin of the forearms and hands.

5. *Axillary nerves* supply muscles and skin of the upper, lateral, and posterior regions of the arm (figure 9.53).

Other nerves associated with the brachial plexus that innervate various skeletal muscles include:

1. *Lateral* and *medial pectoral nerves* supply the pectoralis major and pectoralis minor muscles.
2. *Dorsal scapular nerves* supply the rhomboideus major and minor, and levator scapulae muscles.
3. *Lower scapular nerves* supply the subscapularis and teres major muscles.
4. *Thoracodorsal nerves* supply the latissimus dorsi muscles.
5. *Suprascapular nerves* supply the supraspinatus and infraspinatus muscles.

The muscles of the hands and fingers are innervated primarily by the radial and median nerves. In some individuals, the median nerve supplies most of these muscles. In others, the radial nerve is the major nerve supply. In still others, there is a communicating arch between the median and radial nerves, and both supply the muscles.

In contact sports such as football, a player's shoulder girdle is sometimes depressed at the same time that the head and neck are pushed away from the depressed side. This may result in a painful stretching of the brachial plexus that athletes call a "stinger."

FIGURE 9.53
Nerves of the upper limb.

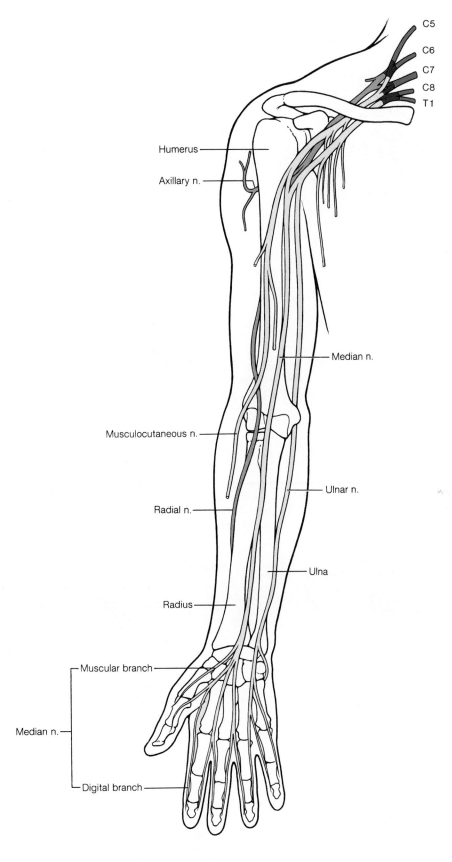

Humerus

Axillary n.

C5
C6
C7
C8
T1

Median n.

Musculocutaneous n.

Ulnar n.

Radial n.

Ulna

Radius

Muscular branch

Median n.

Digital branch

FIGURE 9.54

(*a*) Lumbar and (*b*) sacral portions of the lumbosacral plexus.

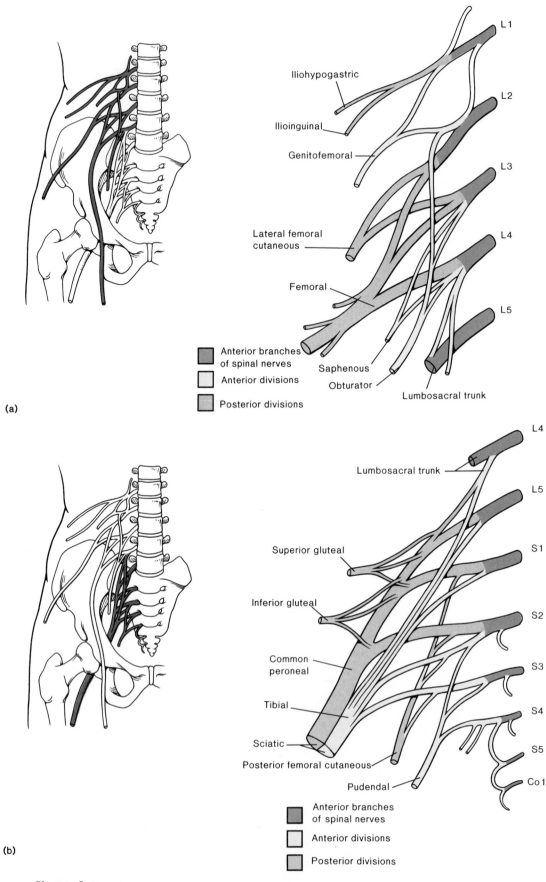

FIGURE 9.55

Nerves of the lower limb. (*a*) Anterior view; (*b*) posterior view.

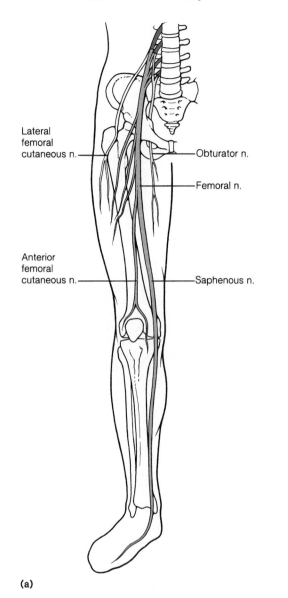

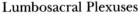

(a)

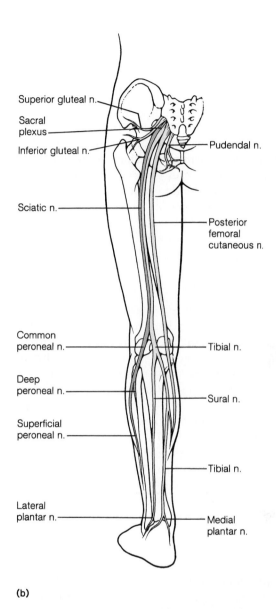

(b)

Lumbosacral Plexuses

The **lumbosacral** (lum″bo-sa′kral) **plexuses** are formed by the last thoracic nerve and the lumbar, sacral, and coccygeal nerves. These networks of nerve fibers extend from the lumbar region of the back into the pelvic cavity, giving rise to a number of motor and sensory fibers associated with the lower abdominal wall, external genitalia, buttocks, thighs, legs, and feet (figure 9.54). The major branches of these plexuses include the following:

1. *Obturator nerves* supply the adductor muscles of the thighs.
2. *Femoral nerves* divide into many branches, supplying motor impulses to muscles of the thighs and legs, and receiving sensory impulses from the skin of the thighs and lower legs.
3. *Sciatic nerves* are the largest and longest nerves in the body. They pass downward into the buttocks

and descend into the thighs, where they divide into *tibial* and *common peroneal nerves.* The many branches of these nerves supply muscles and skin in the thighs, legs, and feet. (See figure 9.55.)

Other nerves associated with the lumbosacral plexus that innervate various skeletal muscles include *pudendal nerves,* which supply the muscles of the perineum; and *inferior* and *superior gluteal nerves,* which supply the gluteal muscles and the tensor fasciae latae muscles.

The anterior branches of the thoracic spinal nerves do not enter a plexus. Instead, they travel into spaces between the ribs and become **intercostal** (in″ter-kos′tal) **nerves.** These nerves supply motor impulses to the intercostal muscles and the upper abdominal wall muscles. They also receive sensory impulses from the skin of the thorax and abdomen.

The Autonomic Nervous System

The autonomic nervous system includes the portions of the peripheral and central nervous systems that function somewhat independently (autonomously) and continuously without conscious effort. This system controls visceral activities by regulating the actions of smooth muscles, cardiac muscle, and various glands. It is concerned with regulating heart rate, blood pressure, breathing rate, body temperature, and other visceral activities. Portions of the autonomic nervous system are also responsive during times of emotional stress, and they prepare the body to meet the demands of strenuous physical activity.

General Characteristics

Autonomic activities are regulated largely by reflexes in which sensory signals originate from receptors within visceral organs and the skin. These signals are transmitted on sensory nerve fibers to nerve centers within the brain or spinal cord. In response, motor impulses then travel out from these centers on motor nerve fibers within cranial and spinal nerves.

Typically, these motor fibers lead to ganglia outside the central nervous system. The impulses they carry are integrated within the ganglia and are relayed to various visceral organs (muscles or glands) that respond by contracting, secreting, or being inhibited. The integrative function of the ganglia provides the autonomic nervous system with some degree of independence from the brain and spinal cord.

The autonomic nervous system includes the **sympathetic** and **parasympathetic divisions,** which act together. For example, some visceral organs are supplied by nerve fibers from each of the divisions. In such cases, impulses on one set of fibers activate an organ, while impulses on the other set inhibit it. Thus, the divisions may act antagonistically, so that the actions of some visceral organs are regulated by alternately being activated or inhibited.

The functions of the autonomic divisions are mixed; that is, each activates some organs and inhibits others. However, the divisions have important functional differences. The sympathetic division is concerned primarily with preparing the body for energy-expending, stressful, or emergency situations. Conversely, the parasympathetic division is most active under ordinary, restful conditions. It also counterbalances the effects of the sympathetic division, and restores the body to a resting state following a stressful experience. For example, during an emergency the sympathetic division will cause the heart and breathing rates to increase, and following the emergency, the parasympathetic division will slow these activities.

Autonomic Nerve Pathways

Unlike the motor pathways of the somatic nervous system, which usually include a single neuron between the brain or spinal cord and a skeletal muscle, those of the autonomic system involve two neurons, as shown in figure 9.56. The cell body of one neuron is located in the brain or spinal cord. Its axon, the **preganglionic fiber,** leaves the CNS and forms a synapse with one or more nerve fibers whose cell bodies are housed within an autonomic ganglion. The axon of such a second neuron is called a **postganglionic fiber,** and it extends to a visceral effector.

The autonomic sensory pathways are similar to the somatic pathways. The cell bodies are found in spinal ganglia, and the fibers extend from the visceral organs, through the ganglia, to the spinal cord or brain (figure 9.56).

In order to control pain or to prepare patients for various clinical procedures, a drug is sometimes injected into the pathway of a sensory nerve to produce a *nerve block.* In addition to somatic sensory pathways, sympathetic sensory pathways may be interrupted to treat pain originating in the visceral organs caused by cancer. A short-acting local anesthetic may be used, or a substance that causes tissue destruction may produce a more permanent effect. Care must be taken that only sensory fibers are affected, because damage to motor fibers may cause permanent motor impairment. Thus, the injection needle must be inserted very carefully. CT scans are often used to help guide the needle along its path.

Sympathetic Division

Within the sympathetic division (thoracolumbar division), the preganglionic fibers originate from neurons within the lateral horn of the spinal cord. These neurons are found in all of the thoracic segments and the upper two or three lumbar segments of the cord. Their axons exit through the ventral roots of spinal nerves along with various somatic motor fibers.

After traveling a short distance, preganglionic fibers leave the spinal nerves through branches called *white rami* (sing. *ramus*) and enter sympathetic ganglia. Two groups of such ganglia, called **paravertebral ganglia,** are located in chains along the sides of the vertebral column. These ganglia, together with the fibers that interconnect them, comprise the **sympathetic trunks.** (See figure 9.57.)

The paravertebral ganglia are found just beneath the parietal pleura in the thorax and beneath the parietal peritoneum in the abdomen. (See chapter 2.) Although these ganglia are located some distance from the visceral organs they help to control, other sympathetic ganglia are positioned closer to the viscera. The *collateral sympathetic ganglia,* for example, are found within the abdomen, closely associated with certain large blood vessels.

Some of the preganglionic fibers that enter paravertebral ganglia synapse with neurons within these ganglia. Other fibers travel through the ganglia and pass up or down the sympathetic trunk, and synapse with neurons in ganglia at higher or lower levels within the chain. Still other

FIGURE 9.56

(*a*) Somatic neuron motor pathways usually have a single neuron between the central nervous system and an effector. (*b*) Autonomic neuron motor pathways involve two neurons between the central nervous system and an effector.

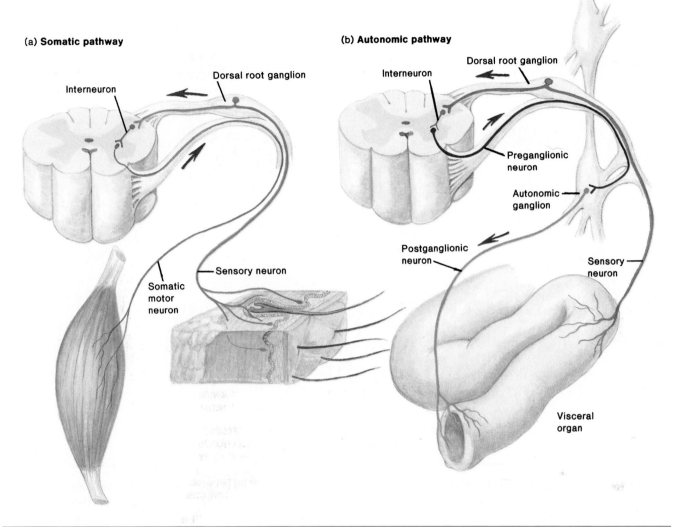

(a) Somatic pathway

Interneuron

Dorsal root ganglion

Sensory neuron

Somatic motor neuron

(b) Autonomic pathway

Interneuron

Dorsal root ganglion

Preganglionic neuron

Autonomic ganglion

Postganglionic neuron

Sensory neuron

Visceral organ

FIGURE 9.57

A chain of paravertebral ganglia extends along each side of the vertebral column.

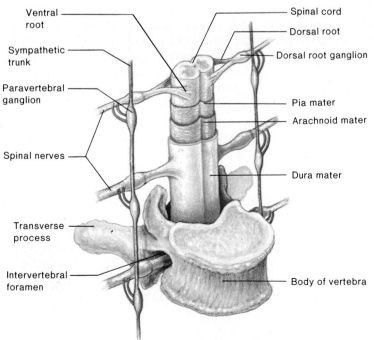

Ventral root

Sympathetic trunk

Paravertebral ganglion

Spinal nerves

Transverse process

Intervertebral foramen

Spinal cord

Dorsal root

Dorsal root ganglion

Pia mater

Arachnoid mater

Dura mater

Body of vertebra

FIGURE 9.58
Sympathetic fibers leave the spinal cord in the ventral roots of spinal nerves, enter sympathetic ganglia, and synapse with other neurons that extend to visceral effectors.

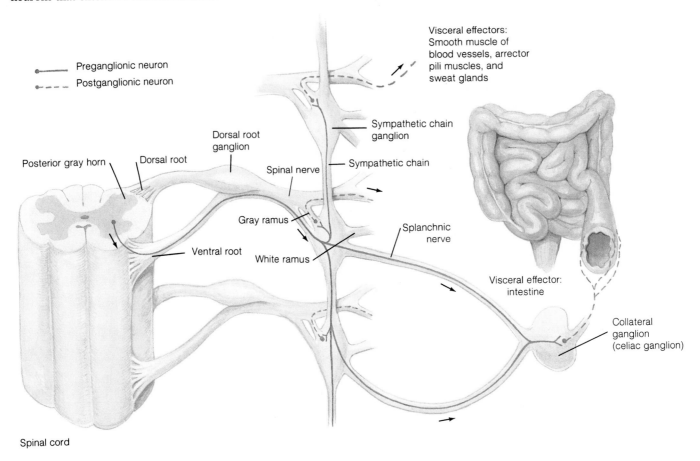

fibers pass through to collateral ganglia before they synapse. Typically, a preganglionic axon will synapse with several other neurons within a sympathetic ganglion, and, therefore, nerve impulses carried by a preganglionic axon will be amplified.

The axons of the second neurons in sympathetic pathways—the postganglionic fibers—extend out from the sympathetic ganglia to visceral effectors. Those leaving paravertebral ganglia usually pass through branches called **gray rami** and return to a spinal nerve before proceeding to an effector. (See figure 9.58.) These branches appear gray because the postganglionic axons generally are unmyelinated, whereas the preganglionic axons in the white rami are nearly all myelinated. An important exception to the usual arrangement of sympathetic fibers occurs in a set of preganglionic fibers that pass through the sympathetic ganglia and extend out to the medulla of each adrenal gland.

Parasympathetic Division

The preganglionic fibers of the parasympathetic division (craniosacral division) arise from neurons in the midbrain,
pons, and medulla oblongata of the brain stem and from the sacral region of the spinal cord. From there, they lead outward on cranial or sacral nerves to ganglia located near or within various visceral organs (terminal ganglia). The relatively short postganglionic fibers continue from the ganglia to specific muscles or glands within these visceral organs. As in the case of the sympathetic fibers, the parasympathetic preganglionic axons are usually myelinated, and the parasympathetic postganglionic fibers are unmyelinated.

The parasympathetic preganglionic fibers associated with parts of the head are included in the oculomotor, facial, and glossopharyngeal nerves. Those that innervate organs of the thorax and upper abdomen are parts of the vagus nerves. (The vagus nerves carry about 75% of all parasympathetic fibers.) Preganglionic fibers arising from the sacrum are found within the branches of the second through the fourth sacral spinal nerves, and they carry impulses to visceral organs within the pelvis. Figures 9.59 and 9.60 compare the distribution of nerve fibers in the sympathetic division with that in the parasympathetic division.

The effects of sympathetic and parasympathetic stimulation on visceral effectors are summarized in chart 9.6.

FIGURE 9.59

The preganglionic fibers of the sympathetic division of the autonomic nervous system arise from the thoracic and lumbar regions of the spinal cord.

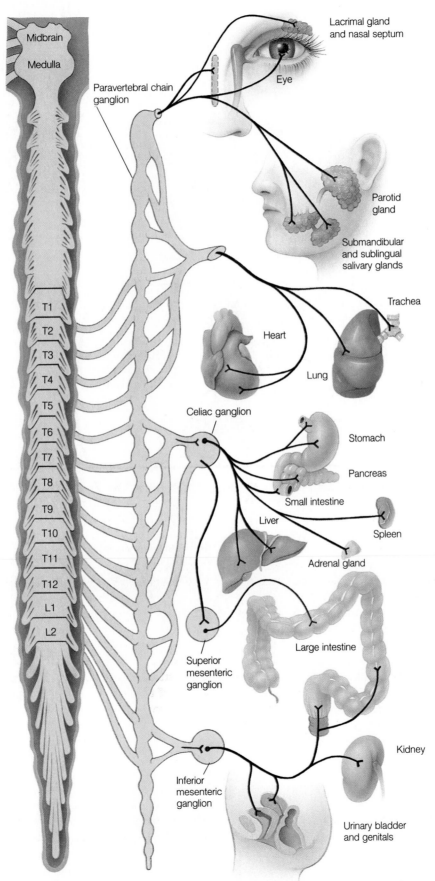

319

FIGURE 9.60

The preganglionic fibers of
the parasympathetic division
of the autonomic nervous
system arise from the brain
and sacral region of the spinal
cord.

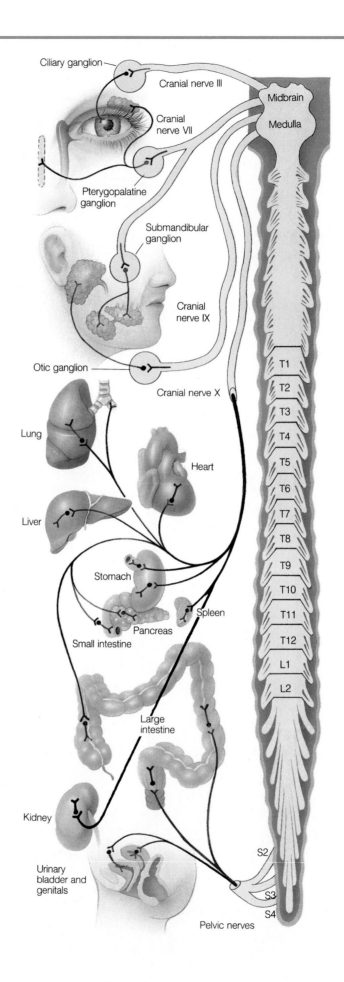

Ciliary ganglion

Cranial nerve III

Midbrain

Medulla

Cranial
nerve VII

Pterygopalatine
ganglion

Submandibular
ganglion

Cranial
nerve IX

Otic ganglion

Cranial nerve X

T1
T2
T3
T4
T5
T6
T7
T8
T9
T10
T11
T12
L1
L2

Lung

Heart

Liver

Stomach

Spleen

Pancreas

Small intestine

Large
intestine

Kidney

S2

Urinary
bladder and
genitals

S3

S4

Pelvic nerves

Chart 9.6 Effects of autonomic stimulation on various effectors

Effector location	Response to sympathetic stimulation	Response to parasympathetic stimulation
Integumentary system		
Apocrine glands	Increased secretion	No action
Eccrine glands	Increased secretion	No action
Special senses		
Iris of eye	Dilation	Constriction
Tear gland	Slightly increased secretion	Greatly increased secretion
Endocrine system		
Adrenal cortex	Increased secretion	No action
Adrenal medulla	Increased secretion	No action
Digestive system		
Muscle of gallbladder wall	Relaxation	Contraction
Muscle of intestinal wall	Decreased peristaltic action	Increased peristaltic action
Muscle of internal anal sphincter	Contraction	Relaxation
Pancreatic glands	Reduced secretion	Greatly increased secretion
Salivary glands	Reduced secretion	Greatly increased secretion
Respiratory system		
Muscles in walls of bronchioles	Dilation	Constriction
Cardiovascular system		
Blood vessels supplying muscles	Constriction of some and dilation of others	No action
Blood vessels supplying skin	Constriction	No action
Blood vessels supplying heart (coronary arteries)	Dilation of some and constriction of others	Dilation
Muscles in wall of heart	Increased contraction rate	Decreased contraction rate
Urinary system		
Muscle of bladder wall	Relaxation	Contraction
Muscle of internal urethral sphincter	Contraction	Relaxation
Reproductive systems		
Blood vessels to clitoris and penis	No action	Dilation leading to erection
Muscles associated with male internal reproductive organs	Ejaculation	

---

1. What is the general function of the autonomic nervous system?
2. How are the subdivisions of the autonomic system distinguished?
3. What functions are generally controlled by the sympathetic division? By the parasympathetic division?
4. Describe a sympathetic motor nerve pathway and a parasympathetic motor nerve pathway.

Clinical Terms Related to the Nervous System

analgesia (an″al-je′ze-ah)   loss or reduction in the ability to sense pain, but without loss of consciousness.

anesthesia (an″es-the′ze-ah)   a loss of feeling.

aphasia (ah-fa′ze-ah)   a disturbance or loss in the ability to use words or to understand them, usually due to damage to cerebral association areas.

apraxia (ah-prak′se-ah)   an impairment in a person's ability to make correct use of objects.

ataxia (ah-tak′se-ah)   a partial or complete inability to coordinate voluntary movements.

cerebral palsy (ser′e-bral pawl′ze)   a condition characterized by partial paralysis and lack of muscular coordination.

coma (ko′mah)   an unconscious condition in which a person does not respond to stimulation.

cordotomy (kor-dot′o-me)   a surgical procedure in which a nerve tract within the spinal cord is severed, usually to relieve intractable pain.

craniotomy (kra″ne-ot′o-me)   a surgical procedure in which part of the skull is opened.

encephalitis (en″sef-ah-li′tis)   an inflammation of the brain and meninges characterized by drowsiness and apathy.

hemiplegia (hem″i-ple′je-ah)   paralysis on one side of the body and the limbs on that side.

laminectomy (lam″i-nek′to-me)   surgical removal of the posterior arch of a vertebra, usually to relieve the symptoms of a ruptured intervertebral disk.

monoplegia (mon″o-ple′je-ah)   paralysis of a single limb.

multiple sclerosis (mul′ti-pl skle-ro′sis)   a disease of the central nervous system characterized by loss of myelin, and the appearance of scarlike patches throughout the brain and spinal cord or throughout both.

neuralgia (nu-ral′je-ah)   a sharp, recurring pain associated with a nerve, usually caused by inflammation or injury.

neuritis (nu-ri′tis)   an inflammation of a nerve.

paraplegia (par″ah-ple′je-ah)   paralysis of both legs.

quadriplegia (kwod″ri-ple′je-ah)   paralysis of all four limbs.

vagotomy (va-got′o-me)   surgical severing of a vagus nerve.

Chapter Summary

Introduction (page 266)

Organs of the nervous system are divided into the central and peripheral nervous systems. These parts provide sensory, integrative, and motor functions.

General Functions of the Nervous System (page 266)

1. Sensory functions employ receptors that detect changes in internal and external body conditions.
2. Integrative functions bring sensory information together and make decisions that are acted upon by using motor functions.
3. Motor functions use effectors that respond when they are stimulated by motor impulses.

Nerve Tissue (page 266)

1. Neuron structure
   a. A neuron includes a cell body, cell processes, and other organelles usually found in cells.
   b. Dendrites and the cell body provide receptive surfaces.
   c. A single axon arises from the cell body and may be enclosed in a myelin sheath and a neurilemma.
2. Neuroglial cells
   a. Neuroglial cells are accessory cells.
   b. They fill spaces, support neurons, hold nerve tissue together, produce myelin, and destroy cellular debris.

The Synapse (page 272)

A synapse is a junction between two neurons.

1. A synaptic cleft is the gap between parts of two neurons at a synapse.
2. Axons have synaptic knobs at their ends that secrete neurotransmitters.

Organization of Neurons (page 272)

The way impulses are processed reflects the organization of the neurons in the brain and spinal cord.

1. Neuronal pools
   a. Neurons are organized into pools within the central nervous system.
   b. Each pool receives impulses, processes them, and conducts impulses away.
2. Convergence
   a. Impulses from two or more incoming fibers may converge on a single neuron.
   b. Convergence makes it possible for a neuron to bring together impulses from different sources.
3. Divergence
   a. Impulses leaving a pool may diverge by passing onto several output fibers.
   b. Divergence allows impulses to be amplified.

Classification of Neurons and Nerves (page 275)

Neurons can be classified according to structure or function.

1. Classification of neurons
   a. On the basis of structure, neurons can be classified as bipolar, unipolar, and multipolar.
   b. On the basis of function, neurons can be classified as sensory neurons, interneurons, or motor neurons.
2. Types of nerves
   a. Nerves are cordlike bundles of nerve fibers.
   b. Nerves can be classified as sensory, motor, or mixed, depending upon the type of fibers they contain.

Nerve Pathways (page 276)

A nerve pathway is a route followed by an impulse as it travels through the nervous system.

1. Reflex arcs
   a. A reflex arc includes a sensory neuron, a reflex center composed of interneurons, and a motor neuron.
   b. The reflex arc is the behavioral unit of the nervous system.
2. Reflex behavior
   Reflexes are automatic, unconscious responses to changes and help control body processes.

The Meninges (page 278)

The brain and spinal cord are surrounded by bone and protective membranes called meninges.

1. The meninges consist of a dura mater, arachnoid mater, and pia mater.
2. Cerebrospinal fluid occupies the space between the arachnoid and pia maters.

The Spinal Cord (page 281)

The spinal cord is a nerve column that extends from the brain into the vertebral canal. It terminates at the level between the first and second lumbar vertebrae.

1. Structure of the spinal cord
   a. The spinal cord is composed of thirty-one segments, each of which gives rise to a pair of spinal nerves.
   b. It is characterized by a cervical enlargement, a lumbar enlargement, and two deep longitudinal grooves that divide it into right and left halves.
   c. It has a central core of gray matter that is surrounded by white matter.
2. Functions of the spinal cord
   a. The cord provides a two-way communication system between the brain and body parts outside the nervous system.
   b. Ascending tracts carry sensory impulses to the brain; descending tracts carry motor impulses to muscles and glands.
   c. Many of the fibers in the ascending and descending tracts cross over in the spinal cord or brain.

The Brain (page 286)

The brain is the largest and most complex part of the nervous system. It contains nerve centers that are associated with sensations, issue motor commands, and carry on higher mental functions. It develops from a tubular part with cavities that persist as ventricles, and walls that give rise to the cerebrum, cerebellum, and brain stem.

1. Structure of the cerebrum
   a. The cerebrum consists of two cerebral hemispheres connected by the corpus callosum.

    b. Its surface is marked by ridges and grooves; sulci divide each hemisphere into lobes.

    c. The cerebral cortex is a thin layer of gray matter near the surface.

    d. White matter consists of myelinated nerve fibers that interconnect neurons within the nervous system and with other body parts.

2. Functions of the cerebrum

    a. The cerebrum is concerned with higher brain functions, such as interpretation of sensory impulses, control of voluntary muscles, and storage of memory, thought, and reasoning.

    b. The cerebral cortex can be divided into sensory, motor, and association areas.

    c. The primary motor regions lie in the frontal lobes near the central sulcus and are aided by other areas of the frontal lobes that control special motor functions.

    d. Areas responsible for interpreting sensory impulses from the skin are located in the parietal lobes near the central sulcus; other specialized sensory areas occur in the temporal and occipital lobes.

    e. Association areas analyze and interpret sensory impulses and are involved with memory, reasoning, verbalizing, judgment, and emotional feelings.

3. Basal nuclei

    a. Basal nuclei are masses of gray matter located deep within the cerebral hemispheres.

    b. They function as relay stations for motor impulses originating in the cerebral cortex, and they aid in the control of motor activities.

4. The ventricles and cerebrospinal fluid

    a. Ventricles are interconnected cavities within the cerebral hemispheres and brain stem.

    b. These spaces are filled with cerebrospinal fluid.

    c. Cerebrospinal fluid is secreted by choroid plexuses in the walls of the ventricles; it circulates through the ventricles and is reabsorbed into the blood of the dural sinuses.

5. The brain stem

    a. The brain stem extends from the base of the cerebrum to the spinal cord.

    b. The brain stem consists of the diencephalon, midbrain, pons, and medulla oblongata.

    c. The diencephalon contains the thalamus, which serves as a central relay station for incoming sensory impulses; and the hypothalamus, which plays an important role in maintaining stable internal conditions.

    d. The limbic system functions to produce emotional feelings and to modify behavior.

    e. The midbrain contains reflex centers associated with eye and head movements.

    f. The pons transmits impulses between the cerebrum and other parts of the nervous system, and contains centers that help regulate the rate and depth of breathing.

    g. The medulla oblongata transmits all ascending and descending impulses, and contains several vital and nonvital reflex centers.

    h. The reticular formation arouses the cerebral cortex into wakefulness whenever significant impulses are received.

6. The cerebellum

    a. The cerebellum consists of two hemispheres connected by the vermis.

    b. It is composed of white matter surrounded by a thin cortex of gray matter.

    c. The cerebellum functions primarily as a reflex center in the coordination of skeletal muscle movements and the maintenance of equilibrium.

The Peripheral Nervous System (page 299)

The peripheral nervous system consists of cranial and spinal nerves that branch out from the brain and spinal cord to all body parts. It can be divided into somatic and autonomic portions.

1. Structure of peripheral nerves

    a. A nerve consists of a bundle of nerve fibers surrounded by connective tissues.

    b. The connective tissues form an outer epineurium, a perineurium enclosing bundles of nerve fibers, and an endoneurium surrounding each fiber.

2. The cranial nerves

    a. Twelve pairs of cranial nerves connect the brain to parts in the head, neck, and trunk.

    b. Although most cranial nerves are mixed, some are pure sensory, and others are primarily motor.

    c. The names of cranial nerves indicate their primary functions or the general distributions of their fibers.

    d. Some cranial nerve fibers are somatic and others are autonomic.

3. The spinal nerves

    a. Thirty-one pairs of spinal nerves originate from the spinal cord.

    b. These mixed nerves provide a two-way communication system between the spinal cord and parts in the arms, legs, neck, and trunk.

    c. Spinal nerves are grouped according to the levels from which they arise, and they are numbered in sequence.

    d. Each nerve emerges by a dorsal and a ventral root.

        (1) A dorsal root contains sensory fibers and is characterized by the presence of a dorsal root ganglion.

        (2) A ventral root contains motor fibers.

    e. Just beyond its foramen, each spinal nerve divides into several branches.

    f. Most spinal nerves combine to form plexuses in which nerve fibers are sorted and recombined so that those fibers associated with a particular part reach it together.

The Autonomic Nervous System (page 316)

The autonomic nervous system consists of the portions of the nervous system that function without conscious effort. It is concerned primarily with the regulation of visceral activities that aid in maintaining constant conditions.

1. General characteristics

    a. Autonomic functions operate as reflex actions controlled from centers in the hypothalamus, brain stem, and spinal cord.

    b. Autonomic nerve fibers are associated with ganglia in which impulses are integrated before passing out to effectors.

c. The integrative function of the ganglia provides a degree of independence from the central nervous system.

d. The autonomic nervous system consists of the visceral efferent fibers associated with these ganglia.

e. The autonomic nervous system is subdivided into two divisions—sympathetic and parasympathetic.

f. The sympathetic division prepares the body for stressful and emergency conditions.

g. The parasympathetic division is most active under ordinary conditions.

2. Autonomic nerve pathways
   a. Sympathetic motor fibers leave the spinal cord and synapse in ganglia.
      (1) Preganglionic fibers pass through white rami to reach paravertebral ganglia.
      (2) Paravertebral ganglia and interconnecting fibers comprise the sympathetic trunks.
      (3) Preganglionic fibers synapse within paravertebral or collateral ganglia.
      (4) Postganglionic fibers usually pass through gray rami to reach spinal nerves before passing to effectors.
      (5) A special set of sympathetic preganglionic fibers passes through ganglia and extends to the adrenal medulla.
   b. Parasympathetic fibers begin in the brain stem and sacral region of the spinal cord, and synapse in ganglia near visceral organs.

Clinical Application of Knowledge

1. How would you explain the following observations?
   a. When motor nerve fibers in the leg are severed, the muscles they innervate become paralyzed; however, in time, control over the muscles returns.
   b. When motor nerve fibers in the spinal cord are severed, the muscles they control become paralyzed permanently.

2. Multiple sclerosis is a disease in which nerve fibers in the central nervous system lose their myelin. Why would this loss be likely to affect the person's ability to control skeletal muscles?

3. What functional losses would you expect to observe in a patient who has suffered injury to the right occipital lobe of the cerebral cortex? To the right temporal lobe?

4. Based on your knowledge of the cranial nerves, devise a set of tests to assess the normal functions of each of these nerves.

5. The Brown-Sequard syndrome is due to an injury on one side of the spinal cord. It is characterized by paralysis below the injury and on the same side as the injury, and by loss of sensations of temperature and pain on the opposite side. How would you explain these symptoms?

6. Why are rapidly growing cancers originating in nerve tissue more likely to be composed of neuroglial cells than of neurons?

7. The biceps-jerk reflex employs motor neurons that exit from the spinal cord in the 5th spinal nerve (C5), that is, fifth from the top of the cord. The triceps-jerk reflex involves motor neurons in the 7th spinal nerve (C7). How might these reflexes be used to help locate the site of spinal cord damage in a patient with a neck injury?

Review Activities

Part A
1. Explain the relationship between the central nervous system and the peripheral nervous system.
2. List three general functions of the nervous system.
3. Distinguish between neurons and neuroglial cells.
4. Describe the generalized structure of a neuron.
5. Describe the location of myelin.
6. Distinguish between myelinated and unmyelinated nerve fibers.
7. Discuss the functions of each type of neuroglial cell.
8. Define *synapse*.
9. Sketch a sensory neuron and a motor neuron synapsed in the correct manner.
10. Distinguish between convergent and divergent neuronal pools.
11. Explain how the organization of neurons can result in an amplified nerve impulse.
12. Explain how neurons can be classified on the basis of their structure.
13. Explain how neurons can be classified on the basis of their function.
14. Distinguish between sensory, motor, and mixed nerves.
15. Describe a reflex arc.
16. Define *reflex*.
17. Describe a withdrawal reflex.
18. Name the layers of the meninges and explain their functions.
19. Describe the location of cerebrospinal fluid within the meninges.
20. Describe the structure of the spinal cord.
21. Name the major ascending and descending tracts of the spinal cord, and list the functions of each.
22. Explain the consequences of nerve fibers crossing over.
23. Describe the structure of the cerebrum.
24. Define *cerebral cortex*.
25. Describe the location and function of the primary motor areas of the cortex.
26. Describe the location and function of Broca's area.
27. Describe the location and function of the sensory areas of the cortex.
28. Distinguish between association areas and association tracts of the cerebrum.
29. Explain the function of the corpus callosum.
30. Describe the location and function of the basal nuclei.
31. Describe the location of the ventricles of the brain.
32. Explain how cerebrospinal fluid is produced and how it functions.

33. Name the parts of the brain stem and describe the general functions of each.
34. Define the limbic system and explain its functions.
35. Name the parts of the midbrain and describe the general functions of each.
36. Describe the pons and its functions.
37. Describe the medulla oblongata and its functions.
38. Describe the location and function of the reticular formation.
39. Describe the functions of the cerebellum.
40. Distinguish between somatic and autonomic nervous systems.
41. Describe the structure of a peripheral nerve.
42. Name, locate, and describe the major functions of each pair of cranial nerves.
43. Explain how the spinal nerves are grouped and numbered.
44. Define *cauda equina.*
45. Describe the structure of a spinal nerve.
46. Define *plexus* and locate the major plexuses of the spinal nerves.
47. Distinguish between the sympathetic and parasympathetic divisions of the autonomic nervous system.
48. Explain how autonomic ganglia provide a degree of independence from the central nervous system.
49. Distinguish between a preganglionic fiber and a postganglionic fiber.
50. Define *paravertebral ganglion.*
51. Trace a sympathetic motor nerve pathway through a ganglion to an effector.

Part B
Match the term in column I with the definition in column II.

I	II
1. Sulcus	A. Supportive and protective cells in nerve tissue
2. Convolution	B. Group of neuron cell bodies in the central nervous system
3. Nerve fiber	C. Bundle of nerve fibers within the central nervous system
4. Neuron	D. Extensions from neuron cell body
5. Nerve	E. Fold of the cerebral cortex
6. Tract	F. Depression between convolutions of cerebral cortex
7. Nucleus	G. Nerve cell
8. Ganglion	H. Bundle of nerve fibers within the peripheral nervous system
9. Neuroglia	I. Group of neuron cell bodies within peripheral nervous system
10. Plexus	J. Network of branching spinal nerves

REFERENCE PLATES

Human Brain

The following series of reference plates is presented to help you locate some of the more important features revealed in sections and MRI scans of the brain.

PLATE 32
Median section of the brain.

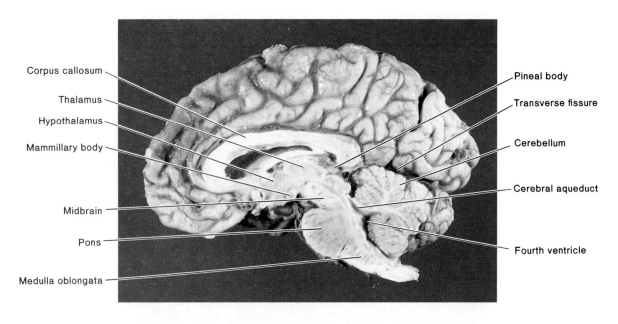

Corpus callosum
Thalamus
Hypothalamus
Mammillary body
Midbrain
Pons
Medulla oblongata

Pineal body
Transverse fissure
Cerebellum
Cerebral aqueduct
Fourth ventricle

PLATE 33
Sagittal section of the brain, 6 mm to the right of the midline.

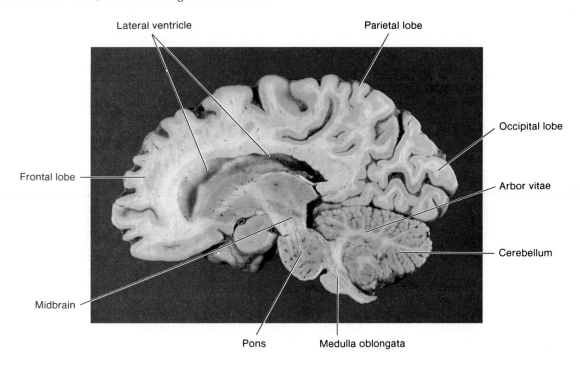

Lateral ventricle
Parietal lobe
Frontal lobe
Occipital lobe
Arbor vitae
Cerebellum
Midbrain
Pons
Medulla oblongata

PLATE 34

What features do you recognize in this MRI scan of the brain (sagittal section)?

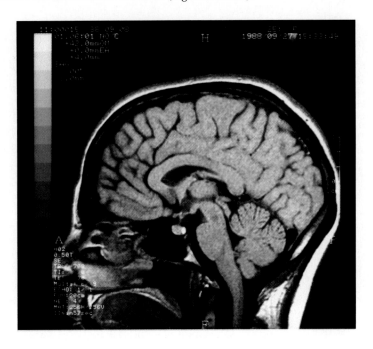

PLATE 35

Frontal section of the brain revealing the basal nuclei.

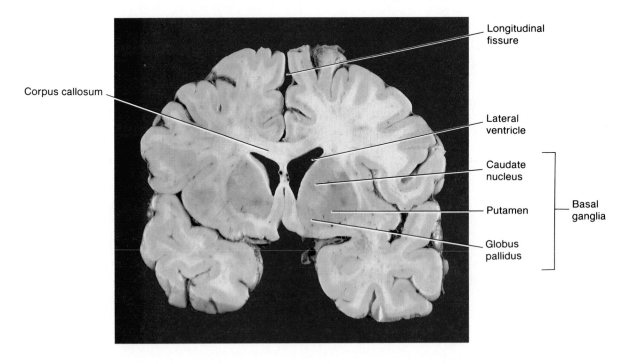

Corpus callosum

Longitudinal fissure

Lateral ventricle

Caudate nucleus

Putamen

Globus pallidus

Basal ganglia

PLATE 36
Frontal section of the brain revealing the insula.

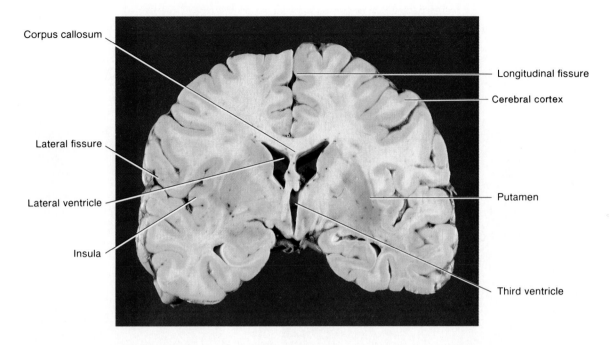

Corpus callosum

Longitudinal fissure

Cerebral cortex

Lateral fissure

Lateral ventricle

Putamen

Insula

Third ventricle

PLATE 37
Frontal section of the brain through the thalamus and hypothalamus.

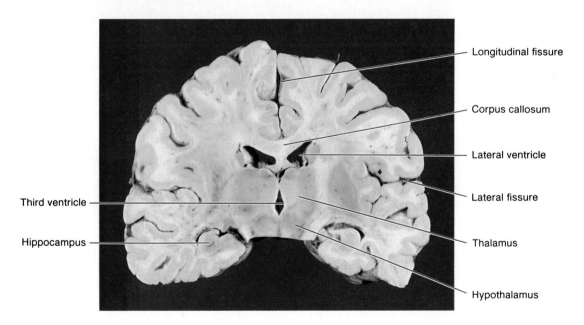

Longitudinal fissure

Corpus callosum

Lateral ventricle

Lateral fissure

Third ventricle

Hippocampus

Thalamus

Hypothalamus

PLATE 38

What features do you recognize in this MRI scan of the brain (frontal section)?

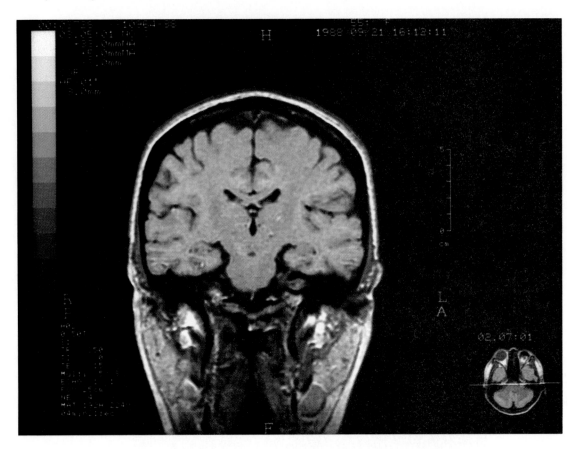

C H A P T E R 1 0

Somatic and Special Senses

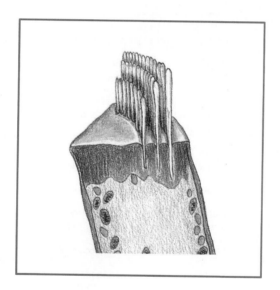

Before parts of the nervous system can act to control body functions, they must detect what is happening inside and outside the body. This information is gathered by sensory receptors that are sensitive to changes occurring in their surroundings.

Although receptors vary greatly in their individual characteristics, they can be grouped into two major categories. The receptors of one group are widely distributed throughout the skin and deeper tissues, and generally have simple forms. These receptors are associated with the somatic senses of touch, pressure, temperature, and pain. Receptors of the second group are parts of complex, specialized sensory organs that are responsible for the special senses of smell, taste, hearing, equilibrium, and vision.

Chapter Objectives

After you have studied this chapter, you should be able to

1. Name five kinds of receptors and explain the function of each kind.

2. Distinguish between somatic and special senses.

3. Describe the receptors associated with the senses of touch and pressure, temperature, and pain.

4. Explain the importance of stretch receptors in muscles and tendons.

5. Describe the structure of the organs associated with the senses of smell and taste.

6. Name the parts of the ear and explain the function of each part.

7. Describe the organs of equilibrium.

8. Name the parts of the eye and explain the function of each part.

9. Describe the visual nerve pathway.

10. Complete the review activities at the end of this chapter. Note that the items are worded in the form of specific learning objectives. You may want to refer to them before reading the chapter.

Aids to Understanding Words

aud-, to hear: *aud*itory—pertaining to hearing.

choroid, skinlike: *choroid* coat—middle, vascular layer of the eye.

cochlea, snail: *cochlea*—coiled tube within the inner ear.

corn-, horn: *corn*ea—transparent outer layer in the anterior portion of the eye.

gust-, taste: *gust*atory—pertaining to the sense of taste.

iris, rainbow: *iris*—colored, muscular part of the eye.

labyrinth, maze: *labyrinth*—complex system of interconnecting chambers and tubes of the inner ear.

lacri-, tears: *lacri*mal gland—tear gland.

lut-, yellow: macula *lut*ea—yellowish spot on the retina.

macula, spot: *macula* lutea—yellowish spot on the retina.

oculi-, eye: orbicularis *oculi*—muscle associated with the eyelid.

olfact-, to smell: *olfact*ory—pertaining to the sense of smell.

palpebra, eyelid: levator *palpebrae* superioris—muscle associated with the eyelid.

scler-, hard: *scler*a—tough, outer protective layer of the eye.

therm-, heat: *therm*oreceptor—receptor sensitive to changes in temperature.

tympan-, drum: *tympan*ic membrane—the eardrum.

vitre-, glass: *vitre*ous humor—clear, jellylike substance within the eye.

Introduction

As changes occur within the body and its surroundings, sensory receptors are stimulated. They, in turn, trigger nerve impulses, which travel on sensory pathways into the central nervous system to be processed and interpreted. The result is a particular feeling or sensation.

Types of Receptors

Most receptors are the terminal ends of sensory nerve fibers, although a few receptors are composed of other kinds of specialized cells. In any case, when receptors are stimulated, changes occur in the cells that trigger nerve impulses. Although there are many kinds of sensory receptors, they have features in common. For example, each type of receptor is particularly sensitive to a distinct kind of environmental change and is much less sensitive to other forms of stimulation.

On the basis of their sensitivities, receptors can be placed into five general groups.

1. **Chemoreceptors** are stimulated by changes in concentration of chemical substances. Receptors associated with the senses of smell and taste are of this type.
2. **Pain receptors** (nociceptors) are likely to be stimulated whenever tissues are damaged in any way. These receptors may be triggered by exposure to excessive mechanical, heat, or chemical energy.
3. **Thermoreceptors** are sensitive to temperature change.
4. **Mechanoreceptors** detect changes that cause the receptors to become deformed. These sensory receptors are sensitive to mechanical forces, such as changes in pressure or movement of fluids. For example, *proprioceptors* are sensitive to changes in the tensions of muscles and tendons.
5. **Photoreceptors** occur only in the eyes, and they respond whenever they are exposed to light energy of sufficient intensity.

Receptors can also be divided into groups on the basis of their locations, as follows:

1. Receptors associated with changes occurring at the body surface (exteroceptors), which include the receptors of touch, pressure, and temperature in the skin and in the special sense receptors.
2. Receptors associated with changes occurring in muscles, tendons, and body position (proprioceptors).
3. Receptors associated with changes occurring in visceral organs (interoreceptors).

Sensory impulses enter the central nervous system by means of peripheral nerves, and are analyzed and interpreted by the brain (see chapter 9).

A **sensation** is a feeling that occurs when sensory impulses are interpreted by the brain. Because all nerve impulses that travel from sensory receptors to the central nervous system are alike, different kinds of sensations must be due to the way the brain interprets the impulses rather than to differences in the receptors. In other words, when a receptor is stimulated, the resulting sensation depends on what region of the cerebral cortex receives the impulse. For example, impulses reaching one region are always interpreted as sounds, and those reaching another portion are always sensed as touch. Impulses reaching still other regions of the brain are always interpreted as pain.

At the same time a sensation is created, the brain causes it to seem to come from the receptors being stimulated. This process is called **projection,** because the brain projects the sensation back to its apparent source. Projection allows the person to pinpoint the region of stimulation. Thus, the eyes appear to see, and the ears appear to hear, and the skin appears to itch.

---

1. List five general types of sensory receptors.
2. What do these receptors have in common?

Somatic Sense Receptors

Somatic sense receptors are those associated with the skin, muscles, joints, and visceral organs. Many of these receptors are *free nerve endings* of sensory nerve fibers. Others are sensory nerve endings enclosed in sheaths of connective tissue cells.

Touch and Pressure Receptors

The senses of touch and pressure employ three kinds of receptors that are sensitive to mechanical forces that cause tissues to be deformed or displaced (figure 10.1). Touch and pressure receptors include the following:

1. **Sensory nerve fibers.** These receptors are common in connective tissues and in epithelial tissues, where their free ends are between epithelial cells. These free nerve endings may branch and form an interconnected network (plexus). For example, some sensory nerve fibers in the skin may form a plexus that is wrapped around a hair follicle, and these fibers may be activated when the hair is moved.
2. **Meissner's (tactile) corpuscles.** These structures consist of small, oval masses of flattened connective tissue cells surrounded by connective tissue sheaths. Two or more sensory nerve fibers branch into each corpuscle and end within it as tiny knobs.

FIGURE 10.1
Touch and pressure receptors include (*a*) free ends of sensory nerve fibers, (*b*) a Meissner's corpuscle, and (*c*) a pacinian corpuscle.

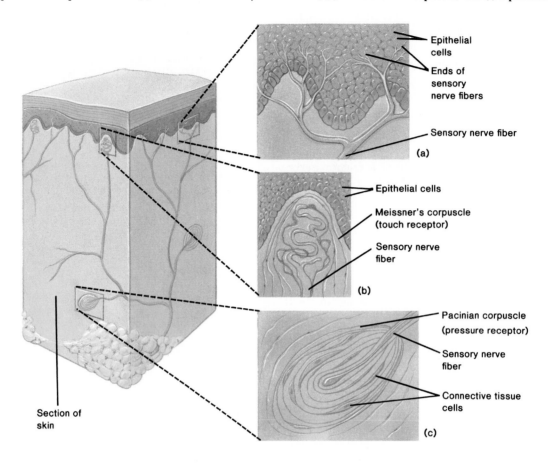

Meissner's corpuscles occur in the papillary layer of the dermis. They are especially numerous in the hairless portions of the skin, such as the lips, fingertips, palms, soles, nipples, and external genital organs. They are sensitive to the motion of objects that barely contact the skin, and impulses from them are interpreted as the sensation of light touch. They are also used when a person touches something to judge its texture. (See figure 10.2.)

3. **Pacinian (lamellated) corpuscles.** These sensory bodies are relatively large, ellipsoidal structures composed of many layers of connective tissue fibers and cells that surround a nerve fiber. They are common in the deeper subcutaneous tissues of such organs as the hands, feet, penis, clitoris, urethra, and breasts, and also occur in tendons of muscles and the ligaments of joints (figure 10.3).

Pacinian corpuscles are stimulated by heavy pressure and are thought to be associated with the sensation of deep pressure. They may also detect vibrations in tissues.

FIGURE 10.2
Light micrograph of a Meissner's corpuscle from the skin of the palm (×400).

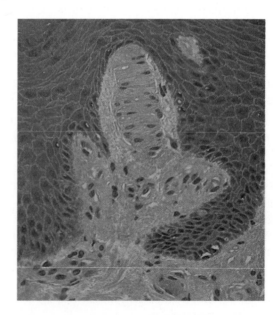

FIGURE 10.3

Light micrograph of a pacinian corpuscle (×25).

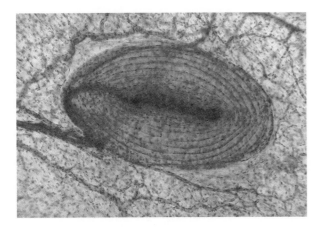

Temperature Receptors

The temperature senses employ two kinds of thermoreceptors. These receptors include two types of sensory nerve endings located in the skin called *heat receptors* and *cold receptors*. The heat receptors are most sensitive to temperatures above 25° C (77° F). Cold receptors are most sensitive to temperatures below 20° C (68° F).

Pain Receptors

The sense of pain also involves receptors that consist of sensory nerve fiber endings. These receptors are widely distributed throughout the skin and internal tissues, except in the nerve tissue in the brain, which lacks pain receptors.

Pain receptors are stimulated whenever tissues are being damaged. The resulting sensory impulses are likely to stimulate the reticular formation and, thus, activate the brain. The pain sensation is usually perceived as unpleasant, and serves as a signal that something should be done to remove the source of stimulation.

Although most pain receptors can be stimulated by more than one type of change, some are most sensitive to mechanical damage while others are particularly sensitive to extremes in temperature. Still other pain receptors are most responsive to various chemicals.

Pain Nerve Pathways

The nerve fibers that conduct impulses away from pain receptors include two main types: acute pain fibers and chronic pain fibers.

The *acute pain fibers* (also known as A-delta fibers) are relatively thin, myelinated nerve fibers. They conduct nerve impulses rapidly, at velocities up to 30 meters per second. These impulses are associated with the sensation of "sharp" pain, which typically seems to originate in the skin and is restricted to a local area. This type of pain seldom continues after its stimulus is discontinued.

A common form of pain is headache. Although the brain tissue itself lacks pain receptors, nearly all other tissues of the head, including the meninges and blood vessels associated with the brain, are well supplied with them.

Most headaches seem to be related to stressful life situations that result in fatigue, emotional tension, anxiety, or frustration. These conditions are reflected in various physiological changes. For example, they may cause prolonged contraction of skeletal muscles in the forehead, sides of the head, or back of the neck. Such contractions may stimulate pain receptors and produce what is often called a *tension headache*.

Still another form of headache is called *migraine*. In this disorder, certain cranial blood vessels seem to constrict, producing a localized cerebral blood deficiency. As a result, the person may experience a variety of symptoms, such as seeing patterns of bright light that interfere with vision or feeling numbness in the limbs or face. Typically, the vasoconstriction is followed by vasodilation of the cranial vessels and a severe headache, which is usually limited to one side of the head and lasts for several hours. Migraine headaches tend to run in families and generally begin in adolescence. They are also more common in women than in men.

The *chronic pain fibers* (C fibers) are thin, unmyelinated nerve fibers. They conduct impulses more slowly than the acute pain fibers, at velocities up to 2 meters per second. These impulses are related to the dull, aching pain that may be widespread and difficult to pinpoint. Such pain may continue for some time after the original stimulus has been eliminated. Although acute pain usually is sensed as coming from the surface, chronic pain is likely to be felt in deeper tissues as well as in the skin.

Commonly, an event that stimulates pain receptors will trigger impulses on both types of pain fibers. This causes a dual sensation—a sharp, pricking pain soon followed by a dull, aching pain. The aching pain is usually more intense and may become even more painful with time. It is this chronic pain that sometimes gives rise to prolonged suffering that is very resistant to relief and control.

Pain impulses that originate from tissues of the head reach the brain on sensory fibers of the 5th, 7th, 9th, and 10th cranial nerves. All other pain impulses travel on sensory fibers of the spinal nerves, and they pass into the spinal cord by way of the dorsal roots of these spinal nerves.

Upon reaching the spinal cord, pain impulses enter the gray matter of the dorsal horn, where they are processed (see chapter 9). The fast-conducting fibers synapse with long nerve fibers that cross over to the opposite side of the spinal cord and ascend in the lateral spinothalamic tracts. The impulses carried on the slow-conducting fibers pass through one or more interneurons before reaching the long fibers that cross over and ascend to the brain.

Within the brain, most of the pain fibers terminate in the reticular formation and from there are conducted on still other neurons to the thalamus, hypothalamus, and cerebral cortex.

Visceral Pain

As a rule, pain receptors are the only receptors in visceral organs whose stimulation produces sensations. Pain receptors in these organs seem to respond differently to stimulation than those associated with surface tissues. For example, localized damage to intestinal tissue during surgical procedures may not elicit any pain sensations even in a conscious person. However, when visceral tissues are subjected to more widespread stimulation, as when intestinal tissues are stretched or when the smooth muscles in the intestinal walls undergo spasms, a strong pain sensation may follow. The resulting pain seems to be related to the stimulation of mechanical-sensitive receptors and to a decreased blood flow.

Another characteristic of visceral pain is that it may feel as if it is coming from some part of the body other than the part being stimulated—a phenomenon called **referred pain.** Pain originating from the heart, for example, may be referred to the left shoulder or the inside of the left arm. Pain from the lower esophagus, stomach, or small intestine may seem to be coming from the upper central (epigastric) region of the abdomen; pain from the urogenital tract may be referred to the lower central (hypogastric) region of the abdomen or to the sides between the ribs and the hip (figure 10.4).

The occurrence of referred pain seems to be related to *common nerve pathways* that are used by sensory impulses coming both from skin areas and from visceral organs. For example, pain impulses from the heart travel to the spinal cord through a sympathetic pathway, through a paravertebral ganglion, and into the dorsal root of a spinal nerve. The sensory pathway from the skin of the shoulder and medial surface of the left arm leads

FIGURE 10.4
Surface regions to which visceral pain may be referred.

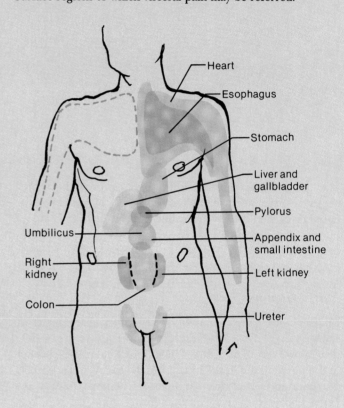

1. Describe three types of touch and pressure receptors.
2. Describe the thermoreceptors.
3. What types of receptors function as pain receptors?

Stretch Receptors

Stretch receptors are proprioceptors that provide information to the spinal cord and brain concerning the lengths and tensions of muscles. The two main kinds of stretch receptors are muscle spindles and Golgi tendon organs. No sensation results when these receptors are stimulated.

Muscle spindles are located in skeletal muscles near their junctions with tendons. Each spindle consists of one or more small, modified skeletal muscle fibers (intrafusal fibers) enclosed in a connective tissue sheath. Near its center, each fiber has a specialized nonstriated region with the end of a sensory nerve fiber wrapped around it (figure 10.6).

The striated portions of the muscle fiber can contract, and they keep the spindle taut. However, if the entire muscle becomes relaxed and is stretched longer than usual, the muscle spindle detects this change and sensory nerve impulses may be triggered on its nerve fiber. Such sensory impulses travel into the spinal cord and onto motor fibers

FIGURE 10.5
Pain originating in the heart may feel as if it is coming from the skin because sensory impulses from these two regions follow common nerve pathways to the brain.

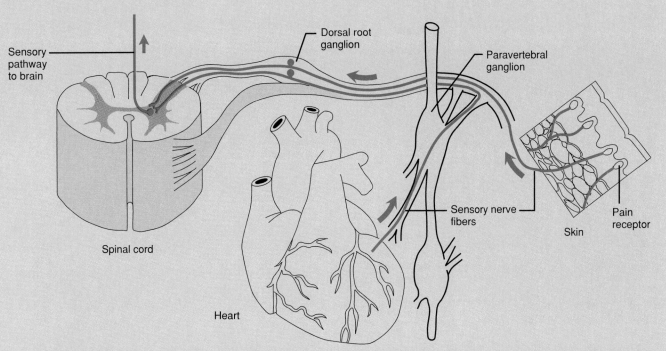

through sensory fibers in the anterior branch of the same spinal nerve and then through its dorsal root. (See chapter 9.) Thus, impulses from the heart, skin of the shoulder, and left arm seem to converge and are conducted over the same nerve pathways in the spinal cord and to the brain (figure 10.5). Consequently, the cerebral cortex may incorrectly interpret the source of the impulses as the shoulder or arm rather than the heart.

Pain originating from the parietal layers of thoracic and abdominal membranes—parietal pleura, pericardium, or peritoneum—is usually not referred; instead, such pain is likely to be felt directly over the area being stimulated.

leading back to the same muscle, causing it to contract. This action, called a **stretch reflex,** opposes the lengthening of the muscle and helps to maintain the desired position of a limb in spite of gravitational or other forces tending to move it (see chapter 9).

Golgi tendon organs are found in tendons close to their attachments to muscles. Each is connected to a set of skeletal muscle fibers and is innervated by a sensory neuron (figure 10.6). These receptors are stimulated by increased tension. Sensory impulses from these receptors produce a reflex that inhibits contraction of the muscle whose tendon they occupy. Thus, Golgi tendon organs stimulate an opposite reflex than that of a stretch reflex. This reflex also helps to maintain posture and protects muscle attachments from being pulled away from their insertions by excessive tension. Chart 10.1 summarizes the somatic receptors and their functions.

Chart 10.1 Somatic receptors

Type	Function	Sensation
Free nerve endings (mechanoreceptors)	Detect changes in pressure	Touch, pressure
Meissner's corpuscles (mechanoreceptors)	Detect objects moving over the skin	Touch, texture
Pacinian corpuscles (mechanoreceptors)	Detect changes in pressure	Deep pressure, vibrations
Free nerve endings (thermoreceptors for heat)	Detect changes in temperature	Heat
Free nerve endings (thermoreceptors for cold)	Detect changes in temperature	Cold
Free nerve endings (pain receptors)	Detect tissue damage	Pain
Muscle spindle (mechanoreceptor)	Detect changes in muscle length	None
Golgi tendon organ (mechanoreceptor)	Detect changes in muscle tension	None

FIGURE 10.6
(*a*) Muscle spindles, which are modified muscle fibers, are stimulated by changes in muscle length; (*b*) Golgi tendon organs inhibit the contraction of muscles whose tendons they occupy.

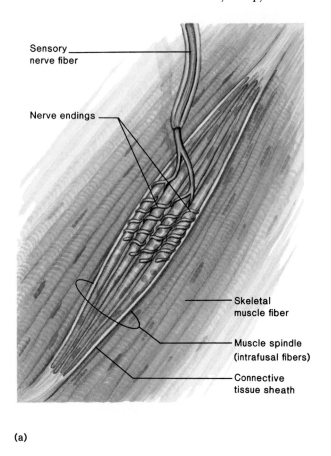

Sensory nerve fiber

Nerve endings

Skeletal muscle fiber

Muscle spindle (intrafusal fibers)

Connective tissue sheath

(a)

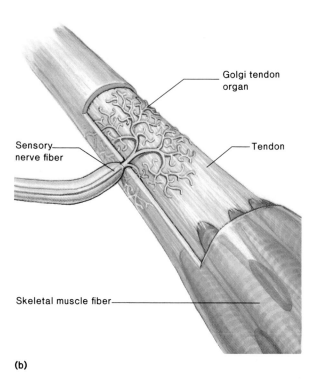

Golgi tendon organ

Sensory nerve fiber

Tendon

Skeletal muscle fiber

(b)

1. Describe a muscle spindle.
2. Explain how muscle spindles help maintain posture.
3. Where are Golgi tendon organs located?
4. What is the function of Golgi tendon organs?

Special Sense Receptors

Special sense receptors occur within large, complex sensory organs in the head. These organs include the olfactory organs, taste buds, ears, and eyes, which are associated with the senses of smell, taste, hearing and equilibrium, and sight, respectively.

Olfactory Organs

The sense of smell is associated with sensory receptors in the upper nasal cavity.

The smell, or olfactory (ol-fak′to-re), receptors are similar to those for taste (discussed in a subsequent section of this chapter) in that they are chemoreceptors. These two senses function together and aid in food selection.

Olfactory Organs and Receptors

The **olfactory organs,** which contain the olfactory receptors, also include various epithelial supporting cells. These organs appear as yellowish-brown masses surrounded by pinkish mucous membrane. They cover the upper parts of the nasal cavity, the superior nasal conchae, and a portion of the nasal septum (figure 10.7).

The **olfactory receptor cells** are bipolar neurons surrounded by columnar epithelial supporting cells. These neurons have knobs at the distal ends of their dendrites that are covered by hairlike cilia. The cilia project into the nasal cavity and are thought to be the sensitive portions of the receptors (figure 10.8).

FIGURE 10.7

The olfactory receptor cells, which have cilia at their distal ends, are supported by columnar epithelial cells.

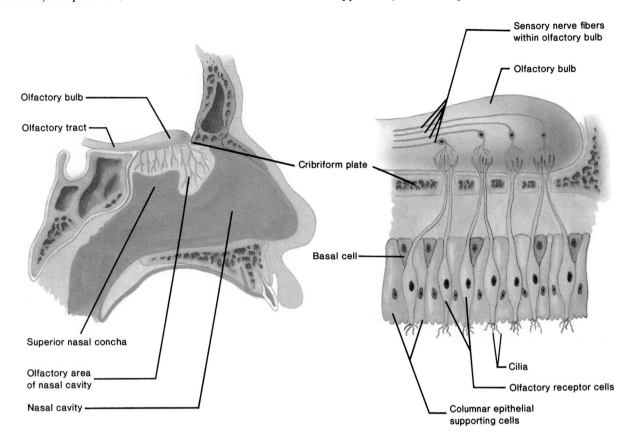

Chemicals that stimulate olfactory receptors enter the nasal cavity as gases, but they must dissolve in the watery fluids that surround the cilia before they can be detected.

The olfactory receptor neurons are the only parts of the nervous system that are in direct contact with the outside environment. Because of their exposed positions, these neurons are subject to damage, and people typically experience a progressive diminishing of olfactory sense with age. In fact, some investigators have estimated that a person loses about 1% of the olfactory receptors every year.

Small *basal cells,* located deep in the olfactory epithelial layer, are capable of dividing and differentiating into olfactory receptor cells. These cells act as a group of neuron stem cells and provide an exception to the usual pattern for neurons, since neurons usually do not divide. (See chapter 3.) As one of these stem cells differentiates, it produces a dendrite and an axon, and the axon must then form a synapse with a neuron in the olfactory bulb before it becomes functional. Thus, injured olfactory cells may be replaced.

FIGURE 10.8

Light micrograph of the olfactory membrane (×400).

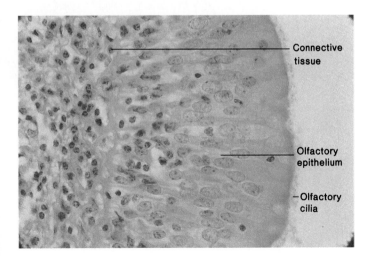

Olfactory Nerve Pathways

Once the olfactory receptors have been stimulated, nerve impulses are triggered, which travel along the axons of the receptor cells that are the fibers of the olfactory nerves. These nerve fibers pass through tiny openings in the cribriform plates of the ethmoid bone and lead to neurons located in enlargements called **olfactory bulbs.** These structures lie on either side of the crista galli of the ethmoid bone. (See figure 6.25.) From the olfactory bulbs, the impulses travel along the **olfactory tracts** to interpreting centers located in the base of the frontal lobes (olfactory cortex).

Partial or complete loss of smell is called *anosmia.* This condition may be caused by a variety of factors including inflammation of the nasal cavity lining, as occurs during a head cold. It may also result from excessive tobacco smoking, or from the use of certain drugs such as epinephrine or cocaine. Persons who have injured their olfactory bulbs, olfactory tracts, or cerebral olfactory interpreting centers will experience some degree of anosmia.

Elderly persons may require special stimulation to encourage eating because their olfactory sensitivities have diminished. For this reason, it is important that their foods be visibly attractive and that mealtimes be pleasant experiences. Otherwise, disinterest in eating may contribute to malnutrition.

1. Where are the olfactory receptors located?
2. Describe an olfactory receptor cell.
3. Trace the pathway of an olfactory impulse from a receptor to the cerebrum.

Gustatory Organs

Taste buds are the special organs of taste. They occur primarily on the surface of the tongue where they are associated with tiny elevations called **papillae** (figure 10.9). They are also found in smaller numbers in the roof of the mouth and the walls of the pharynx.

FIGURE 10.9

(*a*) Taste buds on the surface of the tongue are associated with nipplelike elevations called papillae. (*b*) A taste bud contains taste cells and has an opening, the taste pore, at its free surface.

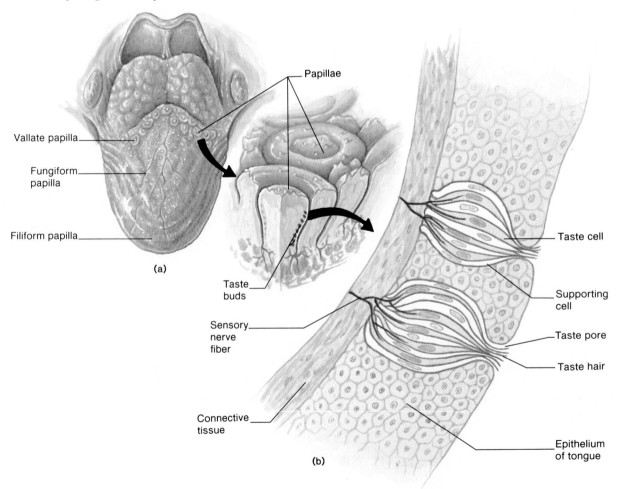

FIGURE 10.10

Scanning electron micrograph of a portion of the tongue, showing papillae.

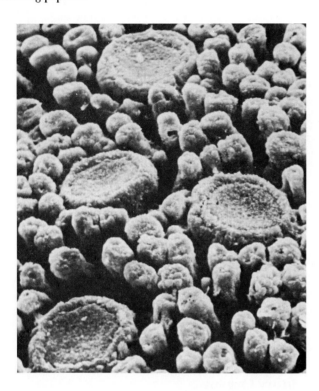

FIGURE 10.11

A light micrograph of taste buds, indicated by arrows.

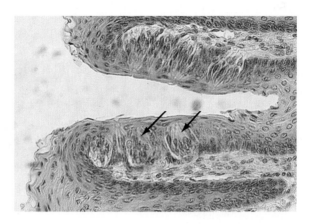

FIGURE 10.12

A scanning electron micrograph of a taste bud (×355). The arrow indicates a taste pore.
R. G. Kessel and R. H. Kardon, *Tissues and Organs: A Text Atlas of Scanning Electron Microscopy,* © 1979, W. H. Freeman & Co.

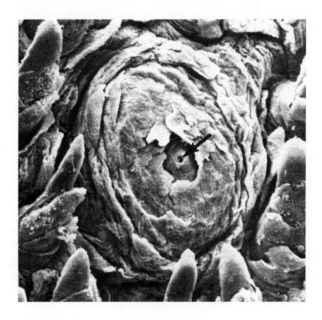

There are three types of papillae—vallate, fungiform, and filiform. The vallate papillae are large (1 to 2 mm in diameter) and are located along the back of the tongue. The fungiform papillae are rounded and found primarily on the sides and tip of the tongue. The filiform papillae are cone-shaped and scattered over the anterior two-thirds of the tongue. The filiform papillae do not have taste buds.

Taste Receptors

Each taste bud includes a group of modified epithelial cells called **taste cells** (gustatory cells), which function as receptors. The taste bud also includes a number of epithelial supporting cells. The entire structure is somewhat spherical, with an opening, the **taste pore,** on its free surface. Tiny projections (microvilli), called **taste hairs,** protrude from the outer ends of the taste cells and jut out through the taste pore (figures 10.10–10.12).

Woven among and wrapped around taste cells is a network of nerve fibers. The ends of these fibers are in close contact with the receptor cell membranes. When a receptor cell is stimulated, an impulse is triggered on a nearby nerve fiber and is carried into the brain.

Although taste cells in all taste buds appear very much alike microscopically, there are at least four types. Each type is sensitive to a particular kind of chemical stimulus, and consequently there are at least four primary taste (gustatory) sensations.

The four *primary taste sensations* are:

1. *Sweet,* as produced by table sugar.
2. *Sour,* as produced by vinegar.
3. *Salty,* as produced by table salt.
4. *Bitter,* as produced by caffeine or quinine.

FIGURE 10.13

Patterns of taste receptor distribution are indicated by color. (*a*) Sweet receptors; (*b*) sour receptors; (*c*) salt receptors; and (*d*) bitter receptors.

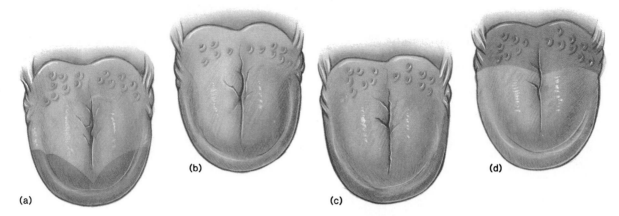

(a)   (b)   (c)   (d)

Each of the four major types of taste receptors is most highly concentrated in certain regions of the tongue's surface (figure 10.13). For example, *sweet receptors* are most plentiful near the tip of the tongue. *Sour receptors* occur primarily along the margins of the tongue. *Salt receptors* are most common in the tip and the upper front portion of the tongue. *Bitter receptors* are located toward the back of the tongue.

Although the taste cells are located very close to the surface of the tongue and are somewhat exposed to damage by environmental factors, the sense of taste is not as likely to diminish with age as the sense of smell. This is because taste cells are epithelial cells that are reproduced continually, so that any one of these cells functions for only about a week before it is replaced.

Taste Nerve Pathways

Sensory impulses from taste receptors located in the anterior two-thirds of the tongue travel on fibers of the facial nerve (VII); impulses from receptors in the posterior one-third of the tongue and the back of the mouth pass along the glossopharyngeal nerve (IX); and impulses from receptors at the base of the tongue and the pharynx travel on the vagus nerve (X) (see chapter 9).

These cranial nerves conduct the impulses into the medulla oblongata. From there, the impulses ascend to the thalamus and are directed to the gustatory cortex, located in the parietal lobe along a deep portion of the lateral sulcus.

The ability to taste certain substances shows great individual variation. Phenylthiocarbamide (PTC) is a substance associated with an inherited variation in taste. Some individuals perceive PTC as having a bitter taste; they are called tasters. Others cannot taste this substance at all; they are called nontasters, or "taste blind."

1. Describe a taste bud.
2. Name the four major types of taste receptors.
3. Describe the distribution of taste receptors on the tongue.
4. Trace a sensory impulse from a taste receptor to the cerebral cortex.

Auditory Organs

The **ear,** the organ of hearing, has external, middle, and inner parts. In addition to making hearing possible, the ear functions in the sense of equilibrium, which will be discussed in a subsequent section of this chapter.

External Ear

The external ear consists of an outer, funnel-like structure called the **auricle,** and an S-shaped tube, called the **external auditory meatus** that leads inward for about 2.5 centimeters (figure 10.14).

The external auditory meatus passes into the temporal bone. Near its opening the tube is guarded by hairs. It is lined with skin that contains numerous modified sweat glands called *ceruminous glands,* which secrete wax (cerumen). The hairs and wax help to keep foreign objects, such as insects, from entering the ear.

Sounds are generally created by vibrating objects, and the vibrations are transmitted through matter in the form of sound waves. For example, the sounds of the voice are created by vibrating vocal folds in the larynx. The auricle of the ear helps collect sound waves traveling through air and directs them into the auditory meatus.

After entering the meatus, the sound waves pass to the end of the tube and cause the eardrum to move back and forth in response.

FIGURE 10.14

Major parts of the ear.

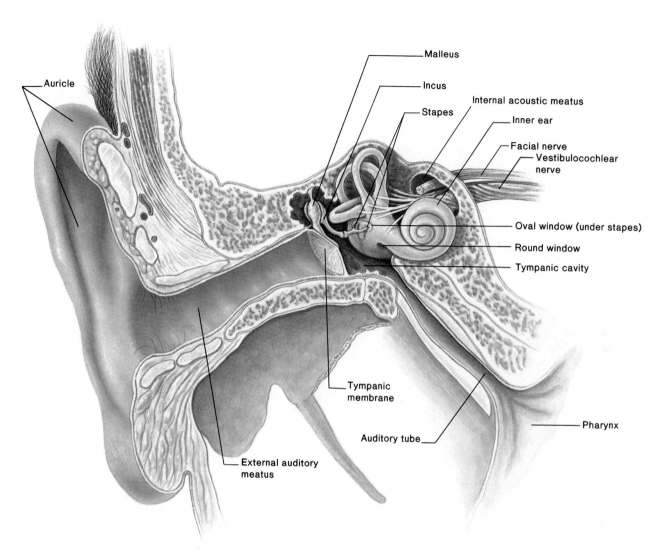

- Malleus
- Incus
- Internal acoustic meatus
- Stapes
- Inner ear
- Facial nerve
- Vestibulocochlear nerve
- Oval window (under stapes)
- Round window
- Tympanic cavity
- Auricle
- Tympanic membrane
- Auditory tube
- Pharynx
- External auditory meatus

Middle Ear

The middle ear is comprised of the tympanic cavity, the tympanic membrane (eardrum), and three small bones called auditory ossicles.

The **tympanic cavity** is an air-filled space in the temporal bone that separates the external and internal ears. The **tympanic membrane** is a semitransparent membrane covered by a thin layer of skin on its outer surface and by a mucous membrane on the inside. It has an oval margin and is cone-shaped, with the apex of the cone directed inward. Its cone shape is maintained by the attachment of one of the auditory ossicles (malleus).

The three **auditory** (aw′di-to″re) **ossicles**—the *malleus* (hammer), *incus* (anvil), and *stapes* (stirrup)—are attached to the wall of the tympanic cavity by tiny ligaments and are covered by mucous membrane. These bones form a bridge connecting the eardrum to the inner ear and

function to transmit vibrations between its parts. Specifically, the malleus is attached to the eardrum, and when the eardrum vibrates, the malleus vibrates in unison with it. The malleus causes the incus to vibrate, which then passes the movement onto the stapes. The stapes is held by ligaments to an opening in the wall of the tympanic cavity called the oval window. Vibration of the stapes, which acts like a piston at the oval window, causes motion of a fluid within the inner ear. These vibrations are responsible for stimulating the hearing receptors (figure 10.14).

In addition to transmitting vibrations, the auditory ossicles form a lever system that helps increase (amplify) the force of the vibrations as they are passed from the eardrum to the oval window.

The middle ear also contains two small skeletal muscles that are attached to the auditory ossicles and controlled involuntarily. One of them, the *tensor tympani*, is

Somatic and Special Senses   343

FIGURE 10.15

Two small muscles attached to the (*a*) malleus and (*b*) stapes, the tensor tympani and the stapedius, serve as effectors in the tympanic reflex.

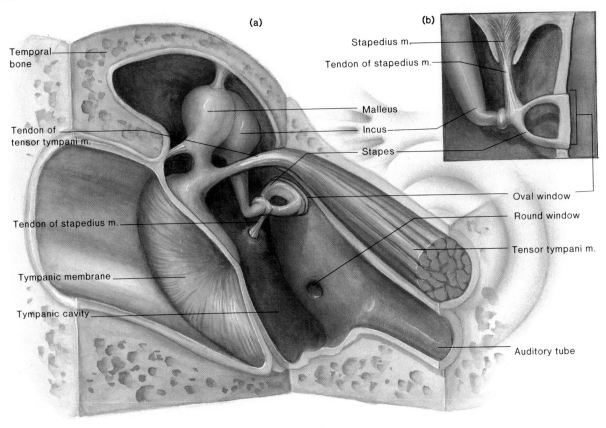

inserted on the medial surface of the malleus and is anchored to the cartilaginous wall of the auditory tube. When it contracts, it pulls the malleus inward. The other muscle, the *stapedius*, is attached to the posterior side of the stapes and the inner wall of the tympanic cavity. It serves to pull the stapes outward (figure 10.15). These muscles are the effectors in the **tympanic reflex,** which is elicited by loud sounds. When this reflex occurs, the muscles contract and the malleus and stapes are moved. As a result, the bridge of ossicles in the middle ear becomes more rigid, and its effectiveness in transmitting vibrations to the inner ear is reduced.

In this instance, the tympanic reflex is a protective mechanism that reduces pressure from loud sounds, which might otherwise damage the hearing receptors. The tympanic reflex is also elicited by ordinary vocal sounds, as when a person speaks or sings, and this action muffles the lower frequencies of such sounds. As a result, the hearing of higher frequency sounds, which are common in human vocal sounds, is improved. In addition, the tensor tympani muscle also maintains a steady pull on the eardrum, which is important because a loose tympanic membrane would not be able to effectively transmit vibrations to the auditory ossicles.

The middle ear muscles require from 100 to 200 milliseconds to contract. For this reason, the tympanic reflex cannot protect the hearing receptors from the effects of loud sounds that occur very rapidly, such as those from an explosion or a gunshot. On the other hand, this protective mechanism can reduce the effects of intense sounds that arise relatively slowly, such as the roar of thunder.

Auditory Tube

An **auditory tube** (eustachian tube) connects each middle ear to the throat. This tube allows air to pass between the tympanic cavity and the outside of the body by way of the throat (pharynx) and mouth. It helps maintain equal air pressure on both sides of the eardrum, which is necessary for normal hearing (figure 10.14).

The function of the auditory tube can be experienced during rapid change in altitude. For example, as a person moves from a high altitude to a lower one, the air pressure on the outside of the membrane becomes greater and greater. As a result, the eardrum may be pushed inward, out of its normal position, and hearing may be impaired.

FIGURE 10.16

The osseous labyrinth of the inner ear is separated from the membranous labyrinth by perilymph. The membranous labyrinth contains endolymph.

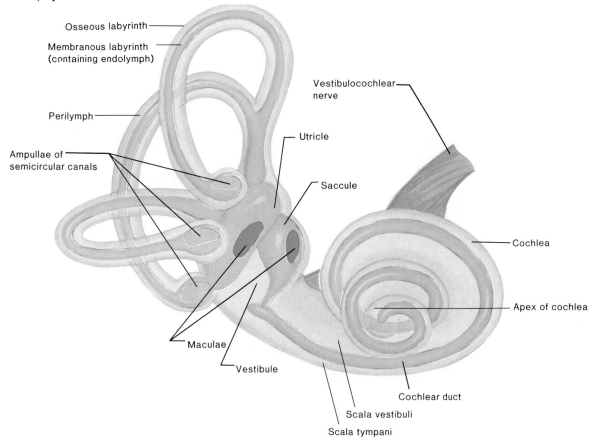

When the air pressure difference is great enough, some air may force its way up through the auditory tube into the middle ear. This allows the pressure on both sides of the eardrum to equalize, and the drum moves back into its regular position. The person usually hears a popping sound at this moment, and normal hearing is restored. A reverse movement of air ordinarily occurs when a person moves from low altitude into a higher one.

The auditory tube is usually closed by valvelike flaps in the throat, which may inhibit air movements into the middle ear. Swallowing, yawning, or chewing may aid in opening the valves; thus, these actions can hasten the equalization of air pressure during altitude changes.

The mucous membranes that line the auditory tubes are continuous with the linings of the middle ears. Consequently, the tubes provide a route by which mucous membrane infections of the throat (pharyngitis) may pass to the ear and cause an infection of the middle ear (otitis media). For this reason, it is poor practice to pinch one nostril when blowing the nose, because pressure in the nasal cavity may force material from the throat up the tube and into the middle ear.

Inner Ear

The inner ear consists of a complex system of intercommunicating chambers and tubes called a **labyrinth.** In fact, there are two such structures in each ear—the *osseous labyrinth* is a bony canal in the temporal bone; the *membranous labyrinth* is a tube that lies within the osseous labyrinth and has a similar shape (figure 10.16). Between the osseous and membranous labyrinths is a fluid called *perilymph,* which is secreted by cells in the wall of the bony canal. The membranous labyrinth contains another fluid, called *endolymph.*

The parts of the labyrinths include a **cochlea** that functions in hearing, and three **semicircular canals** that function in providing a sense of equilibrium. A bony chamber called the **vestibule,** which is located between the cochlea and the semicircular canals, contains membranous structures that serve both hearing and equilibrium.

The **cochlea** (kok′le-ah) is shaped like the coiled shell of a snail. Inside, it contains a bony core (modiolus) and a thin, bony shelf (spiral lamina) that winds around the core like the threads of a screw. The shelf divides the bony labyrinth of the cochlea into upper and lower compartments. The upper compartment, called the *scala vestibuli,* leads from the oval window to the apex of the spiral. The lower

FIGURE 10.17

A cross section of the cochlea shows a bony canal with a membranous tube inside.

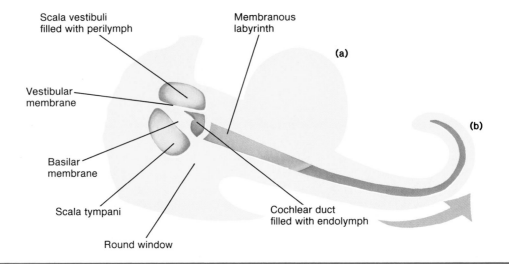

FIGURE 10.18

(*a*) Cross section of the cochlea; (*b*) enlargement of the organ of Corti.

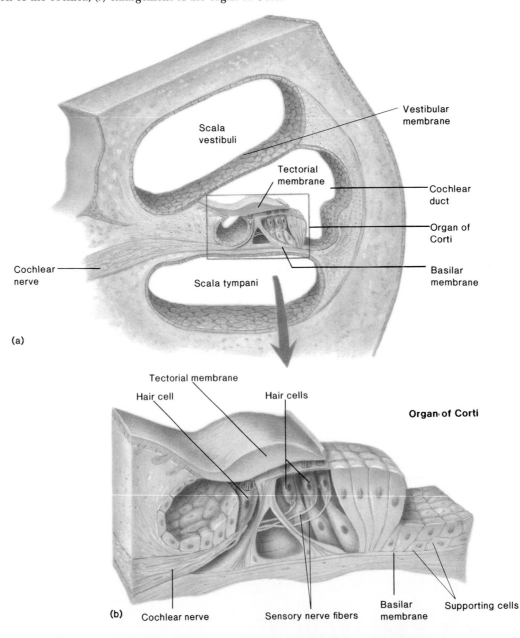

compartment, the *scala tympani*, extends from the apex of the cochlea to a membrane-covered opening in the wall of the inner ear, called the **round window.** These compartments constitute the bony labyrinth of the cochlea, and are filled with perilymph. At the apex of the cochlea, the fluids in the chambers can flow together through a small opening (helicotrema).

A portion of the membranous labyrinth within the cochlea is called the *cochlear duct* (scala media). It is filled with endolymph and lies between the scala vestibuli and the scala tympani. The cochlear duct ends as a closed sac at the apex of the cochlea. The duct is separated from the scala vestibuli by a *vestibular membrane* (Reissner's membrane) and from the scala tympani by a *basilar membrane* (figure 10.17).

The basilar membrane extends from the bony shelf of the cochlea and forms the floor of the cochlear duct. Vibrations entering the perilymph at the oval window travel along the scala vestibuli and pass through the vestibular membrane to enter the endolymph of the cochlear duct, where they cause movements in the basilar membrane.

The **organ of Corti,** which contains about 16,000 hearing receptor cells and many supporting cells, is located on the upper surface of the basilar membrane and stretches from the apex to the base of the cochlea. The receptor cells, which are called **hair cells,** are arranged in four parallel rows and possess numerous microvilli, called *stereocilia,* that extend into the endolymph of the cochlear duct. Above these hair cells is a *tectorial membrane* that is attached to the bony shelf of the cochlea and passes like a roof over the receptor cells, making contact with the tips of their hairs. (See figures 10.18 and 10.19.)

As sound vibrations pass through the inner ear, the hairs shear back and forth against the tectorial membrane, and the mechanical deformation of the hairs stimulates the receptor cells. The stereocilia become progressively longer from the base of the cochlea to its apex. This results in hair cells having slightly different sensitivities to sounds with different frequencies of vibration.

After passing through the basilar membrane, sound vibrations enter the perilymph of the scala tympani, and their forces are dissipated to the air in the tympanic cavity by movement of the membrane covering the round window.

Although the receptor cells are epithelial cells, they act somewhat like neurons (see chapter 9). Hair cells have no axons or dendrites, but have vesicles that contain neurotransmitter in the cytoplasm near the base. The release of neurotransmitter stimulates the ends of nearby sensory nerve fibers, which, in response, transmit nerve impulses along the cochlear branch of the vestibulocochlear nerve to the brain.

Auditory Nerve Pathways

The cochlear branches of the vestibulocochlear nerves enter the auditory nerve pathways, which extend into the medulla oblongata, and proceed through the midbrain to the thalamic regions. From there they pass into the auditory cortices of the temporal lobes of the cerebrum, where they are interpreted. On the way, some of these fibers cross over, so that impulses arising from each ear are interpreted on both sides of the brain. Consequently, damage

Figure 10.19

(*a*) A light micrograph of the organ of Corti (×135); (*b*) a scanning electron micrograph of hair cells in the organ of Corti showing the arrangement of stereocilia (×13,000).

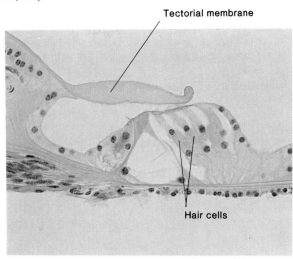

Tectorial membrane

Hair cells

(a)

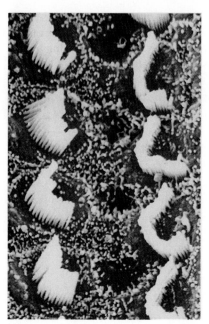

(b)

FIGURE 10.20

The auditory nerve pathway extends into the medulla oblongata, proceeds through the midbrain to the thalamus, and passes into the auditory cortex of the cerebrum.

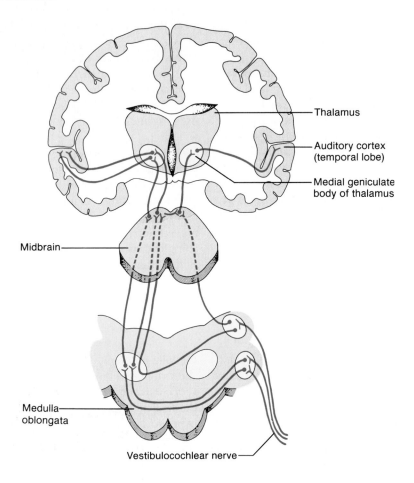

Thalamus

Auditory cortex (temporal lobe)

Medial geniculate body of thalamus

Midbrain

Medulla oblongata

Vestibulocochlear nerve

to a temporal lobe on one side of the brain is not necessarily accompanied by complete hearing loss in the ear on that side. (See figure 10.20.)

Chart 10.2 summarizes the pathway of vibrations through the parts of the middle and inner ears.

1. Describe the external, middle, and inner ears.
2. Explain how sound waves are transmitted through the parts of the ear.
3. Describe the tympanic reflex.
4. Distinguish between the osseous and membranous labyrinths.
5. Explain the function of the organ of Corti.

Chart 10.2 Steps in the generation of sensory impulses from the ear

1. Sound waves enter external auditory meatus.
2. Waves of changing pressures cause the eardrum to reproduce the vibrations coming from the sound wave source.
3. Auditory ossicles amplify and transmit vibrations to the end of the stapes.
4. Movement of the stapes at the oval window transmits vibrations to the perilymph in the scala vestibuli.
5. Vibrations pass through the vestibular membrane and enter the endolymph of the cochlear duct.
6. Vesicles at the base of the receptor cell release neurotransmitter.
7. The neurotransmitter stimulates the ends of nearby sensory neurons.
8. Sensory impulses are triggered on fibers of the cochlear branch of the vestibulocochlear nerve.
9. The auditory cortex of the temporal lobe interprets the sensory impulses.

Deafness

Partial or complete hearing loss can be caused by a variety of factors, including interference with the transmission of vibrations to the inner ear (conductive deafness), or damage to the cochlea, auditory nerve, or auditory nerve pathways (sensorineural deafness).

Conductive deafness may be due to a simple plugging of the external auditory meatus by an accumulation of dry wax or the presence of a foreign object. In other instances, the impairment is related to changes in the eardrum or the auditory ossicles. The eardrum, for example, may harden as a result of disease and thus be less responsive to sound waves, or it may be torn or perforated by disease or injury. The auditory ossicles may also be damaged or destroyed by disease or may lose their mobility.

One of the more common diseases involving the auditory ossicles is *otosclerosis.* In this condition, new bone is deposited abnormally around the base of the stapes, interfering with the motion of the ossicle needed to effectively transmit vibrations to the inner ear. Although the cause of otosclerosis is unknown, a victim's hearing can often be restored by surgical procedures. For instance, the base of the stapes may be freed by chipping away the bone that holds it fixed in position, or the stapes may be removed and replaced with a wire or plastic substitute (prosthesis).

One cause of *sensorineural deafness* is exposure to excessively loud sounds. If the exposure is of short duration, the hearing loss may be temporary; however, when there is repeated and prolonged exposure, such as occurs in some foundries, near jackhammers, or on a firing range, the impairment may be permanent. This is usually due to damage to the hair cells.

Other causes of sensorineural deafness include tumors in the central nervous system, brain damage as a result of vascular accidents, and the use of certain drugs.

Persons over age 65 commonly lose the ability to hear high-frequency sounds and have a decreased ability to discriminate speech sounds as a result of a condition called presbycusis. Thus, it is important to use lower voice tones when speaking to an elderly person. Also, the speaker should face the listener so that some lip reading is possible.

Organs of Equilibrium

The organs of equilibrium are also located in the inner ear. The vestibule and semicircular canals of the inner ear contain receptors that function to sense the position of the head, to detect motion, and to aid in maintaining balance.

Vestibule

The *vestibule* is the bony chamber between the semicircular canals and the cochlea. The membranous labyrinth inside the vestibule consists of two expanded chambers—an **utricle** and a **saccule.** The larger utricle communicates with the saccule and the membranous portions of the semicircular canals; the saccule, in turn, communicates with the cochlear duct (figure 10.16).

Each of these chambers has a small patch of hair cells and supporting cells called a **macula** (mak′u-la) on its wall. When the head is upright, the hairs of the macula in the utricle project vertically, while those in the saccule project horizontally. In each case, the hairs are in contact with a sheet of gelatinous material (otolithic membrane) that has crystals of calcium carbonate (otoliths) embedded on its surface. These particles increase the weight of the gelatinous sheet, making it more responsive to changes in position. The hair cells, which serve as sensory receptors, have sensory nerve fibers wrapped around their bases. These fibers are associated with the vestibular portion of the vestibulocochlear nerve.

The usual stimulus to the hair cells occurs when the head is bent forward, backward, or to one side. Such movements may cause the gelatinous mass of one or more maculae to be tilted, and, as it sags in response to gravity, the hairs projecting into it are bent. This action stimulates the hair cells to release neurotransmitter, which then signals the nerve fibers. The resulting nerve impulses travel into the central nervous system by means of the vestibular branch of the vestibulocochlear nerve. These impulses inform the brain as to the position of the head. The brain may act on this information by sending motor impulses to skeletal muscles, which may contract or relax appropriately so that balance is maintained (figures 10.21 and 10.22).

The maculae also sense certain types of body movements. For example, if the head or body is thrust forward or backward abruptly, the gelatinous mass of the maculae lags slightly behind, and the hair cells are stimulated. In this way, the maculae aid the brain in detecting movements such as falling and in maintaining posture while walking.

FIGURE 10.21
The macula is responsive to changes in the position of the head. (*a*) Macula with the head in an upright position; (*b*) with the head bent forward.

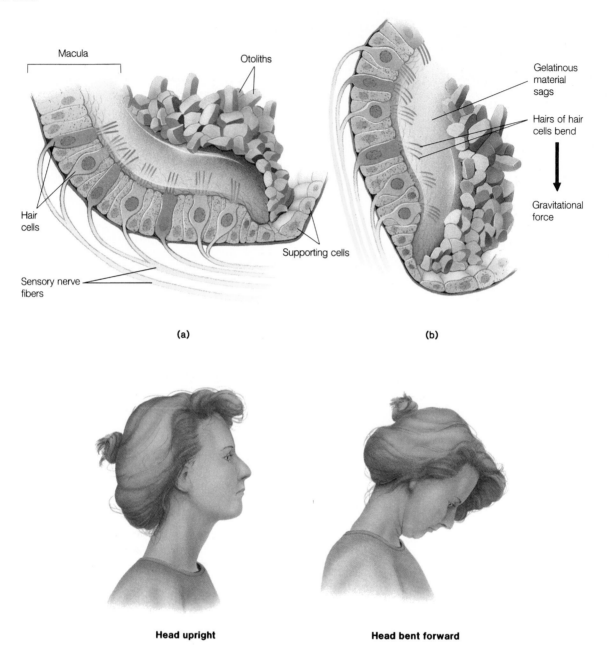

(a) (b)

Head upright **Head bent forward**

Semicircular Canals

Each semicircular canal follows a circular path about six millimeters in diameter. The three bony **semicircular canals** lie at right angles to each other, and each occupies a different plane in space. Two of them, the *superior* and the *posterior canals,* stand vertically, while the third, the *lateral canal* is horizontal (figure 10.16).

Suspended in the perilymph of each bony canal is a membranous, semicircular canal that ends in a swelling called an **ampulla.** The ampullae communicate with the utricle of the vestibule.

Each ampulla contains a **crista ampullaris,** which includes a number of sensory hair cells and supporting cells. The hairs of the hair cells extend upward into a dome-shaped gelatinous mass, called the *cupula.* Also, hair cells are connected at their bases to nerve fibers that make up part of the vestibular branch of the vestibulocochlear nerve (figure 10.23).

Hair cells of the crista are ordinarily stimulated by rapid turns of the head or body. At such times, the semicircular canals move with the head or body, but the fluid inside the membranous canals remains stationary because

FIGURE 10.22

Scanning electron micrograph of "hairs" of hair cells, such as those found in the utricle and saccule.

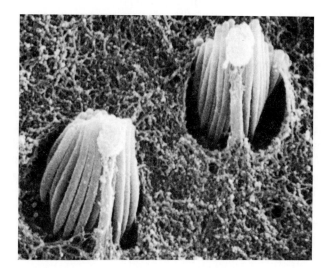

FIGURE 10.23

A crista ampullaris is located within the ampulla of each semicircular canal.

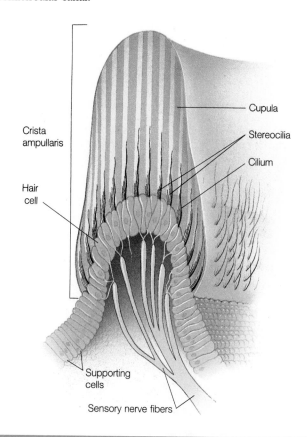

of inertia. This causes the cupula in one or more of the canals to bend in a direction opposite to the movement of the head or body, and the hairs embedded in it are also bent. This bending of the hairs stimulates the hair cells to signal their associated nerve fibers, and, as a result, impulses travel to the brain (figure 10.24).

FIGURE 10.24

(a) When the head is stationary, the cupula of this crista ampullaris remains upright. (b) When the head is moving rapidly, the cupula is bent and sensory receptors are stimulated.

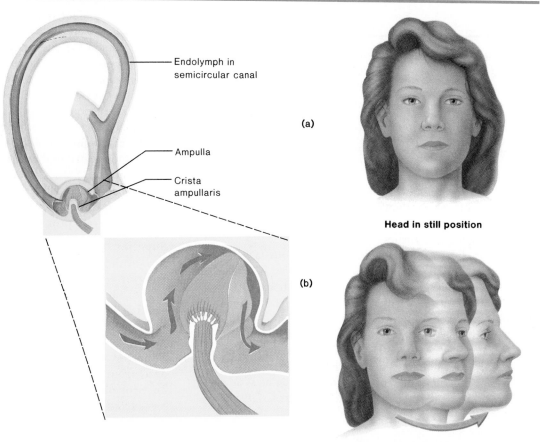

Parts of the cerebellum are particularly important in interpreting impulses from the semicircular canals. Analyzing such information allows the brain to predict the consequences of rapid body movements, and, by stimulating various skeletal muscles, it can prevent loss of balance.

Some people experience a discomfort called *motion sickness* when they are in a moving boat, airplane, or automobile. This discomfort seems to be caused by abnormal and irregular body motions that disturb the organs of equilibrium. Symptoms of motion sickness include nausea, vomiting, dizziness, headache, and prostration.

Other sensory structures also aid in maintaining equilibrium. For example, various proprioceptors (particularly those associated with the joints of the neck) supply the brain with information concerning the position of body parts. In addition, the eyes can detect changes in posture that result from body movements. Visual information is so important that even though a person has suffered damage to the organs of equilibrium he or she may be able to maintain normal balance by keeping the eyes open and moving slowly.

---

1. What structures provide the sense of equilibrium?
2. Which other sensory receptors help maintain equilibrium?

Visual Organs

Although the eye contains the visual receptors, its functions are assisted by a number of *accessory organs*. These include the eyelids and the lacrimal apparatus that help protect the eye, and a set of extrinsic muscles that move it.

Visual Accessory Organs

The eye, lacrimal gland, and the extrinsic muscles of the eye are housed within the pear-shaped orbital cavity of the skull. The orbit, which is lined with the periosteums of various bones, also contains fat, blood vessels, nerves, and a variety of connective tissues.

Each **eyelid** (palpebra) is composed of four layers—skin, muscle, connective tissue, and conjunctiva. The skin of the eyelid, which is the thinnest skin of the body, covers the lid's outer surface and fuses with its inner lining near the margin of the lid (figure 10.25).

The muscles of the eyelids include the *orbicularis oculi* and the *levator palpebrae superioris.* Fibers of the orbicularis oculi encircle the opening between the lids and spread out onto the cheek and forehead. This muscle acts as a sphincter that closes the lids when it contracts.

Fibers of the levator palpebrae superioris muscle arise from the roof of the orbit and are inserted in the connective tissue of the upper lid. When these fibers contract, the upper lid is raised and the eye opens.

The connective tissue layer of the eyelid, which helps give it form, contains numerous modified sebaceous glands (tarsal glands). The oily secretions of these glands are carried by ducts to openings along the borders of the lids. This secretion helps keep the lids from sticking together.

The **conjunctiva** is a mucous membrane that lines the inner surfaces of the eyelids and folds back to cover the anterior surface of the eyeball, except for its central portion (cornea). Although the portion that lines the eyelids is relatively thick, the conjunctiva that covers the eyeball is very thin. It is also freely movable and quite transparent, so that blood vessels are clearly visible beneath it.

The *lacrimal apparatus* (figure 10.26) consists of the **lacrimal gland,** which secretes tears, and a series of *ducts,* which carry the tears into the nasal cavity. The gland is located in the orbit, above and to the lateral side of the eye. It secretes tears continuously, and they pass out through tiny tubules, and flow downward and medially across the eye.

Tears are collected by two small ducts (superior and inferior canaliculi) whose openings (puncta) can be seen on the medial borders of the eyelids. From these ducts, the fluid moves into the *lacrimal sac,* which lies in a deep groove of the lacrimal bone, and then into the *nasolacrimal duct,* which empties into the nasal cavity.

Glandular cells of the conjunctiva also secrete a tear-like liquid that, together with the secretion of the lacrimal gland, keeps the surface of the eye and the lining of the lids moist and lubricated.

When a person experiences strong emotion, such as grief or happiness, or when the conjunctiva is irritated, the tear glands are likely to secrete excessive fluids. Tears may spill over the edges of the eyelids, and the nose may fill with fluid. This response involves motor impulses carried to the lacrimal glands on parasympathetic nerve fibers.

The **extrinsic muscles** of the eye arise from the bones of the orbit and are inserted by broad tendons on the eye's tough outer surface. Six such muscles move the eye in various directions (figure 10.27). Although any given eye movement may involve more than one of them, each muscle is associated with one primary action, as follows:

1. **Superior rectus**—rotates the eye upward and toward the midline.
2. **Inferior rectus**—rotates the eye downward and toward the midline.
3. **Medial rectus**—rotates the eye toward the midline.
4. **Lateral rectus**—rotates the eye away from the midline.
5. **Superior oblique**—rotates the eye downward and away from the midline.
6. **Inferior oblique**—rotates the eye upward and away from the midline.

FIGURE 10.25

Sagittal section of the eyelids and the anterior portion of the eye.

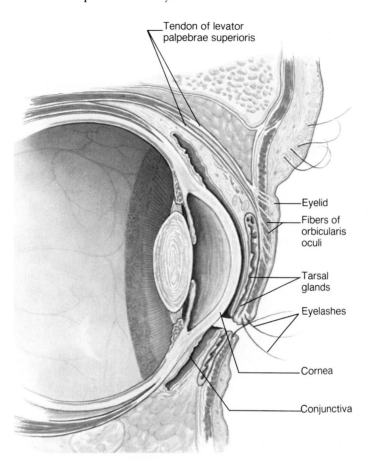

Tendon of levator palpebrae superioris

Eyelid

Fibers of orbicularis oculi

Tarsal glands

Eyelashes

Cornea

Conjunctiva

FIGURE 10.26

The lacrimal apparatus consists of a tear-secreting gland and a series of ducts.

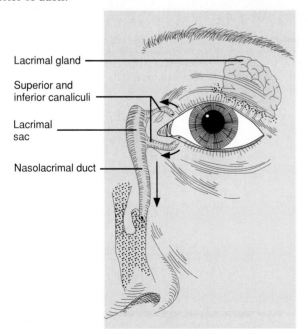

Lacrimal gland

Superior and inferior canaliculi

Lacrimal sac

Nasolacrimal duct

The motor units of the extrinsic eye muscles contain the smallest number of muscle fibers (five to ten) of any muscles in the body. Because of this, the eyes can be moved with great precision. Also, the eyes move together so that they are aligned when looking at something. Such alignment involves complex motor adjustments that result in the contraction of certain eye muscles while their antagonists are relaxed. For example, when the eyes move to the right, the lateral rectus of the right eye and the medial rectus of the left eye must contract. At the same time, the medial rectus of the right eye and the lateral rectus of the left eye must relax. A person whose eyes are not coordinated well enough to produce alignment is said to have *strabismus,* or squint.

Chart 10.3 summarizes the muscles associated with the eye.

FIGURE 10.27

The extrinsic muscles of the eye.

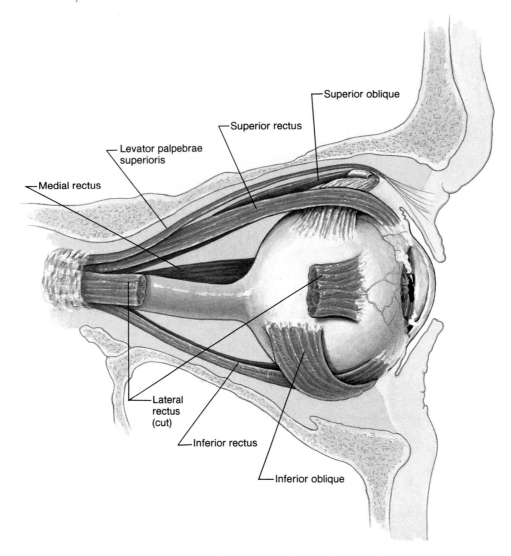

Chart 10.3 Muscles associated with the eye

Skeletal muscles			Smooth muscles		
Name	*Innervation*	*Function*	*Name*	*Innervation*	*Function*
Orbicularis oculi	Facial nerve (VII)	Closes eye	Ciliary muscles	Oculomotor nerve (III) parasympathetic fibers	Causes suspensory ligaments to relax
Levator palpebrae superioris	Oculomotor nerve (III)	Opens eye			
Superior rectus	Oculomotor nerve (III)	Rotates eye upward and toward midline	Iris, circular muscles	Oculomotor nerve (III) parasympathetic fibers	Causes size of pupil to decrease
Inferior rectus	Oculomotor nerve (III)	Rotates eye downward and toward midline	Iris, radial muscles	Sympathetic fibers	Causes size of pupil to increase
Medial rectus	Oculomotor nerve (III)	Rotates eye toward midline			
Lateral rectus	Abducens nerve (VI)	Rotates eye away from midline			
Superior oblique	Trochlear nerve (IV)	Rotates eye downward and away from midline			
Inferior oblique	Oculomotor nerve (III)	Rotates eye upward and away from midline			

FIGURE 10.28
Transverse section of the eye.

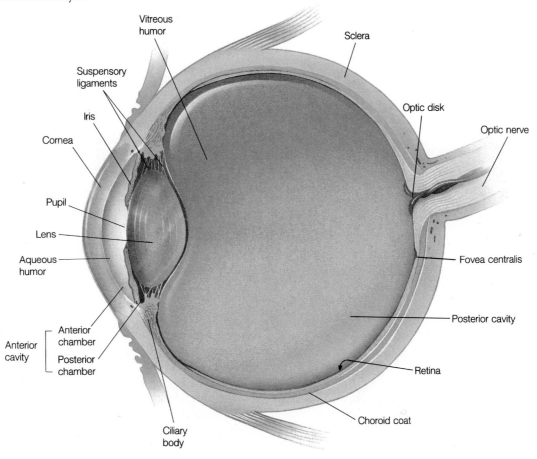

When one eye deviates from the line of vision, the person has double vision (diplopia). If this condition persists, there is danger that changes will occur in the brain to suppress the image from the deviated eye. As a result, the turning eye may become blind (suppression amblyopia). Such monocular blindness can often be prevented if the eye deviation is treated early in life with exercises, glasses, and surgery. For this reason, vision screening programs for preschool children are very important.

1. Explain how the eyelid is moved.
2. Describe the conjunctiva.
3. What is the function of the lacrimal apparatus?
4. Describe the function of each extrinsic eye muscle.

Structure of the Eye

The eye is a hollow, spherical structure about 2.5 centimeters in diameter. Its wall has three distinct layers—an outer *fibrous tunic,* a middle *vascular tunic,* and an inner *nervous tunic.* The spaces within the eye are filled with fluids that provide support for its wall and internal parts, and help maintain its shape. Figure 10.28 shows the major parts of the eye.

The Outer Tunic

The anterior 1/6 of the outer tunic bulges forward as the transparent **cornea** (kor'ne-ah), which serves as the window of the eye and helps focus entering light rays. It is composed largely of connective tissue with a thin layer of epithelium on the surface. The transparency of the cornea is due to the fact that it contains relatively few cells and no blood vessels. Also, the cells and collagenous fibers are arranged in unusually regular patterns.

The cornea is well supplied with nerve fibers that enter its margin and radiate toward its center. These fibers are associated with numerous pain receptors. Cold receptors are also abundant in the cornea, but heat and touch receptors seem to be lacking.

Along its circumference, the cornea is continuous with the **sclera** (skle'rah), the white portion of the eye. This part makes up the posterior 5/6 of the outer tunic and is

FIGURE 10.29
(*a*) Anterior portion of the eye; (*b*) light micrograph of the cornea, iris, and lens.

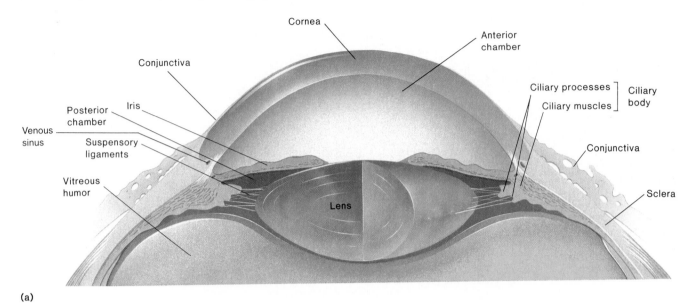

(a)

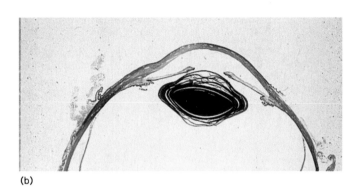

(b)

opaque, due to the presence of many large, irregularly arranged collagenous and elastic fibers. The sclera provides protection and serves as an attachment for the extrinsic muscles of the eye.

In the back of the eye, the sclera is pierced by the **optic nerve** and certain blood vessels, and is attached to the dura mater that encloses these structures as well as other parts of the central nervous system.

The Middle Tunic

The middle or vascular tunic of the eyeball (uveal layer) includes the choroid coat, the ciliary body, the lens, and the iris.

The **choroid coat,** in the posterior 5/6 of the globe, is loosely joined to the sclera and is honeycombed with blood vessels that nourish surrounding tissues. The choroid also contains numerous pigment-producing melano-

cytes that give it a brownish-black appearance. The melanin of these cells absorbs excess light and helps keep the inside of the eye dark.

The **ciliary body,** which is the thickest part of the middle tunic, extends forward from the choroid and forms an internal ring around the front of the eye. Within the ciliary body are many radiating folds called *ciliary processes* and two distinct groups of muscle fibers that constitute the *ciliary muscles.* These structures are shown in figure 10.29.

The transparent **lens** is held in position by a large number of strong but delicate fibers called *suspensory ligaments* (zonular fibers), which extend inward from the ciliary processes. The distal ends of these fibers are attached along the margin of a thin capsule that surrounds the lens. The body of the lens, which contains no blood vessels, lies directly behind the iris and is composed of long, thin epithelial cells. In fact, the cytoplasm of these epithelial cells makes up the transparent substance of the lens. Many of these lens cells are capable of mitosis, and when they divide, they produce new cells that differentiate into columnar cells, or lens "fibers," on the lens surface. Consequently, lens thickness increases with age (figure 10.30).

Because new lens fibers are produced throughout life, the lens thickness (anteroposterior dimension) varies with age. At birth, the lens thickness measures from 3.5 to 4.0 mm; at age 95 it may be 4.75 to 5.0 mm thick. The lens diameter also varies with age, being about 6.5 mm at birth and increasing to 9.0 mm at puberty.

FIGURE 10.30

A scanning electron micrograph of the long, flattened cells of the lens. Note the fingerlike junctions (interdigitations) by which one cell joins to another (×4,800).

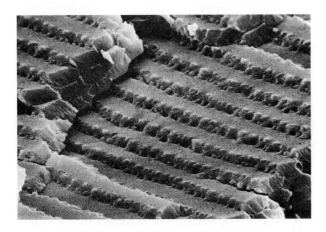

FIGURE 10.31

The lens and ciliary body viewed from behind.

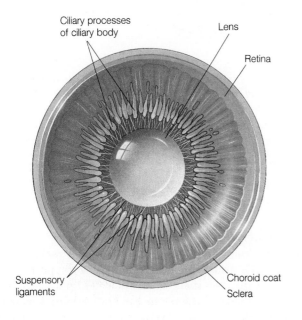

The lens capsule is a clear, membranelike structure composed largely of intercellular material. It is quite elastic, which keeps it under constant tension. As a result, the lens can assume a globular shape. However, the suspensory ligaments attached to the margin of the capsule are also under tension, and as they pull outward, the capsule and the lens inside are kept somewhat flattened (figure 10.31).

If the tension on the suspensory ligaments is relaxed, the elastic capsule rebounds, and the lens surface becomes more convex. Such a change occurs in the lens when the

FIGURE 10.32

(a) How is the focus of the eye affected when the lens becomes thin as the ciliary muscle fibers relax? (b) How is it affected when the lens thickens as the ciliary muscle fibers contract?

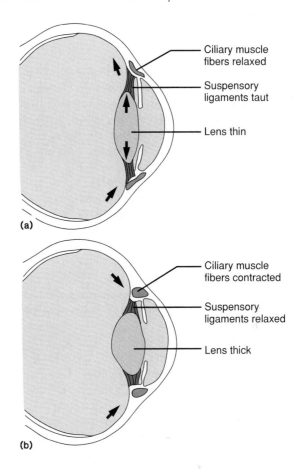

eye is focused to view a close object. This adjustment is called **accommodation.**

The relaxation of the suspensory ligaments during accommodation is a function of the ciliary muscles. One set of these muscle fibers is arranged in a circular pattern, forming a sphincterlike structure around the ciliary processes. The fibers of the other set extend back from fixed points in the sclera to the choroid. When the circular muscle fibers contract, the diameter of the ring formed by the ciliary processes is lessened; when the other fibers contract, the choroid is pulled forward and the ciliary body is shortened. Each of these actions causes the suspensory ligaments to become relaxed, and the lens thickens in response. In this thickened state, the lens is focused for viewing closer objects than before (figure 10.32).

To focus on a more distant object, the ciliary muscles are relaxed, tension on the suspensory ligaments increases, and the lens becomes thinner again.

1. Describe the three layers of the eye.
2. What factors contribute to the transparency of the cornea?
3. Describe the structure of the lens.
4. How does the shape of the lens change during accommodation?

The **iris** is a thin diaphragm composed largely of connective tissue and smooth muscle fibers that is seen as the colored portion of the eye. It extends forward from the periphery of the ciliary body and lies between the cornea and the lens. The iris divides the space separating these parts, which is called the *anterior cavity,* into an *anterior chamber* (between the cornea and the iris) and a *posterior chamber* (between the iris and the lens).

The epithelium on the inner surface of the ciliary body continuously secretes a watery fluid called **aqueous humor** into the posterior chamber. The fluid circulates from this chamber through the **pupil,** a circular opening in the center of the iris, and into the anterior chamber. Aqueous humor fills the space between the cornea and the lens, helps nourish these parts, and aids in maintaining the shape of the front of the eye. The aqueous humor subsequently leaves the anterior chamber through a *venous sinus* (canal of Schlemm) located in its wall (figure 10.29).

The smooth muscle fibers of the iris are arranged into two groups, a circular set and a radial set. These muscles control the size of the pupil, which is the opening that light passes through as it enters the eye. The circular set acts as a sphincter, and when it contracts, the pupil gets smaller and the intensity of the light entering decreases. When the radial muscle fibers contract, the diameter of the pupil increases and the intensity of the light entering it increases.

The size of the pupils change constantly in response to pupillary reflexes that are triggered by such factors as light intensity, gaze, and variations in emotional state. For example, bright light elicits a reflex, and impulses travel along parasympathetic nerve fibers to the *circular muscles* of the irises. The pupils become constricted in response. Conversely, in dim light, impulses travel on sympathetic nerve fibers to the *radial muscles* of the irises, and the pupils become dilated (figure 10.33).

The variations in eye color are largely inherited and range from light blue to dark brown.

The color of the eyes is determined chiefly by the amount and distribution of melanin within the irises. If melanin is present only in the epithelial cells that cover an iris's posterior surface, the iris appears blue. When this condition exists together with denser than usual tissue within the body of the iris, it looks gray, and when melanin is present within the body of the iris, as well as in the epithelial covering, the iris appears brown.

FIGURE 10.33

In dim light, the radial muscles of the iris are stimulated to contract, and the pupil becomes dilated. In bright light, the circular muscles of the iris are stimulated to contract, and the pupil becomes smaller.

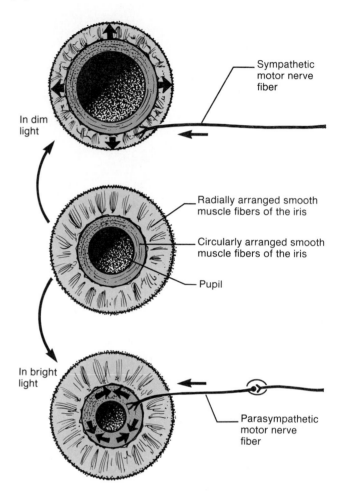

In dim light

Sympathetic motor nerve fiber

Radially arranged smooth muscle fibers of the iris

Circularly arranged smooth muscle fibers of the iris

Pupil

In bright light

Parasympathetic motor nerve fiber

The Inner Tunic

The inner tunic of the eye consists of the **retina,** which contains the visual receptor cells (photoreceptors). This nearly transparent sheet of tissue is continuous with the optic nerve in the back of the eye and extends forward as the inner lining of the eyeball. It ends just behind the margin of the ciliary body.

Although the retina is thin and delicate, its structure is quite complex. It has a number of distinct layers, including pigmented epithelium, neurons, nerve fibers, and limiting membranes (figures 10.34 and 10.35).

There are five major groups of retinal neurons. The nerve fibers of three of these groups—*receptor cells, bipolar neurons,* and *ganglion cells* provide a direct pathway for impulses triggered in the receptors to the optic nerve and brain. The nerve fibers of the other two groups of retinal cells, called *horizontal cells* and *amacrine cells,* pass laterally between the other retinal cells. The horizontal and amacrine cells modify the impulses transmitted on the fibers of the direct pathway.

FIGURE 10.34

The retina consists of several cell layers.

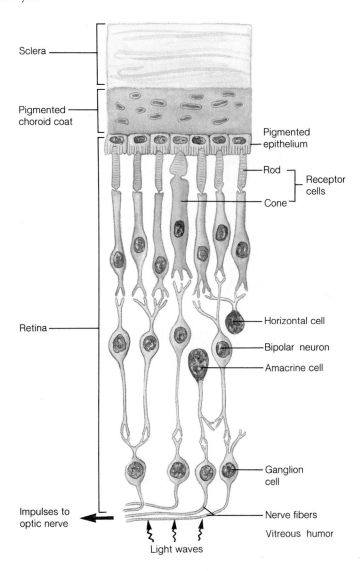

Sclera

Pigmented choroid coat

Pigmented epithelium

Rod

Cone

Receptor cells

Retina

Horizontal cell

Bipolar neuron

Amacrine cell

Ganglion cell

Impulses to optic nerve

Nerve fibers

Vitreous humor

Light waves

FIGURE 10.35

Note the layers of cells and nerve fibers in this light micrograph of the retina.

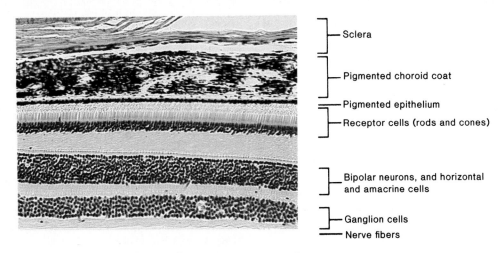

Sclera

Pigmented choroid coat

Pigmented epithelium

Receptor cells (rods and cones)

Bipolar neurons, and horizontal and amacrine cells

Ganglion cells

Nerve fibers

FIGURE 10.36

Nerve fibers leave the eye in the area of the optic disk (arrow) to form the optic nerve.

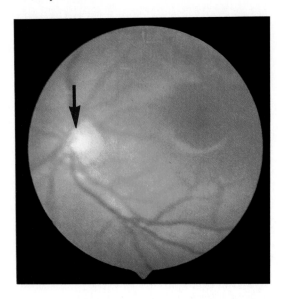

FIGURE 10.37

The retina, as seen through the pupil.

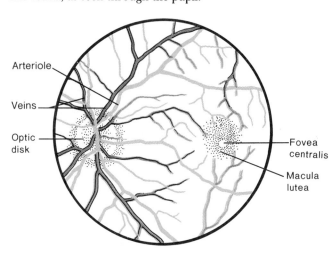

Arteriole

Veins

Optic disk

Fovea centralis

Macula lutea

Chart 10.4 Layers of the eye				
Tunic	Posterior portion	Function	Anterior portion	Function
Outer layer	Sclera	Protection	Cornea	Light transmission
Middle layer	Choroid coat	Blood supply; pigment prevents reflection	Ciliary body, iris	Accommodation, controls light intensity
Inner layer	Retina	Photoreception, impulse transmission	None	

In the central region of the retina is a yellowish spot called the **macula lutea** that occupies about one square millimeter. A depression in its center, called the **fovea centralis,** is in the region of the retina that produces the sharpest vision.

Just medial to the fovea centralis is an area called the **optic disk.** Here the nerve fibers from the retina leave the eye and become parts of the optic nerve. A central artery and vein also pass through at the optic disk. These vessels are continuous with capillary networks of the retina, and together with vessels in the underlying choroid coat, they supply blood to the cells of the inner tunic (figures 10.36 and 10.37). Because there are no receptor cells in the region of the optic disk, it is commonly referred to as the *blind spot* of the eye.

The space bounded by the lens, ciliary body, and retina is the largest compartment of the eye, called the *posterior cavity.* It is filled with a clear, jellylike fluid called **vitreous humor.** This fluid supports the internal parts of the eye and maintains its shape.

In summary, light waves entering the eye must pass through the cornea, aqueous humor, lens, vitreous humor, and several layers of the retina before they reach the photoreceptors. The layers of the eye are summarized in chart 10.4.

Commonly, as a person ages, tiny dense clumps of gel or deposits of crystal-like substances form in the vitreous humor. These clumps may cast shadows on the retina, and as a result, the person sees small moving specks in the field of vision. Such specks are known as *floaters,* and they are most apparent when looking at a plain background, such as the sky or blank wall.

Also with age, the vitreous humor tends to shrink and pull away from the retina. As this occurs, receptor cells of the retina may be mechanically stimulated, and the person may see flashes of light. The presence of floaters or light flashes usually does not indicate a serious eye problem; however, if they develop suddenly or seem to be increasing in number or frequency, the eye should be examined by an ophthalmologist.

1. Explain the origin of aqueous humor and trace its path through the eye.
2. How is the size of the pupil regulated?
3. Describe the structure of the retina.

FIGURE 10.38

(a) Rod cells have long, thin projections; (b) cone cells have short, blunt projections; (c) a scanning electron micrograph of rod and cone cells.

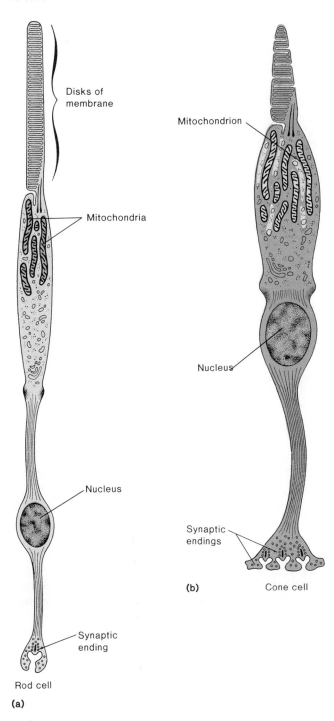

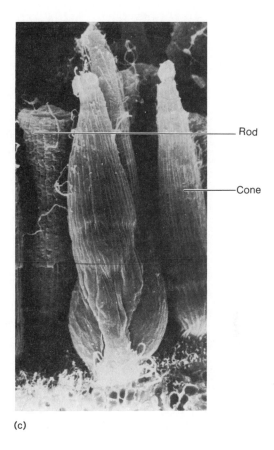

(c)

Visual Receptors

The photoreceptors of the eye are actually two distinct kinds of modified neurons. One group of receptor cells has long, thin projections at their terminal ends and are called **rods.** There are about 100 million of them in a human retina. The cells of the other group have short, blunt projections and are called **cones.** They number about three million (figure 10.38).

Instead of being located in the surface layer of the retina, rods and cones are found in a deep portion, closely associated with a layer of pigmented epithelium. The projections from these receptors extend into the pigmented layer and contain hundreds of tiny disks loaded with visual pigments.

The epithelial pigment of the retina absorbs light waves that are not absorbed by the receptor cells, and together with the pigment of the choroid coat, it keeps light from reflecting off the surfaces inside the eye. The pigment layer also stores vitamin A, which can be used by the receptor cells to synthesize visual pigments. Albinos, who lack melanin in all parts of their bodies, including their eyes, suffer a considerable loss in visual sharpness (acuity). This is because light reflects from inside their eyes and stimulates their visual receptors excessively.

The visual receptors are only stimulated when light reaches them. Thus, when a light image is focused on an area of the retina, some receptors are stimulated, and impulses travel away from them to the brain.

Rods and cones function differently. For example, rods are hundreds of times more sensitive to light than cones, and, as a result, they enable persons to see in relatively dim light. In addition, the rods produce colorless vision, while cones can detect colors.

FIGURE 10.39

(*a*) Impulses from several rods may be transmitted to the brain on a single nerve fiber; (*b*) impulses from cones are often transmitted to the brain on separate sensory nerve fibers.

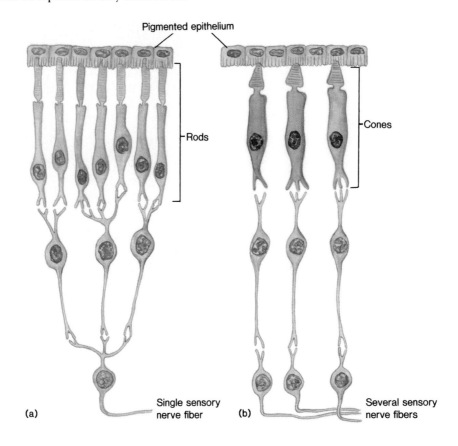

Pigmented epithelium

Rods

Cones

(a)   Single sensory nerve fiber

(b)   Several sensory nerve fibers

Still another difference involves the sharpness of the images perceived. Cones allow a person to see sharp images, while rods enable one to see more general outlines of objects. This characteristic is related to the fact that nerve fibers from many rods may converge, and their impulses may be transmitted to the brain on the same nerve fiber (see chapter 9). Thus, if a point of light stimulates a rod, the brain cannot tell which one of many receptors has actually been stimulated. Such a convergence of fibers occurs to a much lesser degree among cones, so when a cone is stimulated, the brain is able to pinpoint the stimulation more accurately (figure 10.39).

As was mentioned, the area of sharpest vision is the fovea centralis in the macula lutea. This area lacks rods, but contains densely packed cones with few or no converging fibers. Also, the overlying layers of the retina, as well as the retinal blood vessels, are displaced to the sides.

This displacement more fully exposes the receptors to incoming light. Consequently, to view something in detail, one moves the eyes so the important part of an image falls upon the fovea centralis.

The concentration of cones decreases in areas farther away from the macula lutea, while the concentration of rods increases in these areas. Also, the amount of convergence among the rods and cones increases toward the periphery of the retina. As a result, the visual sensations from images focused on the sides of the retina tend to be blurred compared with those focused on the central portion of the retina.

Some persons have inherited defective color vision, due to a decreased sensitivity in one or more cone sets. Such people perceive colors differently from those with normal vision and are said to be *color-blind*.

Disorders of the Eyes

Impairments or loss of vision can occur as a result of disorders involving the cornea or lens, or injury to the receptors.

The visual disorder *astigmatism* usually results from a defect in the curvature of the cornea. The normal cornea has a spherical curvature, like the inside of a ball; an astigmatic cornea usually has an elliptical curvature, like the bowl of a spoon. As a result, some portions of an image are in focus on the retina, but other portions are blurred, and vision is distorted.

Worldwide, the most common cause of blindness is corneal disease, in which the transparency of the cornea is lost. Treatment for this condition may involve *corneal transplantation* (penetrating keratoplasty). In this procedure, the central 2/3 of the defective cornea is removed and replaced by a similar-sized portion of cornea from a donor eye. Because corneal tissues lack blood vessels, the transplanted tissue is usually not rejected by the recipient's immune system and the success rate of this procedure is very high. Unfortunately for many persons in need of corneal transplantation, the supply of donor eyes remains inadequate.

The elastic quality of the lens capsule tends to lessen with age, and persons over 45 years of age are often unable to accommodate sufficiently to read the fine print in books and newspapers. Their eyes remain focused for distant vision. This condition is termed *presbyopia,* or farsightedness of age, and can usually be corrected with eyeglasses or contact lenses.

A relatively common eye disorder, particularly in older people, is called *cataract.* In this condition, the lens or its capsule slowly loses its transparency and becomes cloudy, discolored, and opaque. As a result, clear images cannot be focused on the retina, and in time the person may become blind.

Cataract is often treated by surgically removing the lens and replacing it with an artificial one (intraocular lens implant). Sometimes the loss of focusing power following removal of the lens may be corrected with eyeglasses or contact lenses.

A disorder called *glaucoma* sometimes develops in the eyes as a person ages. This condition occurs when the rate of aqueous humor formation exceeds the rate of its removal. As a result, fluid accumulates in the anterior chamber of the eye, and the fluid pressure rises.

Because liquids cannot be compressed, the increasing pressure from the anterior chamber is transmitted to all parts of the eye, and, in time, the blood vessels that supply the receptor cells of the retina may be squeezed closed. If this happens, cells that fail to receive needed nutrients and oxygen may die, and permanent blindness may result.

Glaucoma often can be controlled. It is relatively easy to measure the pressure of the fluids within the eyes, and if the pressure is reaching a dangerous level, steps can be taken to reduce it. For example, drugs that reduce the formation of aqueous humor by the ciliary body may be used, or an opening may be created surgically to allow excess aqueous humor to drain into the tissues beneath the conjunctiva.

Although the eye is well protected by the bony orbit, it is sometimes injured by a forceful blow. If the eye is jarred sufficiently, some of its contents may be displaced; for example, the suspensory ligaments may be torn and the lens dislocated into the posterior cavity. Similarly, a blow to the eye (or to the head) may cause the retina to pull away from the underlying vascular choroid coat. Once the retina is detached, there is danger that photoreceptor cells will die because of lack of oxygen and nutrients. A *detached retina* can be repaired surgically, or by using a laser beam to reattach the retina. Without treatment, this injury may result in varying degrees of visual loss or blindness. Such injuries to the eye can usually be prevented by wearing protective devices such as face masks or goggles.

Visual Nerve Pathways

As mentioned in chapter 9, the axons of the ganglion cells in the retina leave the eyes to form the *optic nerves.* Just anterior to the pituitary gland, these nerves give rise to the X-shaped *optic chiasma,* and within the chiasma some of the fibers cross over. More specifically, the fibers from the nasal (medial) half of each retina cross over, while those from the temporal (lateral) sides do not. Thus, fibers from the nasal half of the left eye and the temporal half of the right eye form the right *optic tract;* and fibers from the nasal half of the right eye and the temporal half of the left eye form the left optic tract.

The nerve fibers continue in the optic tracts, and just before they reach the thalamus, a few of them leave to enter nuclei that function in various visual reflexes. Most of the fibers, however, enter the thalamus and synapse in its posterior portion (lateral geniculate body). From this region, the visual impulses enter nerve pathways called *optic radiations,* and these pathways lead to the visual cortex of the occipital lobes (figure 10.40).

Other fibers conducting visual impulses pass downward into various regions of the brain stem. These impulses are important for controlling head and eye

FIGURE 10.40

The visual pathway includes the optic nerve, optic chiasma, optic tract, and optic radiations.

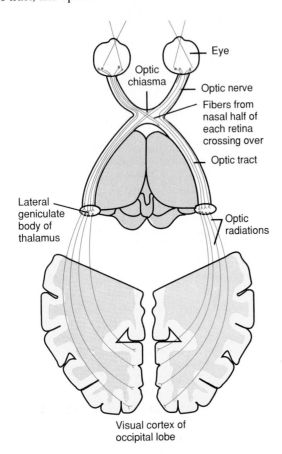

movements associated with tracking an object visually, for controlling the simultaneous movements of both eyes, and for controlling certain visual reflexes, such as those involved with movements of the iris muscles.

Since each visual cortex receives impulses from each eye, a person may develop partial blindness in both eyes if either visual cortex is injured. For example, if the right visual cortex (or the right optic tract) is injured, sight may be lost in the temporal side of the right eye and the nasal side of the left eye. Similarly, if the central portion of the optic chiasma, where fibers from the nasal sides of the eyes cross over, is damaged, the nasal sides of both eyes are blinded.

1. Distinguish between the rods and the cones of the retina.
2. Trace the pathway of visual impulses from the retina to the occipital cortex.

Clinical Terms Related to the Senses

ametropia (am″ĕ-tro′pe-ah) an eye condition characterized by inability to focus images sharply on the retina.

anopia (an-o′pe-ah) absence of the eye.

blepharitis (blef″ah-ri′tis) an inflammation of the margins of the eyelids.

causalgia (kaw-zal′je-ah) a persistent, burning pain usually associated with injury to a limb.

conjunctivitis (kon-junk″tĭ-vi′tis) an inflammation of the conjunctiva.

diplopia (dĭ-plo′pe-ah) double vision, or the sensation of seeing two objects when only one is viewed.

emmetropia (em″ĕ-tro′pe-ah) normal condition of the eyes; eyes with no defects of focusing ability.

enucleation (e-nu″kle-a′shun) removal of the eyeball.

exophthalmos (ek″sof-thal′mos) condition in which the eyes protrude abnormally.

hemianopsia (hem″e-an-op′se-ah) defective vision affecting half of the visual field.

hyperalgesia (hi″per-al-je′ze-ah) an abnormally increased sensitivity to pain.

iridectomy (ir″ĭ-dek′to-me) the surgical removal of part of the iris.

iritis (i-ri′tis) an inflammation of the iris.

keratitis (ker″ah-ti′tis) an inflammation of the cornea.

labyrinthectomy (lab″ĭ-rin-thek′to-me) the surgical removal of the labyrinth.

labyrinthitis (lab″ĭ-rin-thi′tis) an inflammation of the labyrinth.

Meniere's disease (men″e-ārz′ dĭ-zēz) an inner ear disorder characterized by ringing in the ears, increased sensitivity to sounds, dizziness, and loss of hearing.

neuralgia (nu-ral′je-ah) pain resulting from inflammation of a nerve or a group of nerves.

neuritis (nu-ri′tis) an inflammation of a nerve.

nystagmus (nis-tag′mus) an involuntary oscillation of the eyes.

otitis media (o-ti′tis me′de-ah) an inflammation of the middle ear.

otosclerosis (o″to-skle-ro′sis) a formation of spongy bone in the inner ear, which often causes deafness by fixing the stapes to the oval window.

pterygium (tĕ-rij′e-um) an abnormally thickened patch of conjunctiva that extends over part of the cornea.

retinitis pigmentosa (ret″ĭ-ni′tis pig″men-to′sa) a progressive retinal sclerosis characterized by deposits of pigment in the retina and by atrophy of the retina.

retinoblastoma (ret″ĭ-no-blas-to′mah) an inherited, highly malignant tumor arising from immature retinal cells.

tinnitus (ti-ni′tus) a ringing or buzzing noise in the ears.

tonometry (to-nom′ĕ-tre) the measurement of fluid pressure within the eyeball.

tympanoplasty (tim″pah-no-plas′te) the surgical reconstruction of the middle ear bones and establishment of continuity from the tympanic membrane to the oval window.

uveitis (u″ve-i′tis) an inflammation of the uvea, which includes the iris, the ciliary body, and the choroid coat.

vertigo (ver′tĭ-go) a sensation of dizziness.

Chapter Summary

Introduction (page 333)
Sensory receptors are sensitive to environmental changes and initiate impulses to the brain and spinal cord.

Types of Receptors (page 333)
1. Each type of receptor is sensitive to a distinct type of stimulus.
2. The major types of receptors include the following:
   a. Chemoreceptors, sensitive to changes in chemical concentration.
   b. Pain receptors, sensitive to tissue damage.
   c. Thermoreceptors, sensitive to temperature changes.
   d. Mechanoreceptors, sensitive to mechanical forces.
   e. Photoreceptors, sensitive to light.
3. Receptors can also be grouped as exteroceptors, proprioceptors, and interoceptors.

Somatic Sense Receptors (page 333)
Somatic senses are those involved with receptors in skin, muscles, joints, and visceral organs.

1. Touch and pressure receptors
   a. Free ends of sensory nerve fibers are responsible for the sensations of touch and pressure.
   b. Meissner's corpuscles are responsible for the sensations of light touch.
   c. Pacinian corpuscles are responsible for the sensations of heavy pressure and vibrations.
2. Thermoreceptors include two sets of free nerve endings that serve as heat and cold receptors.
3. Pain receptors are free nerve endings stimulated by tissue damage. These receptors can be stimulated by changes in temperature, mechanical force, and chemical concentration.
4. Acute pain fibers and chronic pain fibers transmit pain impulses to sensory fibers of spinal and cranial nerves.
5. Stretch receptors provide information about the condition of muscles and tendons.
   a. Muscle spindles are stimulated when a muscle is relaxed, and they initiate a reflex that causes the muscle to contract.
   b. Golgi tendon organs are stimulated when muscle tension increases, and they initiate a reflex that causes muscle relaxation.

Special Sense Receptors (page 338)
Special sense receptors are those that occur in large, complex organs of the head.

Olfactory Organs (page 338)
Olfactory receptors are chemoreceptors stimulated by chemicals dissolved in liquid. They function together with taste receptors and aid in food selection.

1. Olfactory organs and receptors
   a. The olfactory organs consist of receptors and supporting cells in the nasal cavity.
   b. Olfactory receptors are neurons with cilia.
   c. Olfactory receptors are often damaged by environmental factors, but are not replaced.
2. Olfactory nerve pathways
   Nerve impulses travel from the olfactory receptors through the olfactory nerves, olfactory bulbs, and olfactory tracts to interpreting centers in the frontal lobes of the cerebrum.

Gustatory Organs (page 340)
1. Taste receptors
   a. Taste buds consist of receptor cells and supporting cells.
   b. Taste cells are sensitive to particular chemicals dissolved in water.
   c. There are four primary kinds of taste cells, each of which are particularly sensitive to a certain group of chemicals.
   d. Sweet receptors are most plentiful near the tip of the tongue, sour receptors along the margins, salt receptors in the tip and upper front, and bitter receptors toward the back.
2. Taste nerve pathways
   a. Sensory impulses from taste receptors travel on fibers of the facial, glossopharyngeal, and vagus nerves.
   b. These impulses are carried to the medulla and ascend to the thalamus. From there they are directed to the gustatory cortex in the parietal lobes.

Auditory Organs (page 342)
1. The external ear collects sound waves created by vibrating objects.
2. Middle ear
   a. Auditory ossicles of the middle ear conduct sound waves from the tympanic membrane to the oval window of the inner ear. They also increase the force of these waves.
   b. Skeletal muscles attached to the auditory ossicles act in the tympanic reflex to protect the inner ear from the effects of loud sounds.
3. Auditory tubes connect the middle ears to the throat, and function to help maintain equal air pressure on both sides of the eardrums.
4. Inner ear
   a. The inner ear consists of a complex system of interconnected tubes and chambers—the osseous and membranous labyrinths. It includes the cochlea, which houses the organ of Corti.
   b. The organ of Corti contains the hearing receptors that are stimulated by vibrations in the fluids of the inner ear.
5. Auditory nerve pathways
   a. The nerve fibers from hearing receptors travel in the cochlear branch of the vestibulocochlear nerves.
   b. Auditory impulses travel into the medulla oblongata, midbrain, and thalamus, and are interpreted in the temporal lobes of the cerebrum.

Organs of Equilibrium (page 349)

1. The vestibule includes the utricle and saccule, which each contain maculae with receptors.
2. The organs located in the ampullae of the semicircular canals contain hair cells and detect rotation.
3. Other parts that help with the maintenance of equilibrium include the eyes and the proprioceptors associated with certain joints.

Visual Organs (page 352)

1. Visual accessory organs include the eyelids and lacrimal apparatus that function to protect the eye, and the extrinsic muscles that move the eye.
2. Structure of the eye
   a. The wall of the eye has an outer, a middle, and an inner tunic that function as follows:
      (1) The outer layer (sclera) is protective, and its transparent anterior portion (cornea) refracts light entering the eye.
      (2) The middle layer (choroid) is vascular and contains pigments that help to keep the inside of the eye dark.
      (3) The inner layer (retina) contains the visual receptor cells.
   b. The lens is a transparent, elastic structure whose shape is controlled by the action of ciliary muscles.
   c. The iris is a muscular diaphragm that controls the amount of light entering the eye; the pupil is an opening in the iris.
   d. Spaces within the eye are filled with fluids (aqueous and vitreous humors) that help to maintain its shape.
3. Visual receptors are called rods and cones.
   a. Rods are more numerous and are responsible for colorless vision in relatively dim light.
   b. Cones are responsible for color vision and produce sharper images.
4. Visual nerve pathways
   a. Nerve fibers from the retina form the optic nerves.
   b. Some fibers cross over in the optic chiasma.
   c. Most of the fibers enter the thalamus and synapse with others that continue to the visual cortex.
   d. Other impulses pass into the brain stem and function in various visual reflexes.

Clinical Application of Knowledge

1. Why is it that some serious injuries, such as those produced by a bullet entering the abdomen, may be relatively painless, while others such as those involving a crushing of the skin may produce considerable discomfort?
2. Sometimes, as a result of an injury to the eye, the retina becomes detached from its pigmented epithelium. Assuming that the retinal tissues remain functional, what is likely to happen to the person's vision if the retina moves unevenly toward the interior of the eye?
3. The auditory tubes of a child are shorter and are directed more horizontally than those of an adult. How might this be related to the observation that children have middle ear infections more frequently than do adults?

4. A patient with heart disease experiences pain at the base of the neck, and in the left shoulder and arm after exercise. How would you explain to the patient the origin of the pain?
5. Which sense(s) might be affected in the disorder called labyrinthitis, in which the canals of the inner ear are inflamed and their functions impaired?

Review Activities

1. List five groups of sensory receptors and name the kind of change to which each is sensitive.
2. Explain how sense receptors can be grouped.
3. Describe the structures and functions of free nerve endings, Meissner's corpuscles, and pacinian corpuscles.
4. Distinguish between muscle spindles and Golgi tendon organs.
5. Describe the olfactory organ and its function.
6. Trace a nerve impulse from the olfactory receptor to the interpreting center of the cerebrum.
7. Name the four main types of taste receptors and describe the patterns in which the taste receptors are distributed on the tongue.
8. Explain why taste sensation is less likely to diminish with age than olfactory sensation.
9. Trace the pathway of a taste impulse from the receptor to the cerebral cortex.
10. Distinguish between the external, middle, and inner ears.
11. Trace the path of a sound vibration from the tympanic membrane to the hearing receptors.
12. Name and describe the functions of the auditory ossicles.
13. Describe the tympanic reflex, and explain its importance.
14. Explain the function of the auditory tubes.
15. Distinguish between the osseous and the membranous labyrinths.
16. Describe the cochlea and its function.
17. Describe a hearing receptor.
18. Trace a nerve impulse from the organ of Corti to the interpreting centers of the cerebrum.
19. Locate the organs of equilibrium and describe their functions.
20. Explain how the sense of vision helps maintain equilibrium.
21. List the visual accessory organs and describe the functions of each.
22. Name the three layers of the eye wall and describe the functions of each.
23. Describe how accommodation is accomplished.
24. Explain how the iris functions.
25. Distinguish between aqueous and vitreous humor.
26. Distinguish between the macula lutea and the optic disk.
27. Distinguish between rods and cones.
28. Explain why cone vision is generally more acute than rod vision.
29. Trace a nerve impulse from the retina to the visual cortex.

CHAPTER 11

The Endocrine System

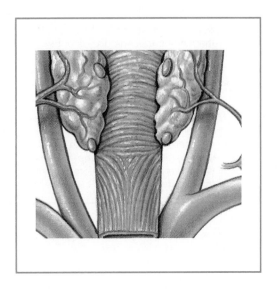

The endocrine system consists of a variety of loosely related cells, tissues, and organs that act together with parts of the nervous system to control body activities and maintain stable internal conditions. The endocrine system and nervous system each provide a means by which body parts can communicate with one another and adjust to changing needs. Whereas the parts of the nervous system communicate with various cells by means of nerve impulses carried on nerve fibers, the parts of the endocrine system use hormones that act as chemical messengers to their target cells.

Chapter Objectives

After you have studied this chapter, you should be able to

1. Distinguish between endocrine and exocrine glands.

2. Name and describe the location of the major endocrine glands of the body.

3. Describe the structures of the major endocrine glands.

4. Complete the review activities at the end of this chapter. Note that the items are worded in the form of specific learning objectives. You may want to refer to them before reading the chapter.

Aids to Understanding Words

-crin, to secrete: endo*crine*—pertaining to internal secretions.

endo-, within: *endo*crine gland—a gland that releases its secretion internally into a body fluid.

exo-, outside: *exo*crine gland—a gland that releases its secretion to a free surface through a duct.

lact-, milk: pro*lact*in—a hormone that promotes milk production.

para-, beside: *para*thyroid glands—a set of glands located near the surface of the thyroid gland.

-tropic, influencing: adrenocortico*tropic* hormone—a hormone secreted by the anterior pituitary gland that stimulates the adrenal cortex.

Introduction

The term *endocrine* describes cells, tissues, and organs that secrete hormones into body fluids. In contrast, the term *exocrine* refers to those parts whose secretions are carried by tubes or ducts to internal or external body surfaces. Thus, the thyroid and parathyroid glands, which secrete hormones into the blood, are endocrine glands (ductless glands), while the sweat glands and salivary glands are exocrine glands (figure 11.1). (Recall that a *gland* is one or more cells specialized to secrete substances.)

General Characteristics of the Endocrine System

As a group, endocrine structures help regulate body processes. They control the rates of certain chemical reactions, aid in the transport of substances through membranes, and help regulate water and electrolyte balances. They also play vital roles in reproductive processes, and in development and growth.

The larger **endocrine glands** are described in this chapter. These glands include the pituitary gland, thyroid gland, parathyroid glands, adrenal glands, and pancreas. Other hormone-secreting glands and tissues, including those involved in the processes of immunity and reproduction, are discussed briefly (figure 11.2).

Other organs, such as the heart, kidneys, stomach, intestines, and placenta, contain cells that secrete hormones. These cells, called *diffuse endocrine structures,* have endocrine functions.

A **hormone** is a substance secreted by a gland that has an effect on the functions of other cells. Such substances are released into the extracellular spaces surrounding the endocrine cells. Some of them travel only short distances and produce their effects locally. Other hormones are transported in the blood to all parts of the body and may produce rather general effects. In either case, the action of a particular hormone is restricted to its *target cells*—those cells that respond to the hormone molecules.

---

1. What is the difference between an endocrine gland and an exocrine gland?
2. What is a hormone?

The Pituitary Gland

The **pituitary** (pi-tu′i-tar″e) **gland** (hypophysis) is about 1 centimeter in diameter and is located at the base of the brain. It is attached to the hypothalamus by the pituitary stalk, or *infundibulum,* and lies in the sella turcica of the sphenoid bone, as shown in figure 11.3.

FIGURE 11.1

Endocrine glands, such as (*a*) the thyroid gland, release hormones into body fluids, while exocrine glands, such as (*b*) sweat glands, release their secretions into ducts that lead to body surfaces.

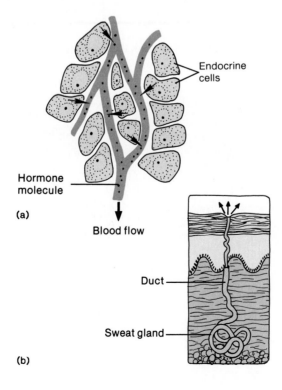

FIGURE 11.2

Locations of major endocrine glands.

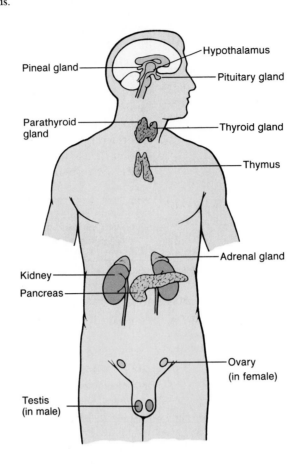

Hypothalamus
Pineal gland
Pituitary gland
Parathyroid gland
Thyroid gland
Thymus
Adrenal gland
Kidney
Pancreas
Ovary (in female)
Testis (in male)

FIGURE 11.3

The pituitary gland is attached to the hypothalamus and lies in the sella turcica of the sphenoid bone.

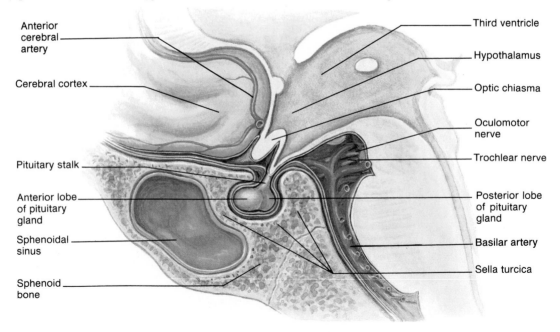

Anterior cerebral artery
Cerebral cortex
Pituitary stalk
Anterior lobe of pituitary gland
Sphenoidal sinus
Sphenoid bone
Third ventricle
Hypothalamus
Optic chiasma
Oculomotor nerve
Trochlear nerve
Posterior lobe of pituitary gland
Basilar artery
Sella turcica

FIGURE 11.4
Axons in the posterior lobe of the pituitary gland are stimulated to release hormones by nerve impulses originating in the hypothalamus; cells of the anterior lobe are stimulated by substances secreted by hypothalamic neurons.

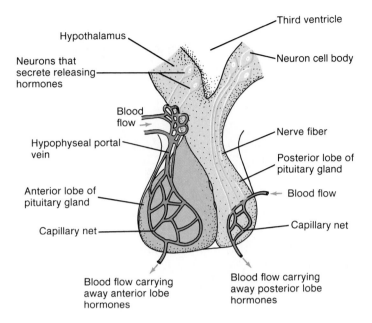

The gland consists of two distinct portions: an anterior lobe (adenohypophysis) and a posterior lobe (neurohypophysis). The *anterior lobe* secretes a number of hormones. Although the *posterior lobe* does not synthesize any hormones, two important ones are secreted by nerve fibers within its tissues.

> During fetal development, a narrow region appears between the anterior and posterior lobes of the pituitary gland. This part is called the *intermediate lobe* (pars intermedia). It produces melanocyte-stimulating hormone (MSH), which regulates the formation of melanin—the pigment found in the skin—and portions of the eyes and brain. This region atrophies during prenatal development, and appears only as a vestige in adults.

Most of the pituitary activities are controlled by the brain. For example, the release of hormones from the posterior lobe occurs when nerve impulses from the *hypothalamus* signal the axon ends of neurosecretory cells in the posterior lobe. On the other hand, secretions from the anterior lobe are typically controlled by substances produced by the hypothalamus (figure 11.4). These substances are transmitted by blood, in the vessels of a capillary net associated with the hypothalamus. These vessels merge to form the **hypophyseal portal veins** that pass downward along the pituitary stalk and give rise to a capillary net in the anterior lobe. Thus, substances released into the blood from the hypothalamus are carried directly to the anterior lobe.

The hypothalamus (described in chapter 9) receives information from nearly all parts of the nervous system. This information includes data concerning a person's emotional state, body temperature, blood nutrient concentrations, and so forth. The hypothalamus sometimes acts on such information by signaling the pituitary gland to release hormones.

> 1. Where is the pituitary gland located?
> 2. Explain how the hypothalamus controls the actions of the pituitary gland.

Anterior Lobe

The anterior lobe of the pituitary gland is enclosed in a dense capsule of collagenous connective tissue and consists largely of epithelial tissue arranged in blocks around many thin-walled blood vessels. Within the epithelial tissue, five types of secretory cells have been identified: *somatotropes* that secrete growth hormone (GH), *mammatropes* that secrete prolactin (PRL), *thyrotropes* that secrete thyroid-stimulating hormone (TSH), *corticotropes* that secrete adrenocorticotropic hormone (ACTH), and *gonadotropes* that secrete follicle-stimulating hormone (FSH) and luteinizing hormone (LH). (See figures 11.5 and 11.6.)

FIGURE 11.5

Hormones released from the anterior lobe of the pituitary gland and their target organs.

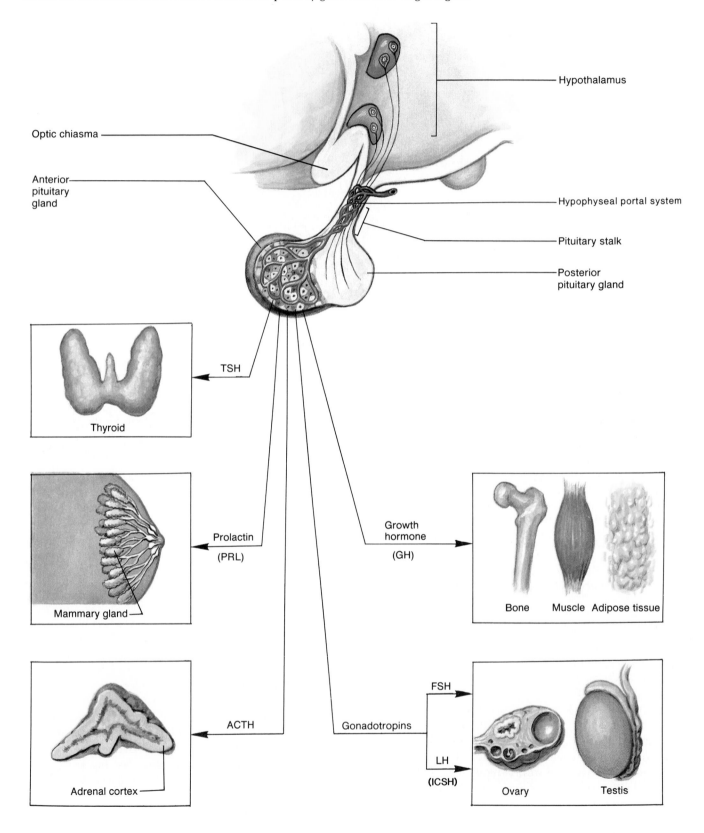

FIGURE 11.6

A light micrograph of the anterior pituitary gland (×320).

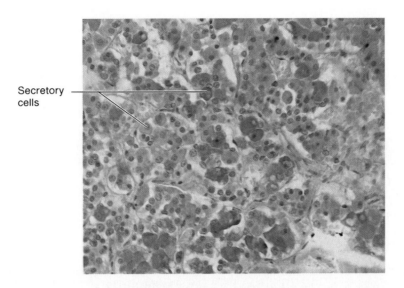

Secretory cells

The Pituitary Gland and Growth

One of the more obvious effects of growth hormone results from its ability to stimulate the growth of cartilage in the epiphyseal disks of long bones and thus promote their elongation. Thus, the amount of growth hormone produced is a major factor determining an individual's adult height. Human heights vary considerably and are a result of growth hormone production and other inherited and environmental factors (figure 11.7). Pathological conditions may result in heights outside the range of normal variation.

If growth hormone is not secreted in sufficient amounts during childhood, body growth is limited, and a type of *dwarfism* (hypopituitary dwarfism) results. In this condition, body parts are usually correctly proportioned and mental development is normal. However, an abnormally low secretion of growth hormone is usually accompanied by lessened secretions from other anterior lobe hormones, leading to additional hormone deficiency symptoms. For example, a hypopituitary dwarf often fails to develop adult sexual features unless hormone therapy is provided.

Hypopituitary dwarfism is sometimes treated by administering growth hormone, and this treatment may stimulate a rapid increase in height. The procedure, however, must be started before the epiphyseal disks of the person's long bones have become ossified; otherwise, growth in height is not possible.

An oversecretion of growth hormone during childhood may result in *gigantism*—a condition in which the person's height may exceed 8 feet. Gigantism, which is relatively rare, is usually accompanied by a tumor of the pituitary gland. In such cases, various pituitary hormones in addition to GH are likely to be secreted excessively, so that a giant often suffers from a variety of disorders and has a shortened life expectancy.

If growth hormone is secreted excessively in an adult, after the epiphyses of the long bones have ossified, the person does not grow taller. The soft tissues, however, may continue to enlarge and the bones may become thicker. As a consequence, an affected individual may develop greatly enlarged hands and feet, a protruding jaw, and a large tongue and nose. This condition is called *acromegaly*, and, like gigantism, it is often associated with a pituitary tumor (figure 11.8).

Continued on next page

FIGURE 11.7

Variation in growth hormone release influences height. Height variation in 175 men (photograph was taken about 1900).

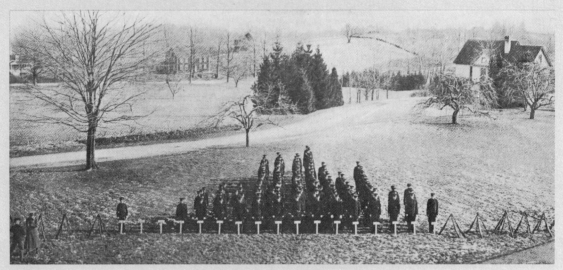

Number of individuals	1	0	0	1	5	7	7	22	25	26	27	17	11	17	4	4	1
Height in inches	58	59	60	61	62	63	64	65	66	67	68	69	70	71	72	73	74

FIGURE 11.8

Acromegaly is caused by an oversecretion of growth hormone in adulthood. Note the changes in facial features of this individual from ages (*a*) nine, (*b*) sixteen, (*c*) thirty-three, and (*d*) fifty-two.

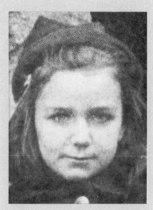
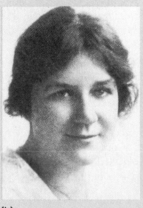
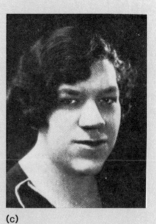
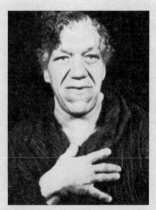

(a)   (b)   (c)   (d)

Posterior Lobe

Unlike the anterior lobe of the pituitary gland, which is composed primarily of glandular epithelial cells, the posterior lobe consists largely of nerve fibers and neuroglial cells (pituicytes). The neuroglial cells function to support the nerve fibers that originate in the hypothalamus.

The two hormones associated with the posterior lobe—antidiuretic hormone (ADH) and oxytocin (OT)—are produced by specialized neurons in the hypothalamus (figure 11.4). These hormones travel down axons through the pituitary stalk to the posterior lobe and are stored in vesicles (secretory granules) near the ends of the axons. The hormones are released into the blood in response to nerve impulses coming from the hypothalamus.

The different types of tissues present in the pituitary gland reflect the embryonic development of its two lobes. The anterior lobe, composed of epithelial tissue, forms as a pouch that grows upward from the developing oral cavity. Eventually, the connection between the oral cavity and the gland is lost. The posterior lobe, composed of nerve fibers, forms from the embryonic brain. As this lobe develops, it grows downward toward the anterior lobe, but retains its connection to the hypothalamus by means of its nerve fibers.

The Thyroid Gland

The **thyroid** (thi'roid) **gland,** shown in figure 11.9, is a very vascular structure that consists of two large lobes connected by a broad isthmus. It is located just below the larynx on either side and in front of the trachea.

The thyroid gland is covered by a capsule of connective tissue and is made up of many secretory parts called *follicles.* The cavities of the follicles are lined with a single layer of cuboidal epithelial cells and are filled with a clear, viscous substance called *colloid.* The follicle cells have the ability to remove iodine from the blood. The iodine is then used to produce and secrete hormones that may be stored in the colloid or released into the blood of nearby capillaries (figure 11.10). Other hormone-secreting cells, called *parafollicular cells* (C cells), occur outside the follicles.

There is great variation in the size of the thyroid follicles (from 0.02 mm to 0.9 mm in diameter). In most individuals, there are more small follicles than large ones.

One of the common variations in the structure of the thyroid gland is the presence of a third lobe. This extra lobe is usually attached to the isthmus.

The thyroid gland produces several hormones. Those hormones synthesized by the follicular cells (thyroxine and triiodothyronine) have marked effects on the energy use by body cells. Another hormone produced by the parafollicular cells, *calcitonin,* influences the blood concentrations of calcium and phosphate.

FIGURE 11.9

(a) The thyroid gland consists of two lobes connected anteriorly by an isthmus; (b) thyroid hormones are secreted by follicle cells.

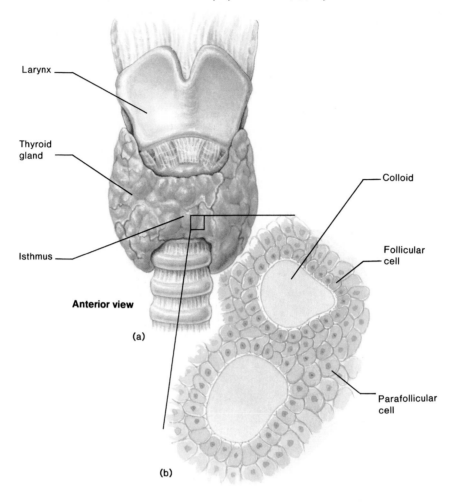

Larynx

Thyroid gland

Isthmus

Anterior view

(a)

Colloid

Follicular cell

Parafollicular cell

(b)

FIGURE 11.10

A micrograph of thyroid gland tissue (×40). The open spaces surrounded by follicle cells are filled with colloid.

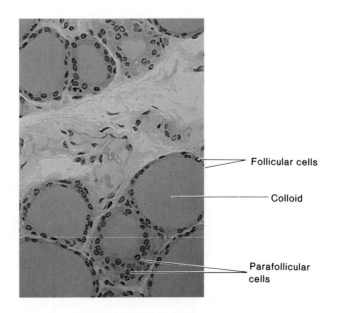

Follicular cells

Colloid

Parafollicular cells

Disorders of the Thyroid Gland

Most functional disorders of the thyroid gland are characterized by *overactivity* (hyperthyroidism) or *underactivity* (hypothyroidism) of the gland cells.

A thyroid disorder may develop at any time during a person's life as a result of a developmental problem, an injury, a disease, or a dietary deficiency. One form of **hypothyroidism** appears in infants when their thyroid glands fail to function normally. An affected child may appear normal at birth because it has received an adequate supply of thyroid hormones from its mother during pregnancy. When its own thyroid gland fails to produce sufficient quantities of these hormones, the child soon develops a condition called *cretinism*. Cretinism is characterized by severe symptoms including stunted growth, abnormal bone formation, retarded mental development, low body temperature, and sluggishness. Without treatment, within a month or so of birth, the child is likely to suffer from permanent mental retardation.

If a person develops hypothyroidism later in life, the symptoms include an abnormal sensitivity to cold, physical sluggishness, and poor appetite. The person also may appear mentally dull and may develop swollen tissues due to an accumulation of body fluid in the subcutaneous tissue—a condition called *myxedema*.

On the other hand, a person with hyperthyroidism is sensitive to heat, is restless or overactive, eats excessively, and appears mentally alert. Also, the person's eyes are likely to protrude (exophthalmos) because of edematous swelling in the tissues behind them (figure 11.11). At the same time, the thyroid gland is likely to enlarge, producing a bulge in the neck called a *goiter*. A goiter associated with hyperthyroidism is said to be a *toxic goiter*.

Another disorder of the thyroid gland is called *simple*, or *endemic, goiter*, which sometimes affects persons who live in regions where iodine is lacking in the soil and drinking water. Such a person is likely to develop an iodine deficiency, which is reflected in an inability to produce thyroid hormones. Since these hormones normally exert an inhibiting effect on the secretion of TSH, without such inhibition, the anterior lobe of the pituitary gland releases TSH excessively. The resulting overstimulation of the thyroid gland causes it to enlarge, but since the gland is unable to manufacture hormones, the condition is accompanied by the symptoms of hypothyroidism (figure 11.12).

Simple goiter usually can be prevented in regions where iodine deficiencies occur if people use table salt containing iodides—*iodized salt*.

FIGURE 11.11
Hyperthyroidism may produce a protrusion of the eyes.

FIGURE 11.12
Endemic goiter is caused by an iodine deficiency.

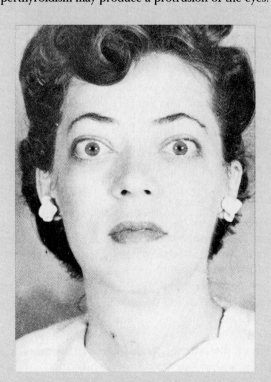

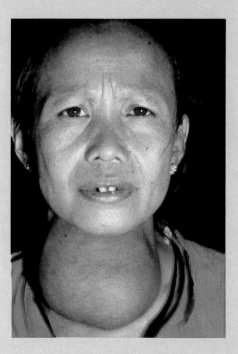

The Endocrine System   377

FIGURE 11.13
The parathyroid glands are embedded in the posterior surface of the thyroid gland.

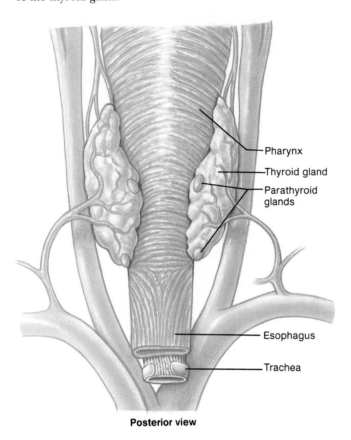

Posterior view

FIGURE 11.14
Light micrograph of the parathyroid gland (×50).

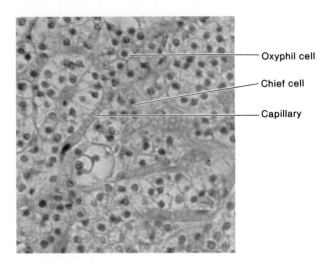

(principal cells), the hormone-producing cells, and *oxyphil cells,* whose function is not well understood (figure 11.14).

1. Where are the parathyroid glands located?
2. What are the two major cell types in the parathyroid gland?

The Parathyroid Glands

The **parathyroid glands** are located on the posterior surface of the thyroid gland, as shown in figure 11.13. Usually there are four of them—two associated with each of the thyroid's lateral lobes. These glands secrete parathyroid hormone (PTH) that functions in the regulation of blood calcium and phosphate levels.

Although the usual number of parathyroid glands is four, there may be only three. Some individuals may lack distinct glands and instead have many small islands of parathyroid tissue scattered throughout the area where a gland would be found.

Structure of the Glands

Each parathyroid gland is a small, yellowish brown structure covered by a thin capsule of connective tissue. The body of the gland consists of numerous tightly packed secretory cells that are closely associated with capillary networks. The two major cell types are called *chief cells*

The Adrenal Glands

The **adrenal** (ah-dre′nal) **glands** (suprarenal glands) are closely associated with the kidneys. A gland sits atop each kidney like a cap and is embedded in the mass of fat that encloses the kidney.

Although the adrenal glands may differ somewhat in size and shape, they are generally pyramidal. Each adrenal gland is very vascular and consists of two parts, as shown in figure 11.15. The central portion is the adrenal medulla, and the outer part is the adrenal cortex. Although these regions are not sharply divided, they represent distinct glands that secrete different hormones.

Adrenal Medulla

The **adrenal medulla** consists of irregularly shaped cells that are arranged in groups around blood vessels. These cells are intimately connected with the sympathetic division of the autonomic nervous system. In fact, these medullary cells are modified postganglionic neurons, and preganglionic autonomic nerve fibers lead to them from the central nervous system without synapsing (see chapter 9).

Cells of the adrenal medulla (chromaffin cells) produce, store, and secrete two closely related hormones, **epinephrine** (adrenalin) and **norepinephrine** (noradrenalin) (figure 11.16). These hormones produce effects similar to

FIGURE 11.15

(*a*) An adrenal gland consists of an outer cortex and an inner medulla; (*b*) the cortex consists of three layers or zones of cells.

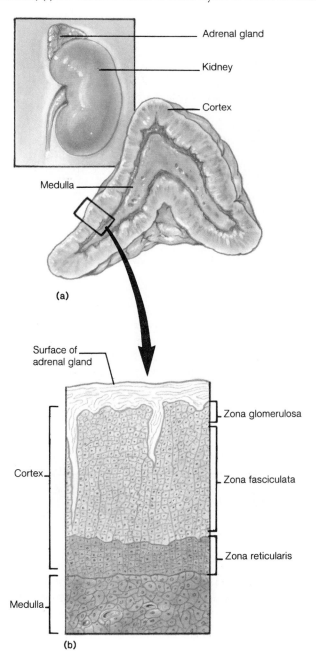

(a)

(b)

FIGURE 11.16

Light micrograph of the adrenal medulla (×45).

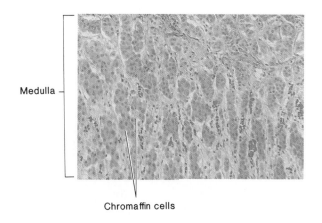

As in the case of the cells of the adrenal medulla, the cells of the adrenal cortex are well supplied with blood vessels (figure 11.17).

The cells of the adrenal cortex produce several hormones. Unlike the adrenal medullary hormones, which a person can survive without, some of those released by the cortex are vital. In fact, in the absence of cortical secretions, a person usually dies within a week unless medical attention is provided. The most important cortical hormones are aldosterone, cortisol, and sex hormones.

Aldosterone is synthesized by cells in the outer zone (zona glomerulosa) of the adrenal cortex. **Cortisol** (hydrocortisone) is produced in the middle zone (zona fasciculata). Adrenal sex hormones are produced by cells in the inner zone (zona reticularis) of the cortex.

1. Describe the location and structure of an adrenal gland.
2. What is the usual stimulus for the release of epinephrine and norepinephrine?
3. Name the three layers of the adrenal cortex.

The Pancreas

The **pancreas** contains two major types of secretory tissues, reflecting its dual function as an exocrine gland that secretes digestive juice through a duct, and an endocrine gland that releases hormones. It is an elongated, somewhat flattened organ that is posterior to the stomach and behind the parietal peritoneum (figure 11.18). It is attached to the first section of the small intestine (duodenum) by a duct that transports its digestive chemicals into the intestine.

The endocrine portion of the pancreas consists of groups of cells closely associated with blood vessels. These

those of the sympathetic nervous system, and their secretion is stimulated by sympathetic impulses originating from the hypothalamus.

Adrenal Cortex

The **adrenal cortex,** which makes up the bulk of the adrenal gland, is composed of closely packed masses of epithelial cells that are arranged in layers. These layers form an outer zone (*zona glomerulosa*), a middle zone (*zona fasciculata*), and an inner zone (*zona reticularis*) of the cortex.

FIGURE 11.17
Light micrograph of the adrenal cortex (×100).

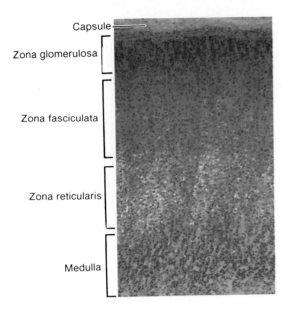

FIGURE 11.19
Light micrograph of an islet of Langerhans within the pancreas.

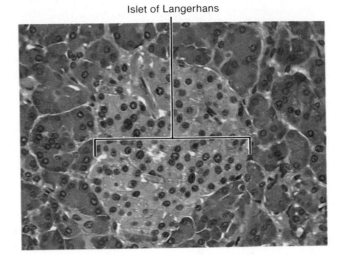

FIGURE 11.18
The hormone-secreting cells of the pancreas are arranged in clusters or islets that are closely associated with blood vessels. Other pancreatic cells secrete digestive chemicals into ducts.

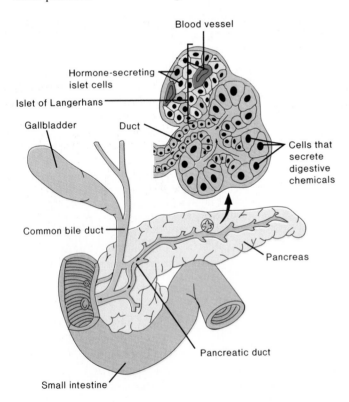

groups, called *islets of Langerhans,* include three distinct types of hormone-secreting cells—*alpha cells* that secrete glucagon, *beta cells* that secrete insulin, and *delta cells* that secrete somatostatin (figure 11.19). All three of these hormones are involved with the regulation of blood sugar concentration. The digestive functions of the pancreas are discussed in chapter 12.

1. What is the name of the endocrine portion of the pancreas?
2. What types of endocrine cells are found in the pancreas?

Other Endocrine Glands

Other organs that produce hormones and, therefore, are parts of the endocrine system include the pineal gland, thymus gland, reproductive glands, and certain glands of the digestive tract.

The Pineal Gland

The **pineal** (pin′e-al) **gland** is a small, oval structure located deep between the cerebral hemispheres, where it is attached to the upper portion of the thalamus near the roof of the third ventricle. Its body consists largely of specialized *pineal cells* and *neuroglial cells* that provide support for the pineal cells (see figure 9.33).

The pineal gland secretes one hormone called *melatonin*. This substance is thought to inhibit the secretion of gonadotropins from the anterior pituitary gland. The pineal gland seems to be controlled by varying light conditions outside the body. Information concerning such conditions reaches the gland by means of nerve impulses originating from the retinas of the eyes. During the night, as the amount of light exposure decreases, the secretion of melatonin increases; during the day, secretion decreases. This mechanism is involved in the regulation of some **circadian rhythms**—patterns of repeated activity associated with environmental cycles of day and night—such as sleep/wake and various hormonal rhythms.

The Thymus Gland

The **thymus gland,** which lies in the mediastinum behind the sternum and between the lungs, is relatively large in young children but diminishes in size with age. It is believed that this gland secretes a group of hormones, including one called *thymosin,* that affects the production of certain white blood cells (lymphocytes). This gland plays an important role in the immune mechanism and is discussed in chapter 15.

The Reproductive Glands

The reproductive organs that secrete important hormones include the **ovaries,** which produce estrogens and progesterone; the **placenta,** which produces estrogens, progesterone, and a gonadotropin; and the **testes,** which produce testosterone. These glands are discussed in chapters 17 and 18.

1. Where is the pineal gland located?
2. What seems to be the function of the pineal gland?
3. Where is the thymus gland located?
4. Which reproductive organs secrete hormones?

Clinical Terms Related to the Endocrine System

adrenalectomy (ah-dre″nah-lek′to-me)   surgical removal of the adrenal glands.

adrenogenital syndrome (ah-dre″no-jen′i-tal sin′drom)   a group of symptoms associated with changes in sexual characteristics as a result of increased secretion of adrenal sex hormones.

exophthalmos (ek″sof-thal′mos)   an abnormal protrusion of the eyes.

hypophysectomy (hi-pof″ĭ-sek′to-me)   surgical removal of the pituitary gland.

parathyroidectomy (par″ah-thi″roi-dek′to-me)   surgical removal of the parathyroid glands.

pheochromocytoma (fe-o-kro″mo-si-to′mah)   a type of tumor found in the adrenal medulla.

thymectomy (thi-mek′to-me)   surgical removal of the thymus gland.

thyroidectomy (thi″roi-dek′to-me)   surgical removal of the thyroid gland.

thyroiditis (thi″roi-di′tis)   inflammation of the thyroid gland.

Chapter Summary

Introduction (page 369)
Endocrine glands secrete their products into body fluids; exocrine glands secrete into ducts that lead outside the body.

General Characteristics of the
Endocrine System (page 369)
1. As a group, endocrine glands are concerned with the regulation of body processes.
2. Some hormones have localized effects, while others produce general actions.
3. Endocrine glands secrete hormones that have effects on specific target cells.

The Pituitary Gland (page 369)
The pituitary gland, which is attached to the base of the brain, has an anterior lobe and a posterior lobe. Most pituitary secretions are controlled by the hypothalamus.

1. The anterior lobe consists largely of epithelial cells that secrete several hormones.
2. The posterior lobe consists largely of neuroglial cells and nerve fibers that originate in the hypothalamus. The two hormones associated with the posterior lobe are produced in the hypothalamus.

The Thyroid Gland (page 375)
The thyroid gland is located in the neck.

1. The thyroid gland consists of many hollow secretory parts called follicles.
2. The follicles are fluid-filled and store the hormones secreted by the follicle cells.

The Parathyroid Glands (page 378)
1. The parathyroid glands are located on the posterior surface of the thyroid.
2. Each gland consists of secretory cells that are well supplied with capillaries.

The Adrenal Glands (page 378)
1. The adrenal glands are located atop the kidneys.
   a. Each gland consists of an inner medulla and an outer cortex.
   b. These parts represent distinct glands that secrete different hormones.
2. Adrenal medulla
   a. The adrenal medulla secretes epinephrine and norepinephrine.
   b. These hormones produce effects similar to those of the sympathetic nervous system.
   c. The secretion of these hormones is stimulated by sympathetic impulses originating from the hypothalamus.

3. Adrenal cortex
   The adrenal cortex is made up of three layers of cells
   and produces a variety of hormones.

The Pancreas (page 379)
The pancreas secretes digestive juices as well as hormones.

1. The pancreas is located in back of the stomach and is
   attached to the small intestine.
2. The endocrine portion, which is called the islets of
   Langerhans, secretes glucagon, insulin, and somatostatin.

Other Endocrine Glands (page 380)
1. The pineal gland
   a. The pineal gland is attached to the thalamus near
      the roof of the third ventricle.
   b. It secretes melatonin, which seems to inhibit the
      secretion of gonadotropins.
2. The thymus gland
   a. The thymus lies behind the sternum and between
      the lungs.
   b. Its size diminishes with age.
   c. It secretes thymosin that affects the production of
      lymphocytes.
3. The reproductive glands
   a. The ovaries secrete estrogens and progesterone.
   b. The placenta secretes estrogens, progesterone, and a
      gonadotropin.
   c. The testes secrete testosterone.

Clinical Application of Knowledge

1. How might an enlarged thyroid gland affect other organs
   near the gland?
2. In some cases of hyperthyroidism and enlargement of the
   thyroid gland, part of the gland may be removed
   surgically. In such cases, why is it important to leave the
   posterior portions of each lobe intact?

Review Activities

1. Explain what is meant by an endocrine gland.
2. Define *hormone* and *target cell.*
3. Describe the location and structure of the pituitary
   gland.
4. List the secretory cells found in the anterior lobe of the
   pituitary gland.
5. Explain how pituitary gland activity is controlled by the
   brain.
6. Compare the cellular structures of the anterior and
   posterior lobes of the pituitary gland.
7. Describe how the hormones associated with the posterior
   pituitary gland are produced.
8. Describe the location and structure of the thyroid gland.
9. Name the hormones secreted by the thyroid gland and
   list the general functions of each.
10. Describe the location and structure of the parathyroid
    glands.
11. Distinguish between the adrenal medulla and the adrenal
    cortex.
12. List the hormones produced by the adrenal medulla.
13. Name the three zones of the adrenal cortex.
14. Describe the location and structure of the pancreas.
15. List the cell types of the islets of Langerhans.
16. Describe the location and general function of the pineal
    gland.
17. Describe the location and general function of the thymus
    gland.

U N I T 4
Processing and Transporting

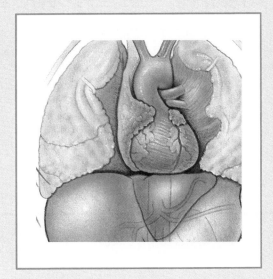

The chapters of unit 4 are concerned with the digestive, respiratory, circulatory, lymphatic, and urinary systems. They describe how organs of these systems obtain nutrients and oxygen from outside the body, and how the nutrients are altered and absorbed into body fluids. They also describe the organs that eliminate wastes.

CHAPTER 12

The Digestive System

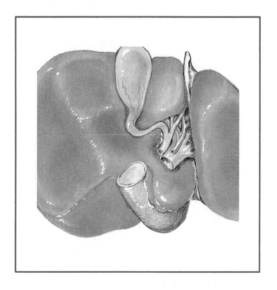

The *digestive system* ingests foods, breaks large particles into smaller ones, secretes substances (enzymes) that decompose food molecules, absorbs the products of this digestive action, and eliminates the unused residues.

Foods are moved through the digestive tract by muscular contractions in the wall of the tubular alimentary canal, and digestive juices are secreted into this canal by various glands and accessory organs. These functions are controlled largely by interactions between the digestive, nervous, and endocrine systems.

Chapter Objectives

After you have studied this chapter, you
should be able to

1. Name and describe the location of
the organs of the digestive system
and their major parts.

2. Describe the structure and general
functions of each digestive organ
and the liver.

3. Describe the structure of the wall of
the alimentary canal.

4. Explain how the contents of the
alimentary canal are mixed and
moved.

5. Describe the mechanism of
swallowing.

6. Explain how the products of
digestion are absorbed.

7. Complete the review activities at the
end of this chapter. Note that the
items are worded in the form of
specific learning objectives. You may
want to refer to them before reading
the chapter.

Aids to Understanding Words

aliment-, food: *aliment*ary canal—the
tubelike portion of the digestive
system.

cari-, decay: dental *cari*es—tooth
decay.

cec-, blindness: *cec*um—blind-ended
sac at the beginning of the large
intestine.

chym-, juice: *chym*e—semifluid paste
of food particles and gastric juice
formed in the stomach.

decidu-, falling off: *decidu*ous teeth—
teeth shed during childhood.

frenul-, a restraint: *frenul*um—
membranous fold that anchors the
tongue to the floor of the mouth.

gastr-, stomach: *gastr*ic gland—
portion of the stomach that secretes
gastric juice.

hepat-, liver: *hepat*ic duct—duct that
carries bile from the liver to the
common bile duct.

hiat-, an opening: esophageal *hiat*us—
opening through which the
esophagus penetrates the
diaphragm.

lingu-, the tongue: *lingu*al tonsil—mass
of lymphatic tissue at the root of the
tongue.

peri-, around: *peri*stalsis—wavelike
ring of contraction that moves
material along the alimentary canal.

pylor-, gatekeeper: *pylor*ic sphincter—
muscle that serves as a valve
between the stomach and small
intestine.

vill-, hairy: *vill*i—tiny projections of
mucous membrane in the small
intestine.

Introduction

Digestion is the process by which food substances are changed into forms that can be absorbed through cell membranes. The **digestive system** includes the organs that promote digestion and absorb the products of this process. It consists of an *alimentary canal* that extends from the mouth to the anus, and several *accessory organs* that release secretions into the canal. The alimentary canal includes the mouth, pharynx, esophagus, stomach, small intestine, and large intestine; and the accessory organs include the salivary glands, liver, gallbladder, and pancreas. The major organs of this system are shown in figure 12.1.

General Characteristics of the Alimentary Canal

The **alimentary canal** is a muscular tube about 9 meters long that passes through the body's anterior cavity. Although it is specialized in various regions to carry on

---

FIGURE 12.1

Major organs of the digestive system. What are the general functions of this system?

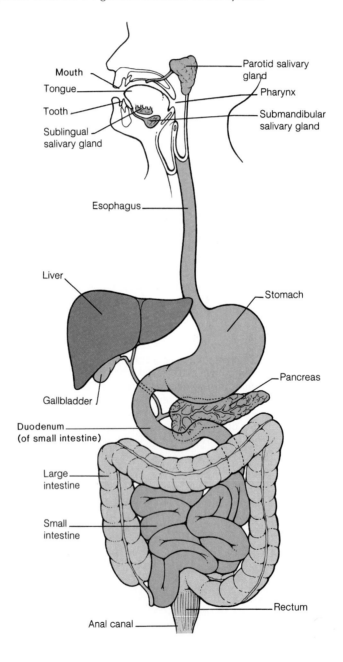

particular functions, the structure of its wall, the method by which it moves food, and its type of innervation are similar throughout its length (figure 12.2).

Structure of the Wall

The wall of the alimentary canal consists of four distinct layers, although the degree to which they are developed varies from region to region. Beginning with the innermost tissues, these layers, shown in figure 12.3, include the following:

1. **Mucous membrane** (mucosa). This layer is formed of surface epithelium, underlying connective tissue (lamina propria), and a small amount of smooth muscle. In some regions, it develops folds and tiny projections that extend into the lumen of the digestive tube and increase its absorptive surface area. It may also contain glands that are tubular invaginations into which the lining cells secrete mucus and digestive chemicals. The mucosa protects the tissues beneath it and carries on absorption and secretion.

2. **Submucosa.** The submucosa contains considerable loose connective tissue as well as blood vessels, lymphatic vessels, and nerves. Its vessels nourish the surrounding tissues and carry away absorbed materials.

3. **Muscular layer.** This layer, which is responsible for the movements of the tube, consists of two coats of smooth muscle tissue. The fibers of the inner coat are arranged so that they encircle the tube, and when these *circular fibers* contract, the diameter of the tube is decreased. The fibers of the outer muscular coat run lengthwise, and when these *longitudinal fibers* contract, the tube is shortened.

4. **Serous layer** (serosa). The serous layer or outer covering of the tube is composed of the *visceral peritoneum,* which is formed of epithelium on the outside and connective tissue beneath. The cells of the serosa secrete serous fluid that keeps the tube's outer surface moist. This lubricates the surface so that the organs within the abdominal cavity slide freely against one another.

The visceral peritoneum is continuous with the parietal peritoneum, which covers the inner wall of the abdominal cavity. (See chapter 2.) The visceral peritoneum forms double-layered folds called *mesentery* and *omenta.* The mesentery suspends organs from the posterior wall of the abdominal cavity and the omenta hang in front of certain abdominal organs, somewhat like a curtain.

The characteristics of these layers of the alimentary canal are summarized in chart 12.1.

Movements of the Tube

The motor functions of the alimentary canal are of two basic types—mixing movements and propelling movements. Mixing occurs when smooth muscles in relatively small segments of the tube undergo rhythmic contractions. For example, when the stomach is full, waves of muscular contractions move along its wall from one end to the other. These waves occur every 20 seconds or so, and their action mixes food substances with digestive juices secreted by the mucosa.

Propelling movements include a wavelike motion called **peristalsis** (per″i-stal′sis). When peristalsis occurs, a ring of contraction appears in the wall of the tube. At the same time, the muscular wall just ahead of the ring relaxes—a phenomenon called *receptive relaxation.* As the wave moves

FIGURE 12.2
The alimentary canal is about nine meters long.

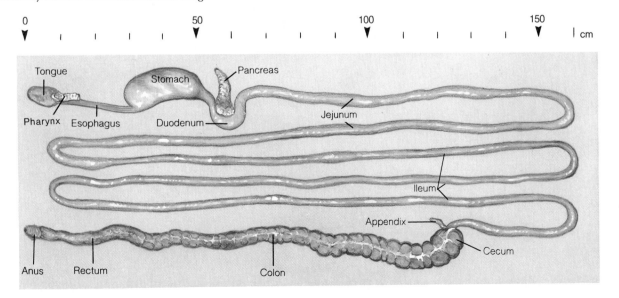

FIGURE 12.3
The wall of the small intestine, as in other portions of the alimentary canal, includes four layers: inner mucous membrane, submucosa, muscular layer, and outer serous layer.

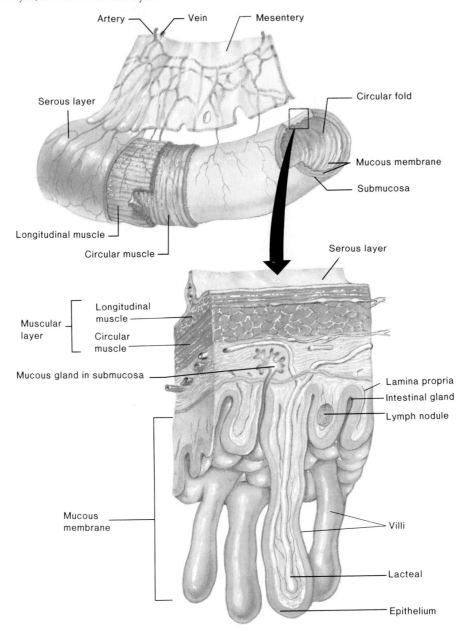

Chart 12.1 Layers in the wall of the alimentary canal

Layer	Composition	Function
Mucous membrane	Epithelium, connective tissue, smooth muscle	Protection, absorption, secretion
Submucosa	Loose connective tissue, blood vessels, lymphatic vessels, nerves	Nourishes surrounding tissues, transports absorbed materials
Muscular layer	Smooth muscle fibers arranged in circular and longitudinal groups	Movements of the tube and its contents
Serous layer	Epithelium, connective tissue	Protection

along, it pushes the tubular contents ahead of it. The usual stimulus for peristalsis is an expansion of the tube due to accumulation of food inside. Such movements create sounds that can be heard through a stethoscope applied to the abdominal wall.

Innervation of the Tube

The alimentary canal is innervated extensively by branches of the sympathetic and parasympathetic divisions of the autonomic nervous system. These nerve fibers are associated mainly with the tube's muscular layer, and they are responsible for maintaining muscle tone and regulating the strength, rate, and velocity of muscular contractions.

Parasympathetic impulses generally cause an increase in the activities of the digestive system. Some of these impulses originate in the brain and are conducted on branches of the vagus nerves to the esophagus, stomach, pancreas, gallbladder, small intestine, and proximal half of the large intestine. Other parasympathetic impulses arise in the sacral region of the spinal cord and supply the distal half of the large intestine.

The effects produced by sympathetic nerve impulses are usually opposite those of the parasympathetic division—they inhibit various digestive actions. Sympathetic impulses are responsible for the contraction of certain sphincter muscles in the wall of the alimentary canal. When they are contracted, these muscles effectively block the movement of materials through the tube.

---

1. What organs constitute the digestive system?
2. Describe the wall of the alimentary canal.
3. Name the two types of movements that occur in the alimentary canal.
4. What effect do parasympathetic nerve impulses have on digestive actions? What effect do sympathetic nerve impulses have?

The Mouth

The **mouth,** which is the first portion of the alimentary canal, is adapted to receive food and prepare it for digestion by mechanically reducing the size of solid particles and mixing them with saliva (mastication). It is also an organ of speech and of pleasure. The mouth is surrounded by the lips, cheeks, tongue, and palate, and includes a chamber between the palate and tongue called the *oral cavity,* as well as a narrow space between the teeth, cheeks, and lips called the *vestibule* (figure 12.4).

The Cheeks and Lips

The **cheeks** form the lateral walls of the mouth. They consist of outer layers of skin, pads of subcutaneous fat, certain muscles associated with expression and chewing, and inner linings of stratified squamous epithelium.

FIGURE 12.4
The mouth is adapted for ingesting food and preparing it for digestion.

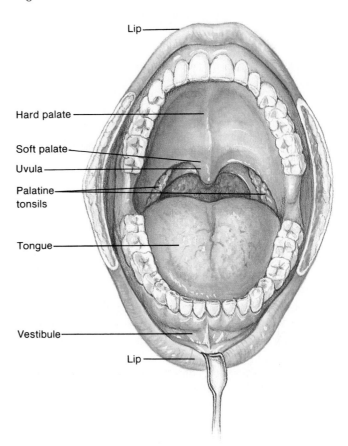

The **lips** are highly mobile structures that surround the mouth opening. They contain skeletal muscles and a variety of sensory receptors useful in judging the temperature and texture of foods. Their normal reddish color is due to an abundance of blood vessels near their surfaces. The external borders of the lips mark the boundaries between the skin of the face and the mucous membrane that lines the alimentary canal.

The Tongue

The **tongue** is a thick, muscular organ that occupies the floor of the mouth and nearly fills the oral cavity when the mouth is closed. It is covered by mucous membrane and is connected in the midline to the floor of the mouth by a membranous fold called the **frenulum.**

A person whose frenulum is too short is said to be tongue-tied. Infants with this condition may have difficulty sucking, and older children may be unable to make the tongue movements needed for normal speech. A short frenulum is sometimes corrected in early infancy by surgery.

FIGURE 12.5

The surface of the tongue, as viewed from above.

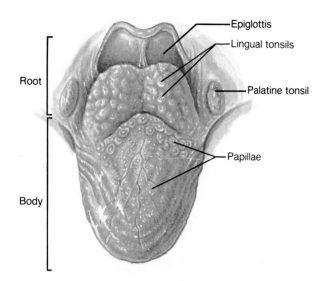

The palatine tonsils themselves are common sites of infections, and if they become inflamed, the condition is termed *tonsillitis.* Infected tonsils may become so swollen that they block the passageways of the pharynx and interfere with breathing and swallowing. Because the mucous membranes of the pharynx, auditory tubes, and middle ears are continuous, there is danger that such an infection may travel from the throat into the middle ears (otitis media).

When tonsillitis occurs repeatedly and remains unresponsive to antibiotic treatment, the tonsils are often removed. This surgical procedure is called *tonsillectomy.*

Still other masses of lymphatic tissue, called **pharyngeal tonsils,** or *adenoids,* occur on the posterior wall of the pharynx, above the border of the soft palate. If these parts become enlarged and block the passage between the pharynx and the nasal cavity, they also may be removed surgically (figure 12.6).

1. What is the function of the mouth?
2. How does the tongue contribute to the function of the digestive system?
3. What is the role of the soft palate in swallowing?
4. Where are the tonsils located?

The *body* of the tongue is composed largely of skeletal muscle whose fibers run in several directions. These muscles aid in mixing food particles with saliva during chewing and in moving food toward the pharynx during swallowing. Rough projections on the surface of the tongue, called **papillae,** provide friction useful in handling food. These papillae also contain taste buds (figure 12.5).

The posterior region, or *root,* of the tongue is anchored to the hyoid bone and covered with rounded masses of lymphatic tissue called **lingual tonsils.**

The Palate

The **palate** forms the roof of the oral cavity and consists of a hard anterior part and a soft posterior part. The *hard palate* is formed by the palatine processes of the maxillary bones in front and the horizontal portions of the palatine bones in back. The *soft palate* forms a muscular arch that extends posteriorly and downward as a cone-shaped projection called the **uvula.**

During swallowing, muscles draw the soft palate and the uvula upward. This action closes the opening between the nasal cavity and the pharynx, preventing food from entering the nasal cavity.

In the back of the mouth, on either side of the tongue and closely associated with the palate, are masses of lymphatic tissue called **palatine tonsils.** These structures lie beneath the epithelial lining of the mouth, and like other lymphatic tissues, they protect the body against infections. (See chapter 15.)

The Teeth

The **teeth** develop in sockets along the alveolar borders of the mandibular and maxillary bones. Teeth are unique structures in that two sets form during development. The members of the first set, the *primary teeth* (deciduous teeth), usually erupt through the gums (gingiva) at regular intervals between the ages of 6 months and 2 years. There are twenty primary teeth—ten in each jaw—and they occur from the midline toward the sides in the following sequence: central incisor, lateral incisor, cuspid (canine), first molar, and second molar.

The primary teeth are usually shed in the same order they appeared. Before this happens, though, their roots are resorbed. The teeth are then pushed out of their sockets by pressure from the developing *secondary teeth* (permanent teeth) (figure 12.7). This second set consists of thirty-two teeth—sixteen in each jaw—arranged from the midline as follows: central incisor, lateral incisor, cuspid (canine), first bicuspid (premolar), second bicuspid, first molar, second molar, and third molar (figure 12.8 and chart 12.2).

FIGURE 12.6

A sagittal section of the mouth, nasal cavity, and pharynx.

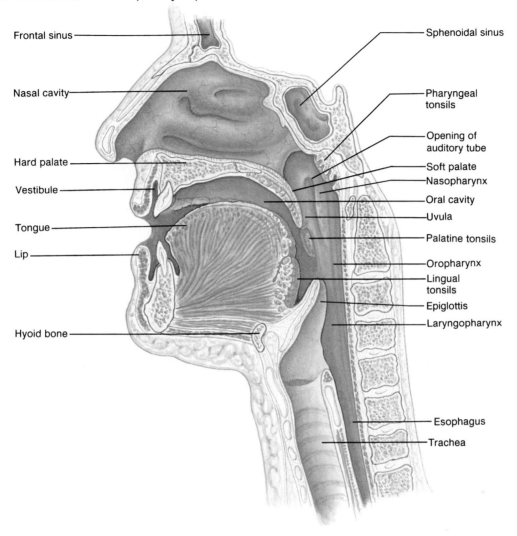

Frontal sinus

Nasal cavity

Hard palate

Vestibule

Tongue

Lip

Hyoid bone

Sphenoidal sinus

Pharyngeal tonsils

Opening of auditory tube

Soft palate

Nasopharynx

Oral cavity

Uvula

Palatine tonsils

Oropharynx

Lingual tonsils

Epiglottis

Laryngopharynx

Esophagus

Trachea

FIGURE 12.7

Secondary teeth developing in the maxilla and mandible are revealed in this skull of a child.

Primary teeth   Secondary teeth

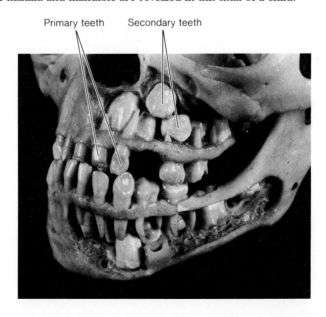

FIGURE 12.8

The permanent teeth of the upper jaw and lower jaw.

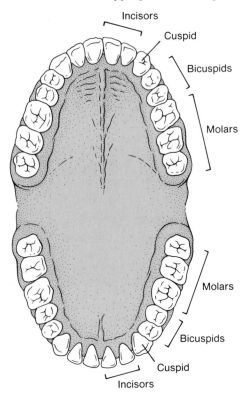

FIGURE 12.9

A section of a cuspid tooth.

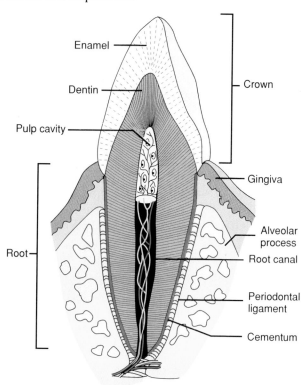

Chart 12.2 Primary and secondary teeth			
Primary teeth (deciduous)		**Secondary teeth (permanent)**	
Type	*Number*	*Type*	*Number*
Incisor		Incisor	
central	4	central	4
lateral	4	lateral	4
Cuspid	4	Cuspid	4
		Bicuspid	
		first	4
		second	4
Molar		Molar	
first	4	first	4
second	4	second	4
		third	4
Total	20	Total	32

The permanent teeth usually begin to appear at age 6, but the set may not be completed until the third molars appear, between 17 and 25 years of age. Sometimes these third molars, also called wisdom teeth, become wedged in abnormal positions within the jaws and fail to erupt. Such teeth are said to be *impacted.*

The teeth mechanically break pieces of food into smaller pieces. This increases the surface area of the food particles and thus makes it possible for digestive juices to react more effectively with food molecules.

Different teeth are adapted to handle food in different ways. The *incisors* are chisel-shaped, and their sharp edges bite off relatively large pieces of food. The *cuspids* are cone-shaped, and are useful in grasping or tearing food. The *bicuspids* and *molars* have somewhat flattened surfaces and are specialized for grinding food particles.

Each tooth consists of two main portions—the *crown,* which projects beyond the gum, and the *root,* which is anchored to the alveolar bone of the jaw. The region where these portions meet is called the *neck* of the tooth. The crown is covered by glossy, white *enamel.* Enamel consists mainly of calcium compounds and is the hardest substance in the body. Unfortunately, if enamel is damaged by abrasive action or injury, it is not replaced. It also tends to wear away with age.

The bulk of a tooth beneath the enamel is composed of *dentin,* a substance much like bone, but somewhat harder. The dentin, in turn, surrounds the tooth's central cavity (pulp cavity), which contains blood vessels, nerves, and connective tissue (*pulp*). The blood vessels and nerves reach this cavity through tubular *root canals* that extend upward into the root.

The root is enclosed by a thin layer of bonelike material called *cementum,* which is surrounded by a *periodontal ligament* (membrane). This ligament contains bundles of thick collagenous fibers that pass between the cementum and the alveolar process, firmly attaching the tooth to the jaw. It also contains blood vessels and nerves near the surface of the cementum-covered root (figure 12.9).

The mouth parts and their functions are summarized in chart 12.3.

Dental Caries

Dental caries (decay) involves the decalcification of tooth enamel and is usually followed by destruction of the enamel and its underlying dentin. The result is a cavity, which must be cleaned and filled to prevent further erosion of the tooth.

Although the cause or causes of dental caries are not well understood, a lack of dental cleanliness and a diet high in sugar and starch seem to contribute to the problem. Accumulations of food particles on the surfaces and between the teeth are thought to aid the growth of certain kinds of bacteria. These microorganisms utilize food particles and produce acid by-products. The acids then begin the process of destroying tooth enamel.

Preventing dental caries requires brushing the teeth at least once a day, using dental floss or tape regularly to remove debris from between the teeth, and limiting the intake of sugar and starch, especially between meals. Fluoridated drinking water or the application of fluoride solution to teeth also help prevent dental decay.

Loss of teeth is most commonly associated with diseases of the gums and the dental pulp (endodontitis). Such diseases can usually be avoided by practicing good oral hygiene and obtaining regular dental treatment.

Chart 12.3 Mouth parts and their functions

Part	Location	Function
Cheeks	Form lateral walls of mouth	Hold food in mouth, muscles function in chewing
Lips	Surround mouth opening	Contain sensory receptors used to judge characteristics of foods
Tongue	Occupies floor of mouth	Aids in mixing food with saliva, moves food toward pharynx, contains taste receptors
Palate	Forms roof of mouth	Holds food in mouth, directs food to pharynx
Teeth	In sockets of mandibular and maxillary bones	Break food particles into smaller pieces, help mix food with saliva during chewing

Teeth of individuals vary in structure and in number. For example, the lower canine and second bicuspid teeth may have two roots, even though one is the usual number. The second bicuspid teeth normally have two roots, but may have one or three.

In some individuals, teeth may be missing. The most common missing teeth are the third molars. One or more of these may be absent in one out of four people.

1. How do primary teeth differ from secondary teeth?
2. How are various types of teeth adapted to provide specialized functions?
3. Describe the structure of a tooth.
4. Explain how a tooth is attached to the bone of the jaw.

The Salivary Glands

The **salivary glands** secrete saliva. This fluid moistens food particles, helps bind them together, and begins the digestion of certain food molecules. Saliva also acts as a solvent, dissolving various food chemicals so they can be tasted, and it helps cleanse the mouth and teeth.

Many small salivary glands are scattered throughout the mucosa of the tongue, palate, and cheeks. They secrete fluid continuously so that the lining of the mouth remains moist. In addition, there are three pairs of major salivary glands: the parotid glands, the submandibular glands, and the sublingual glands.

FIGURE 12.10
Locations of the major salivary glands.

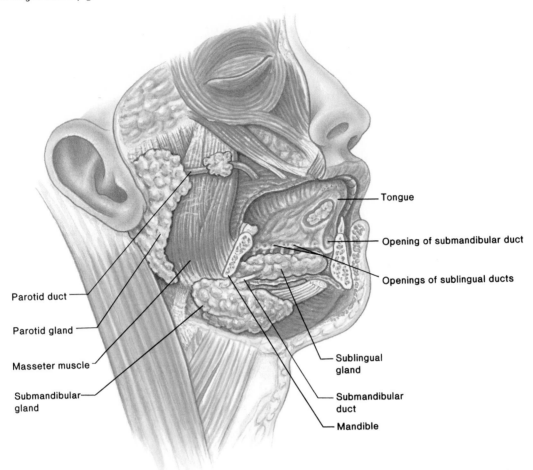

Tongue

Opening of submandibular duct

Openings of sublingual ducts

Parotid duct

Parotid gland

Masseter muscle

Submandibular gland

Sublingual gland

Submandibular duct

Mandible

Salivary Secretions

Within a salivary gland are two types of secretory cells, called *serous cells* and *mucous cells*. These cells occur in varying proportions within different glands. The serous cells produce a watery fluid that contains a digestive chemical. Mucous cells secrete the thick, stringy liquid called **mucus** that binds food particles together and acts as a lubricant during swallowing.

Like other digestive structures, the salivary glands are innervated by branches of both sympathetic and parasympathetic nerves. Impulses arriving on sympathetic fibers stimulate the gland cells to secrete a small quantity of viscous saliva. Parasympathetic impulses, on the other hand, elicit the secretion of a large volume of watery saliva. Such parasympathetic impulses are activated reflexly when a person sees, smells, tastes, or even thinks about pleasant foods. Conversely, if food looks, smells, or tastes unpleasant, parasympathetic activity is inhibited so that less saliva is produced, and swallowing may become difficult.

Major Salivary Glands

The **parotid glands** are the largest of the major salivary glands. One lies in front of and somewhat below each ear, between the skin of the cheek and the masseter muscle. *A parotid duct* (Stensen's duct) passes from the gland inward through the buccinator muscle, entering the mouth just opposite the upper second molar on either side of the jaw. The parotid glands secrete a clear, watery fluid rich in the digestive chemical amylase (figure 12.10).

The **submandibular** (submaxillary) **glands** are located in the floor of the mouth on the inside surface of the lower jaw. The secretory cells of these glands are predominantly serous, although some mucous cells are present. Consequently, the submandibular glands secrete a more viscous fluid than the parotid glands. The submandibular ducts (Wharton's ducts) open under the tongue, near the frenulum (figure 12.10).

The **sublingual glands** are the smallest of the major salivary glands. They are found on the floor of the mouth

FIGURE 12.11
Light micrographs of (*a*) the parotid salivary gland (×200), (*b*) the submandibular salivary gland (×150), and (*c*) the sublingual salivary gland (×200).

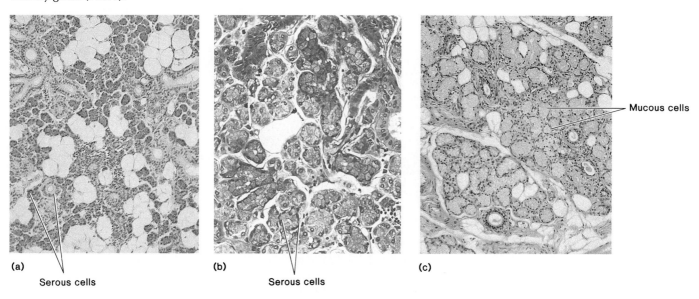

(a)

Serous cells

(b)

Serous cells

(c)

Mucous cells

Chart 12.4 The major salivary glands			
Gland	**Location**	**Duct**	**Type of secretion**
Parotid glands	In front of and somewhat below the ears, between the skin of the cheeks and the masseter muscles	Parotid ducts pass through the buccinator muscles and enter the mouth opposite the upper second molars	Clear, watery serous fluid, rich in amylase
Submandibular glands	In the floor of the mouth on the inside surface of the mandible	Ducts open beneath the tongue near the frenulum	Primarily serous fluid, but with some mucus; more viscous than parotid secretion
Sublingual glands	In the floor of the mouth beneath the tongue	Many separate ducts	Primarily thick, stringy mucus

under the tongue. Their cells are primarily the mucous type; as a result, their secretions, which enter the mouth through many separate ducts, tend to be thick and stringy. (See figures 12.10 and 12.11.)

Chart 12.4 summarizes the characteristics of these glands.

1. What is the function of saliva?
2. What stimulates the salivary glands to secrete saliva?
3. Where are the major salivary glands located?

The Pharynx and Esophagus

The pharynx is a cavity behind the mouth from which the tubular esophagus leads to the stomach. Although neither the pharynx nor the esophagus contributes to the digestive process, both are important passageways, and their muscular walls function in swallowing.

Structure of the Pharynx

The **pharynx** connects the nasal and oral cavities to the larynx and esophagus. (See figure 12.6.) It can be divided into the following parts:

1. The **nasopharynx** is located above the soft palate. It communicates with the nasal cavity and provides a passageway for air during breathing. The auditory tubes, which connect the pharynx with the middle ears, open through the walls of the nasopharynx.
2. The **oropharynx** is behind the mouth. It opens behind the soft palate into the nasopharynx and projects downward to the upper border of the epiglottis. This portion is a passageway for food moving downward from the mouth, and for air moving to and from the nasal cavity.

FIGURE 12.12
Muscles of the pharyngeal wall, as viewed from behind. (Note: the constrictor muscles have been removed on the right side.)

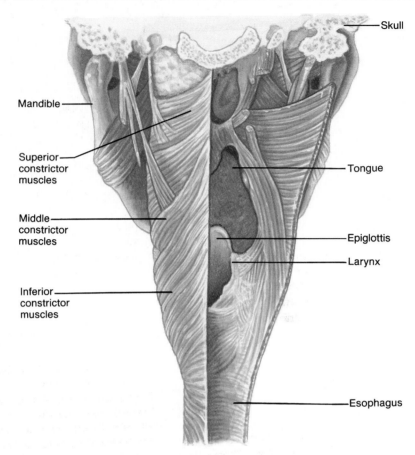

Skull

Mandible

Superior constrictor muscles

Tongue

Middle constrictor muscles

Epiglottis

Larynx

Inferior constrictor muscles

Esophagus

3. The **laryngopharynx** is located just below the oropharynx. It extends from the upper border of the epiglottis downward to the lower border of the cricoid cartilage of the larynx, where it is continuous with the esophagus.

The muscles in the walls of the pharynx are arranged in inner circular and outer longitudinal groups (figure 12.12). The circular muscles, called *constrictor muscles,* serve to pull the walls inward during swallowing. The *superior constrictor muscles,* attached to the bony processes of the skull and mandible, curve around the upper part of the pharynx. The *middle constrictor muscles* arise from projections on the hyoid bone and fan around the middle of the pharynx. The *inferior constrictor muscles* originate from cartilage of the larynx and pass around the lower portion of the cavity. Some of the fibers in the lower part of the inferior constrictor muscles remain contracted most of the time, and this action prevents air from entering the esophagus during breathing.

Although the pharyngeal muscles are skeletal muscles, they generally are not under voluntary control. Instead, they function involuntarily in the swallowing reflex.

The Swallowing Mechanism

The act of swallowing (deglutition) involves a set of complex reflexes and can be divided into three stages. In the first stage, which is initiated voluntarily, food is chewed and mixed with saliva. Then, this mixture is rolled into a mass (bolus) and forced into the pharynx by the tongue. The second stage begins as the food reaches the pharynx and stimulates sensory receptors located around the pharyngeal opening. This triggers the swallowing reflex, illustrated in figure 12.13, which includes the following actions:

1. The soft palate is raised, preventing food from entering the nasal cavity.
2. The hyoid bone and the larynx are elevated, so that food is less likely to enter the trachea.
3. The tongue is pressed against the soft palate, sealing off the oral cavity from the pharynx.
4. The longitudinal muscles in the pharyngeal wall contract, pulling the pharynx upward toward the food.
5. The lower portion of the inferior constrictor muscles relaxes, opening the esophagus.

FIGURE 12.13

Steps in the swallowing reflex: (*a*) the tongue forces food into the pharynx; (*b*) the soft palate, hyoid bone, and larynx are raised; the tongue is pressed against the palate; and inferior constrictor muscles relax so that the esophagus opens; (*c*) superior constrictor muscles contract and force food into the esophagus; (*d*) peristaltic waves move food through the esophagus to the stomach.

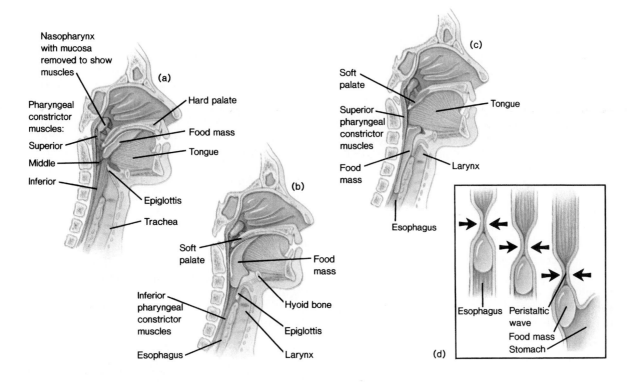

6. The superior constrictor muscles contract, stimulating a peristaltic wave to begin in other pharyngeal muscles. This wave forces the food into the esophagus.

During the third stage of swallowing, the food is transported through the esophagus to the stomach by peristalsis.

The Esophagus

The **esophagus** (e-sof'ă-gus) is a straight, collapsible tube about 25 centimeters long. It provides a passageway for substances from the pharynx to the stomach. It descends through the thorax behind the trachea, passing through the mediastinum. The esophagus penetrates the diaphragm through an opening, the *esophageal hiatus,* and is continuous with the stomach on the abdominal side of the diaphragm.

Mucous glands are scattered throughout the mucosa of the esophagus, and their secretions keep the inner lining of the tube moist and lubricated. The muscle layers propel food toward the stomach (figure 12.14).

FIGURE 12.14

This cross section of the esophagus shows its muscular wall (×10).

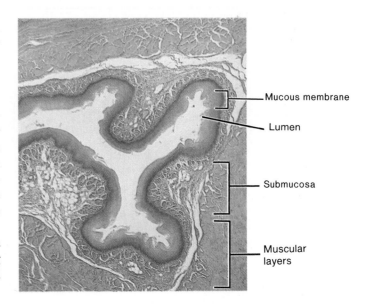

Occasionally there is a weak place in the diaphragm due to a congenital defect or an injury. As a result, a portion of the stomach, large intestine, or some other abdominal organ may protrude upward through the esophageal hiatus and into the thorax. This condition is called *hiatal hernia.*

If gastric juice from the stomach enters the esophagus as a result of such a hernia, or from regurgitation (reflux), the esophageal mucosa may become inflamed. This may lead either to the discomfort commonly called "heartburn," to difficulty in swallowing, or to ulceration accompanied by loss of blood.

In response to the destructive action of gastric juice, the squamous epithelium that normally lines the esophagus may be replaced by columnar epithelium. This condition, called *Barrett's esophagus,* is associated with an increased risk of developing an esophageal cancer.

Just above the point where the esophagus joins the stomach, some of the circular muscle fibers in its wall are thickened. These fibers are usually contracted and function to close the entrance to the stomach. In this way, they help prevent regurgitation of the stomach contents into the esophagus.

When peristaltic waves reach the stomach, the muscle fibers that guard its entrance relax and allow the food to enter.

1. Describe the regions of the pharynx.
2. List the major events that occur during swallowing.
3. Describe the structure and function of the esophagus.

The Stomach

The **stomach** is a J-shaped, pouchlike organ, about 25–30 centimeters long, that hangs under the diaphragm in the upper left portion of the abdominal cavity. It has a capacity of about one liter or more, and its inner lining is marked by thick folds (rugae) that tend to disappear when its wall is distended. The stomach receives food from the esophagus, mixes it with gastric juice, initiates the digestion of some food molecules, carries on a limited amount of absorption, and moves food into the small intestine.

In addition to the two layers of smooth muscle—an inner circular layer and an outer longitudinal layer—found in other regions of the alimentary canal, some parts of the stomach have another inner layer of oblique fibers. This third muscular layer is most highly developed near the opening of the esophagus and in the body of the stomach (figure 12.15).

Parts of the Stomach

The stomach, shown in figures 12.16 and 12.17, can be divided into the cardiac, fundic, body, and pyloric regions. The *cardiac region* is a small area near the esophageal

FIGURE 12.15
Some parts of the stomach have three layers of muscle fibers.

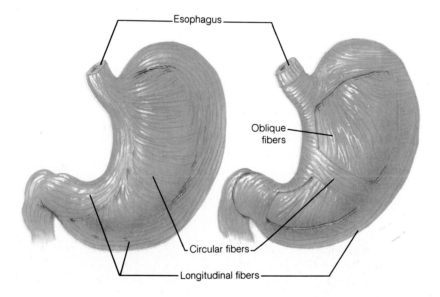

Esophagus

Oblique fibers

Circular fibers

Longitudinal fibers

FIGURE 12.16

Major regions of the stomach.

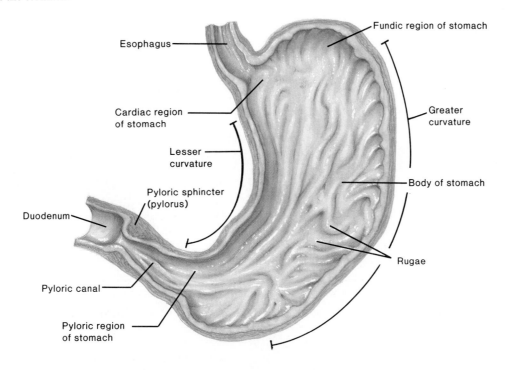

Esophagus

Fundic region of stomach

Cardiac region of stomach

Greater curvature

Lesser curvature

Body of stomach

Pyloric sphincter (pylorus)

Duodenum

Rugae

Pyloric canal

Pyloric region of stomach

FIGURE 12.17

X-ray film of a stomach. (Note: a radiopaque substance that was swallowed by the patient appears white in the X-ray film.)

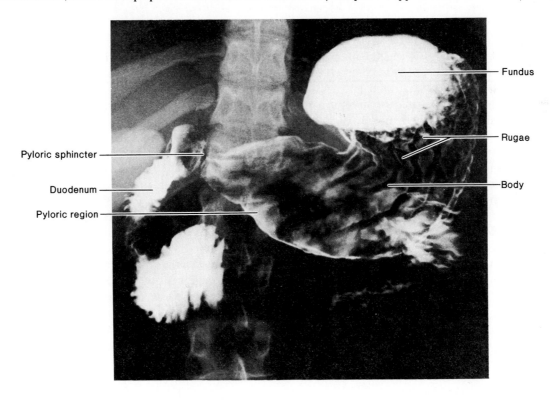

Pyloric sphincter

Fundus

Duodenum

Rugae

Pyloric region

Body

FIGURE 12.18

(*a*) The mucosa of the stomach is studded with gastric pits that are the openings of the gastric glands; (*b*) gastric glands include mucous cells, parietal cells, and chief cells.

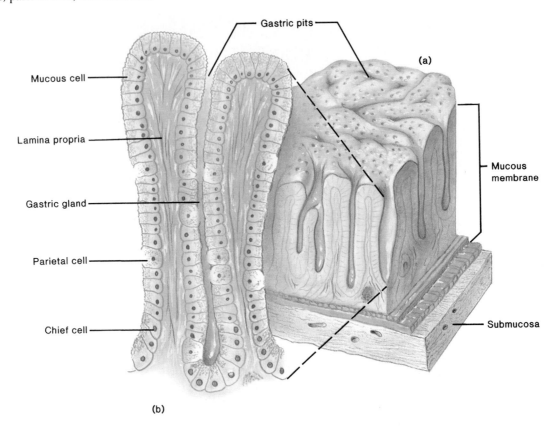

opening (cardia). The *fundic region,* which balloons above the cardiac portion, acts as a temporary storage area and sometimes becomes filled with swallowed air. This produces a gastric air bubble, which may be used as a landmark on an X-ray film of the abdomen. The dilated *body region,* which is the main part of the stomach, is located between the fundic and pyloric portions. The *pyloric region* (antrum) narrows and becomes the *pyloric canal* as it approaches the small intestine.

At the end of the pyloric canal, the circular layer of fibers in its muscular wall is thickened, forming a powerful muscle called the **pyloric sphincter** (pylorus). This muscle serves as a valve that prevents regurgitation of food from the intestine back into the stomach.

Gastric Glands

The mucous membrane that forms the inner lining of the stomach is relatively thick, and its surface is studded with many small openings. These openings, called *gastric pits,*

are located at the ends of tubular **gastric glands** (figure 12.18). Although their structure and the composition of their secretions vary in different parts of the stomach, gastric glands generally contain three types of secretory cells. One type, the *mucous cell,* occurs in the necks of the glands near the openings of the gastric pits. The other types, *chief cells* and *parietal cells,* are found in the deeper parts of the glands (figures 12.18 and 12.19). Chief cells secrete *digestive chemicals* (such as pepsin), and parietal cells release a strong acid (*hydrochloric acid*). The products of mucous cells, chief cells, and parietal cells together form **gastric juice.**

Mucous cells of the gastric glands secrete large quantities of mucus. In addition, the cells of the mucous membrane between these glands release a more viscous secretion that is thought to form a protective coating on the inside of the stomach wall. This coating is especially important because gastric juice is capable of digesting the stomach tissues as well as foods. Thus, the coating normally prevents the stomach from digesting itself.

FIGURE 12.19

Light micrograph of the stomach.

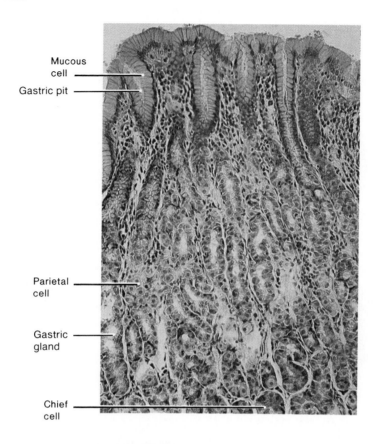

Mucous
cell

Gastric pit

Parietal
cell

Gastric
gland

Chief
cell

An *ulcer* is an open sore in the surface of an organ resulting from a localized breakdown of the tissues. Although ulcers may occur in various parts of the alimentary canal, they often develop in the stomach. Such *gastric ulcers* are most likely to develop in the wall of the lesser curvature.

Ulcers are also common in the first portion of the small intestine, the duodenum. *Duodenal ulcers* occur in regions that are exposed to gastric juice as the contents of the stomach enter the intestine. They often develop in people who are emotionally stressed and whose stomachs secrete excessive amounts of acidic gastric juice between meals.

Fortunately for ulcer victims, the cells of the mucosa are able to reproduce rapidly. In fact, the entire lining of the stomach is replaced every few days.

1. Where is the stomach located?
2. Describe the structure of a gastric gland.

Mixing and Emptying Actions

As more and more food enters the stomach, the smooth muscles in its wall become stretched. A person can eat more than the stomach can comfortably hold, and when this happens, the internal pressure may rise enough so that pain receptors are stimulated. The result is a stomachache.

Following a meal, the mixing movements of the stomach wall aid in producing a semifluid paste of food particles and gastric juice called **chyme** (kīm). Peristaltic waves push the chyme toward the pyloric region of the stomach, and as chyme accumulates near the pyloric sphincter, this muscle begins to relax. The muscular pyloric region then pumps the chyme a little at a time (5–15 ml) into the small intestine. This process is illustrated in figure 12.20.

1. What is chyme?
2. How does chyme leave the stomach?

FIGURE 12.20

(*a*) As the stomach fills, its muscular wall becomes stretched, but the pyloric sphincter remains closed; (*b*) mixing movements combine food and gastric juice, creating chyme; (*c*) peristaltic waves move the chyme toward the pyloric sphincter, which relaxes and allows some chyme to enter the duodenum.

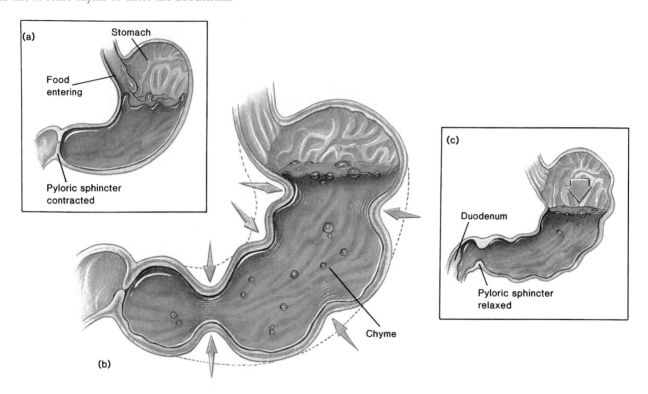

The Pancreas

The shape of the **pancreas** is described in chapter 11, as are its endocrine functions. The pancreas also has an exocrine function—the secretion of digestive juice.

The pancreas is closely associated with the small intestine and is located behind the parietal peritoneum. It extends horizontally across the posterior abdominal wall, with its head in the C-shaped curve of the duodenum and its tail against the spleen (figure 12.21 and reference plate 6).

The cells that produce pancreatic juice are called *pancreatic acinar cells,* and they make up the bulk of the pancreas. These cells are clustered around tiny tubes, into which they release their secretions. The smaller tubes unite to form larger ones, which, in turn, give rise to a *pancreatic duct* extending the length of the pancreas. This duct usually connects with the duodenum at the same place where the bile duct from the liver and gallbladder joins the duodenum. The pancreatic and bile ducts are joined by a short,

dilated tube called the *hepatopancreatic ampulla* (ampulla of Vater). This ampulla is surrounded by a band of smooth muscle, called the *hepatopancreatic sphincter* (sphincter of Oddi) (figures 11.18 and 12.21).

Cystic fibrosis is an inherited condition characterized by the production of very thick, sticky mucus that adversely affects various exocrine glands. For example, this viscid mucus tends to clog the ducts of the pancreas, which interferes with the secretion of pancreatic juice, prevents the pancreatic juice from reaching the duodenum, and leaves the person vulnerable to malnutrition. Cystic fibrosis is also commonly accompanied by excessive secretions of mucous glands within the respiratory tract, which may produce chronic obstruction of airways.

1. Where is the pancreas located?
2. How does pancreatic juice leave the pancreas?

FIGURE 12.21

(*a*) The pancreas is closely associated with the duodenum. (*b*) and (*c*) Pancreatic acinar cells secrete pancreatic juice. (*c*) ×50.

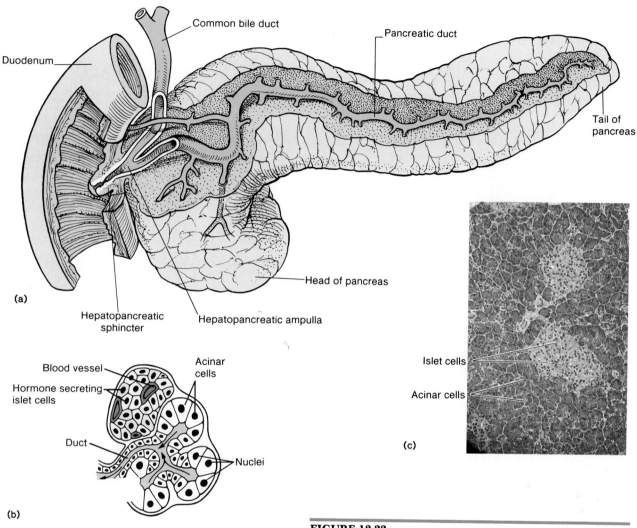

(a)

Common bile duct

Pancreatic duct

Duodenum

Tail of pancreas

Head of pancreas

Hepatopancreatic sphincter

Hepatopancreatic ampulla

Islet cells

Acinar cells

(c)

(b)

Blood vessel

Hormone secreting islet cells

Acinar cells

Duct

Nuclei

The Liver

The **liver** is the largest gland in the body and is located in the upper right and central portions of the abdominal cavity, just below the diaphragm. It is partially surrounded by the ribs and extends from the level of the fifth intercostal space to the lower margin of the ribs. It is reddish brown in color and is well supplied with blood vessels (figure 12.22).

FIGURE 12.22

The liver is partially surrounded by the ribs.

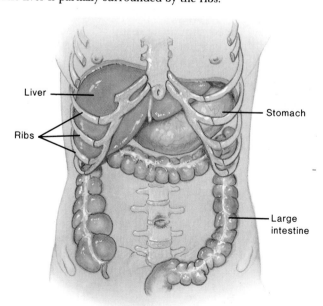

Liver

Ribs

Stomach

Large intestine

FIGURE 12.23
Lobes of the liver as viewed (*a*) from the front and (*b*) from below.

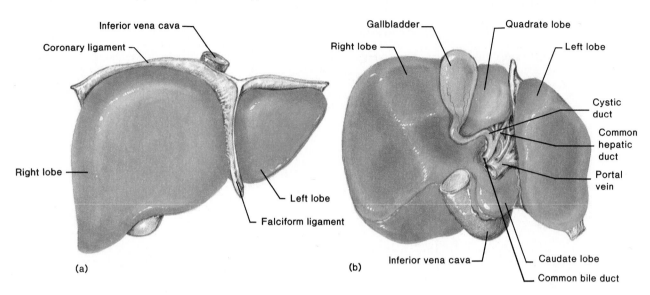

(a)

(b)

Structure of the Liver

The liver is enclosed in a fibrous capsule and is divided by connective tissue into *lobes*—a large right lobe and a smaller left lobe. These lobes are separated by the *falciform ligament,* a fold of visceral peritoneum that also fastens the liver to the abdominal wall, anteriorly. On its superior surface, the liver is attached to the diaphragm by a fold of visceral peritoneum called the *coronary ligament.* As figure 12.23 shows, in addition to the two major lobes, there are two minor ones—the *quadrate lobe* near the gallbladder, and the *caudate lobe* close to the vena cava.

Each lobe is separated into numerous tiny **hepatic lobules,** which are the functional units of the gland (figures 12.24 and 12.25). A lobule consists of numerous *hepatic cells* that radiate outward from a *central vein.* Platelike groups of these cells are separated from each other by blood vessels called **hepatic sinusoids.** The sinusoids are lined with endothelial cells that have large pores, or *fenestrae,* within the cells. Blood from the digestive tract, carried in *portal veins* (see chapter 14), brings newly absorbed nutrients and other substances into the sinusoids. As the blood flows through a sinusoid, these substances reach the hepatic cells by passing through the fenestrae. The hepatic cells destroy certain toxic and waste substances, store nutrients and release nutrients into the blood, and secrete proteins.

Usually the blood in the portal veins contains many bacterial cells that have entered through the intestinal wall. However, large **hepatic macrophages** (Kupffer cells) that are fixed to the endothelium of the hepatic sinusoids engulf and remove most of the bacteria from the blood. The blood then passes into the central veins of the hepatic lobules and moves out of the liver.

Within the liver lobules, are many fine *bile canals* that receive a secretion called bile from the hepatic cells. The canals of neighboring lobules unite to form larger ducts, and these converge to become the **hepatic ducts.** These ducts merge, in turn, to form the *common hepatic duct,* which carries bile out of the liver.

---

1. Describe the location of the liver.
2. Describe an hepatic lobule.
3. Name the ducts in which bile is moved from the hepatic cells out of the liver.

Substances can move readily from the blood in a hepatic sinusoid through the fenestrae, and reach the hepatic cells. However, these substances cannot move between the hepatic cells and into the bile canals. Such movement is prevented by tight junctions that occur on the sides of the hepatic cells and between the bile canals nearest them. Bile is secreted into the bile canals from the hepatic cells. In this way, bile secretions are kept separate from the blood passing through the liver.

The Gallbladder

The **gallbladder** is a pear-shaped sac located in a depression on the inferior surface of the liver. It is connected to the **cystic duct,** which, in turn, joins the common hepatic duct (figure 12.26). The gallbladder has a capacity of 30–50 ml, is lined with columnar epithelial cells, and has a strong muscular layer in its wall. It stores bile between meals, concentrates bile by reabsorbing water, and releases bile into the duodenum of the small intestine.

FIGURE 12.24

(a) A cross section of a hepatic lobule, which is the functional unit of the liver; (b) scanning electron micrograph of a liver section. R. G. Kessel and R. H. Kardon, *Tissues and Organs: A Text Atlas of Scanning Electron Microscopy,* © 1979, W. H. Freeman & Co.

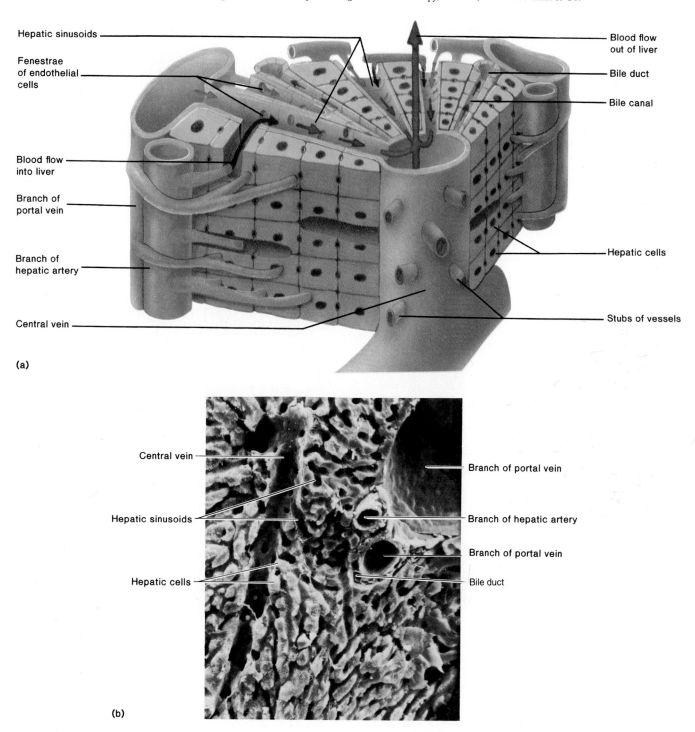

The gallbladder receives bile through the cystic duct. The union of the common hepatic and cystic ducts forms the **common bile duct**. It leads to the duodenum, where its exit is guarded by the hepatopancreatic sphincter. This sphincter normally remains contracted, so that bile collects in the common bile duct and backs up to the cystic duct. When this happens, the bile flows into the gallbladder and is stored there.

During the digestion of food, the gallbladder wall contracts and forces bile into the common bile duct. The hepatopancreatic sphincter relaxes, and bile enters the small intestine.

FIGURE 12.25

A light micrograph of hepatic lobules (×50). What features can you identify?

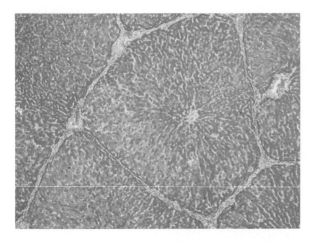

FIGURE 12.26

The gallbladder is located on the inferior surface of the liver.

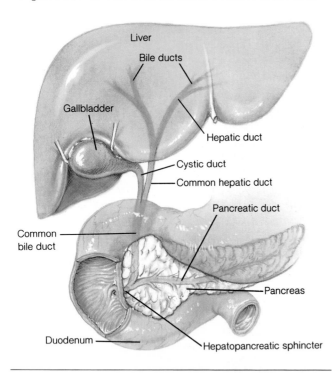

Gallstones form when bile is concentrated excessively, hepatic cells secrete too much cholesterol (which crystallizes), or if there is an inflammation in the gallbladder (cholecystitis). If such stones get into the bile duct, they may block the flow of bile, causing considerable pain and other complications (figure 12.27). Generally, gallstones that cause obstructions are surgically removed. The gallbladder is removed by a surgical procedure called *cholecystectomy*. Following such surgery, the person is unable to produce gallstones or store bile. However, bile continues to reach the intestine by means of the hepatic and common bile ducts.

FIGURE 12.27

X-ray film of a gallbladder that contains gallstones (arrow). What other anatomic features can you identify?

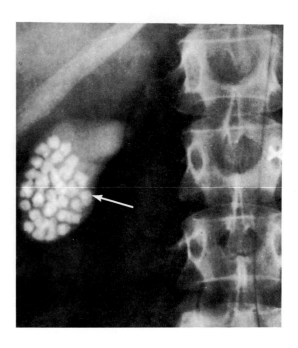

1. Describe the location of the gallbladder.
2. Describe the functions of the gallbladder.
3. Trace the flow of bile from the liver to the small intestine.

The Small Intestine

The **small intestine** is a tubular organ that extends from the pyloric sphincter to the beginning of the large intestine. With its many loops and coils, it fills much of the abdominal cavity. Although it is 5.5– 6.0 meters (18–20 feet) long in a cadaver when the muscular wall is relaxed, the small intestine may be only half this long in a living person.

As mentioned, this portion of the alimentary canal receives secretions from the pancreas and liver. It also completes the digestion of the nutrients in chyme, absorbs the various products of digestion, and transports the remaining residues to the large intestine.

Parts of the Small Intestine

The small intestine, shown in figures 12.28 and 12.29, consists of three portions: the duodenum, the jejunum, and the ileum.

The **duodenum,** (du″o-de′num) which is about 25 centimeters long and 5 centimeters in diameter, lies behind the parietal peritoneum (retroperitoneal). It is the shortest and the most fixed portion of the small intestine. It follows a C-shaped path as it passes in front of the right kidney and the upper three lumbar vertebrae.

FIGURE 12.28

The small intestine includes the duodenum, jejunum, and ileum.

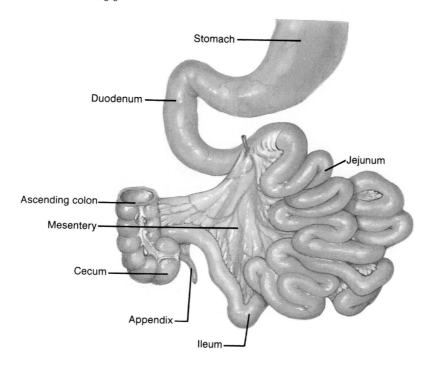

FIGURE 12.29

X-ray film of a normal small intestine.

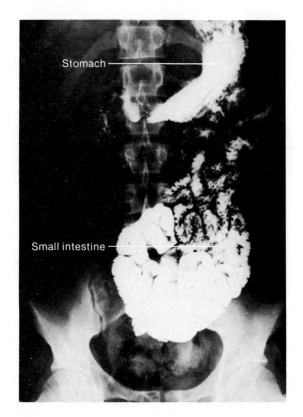

The remainder of the small intestine is mobile and lies free in the peritoneal cavity. The proximal 2/5 of this portion is the **jejunum** (je-ju′num), and the remainder is the **ileum.** Although there is no distinct separation between the jejunum and ileum, the diameter of the jejunum tends to be greater, and its wall is thicker, more vascular, and more active than that of the ileum. The jejunum and ileum are suspended from the posterior abdominal wall by a double-layered fold of peritoneum called mesentery (figure 12.30). This supporting tissue contains the blood vessels, nerves, and lymphatic vessels that supply the intestinal wall.

A filmy fold of peritoneal membrane, called the *greater omentum,* drapes like an apron from the stomach over the transverse colon and the folds of the small intestine (figures 12.30 and 12.31). If infections occur in the wall of the alimentary canal, cells from the omentum may adhere to the inflamed region and help wall it off so that the infection is less likely to enter the peritoneal cavity. The greater omentum also contains a large amount of fat. Another fold of the peritoneum, the *lesser omentum,* connects the stomach and a portion of the duodenum to the liver.

Structure of the Small Intestinal Wall

Throughout its length, the inner wall of the small intestine has a velvety appearance. This is due to the presence of innumerable tiny projections of the mucous membrane called **intestinal villi** (sing. *villus*) (figure 12.32). These

FIGURE 12.30

Portions of the small intestine are suspended from the posterior abdominal wall by mesentery formed by folds of the peritoneal membrane.

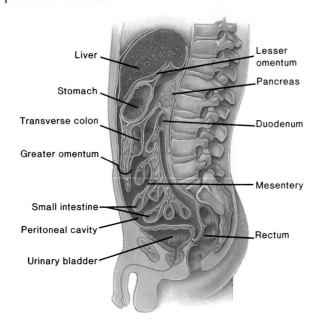

FIGURE 12.31

The greater omentum hangs like an apron over the abdominal organs.

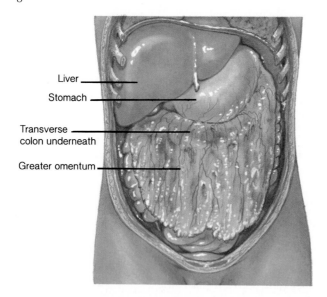

structures are most numerous in the duodenum and the proximal portion of the jejunum. They project into the passageway, or **lumen,** of the alimentary canal contacting the intestinal contents. Villi increase the surface area of the intestinal lining and play an important role in the absorption of digestive products.

Each villus consists of a layer of simple columnar epithelium and a core of connective tissue containing blood

FIGURE 12.32

Structure of a single intestinal villus. What is the function of such projections?

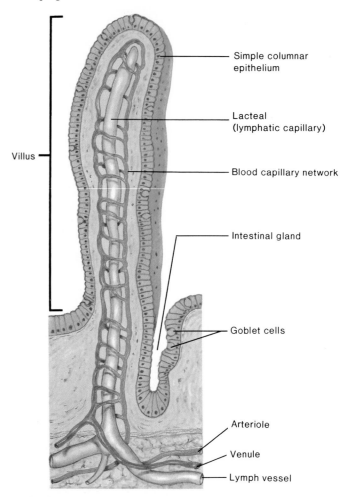

capillaries, a lymphatic capillary called a **lacteal,** and nerve fibers. At their free surfaces, the epithelial cells possess many fine extensions, called *microvilli,* that create a brush-like border and greatly increase the surface area of the intestinal cells (figures 12.33 and 12.34). The presence of microvilli enhances the process of absorption.

Tight junctions are found between the cells of the intestinal mucosa. These junctions prevent food molecules from moving between intestinal cells. The products of digestion are moved through the epithelial cells to the blood vessels or to the lacteal of a villus.

The blood and lymph capillaries carry away substances absorbed by a villus, while the nerve fibers act to stimulate or inhibit its activities.

Between the bases of adjacent villi are tubular *intestinal glands* (crypts of Lieberkühn) that extend downward into the mucous membrane. The deeper layers of the small intestinal wall are much like those of other parts of the alimentary canal in that they include a submucosa, a

FIGURE 12.33

Light micrograph of the small intestine. (*a*) Villi (×50); (*b*) a single villus.

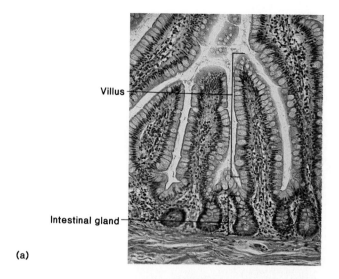

(a)

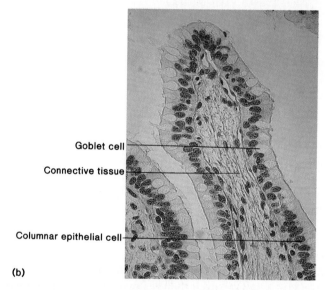

Goblet cell
Connective tissue
Columnar epithelial cell

(b)

FIGURE 12.34

(*a*) Microvilli increase the surface area of intestinal epithelial cells; (*b*) transmission electron micrograph of microvilli at the free surface of the columnar epithelial cells.

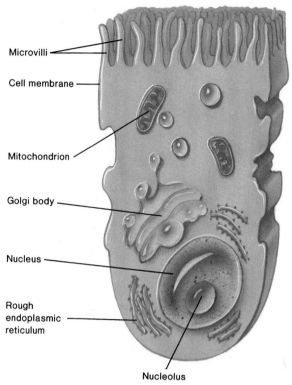

Microvilli
Cell membrane
Mitochondrion
Golgi body
Nucleus
Rough endoplasmic reticulum
Nucleolus

(a)

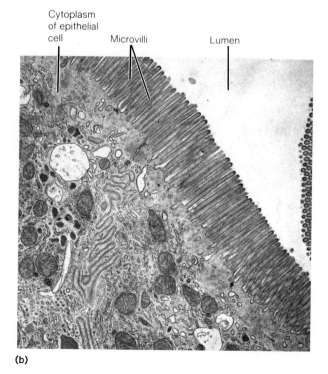

Cytoplasm of epithelial cell
Microvilli
Lumen

(b)

muscular layer, and a serous layer. In addition to the mucous-secreting goblet cells that occur extensively throughout the mucosa, there are many specialized *mucous-secreting glands* (Brunner's glands) that occur in the submucosa within the proximal portion of the duodenum.

The lining of the small intestine also is characterized by the presence of numerous circular folds, called *plicae circulares,* which are especially well-developed in the lower duodenum and upper jejunum. Together with the villi and microvilli, these folds help increase the surface area of the intestinal lining (figure 12.35).

Because villi greatly increase the surface area of the intestinal mucosa, the small intestine is the most important absorbing organ of the alimentary canal. In fact, the small intestine is so effective at absorbing digestive products, water, and electrolytes, that very little absorbable material reaches its distal end.

FIGURE 12.35

(a) The inner lining of the small intestine contains many circular folds, the plicae circulares; (b) a longitudinal section through some of these folds.

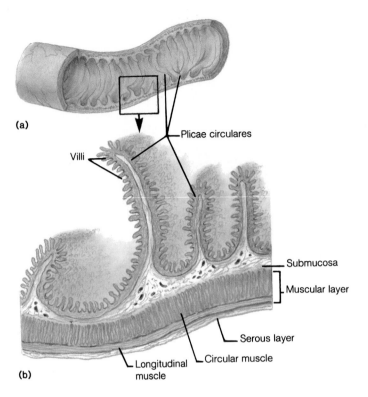

(a)

Plicae circulares

Villi

Submucosa

Muscular layer

Serous layer

Circular muscle

Longitudinal muscle

(b)

The cells of the intestinal glands are undifferentiated columnar epithelial cells. These cells divide and are pushed up along the villi, where they differentiate into absorptive cells and goblet cells. It takes three to five days for these cells to move from the intestinal glands to the tips of the villi, where the cells are shed. (See figure 12.36.) In this way, the small intestine's mucosa is continually replaced. This is important since cells at the tips of the villi are damaged rapidly by their contact with chyme and digestive juices.

1. Describe the parts of the small intestine.
2. Distinguish between intestinal villi and microvilli.
3. What is the function of the intestinal glands?

Movements of the Small Intestine

Like the stomach, the small intestine carries on *mixing movements* and *peristalsis.* The major mixing movement is called *segmentation.* It involves the formation of small, ring-like contractions that occur periodically, cutting the chyme into segments and moving it to and fro. Segmentation also serves to slow the movement of chyme through the intestine.

The chyme is propelled through the small intestine by peristaltic waves. These waves are usually weak and they stop after pushing the chyme a short distance. Consequently, food materials move relatively slowly through the small intestine, taking from three to ten hours to travel its length.

As might be expected, parasympathetic impulses enhance both mixing and peristaltic movements, and sympathetic impulses inhibit them. Reflexes involving parasympathetic impulses to the small intestine sometimes originate in the stomach. For example, as the stomach fills with food and its wall becomes distended, a reflex (gastroenteric reflex) is triggered, and peristaltic activity in the small intestine is greatly increased. Another reflex is initiated when the duodenum is filled with chyme and its wall is stretched. This causes the chyme to be moved through the small intestine more rapidly.

At the distal end of the small intestine, where the ileum joins the cecum of the large intestine, there is a sphincter muscle called the **ileocecal valve.** Normally this sphincter remains constricted, preventing the contents of the small intestine from entering the large intestine. At the same time, it prevents the contents of the large intestine from backing up into the ileum. After a meal, a *gastroileal reflex* is elicited, and peristalsis in the ileum is increased. This action forces some of the contents of the small intestine into the cecum.

FIGURE 12.36

The intestinal mucosa is continually replaced by new cells that originate in the intestinal glands.

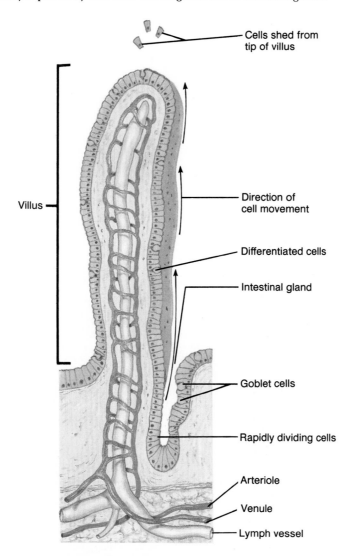

Cells shed from tip of villus

Villus

Direction of cell movement

Differentiated cells

Intestinal gland

Goblet cells

Rapidly dividing cells

Arteriole

Venule

Lymph vessel

---

1. Describe the movements of the small intestine.
2. How are these movements of the small intestine initiated?
3. What stimulus causes the ileocecal valve to relax?

The Large Intestine

The **large intestine** is so named because its diameter is greater than that of the small intestine. This portion of the alimentary canal is about 1.5 meters long and begins in the lower right side of the abdominal cavity, where the ileum joins the cecum. From there, the large intestine travels upward on the right side, crosses obliquely to the left, and descends into the pelvis. At its distal end, the large intestine opens to the outside of the body as the anus.

The large intestine reabsorbs water and electrolytes from the chyme remaining in the alimentary canal. It also forms and stores the feces until defecation occurs.

Parts of the Large Intestine

The large intestine, shown in figure 12.37, consists of the cecum, colon, rectum, and anal canal.

The **cecum,** which represents the beginning of the large intestine, is a dilated, pouchlike structure that hangs slightly below the ileocecal opening. Projecting downward

FIGURE 12.37
Parts of the large intestine (anterior view).

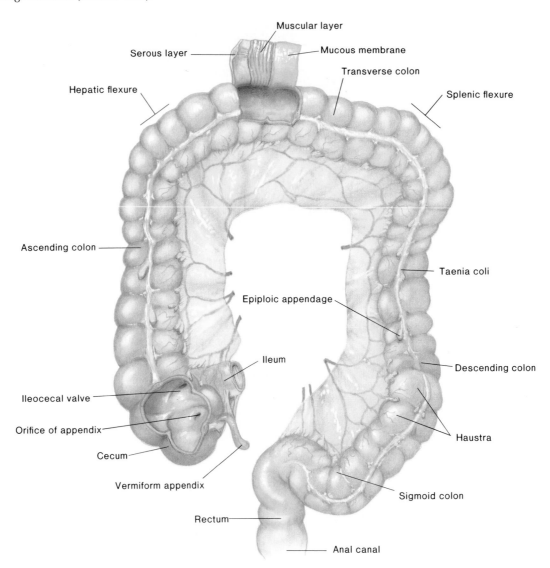

The **colon** is divided into four portions—ascending, transverse, descending, and sigmoid colons. The **ascending colon** begins at the cecum and travels upward against the posterior abdominal wall to a point just below the liver. There it turns sharply to the left (as the hepatic, or right colic, flexure) and becomes the transverse colon. The **transverse colon** is the longest and the most mobile part of the large intestine. It is suspended by a fold of peritoneum (mesocolon) and tends to sag in the middle below the stomach. As the transverse colon approaches the spleen, it turns abruptly downward (as the splenic, or left colic, flexure) and becomes the **descending colon.** At the brim of the pelvis, the descending colon makes an S-shaped curve, called the **sigmoid** colon, and then becomes the rectum. (See figure 1.14.)

from it is a narrow tube with a closed end, called the **vermiform appendix.** Although the human appendix has no digestive function, it does contain lymphatic tissue that can serve to resist infections.

> Occasionally the appendix itself may become infected and inflamed, a condition called *appendicitis*. Inflammation of the appendix results in pain that is often referred to the umbilical region. If the inflammation spreads to the parietal peritoneum, the pain is usually felt directly over the inflamed area. (See chapter 10.) An infected appendix is often removed surgically to prevent it from rupturing. If it does break open, the contents of the large intestine may enter the abdominal cavity and cause a serious infection of the peritoneum, called *peritonitis.*

FIGURE 12.38
The rectum and anal canal are located at the distal end of the alimentary canal.

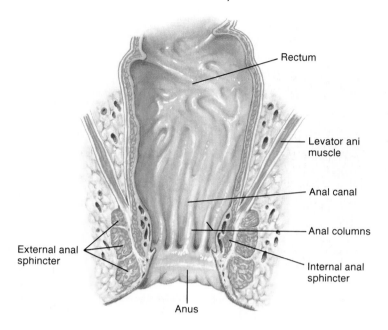

The **rectum** lies next to the sacrum and generally follows its curvature. It is firmly attached to the sacrum by the peritoneum, and ends about 5 centimeters below the tip of the coccyx, where it becomes the anal canal (figure 12.38).

The **anal canal** is formed by the last 2.5 to 4.0 centimeters of the large intestine. The mucous membrane in the canal is folded into a series of six to eight longitudinal *anal columns*. At its distal end, the canal opens to the outside as the anus. This opening is guarded by two sphincter muscles, an *internal anal sphincter* composed of smooth muscle under involuntary control, and an *external anal sphincter* of skeletal muscle, under voluntary control.

Each anal column contains a branch of the rectal vein, and if something interferes with the blood flow in these vessels, the anal columns may become enlarged and inflamed. This condition, called *hemorrhoids,* may be aggravated by bowel movements and may be accompanied by discomfort and bleeding.

---

1. What is the general function of the large intestine?
2. Describe the parts of the large intestine.
3. Distinguish between the internal and external anal sphincters.

Structure of the Large Intestinal Wall

Although the wall of the large intestine includes the same types of tissues found in other parts of the alimentary canal, it has some unique features. For example, it lacks the villi that are characteristic of the small intestine. Also, the layer of longitudinal muscle fibers does not cover its wall uniformly. Instead, the fibers are arranged in three distinct bands (taeniae coli) that extend the entire length of the colon. These bands exert tension on the wall, creating a series of pouches (haustra). The large intestinal wall also is characterized by small collections of fat (epiploic appendages) in the serous layer on its outer surface (figure 12.37).

Functions of the Large Intestine

Unlike the small intestine, which secretes digestive juice and absorbs the products of digestion, the large intestine has little or no digestive function. The mucous membrane that forms the inner lining of the large intestine, however, contains many tubular glands. Structurally, these glands are similar to those of the small intestine, but they are composed almost entirely of goblet cells. Consequently, mucus is the only significant secretion of this portion of the alimentary canal (figures 12.39, 12.40, and 12.41).

Absorption in the large intestine is normally limited to water and a few other substances, which are usually absorbed in the proximal half of the tube.

FIGURE 12.39

A scanning electron micrograph of the large intestine mucosa. Notice the openings of the goblet cells (arrow).
R. G. Kessel and R. H. Kardon, *Tissues and Organs: A Text Atlas of Scanning Electron Microscopy,* © 1979, W. H. Freeman & Co.

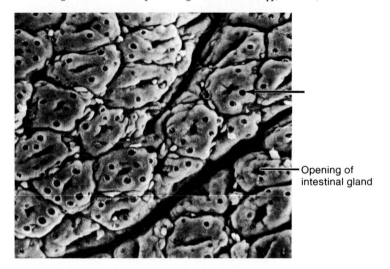

Opening of intestinal gland

FIGURE 12.40

A light micrograph of the large intestine wall (✕10).

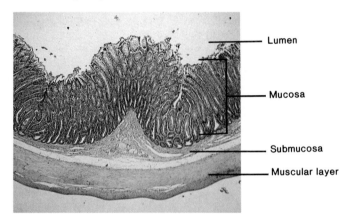

Lumen

Mucosa

Submucosa

Muscular layer

FIGURE 12.41

Light micrograph of the mucosa of the large intestine.

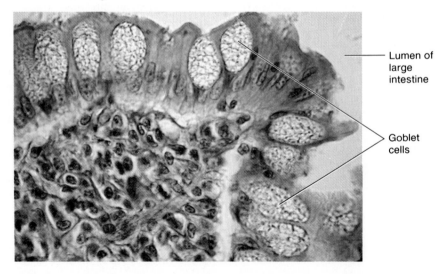

Lumen of large intestine

Goblet cells

Movements of the Large Intestine

The movements of the large intestine—mixing and peristalsis—are similar to those of the small intestine, although they are usually more sluggish. The mixing movements break the fecal matter into segments and turn it so that all portions are exposed to the mucosa. This helps in water and electrolyte absorption.

The peristaltic waves of the large intestine are different from those in the small intestine. Instead of occurring frequently, they come only two or three times each day. These waves produce *mass movements* in which a relatively large section of the colon constricts vigorously, forcing its contents to move toward the rectum. Typically, mass movements occur following a meal, as a result of a reflex that is initiated in the small intestine (duodenocolic reflex). Abnormal irritations of the mucosa can also trigger such movements. For instance, a person suffering from an inflamed colon (colitis) may experience frequent mass movements.

The substances that are discharged from the digestive tube are called *feces;* they are composed largely of materials that were not digested or absorbed, along with water, electrolytes, mucus, and bacteria.

Sometimes the mucosa of the large intestine becomes extensively ulcerated, and the person is said to have *ulcerative colitis.* The cause of this condition is unknown, but it is often associated with prolonged periods of emotional stress. In this condition, the colon becomes very active, mass movements occur frequently, and the person has diarrhea most of the time.

Treatment for ulcerative colitis involves reducing nervous tension, changing the diet, and providing medication. If such measures are unsuccessful, a surgeon may perform an *ileostomy,* in which the colon is removed and a portion of the ileum is connected to an opening in the abdominal wall. As a result, the small intestinal contents can move to the outside of the body without passing through the colon.

A related procedure, called *colostomy,* is sometimes performed in cases of abscesses of the colon or intestinal obstructions, or following removal of the rectum. In this procedure, the colon is connected to an opening on the surface of the abdomen so that the rectum and anus are bypassed.

Clinical Terms Related to the Digestive System

achalasia (ak″ah-la′ze-ah)   failure of the smooth muscle to relax at some junction in the digestive tube, such as that between the esophagus and stomach.

aphagia (ah-fa′je-ah)   an inability to swallow.

cholecystitis (ko″le-sis-ti′tis)   inflammation of the gallbladder.

cholelithiasis (ko″le-lĭ-thi′ah-sis)   the presence of stones in the gallbladder.

cirrhosis (si-ro′sis)   a liver condition in which the hepatic cells degenerate and the surrounding connective tissues thicken.

diverticulitis (di″ver-tik″u-li′tis)   inflammation of small pouches (diverticula) that sometimes form in the lining and wall of the colon.

dysphagia (dis-fa′ze-ah)   difficulty in swallowing.

enteritis (en″tĕ-ri′tis)   inflammation of the intestine.

esophagitis (e-sof″ah-ji′tis)   inflammation of the esophagus.

gastrectomy (gas-trek′to-me)   partial or complete removal of the stomach.

gastritis (gas-tri′tis)   inflammation of the stomach lining.

gastrostomy (gas-tros′to-me)   the creation of an opening in the stomach wall through which food and liquids may be administered when swallowing is not possible.

gingivitis (jin″ji-vi′tis)   inflammation of the gums.

glossitis (glŏ-si′tis)   inflammation of the tongue.

hemorrhoidectomy (hem″ŏ-roi-dek′to-me)   removal of hemorrhoids.

hepatitis (hep″ah-ti′tis)   inflammation of the liver.

ileitis (il″e-i′tis)   inflammation of the ileum.

ileus (il′e-us)   an obstruction of the intestine due to an inhibition of motility or a mechanical cause.

pharyngitis (far″in-ji′tis)   inflammation of the pharynx.

proctitis (prok-ti′tis)   inflammation of the rectum.

pyloric stenosis (pi-lor′ik stĕ-no′sis)   a congenital obstruction at the pyloric sphincter due to an enlargement of the pyloric muscle.

pylorospasm (pi-lor′o-spazm)   a spasm of the pyloric portion of the stomach or the pyloric sphincter.

pyorrhea (pi″o-re′ah)   an inflammation of the dental periosteum.

stomatitis (sto″mah-ti′tis)   inflammation of the lining of the mouth.

vagotomy (va-got′o-me)   sectioning of the vagus nerve fibers.

Chapter Summary

Introduction (page 386)

Digestion is the process of changing food substances into forms that can be absorbed. The digestive system consists of an alimentary canal and several accessory organs.

General Characteristics of the Alimentary Canal (page 386)

Various regions of the canal are specialized to perform specific functions.

1. Structure of the wall
   a. The wall consists of four layers.
   b. These layers are the mucous membrane, submucosa, muscular layer, and serous layer.
   c. The visceral peritoneum forms double-layered folds of mesentery and extends beyond the organs to form curtainlike omenta.
2. Movements of the tube
   a. Motor functions include mixing and propelling movements.
   b. Peristalsis is responsible for propelling movements.
   c. The wall of the tube undergoes receptive relaxation just ahead of a peristaltic wave.
3. Innervation of the tube
   a. The tube is innervated by branches of the sympathetic and parasympathetic divisions of the autonomic nervous system.
   b. Parasympathetic impulses generally cause an increase in digestive activities; sympathetic impulses generally inhibit digestive activities.
   c. Sympathetic impulses are responsible for the contraction of certain sphincter muscles that control movement through the alimentary canal.

The Mouth (page 389)

The mouth is adapted to receive food and begin preparing it for digestion. It also serves as an organ of speech and pleasure.

1. The cheeks and lips
   a. Cheeks form the lateral walls of the mouth.
   b. Lips are highly mobile and possess a variety of sensory receptors useful in judging the characteristics of food.
2. The tongue
   a. The tongue is a thick, muscular organ that aids in mixing food with saliva and moving it toward the pharynx.
   b. Its rough surface aids in handling food and contains taste buds.
   c. Lingual tonsils are located on the root of the tongue.
3. The palate
   a. The palate comprises the roof of the mouth, and includes hard and soft portions.
   b. The soft palate closes the opening to the nasal cavity during swallowing.
   c. Palatine tonsils are located on either side of the tongue in the back of the mouth.
   d. Tonsils consist of lymphatic tissues, but are common sites of infections and may become enlarged so that they interfere with swallowing and breathing.

4. The teeth
   a. Two sets develop in sockets of the mandibular and maxillary bones.
   b. There are twenty primary and thirty-two secondary teeth.
   c. They break food into smaller pieces, thus increasing the surface area exposed to digestive actions.
   d. Different teeth are adapted to handle foods in different ways, such as biting, grasping, or grinding.
   e. Each tooth consists of a crown and root, and is composed of enamel, dentin, pulp, nerves, and blood vessels.
   f. A tooth is attached to the alveolar bone by collagenous fibers of the periodontal ligament.

The Salivary Glands (page 393)

Salivary glands secrete saliva, which moistens food, helps bind food particles together, begins digestion, makes taste possible, and helps cleanse the mouth.

1. Salivary secretions
   a. Salivary glands include serous cells that secrete a digestive chemical and mucous cells that secrete mucus.
   b. Parasympathetic impulses stimulate the secretion of serous fluid.
2. Major salivary glands
   a. The parotid glands are the largest, and they secrete watery saliva.
   b. The submandibular glands in the floor of the mouth produce viscid saliva.
   c. The sublingual glands in the floor of the mouth primarily secrete mucus.

The Pharynx and Esophagus (page 395)

The pharynx and esophagus serve only as passageways.

1. Structure of the pharynx
   a. The pharynx is divided into a nasopharynx, oropharynx, and laryngopharynx.
   b. The muscular walls of the pharynx contain fibers arranged in circular and longitudinal groups.
2. The swallowing mechanism
   a. In the first stage, food is mixed with saliva and forced into the pharynx.
   b. In the second stage, involuntary reflexes move the food into the esophagus.
   c. In the third stage, food is transported to the stomach.
3. The esophagus
   a. The esophagus passes through the mediastinum and penetrates the diaphragm.
   b. Circular muscle fibers at the end of the esophagus help prevent the regurgitation of food from the stomach.

The Stomach (page 398)

The stomach receives food, mixes it with gastric juice, carries on a limited amount of absorption, and moves food into the small intestine.

1. Parts of the stomach
   a. The stomach is divided into cardiac, fundic, body, and pyloric regions.
   b. The pyloric sphincter serves as a valve between the stomach and the small intestine.

2. Gastric glands contain mucous cells, chief cells, and parietal cells, and secrete gastric juice.
3. Mixing and emptying actions
   a. Mixing movements aid in producing chyme; peristaltic waves move the chyme into the pyloric region.
   b. The muscular wall of the pyloric region pumps chyme into the small intestine.

The Pancreas (page 402)
The pancreas is closely associated with the duodenum.

1. It produces pancreatic juice that is secreted into a pancreatic duct.
2. The pancreatic duct leads to the duodenum.

The Liver (page 403)
The liver is the largest gland in the body.

1. Structure of the liver
   a. The liver is a highly vascular organ, enclosed in a fibrous capsule, and divided into lobes.
   b. Each lobe contains hepatic lobules, which are the functional units of the liver.
   c. Bile from the lobules is carried by bile canals to hepatic ducts, which unite to form the common bile duct.
2. The gallbladder
   a. The gallbladder stores bile between meals.
   b. Release of bile from the common bile duct is controlled by a sphincter muscle.

The Small Intestine (page 406)
The small intestine extends from the pyloric sphincter to the large intestine. It receives secretions from the pancreas and liver, completes the digestion of nutrients, absorbs the products of digestion, and transports the residues to the large intestine.

1. Parts of the small intestine
   a. The small intestine consists of the duodenum, jejunum, and ileum.
   b. It is suspended from the posterior abdominal wall by mesentery.
2. Structure of the small intestinal wall
   a. The wall is lined with villi that increase its surface area, and aid in mixing and absorption.
   b. Microvilli on the free ends of epithelial cells greatly increase the surface area.
   c. Intestinal glands are located between the villi.
   d. Circular folds in the lining of the intestinal wall also increase its surface area.
3. Movements of the small intestine
   a. Movements include mixing by segmentation and peristalsis.
   b. The ileocecal valve controls movement from the small intestine into the large intestine.

The Large Intestine (page 411)
The large intestine reabsorbs water and electrolytes, and forms and stores feces.

1. Parts of the large intestine
   a. The large intestine consists of the cecum, colon, rectum, and anal canal.
   b. The colon is divided into ascending, transverse, descending, and sigmoid portions.

2. Structure of the large intestinal wall
   a. Basically, the large intestinal wall is like the wall in other parts of the alimentary canal.
   b. Unique features include a layer of longitudinal muscle fibers that are arranged in distinct bands.
3. Functions of the large intestine
   a. The large intestine has little or no digestive function, although it secretes mucus.
   b. Absorption in the large intestine is generally limited to water and a few other substances.
4. Movements of the large intestine
   a. Movements are similar to those in the small intestine.
   b. Mass movements occur two to three times each day.
5. Feces consist largely of undigested material, water, electrolytes, mucus, and bacteria.

Clinical Application of Knowledge

1. If 95% of a patient's stomach is removed (subtotal gastrectomy), as treatment for severe ulcers or cancer, how would digestion and absorption of foods be affected? How would the patient's eating habits have to be altered? Why?
2. Why is it that a person with inflammation of the gallbladder (cholecystitis) may also develop an inflammation of the pancreas (pancreatitis)?
3. Celiac disease results in destruction of villi. How would this affect a person's digestion and absorption of food?
4. Dentists usually recommend using a soft bristle tooth brush. Explain the reason for this recommendation.

Review Activities

1. List and describe the location of the major parts of the alimentary canal.
2. List and describe the location of the accessory organs of the digestive system.
3. Name the four layers of the wall of the alimentary canal.
4. Distinguish between mixing movements and propelling movements.
5. Define *peristalsis*.
6. Explain the relationship between peristalsis and receptive relaxation.
7. Describe the general effects of parasympathetic and sympathetic impulses on the alimentary canal.
8. Discuss the functions of the mouth and its parts.
9. Distinguish between lingual, palatine, and pharyngeal tonsils.
10. Compare the primary and secondary teeth.
11. Explain how teeth are adapted to perform specialized functions.
12. Describe the structure of a tooth.
13. Explain how a tooth is anchored in its socket.
14. List and describe the locations of the major salivary glands.
15. Explain how the cell types and secretions of the salivary glands differ.

16. Name and locate the three major regions of the pharynx.
17. Describe the mechanism of swallowing.
18. Explain the function of the esophagus.
19. Describe the structure of the stomach.
20. Describe the mechanism that controls the emptying of the stomach.
21. Describe the location of the pancreas and the pancreatic duct.
22. Describe the structure of the liver.

23. List and describe the location of the parts of the small intestine.
24. Distinguish between villi and microvilli, and explain their functions.
25. Explain how the movement of the intestinal contents is controlled.
26. List and describe the location of the parts of the large intestine.
27. Explain the general functions of the large intestine.

CHAPTER 13

The Respiratory System

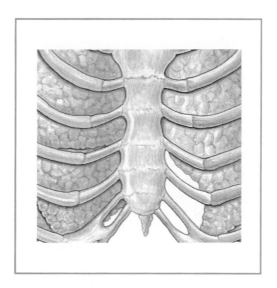

Before body cells can use nutrients and release energy, they must be supplied with oxygen, and the waste product carbon dioxide must be excreted. These two processes—obtaining oxygen and removing carbon dioxide—are the primary functions of the *respiratory system.*

In addition, the respiratory organs filter particles from incoming air, help control the temperature and water content of the air, aid in producing vocal sounds, and play an important role in the sense of smell.

Chapter Outline

Chapter Objectives

After you have studied this chapter, you should be able to

1. List the general functions of the respiratory system.

2. Name and describe the locations of the organs of the respiratory system.

3. Describe the functions of each organ of the respiratory system.

4. Describe the structure and function of the respiratory membrane.

5. Explain how inspiration and expiration are accomplished.

6. Locate the respiratory center and explain how it controls normal breathing.

7. Complete the review activities at the end of this chapter. Note that the items are worded in the form of specific learning objectives. You may want to refer to them before reading the chapter.

Aids to Understanding Words

alveol-, a small cavity: *alveolus*—a microscopic air sac within a lung.

bronch-, the windpipe: *bronchus*—a primary branch of the trachea.

carcin-, a spreading sore: *carcin*oma—a type of cancer.

carin-, keel-like: *carin*a—a ridge of cartilage between the right and left bronchi.

cric-, a ring: *cric*oid cartilage—a ring-shaped mass of cartilage at the base of the larynx.

epi-, upon: *epi*glottis—a flaplike structure that partially covers the opening into the larynx during swallowing.

pulmo-, lung: broncho*pulmo*nary segment—a subdivision of a lung.

tuber-, a swelling: *tuber*culosis—a disease characterized by the formation of fibrous masses within the lungs.

Introduction

The **respiratory system** consists of a group of passages that filter incoming air and transport it from outside the body into the lungs, and numerous microscopic air sacs in which gas exchanges take place. The entire process of exchanging gases between the atmosphere and the body cells is called **respiration.**

Organs of the Respiratory System

The organs of the respiratory system include the nose, nasal cavity, sinuses, pharynx, larynx, trachea, bronchial tree, and lungs.

The parts of the respiratory system, shown in figure 13.1, can be divided into two sets, or *tracts.* Organs outside the thorax constitute the *upper respiratory tract,* and those within the thorax comprise the *lower respiratory tract.*

The Nose

The nose is covered with skin and is supported internally by bone and cartilage (figure 13.2). The *lateral* and *alar cartilages* form most of the framework of the nose. The *septal cartilage* helps divide the nose into two chambers called *nostrils.* Its two nostrils (external nares) provide openings through which air enters and exits the nasal cavity. These openings are guarded by numerous internal hairs that help prevent the entrance of relatively coarse particles sometimes carried in the air.

The Nasal Cavity

The **nasal cavity,** a hollow space within and behind the nose, is divided medially into right and left portions by the bony **nasal septum.** This cavity is separated from the cranial cavity by the cribriform plate of the ethmoid bone and from the mouth by the hard palate.

> The nasal septum is usually straight at birth, although it is sometimes bent as the result of a birth injury. It remains straight throughout early childhood, but as a person ages, the septum tends to bend toward one side or the other. Such a *deviated septum* may create an obstruction in the nasal cavity that makes breathing difficult.

FIGURE 13.1
Organs of the respiratory system.

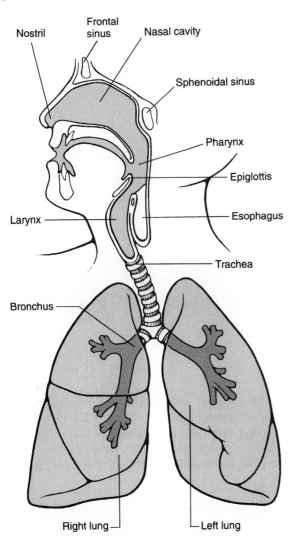

FIGURE 13.2
The nose is supported by cartilage and bone.

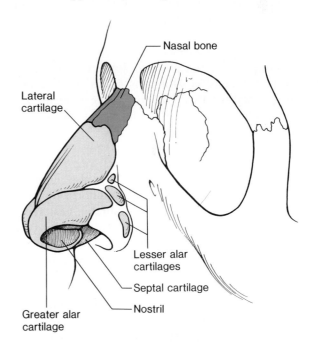

FIGURE 13.3

Major features of the upper respiratory tract.

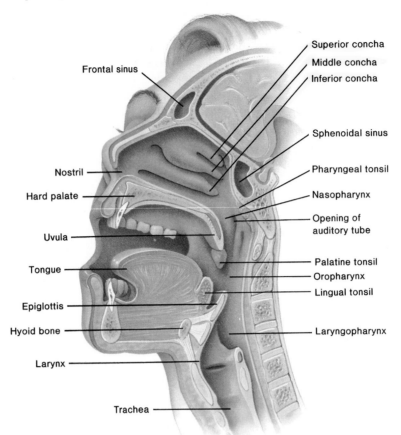

Frontal sinus

Superior concha
Middle concha
Inferior concha

Sphenoidal sinus

Nostril

Hard palate

Pharyngeal tonsil

Nasopharynx

Opening of auditory tube

Uvula

Tongue

Palatine tonsil
Oropharynx
Lingual tonsil

Epiglottis

Hyoid bone

Laryngopharynx

Larynx

Trachea

As figure 13.3 shows, **nasal conchae** (turbinate bones) curl out from the lateral walls of the nasal cavity on each side, dividing the cavity into passageways called the *superior, middle,* and *inferior meatuses* (see figure 6.31). They also support the mucous membrane that lines the nasal cavity and help increase its surface area.

The upper posterior portion of the nasal cavity, below the cribriform plate, is slitlike, and its lining contains the olfactory receptors that function in the sense of smell. The remainder of the cavity conducts air to and from the nasopharynx.

The mucous membrane lining the nasal cavity contains pseudostratified ciliated epithelium, rich in mucus-secreting goblet cells (see chapter 5). It also includes an extensive network of blood vessels, and normally appears pinkish. As air passes over the membrane, heat radiates from the blood and warms the air. In addition, the incoming air becomes moistened by evaporation of water from the mucous lining. The sticky mucus secreted by the mucous membrane entraps dust and other small particles entering with the air.

As the cilia of the epithelial cells move, a thin layer of mucus and any entrapped particles are pushed toward the pharynx (figure 13.4). When the mucus reaches the pharynx, it is swallowed. In the stomach, any microorgan-

FIGURE 13.4

Cilia move mucus and trapped particles from the nasal cavity to the pharynx.

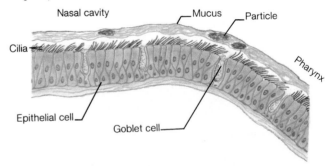

Nasal cavity

Mucus

Particle

Cilia

Pharynx

Epithelial cell

Goblet cell

isms in the mucus, including disease-causing forms, are likely to be destroyed by the action of gastric juice. Thus, the filtering mechanism provided by the mucous membrane not only prevents particles from reaching the lower air passages, but also helps prevent respiratory infections.

1. What is meant by respiration?
2. What organs constitute the respiratory system?
3. What is the function of the mucous membrane that lines the nasal cavity?
4. What is the function of the cilia in the cells that line the nasal cavity?

The Sinuses

As discussed in chapter 6, the **sinuses** (paranasal sinuses) are air-filled spaces located within the *maxillary, frontal, ethmoid,* and *sphenoid bones* of the skull (figure 13.5). These spaces open into the nasal cavity and are lined with mucous membranes that are continuous with the lining of the nasal cavity. Consequently, mucus secretions can drain from the sinuses into the nasal cavity (figure 13.6). If this drainage is blocked by membranes that are inflamed and swollen because of nasal infections or allergic reactions (sinusitis), the accumulating fluids may cause increasing pressure within the sinus, resulting in a painful sinus headache.

Although the sinuses function mainly to reduce the weight of the skull, they also serve as resonant chambers that affect the quality of the voice.

It is possible to illuminate a person's frontal sinus in a darkened room by holding a small flashlight just beneath the eyebrow. Similarly, the maxillary sinuses can be illuminated by holding the flashlight in the mouth.

The sinuses vary considerably from one individual to the next. For example, the frontal, sphenoidal, and maxillary sinuses vary in size and shape. Often, one of a pair of sinuses is larger than the other. The ethmoid sinuses are composed of three to eighteen small sinuses on each side.

1. Where are the sinuses located?
2. What are the functions of the sinuses?

FIGURE 13.5

X-ray film of a skull from the side showing air-filled sinuses (arrows).

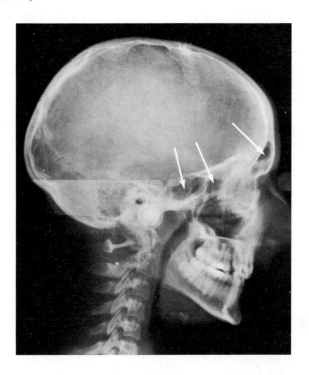

FIGURE 13.6

The sinuses open into the nasal cavity.

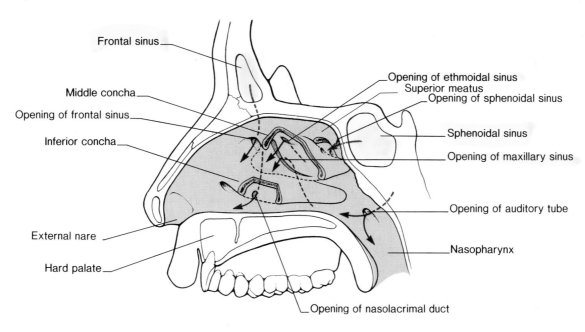

Frontal sinus

Middle concha

Opening of frontal sinus

Inferior concha

External nare

Hard palate

Opening of ethmoidal sinus
Superior meatus
Opening of sphenoidal sinus

Sphenoidal sinus

Opening of maxillary sinus

Opening of auditory tube

Nasopharynx

Opening of nasolacrimal duct

FIGURE 13.7

(a) Anterior view and (b) posterior view of the larynx.

Epiglottic Cartilage

Thyroid ← Arytenoid

Cricoid

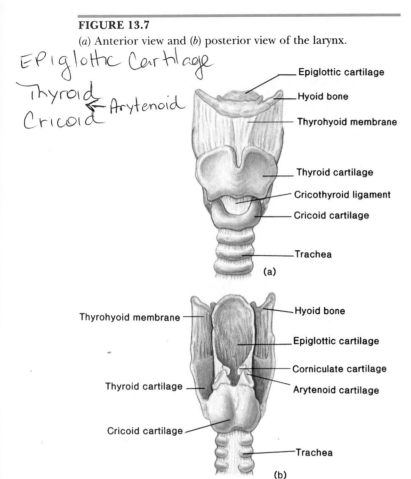

Epiglottic cartilage
Hyoid bone
Thyrohyoid membrane
Thyroid cartilage
Cricothyroid ligament
Cricoid cartilage
Trachea
(a)

Thyrohyoid membrane
Hyoid bone
Epiglottic cartilage
Corniculate cartilage
Thyroid cartilage
Arytenoid cartilage
Cricoid cartilage
Trachea
(b)

The Pharynx

The **pharynx** (throat) is located behind the oral cavity and between the nasal cavity and larynx. It is subdivided into three parts (see chapter 12) and is a passageway for food traveling from the oral cavity to the esophagus and air passing between the nasal cavity and the larynx (figure 13.3). It also aids in speech.

The Larynx

The **larynx** is an enlargement in the airway at the top of the trachea and below the pharynx. It is located opposite the third through sixth cervical vertebrae. The larynx serves as a passageway for air moving in and out of the trachea and prevents foreign objects from entering the trachea. In addition, it houses the *vocal cords.*

The larynx is composed primarily of muscles and cartilages bound together by elastic tissue. The largest of the cartilages (shown in figure 13.7) are the thyroid, cricoid, and epiglottic cartilages. These structures occur singly, and the other laryngeal cartilages—the arytenoid, corniculate, and cuneiform cartilages—are paired.

The **thyroid cartilage** was named for the thyroid gland that covers its lower part. This cartilage is the shieldlike

structure that protrudes in the front of the neck and is sometimes called the Adam's apple. The protrusion typically is more prominent in males than in females because of an effect of male sex hormones on the development of the larynx. The *thyrohyoid membrane* binds the thyroid cartilage to the hyoid bone.

The **cricoid cartilage** lies below the thyroid cartilage and marks the lowermost portion of the larynx.

The *epiglottic cartilage* is attached to the upper border of the thyroid cartilage and is covered by mucous membrane. The entire structure is called the **epiglottis.** The epiglottis usually stands upright and allows air to enter the larynx. During swallowing, however, the larynx is raised by muscular contractions, and the epiglottis is pressed downward by the base of the tongue. As a result, the epiglottis partially covers the opening into the larynx, helping prevent foods and liquids from entering the air passages.

The pyramid-shaped **arytenoid cartilages** are located above and on either side of the posterior portion of the cricoid cartilage. Attached to the tips of the arytenoid cartilages are the tiny, conelike **corniculate cartilages.** These cartilages serve as attachments for muscles that help regulate tension on the vocal cords during speech and aid in closing the larynx during swallowing. The *cricothyroid ligament* joins the cricoid, thyroid, and arytenoid cartilages.

The **cuneiform cartilages** are small, cylindrical parts found in the mucous membrane between the epiglottic and the arytenoid cartilages. They stiffen the soft tissues in this region. (See figure 13.10.)

Inside the larynx, two pairs of horizontal folds in the mucous membrane extend inward from the lateral walls. The upper folds (vestibular folds) are called *false vocal cords* because they do not produce sounds. Muscle fibers within these folds help close the larynx during swallowing.

The lower folds are the *true vocal cords.* They contain elastic fibers and are responsible for vocal sounds, which are created when air forced between the cords causes them to vibrate. This action generates sound waves that can be formed into words by changing the shapes of the pharynx and oral cavity, and by using the tongue and lips. Both pairs of folds are shown in figure 13.8.

The quality of the sound waves produced by vibrating vocal folds is influenced by the length and thickness (mass) of the folds, and the extent to which they are stretched (tension). For example, as the vocal folds are stretched, the pitch (musical tone) of the sound they produce becomes higher, and as the stretch decreases, the pitch becomes lower.

Changes in tension of the vocal folds are brought about by the contraction or relaxation of certain skeletal muscles (laryngeal muscles) associated with the cartilages of the larynx, such as those listed in chart 13.1 and shown in figure 13.9.

FIGURE 13.8

(a) Frontal section and (b) sagittal section of the larynx.

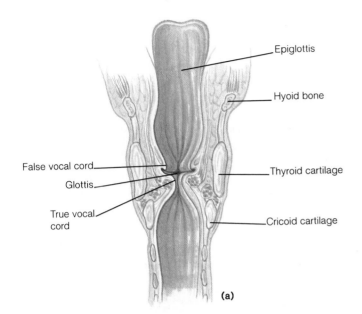

(a)

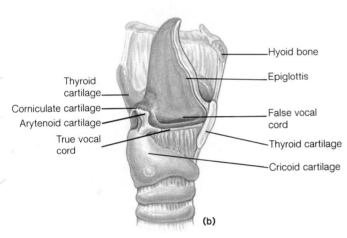

(b)

FIGURE 13.9

The muscles that move parts of the larynx.

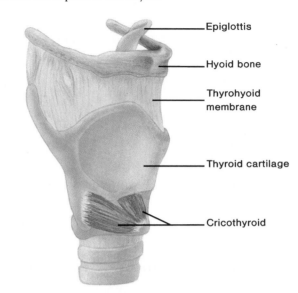

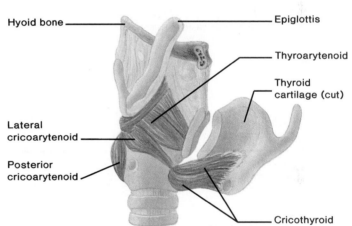

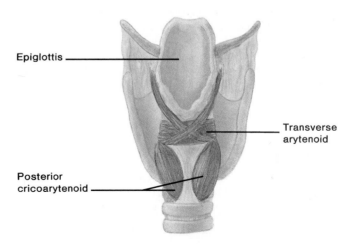

The pitch of a vocal sound is determined by the frequency at which the vocal folds are vibrating in cycles per second (cps). The higher the frequency, the higher the pitch of the sound produced. The frequencies of the vocal sounds used in human speech vary with gender and age, averaging about 100 cps for males, 200 cps for females, and 250 cps for young children.

The *intensity* (loudness) of vocal sound is related to the force of the air passing between the vocal cords. Louder sounds are produced by using stronger blasts of air to cause the vocal cords to vibrate.

During normal breathing, the vocal cords remain relaxed, and the opening between them, called the **glottis,** appears as a triangular slit. However, when food or liquid

Chart 13.1 Laryngeal muscles that influence vocal folds

Muscle	Origin	Insertion	Innervation	Function
Posterior cricoarytenoid muscles	Cricoid cartilage (posterior surface)	Arytenoid cartilage (posterior surface)	Recurrent laryngeal nerve (a branch of the vagus nerve)	Abduct vocal folds; open glottis; lengthen and increase tension of vocal folds
Lateral cricoarytenoid muscles	Cricoid cartilage (superior surface)	Arytenoid cartilage (anterior surface)	Recurrent laryngeal nerve	Adduct vocal folds; close glottis; shorten and decrease tension of vocal folds
Transverse arytenoid muscle	Arytenoid cartilage (posterior surface)	Arytenoid cartilage on the opposite side (posterior surface)	Recurrent laryngeal nerve	Adducts vocal folds; closes glottis; shortens and decreases tension on vocal folds
Cricothyroid muscles	Cricoid cartilage (anterolateral surface)	Thyroid cartilage (anterior border)	Superior laryngeal nerve (a branch of the vagus nerve)	Lengthen and increase tension of vocal folds
Thyroarytenoid muscles	Thyroid cartilage (inferior surface)	Arytenoid cartilage (anterolateral surface)	Recurrent laryngeal nerve	Shorten and decrease tension of vocal folds

is swallowed, the glottis is closed by muscles within the false vocal cords. This prevents foreign substances from entering the trachea (figure 13.10).

The mucous membrane lining the larynx continues to filter the incoming air by entrapping particles and moving them toward the pharynx by ciliary action.

Occasionally, the mucous membrane of the larynx becomes inflamed and swollen as a result of an infection or an irritation from inhaled vapors. When this happens, the vocal cords may not vibrate as freely as before, and the voice may become hoarse. This condition is called *laryngitis,* and although it is usually mild, laryngitis is potentially dangerous because the swollen tissues may obstruct the airway and interfere with breathing. In such cases, it may be necessary to provide a passageway by inserting a tube (endotracheal tube) into the trachea through the nose or mouth.

1. What part of the respiratory tract is shared with the alimentary canal?
2. Describe the structure of the larynx.
3. How do the vocal cords function to produce sounds?
4. What is the function of the glottis? Of the epiglottis?

The Trachea

The **trachea** (windpipe) is a flexible, cylindrical tube about 2.5 centimeters in diameter and 12.5 centimeters in length. It extends downward in front of the esophagus and into the thoracic cavity, where it splits into right and left bronchi (figure 13.11).

FIGURE 13.10

Vocal cords as viewed from above (*a*) with the glottis closed and (*b*) with the glottis open. (*c*) A photograph of the glottis and vocal folds.

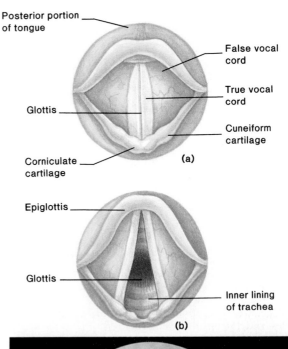

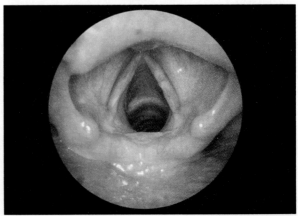

(c)

FIGURE 13.11

The trachea transports air between the larynx and the bronchi.

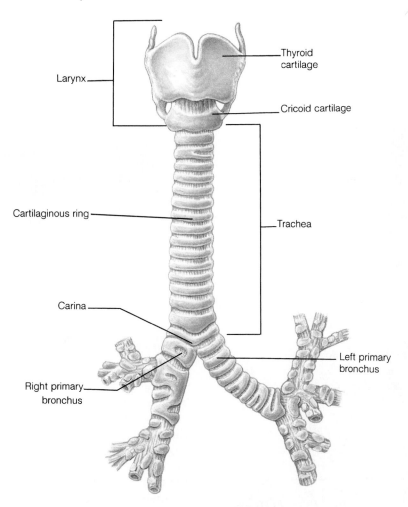

The inner wall of the trachea is lined with a ciliated mucous membrane that contains many goblet cells. This membrane continues to filter the incoming air and to move entrapped particles upward into the pharynx.

Within the tracheal wall are about twenty C-shaped pieces of hyaline cartilage arranged one above the other. The open ends of these incomplete rings are directed posteriorly, and the gaps between their ends are filled with smooth muscle and connective tissues (figures 13.12 and 13.13). These cartilaginous rings prevent the trachea from collapsing and blocking the airway. At the same time, the soft tissues that complete the rings in the back allow the nearby esophagus to expand as food moves through it.

If the trachea becomes obstructed by swollen tissues, excessive secretions, or a foreign object, it may be necessary to create a temporary external opening in the tube so air can bypass the obstruction. This procedure, called a *tracheostomy*, is often a lifesaving procedure because if the trachea is blocked, asphyxiation can occur within a few minutes.

FIGURE 13.12

Cross section of the trachea. What is the significance of the C-shaped rings of hyaline cartilage in its wall?

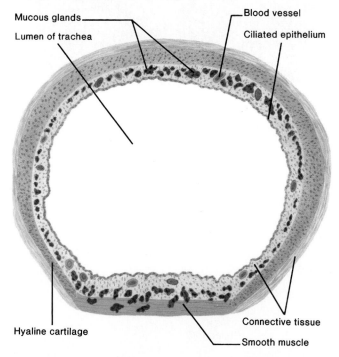

FIGURE 13.13

(*a*) Light micrograph of a section of the tracheal wall (×25); (*b*) magnified view of the epithelial lining (×250); (*c*) scanning electron micrograph of cilia (arrow).

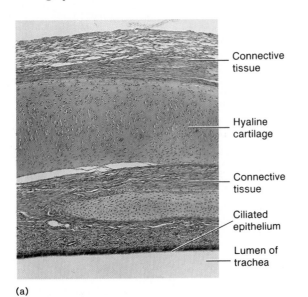

Connective tissue

Hyaline cartilage

Connective tissue

Ciliated epithelium

Lumen of trachea

(a)

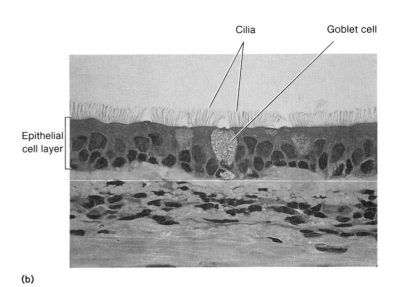

Cilia

Goblet cell

Epithelial cell layer

(b)

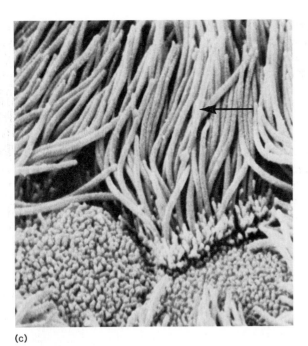

(c)

The Bronchial Tree

The **bronchial tree** consists of the branched airways leading from the trachea to the microscopic air sacs in the lungs. It begins with the right and left **primary bronchi** that arise from the trachea at the level of the fifth thoracic vertebrae. The openings of the primary bronchi are separated by a ridge of cartilage called the *carina*. Each bronchus, accompanied by large blood vessels, enters its respective lung. The right primary bronchus is shorter and wider than the left (figure 13.11).

Branches of the Bronchial Tree

A short distance from its origin, each primary bronchus divides into **secondary,** or **lobar, bronchi** (two on the left; three on the right), which, in turn, branch into finer and finer tubes (figures 13.14, 13.15, and 13.16). The successive divisions of these branches, from the lobar bronchus to the microscopic air sacs, follow:

1. *Tertiary,* or *segmental, bronchi.* Each of these branches supplies a portion of the lung called a *bronchopulmonary segment.* Usually there are ten such segments in the right lung and eight in the left (figure 13.17).

FIGURE 13.14

(a) The bronchial tree consists of the passageways that connect the trachea and the alveoli; (b) light micrograph of a cross section of a primary bronchus.

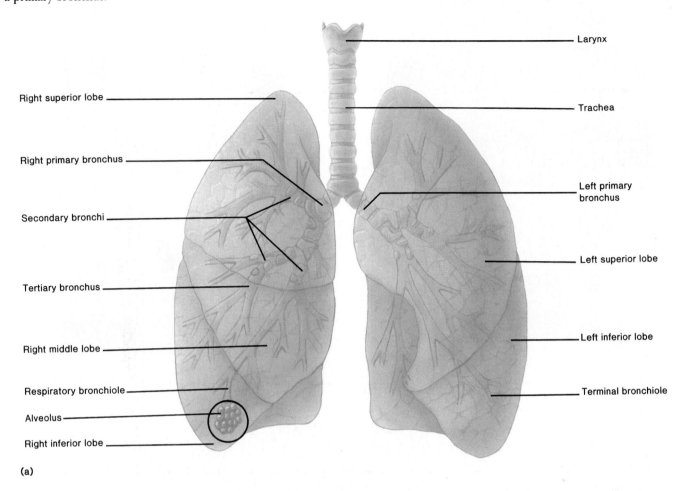

Larynx

Right superior lobe

Trachea

Right primary bronchus

Left primary bronchus

Secondary bronchi

Tertiary bronchus

Left superior lobe

Right middle lobe

Left inferior lobe

Respiratory bronchiole

Terminal bronchiole

Alveolus

Right inferior lobe

(a)

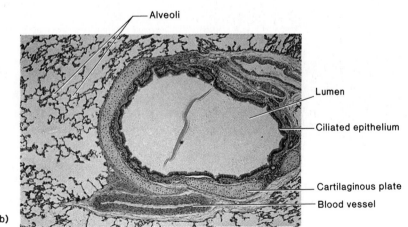

Alveoli

Lumen

Ciliated epithelium

Cartilaginous plate

Blood vessel

(b)

FIGURE 13.15

A plastic cast of the bronchial tree.

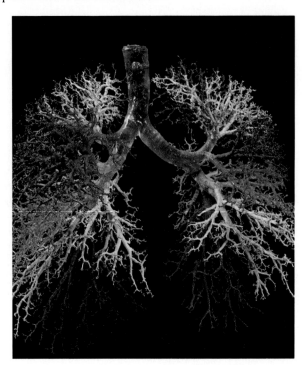

FIGURE 13.16

This 3D computed tomography scan reveals many branches of the bronchial tree.

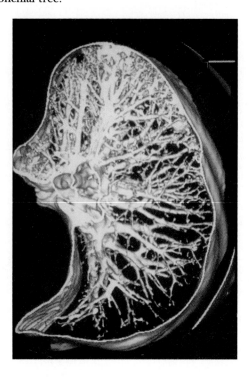

FIGURE 13.17

Each secondary bronchus divides into tertiary bronchi.

From *Basic Human Anatomy*, Second Edition, by Alexander Spence. Copyright © 1986, Benjamin/Cummings Publishing Company, Menlo Park, Calif. Reprinted by permission.

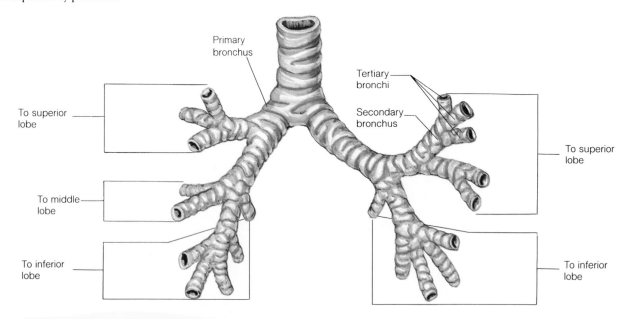

2. *Bronchioles.* These small branches of the segmental bronchi enter the basic units of the lung—the *lobules.*

3. *Terminal bronchioles.* These tubes branch from a bronchiole. There are 50 to 80 terminal bronchioles within a lobule of the lung (figure 13.18).

4. *Respiratory bronchioles.* Two or more respiratory bronchioles branch from each terminal bronchiole. They are relatively short and have diameters of about 0.5 millimeter. They are called "respiratory" because a few air sacs bud from their sides; thus, they are the first structures in the sequence that can engage in gas exchange.

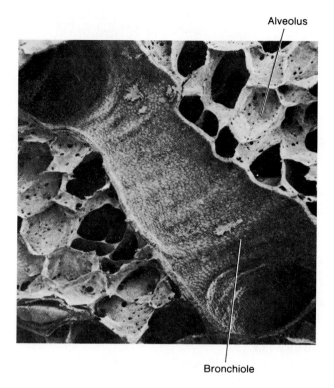

Alveolus

Bronchiole

5. *Alveolar ducts.* There are two to ten long, branching alveolar ducts extending from each respiratory bronchiole (figure 13.19).
6. *Alveolar sacs.* Alveolar sacs are thin-walled, closely packed outpouchings of the alveolar ducts.
7. *Alveoli.* Alveoli are thin-walled, microscopic air sacs that open only on the side communicating with an alveolar sac. Thus, air can move freely from the alveolar ducts, through the alveolar sacs, and into the alveoli (figure 13.20).

Structure of the Respiratory Tubes

The structure of a bronchus is similar to that of the trachea, but the C-shaped cartilaginous rings are replaced with cartilaginous plates where the bronchus enters the lung. These plates are irregularly shaped, and they completely surround the tube, giving it a cylindrical form. However, as finer and finer branched tubes appear, the amount of cartilage decreases, and it finally disappears in the bronchioles, which have diameters of about 1 millimeter.

As the amount of cartilage decreases, the layer of smooth muscle that surrounds the tube just beneath the mucosa becomes more prominent. This muscular layer remains in the wall to the ends of the respiratory bronchioles. Only a few muscle fibers occur in the walls of the alveolar ducts.

Elastic fibers are scattered among the smooth muscle cells and are abundant in the connective tissue that surrounds the respiratory tubes. These fibers play an important role in breathing, as explained in a subsequent section of this chapter.

FIGURE 13.19

The respiratory tubes end in tiny alveoli, each of which is surrounded by a capillary network.

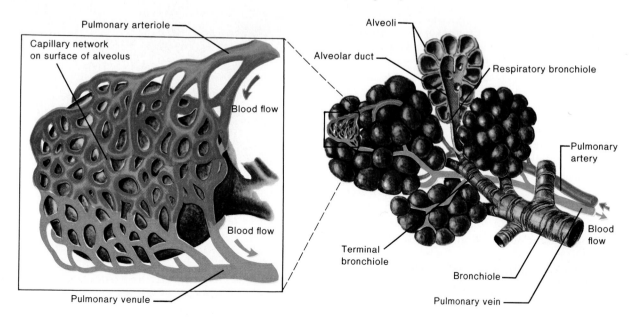

Pulmonary arteriole

Capillary network on surface of alveolus

Blood flow

Blood flow

Pulmonary venule

Alveoli

Alveolar duct

Respiratory bronchiole

Pulmonary artery

Terminal bronchiole

Bronchiole

Pulmonary vein

Blood flow

The Respiratory System   431

FIGURE 13.20

Light micrograph of alveoli (×250).

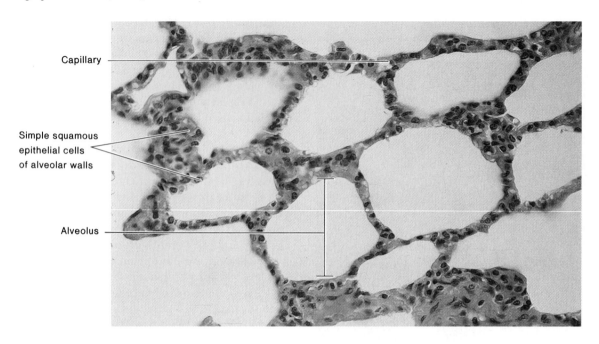

Capillary

Simple squamous
epithelial cells
of alveolar walls

Alveolus

As the tubes become smaller, a change occurs in the type of cells that line them. For example, the lining of the larger tubes consists of pseudostratified, ciliated columnar epithelium and mucus-secreting goblet cells. However, along the way, the number of goblet cells and the height of the other epithelial cells declines, and the abundance of cilia decreases. In the finer tubes, beginning with the respiratory bronchioles, the lining is cuboidal epithelium; and in the alveoli, it is simple squamous epithelium closely associated with a dense network of capillaries.

The trachea and bronchial tree can be examined directly using a flexible, optical instrument called a *fiberoptic bronchoscope*. This procedure, bronchoscopy, is sometimes useful in diagnosing tumors or other pulmonary diseases. It may also be employed to locate and remove aspirated foreign bodies in the air passages.

Functions of the Respiratory Tubes

The branches of the bronchial tree serve as air passages that continue to filter incoming air and distribute it to the alveoli in all parts of the lungs. The alveoli, in turn, provide a large surface area of thin epithelial cells through which gas exchanges can occur. During these exchanges, oxygen moves through the alveolar walls and enters the blood in nearby capillaries, while carbon dioxide moves from the blood through these walls and enters the alveoli (figure 13.21).

It is estimated that there are about 300 million alveoli in an adult lung and that these spaces provide a total surface area of between 70 and 80 square meters.

FIGURE 13.21

Scanning electron micrograph of casts of alveoli and associated capillary networks. These casts were prepared by filling the alveoli and blood vessels with resin and later removing the soft tissues by digestion, leaving only the resin casts (×415).
R. G. Kessel and R. H. Kardon, *Tissues and Organs: A Text Atlas of Scanning Electron Microscopy*, © 1979, W. H. Freeman & Co.

Blood vessel Capillary Alveolus

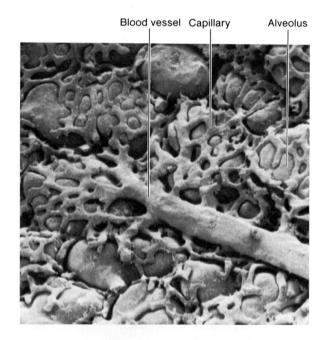

FIGURE 13.22
Locations of the lungs within the thoracic cavity.

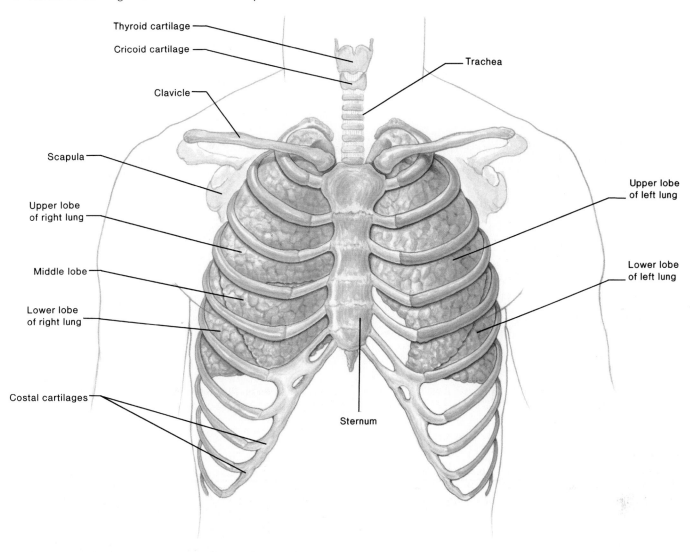

Thyroid cartilage

Cricoid cartilage

Trachea

Clavicle

Scapula

Upper lobe
of left lung

Upper lobe
of right lung

Middle lobe

Lower lobe
of left lung

Lower lobe
of right lung

Costal cartilages

Sternum

1. What is the function of the cartilaginous rings in the tracheal wall?
2. How do the right and left bronchi differ in structure?
3. List the branches of the bronchial tree.
4. Describe the changes in structure that occur in the respiratory tubes as they become smaller and smaller.
5. Describe the structure of an alveolus.

The Lungs

The lungs are soft, spongy, cone-shaped organs located in the thoracic cavity. The right and left lungs are separated medially by the heart and the mediastinum, and they are enclosed by the diaphragm and the thoracic cage (figure 13.22).

Each lung occupies most of the thoracic space on its side and is suspended in the cavity by its attachments, which include a bronchus and large blood vessels. These tubular

parts enter the lung on its medial surface through a region called the **hilus.** A layer of serous membrane, the **visceral pleura,** is firmly attached to the surface of each lung, and this membrane folds back at the hilus to become the **parietal pleura.** The parietal pleura, in turn, forms part of the mediastinum and lines the inner wall of the thoracic cavity.

The potential space between the visceral and parietal pleurae is called the **pleural cavity,** and it contains a thin film of serous fluid (figure 13.23). This fluid lubricates the adjacent pleural surfaces, reducing friction as they move against one another during breathing. It also helps hold the pleural membranes together, as explained in a subsequent section of this chapter.

As figure 13.15 shows, the right lung is larger than the left one. It is divided into the superior, middle, and inferior *lobes.* The left lung consists of a superior and an inferior lobe (figure 13.22).

FIGURE 13.23

Transverse section through the thorax.

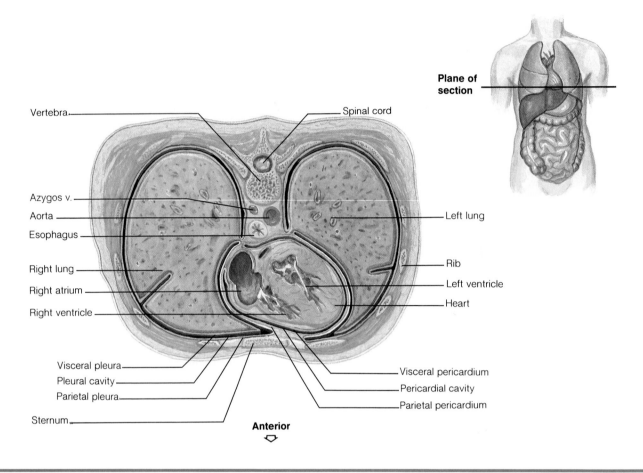

Plane of section

Vertebra

Spinal cord

Azygos v.

Aorta

Esophagus

Right lung

Right atrium

Right ventricle

Left lung

Rib

Left ventricle

Heart

Visceral pleura

Pleural cavity

Parietal pleura

Sternum

Visceral pericardium

Pericardial cavity

Parietal pericardium

Anterior

FIGURE 13.24

Each lung lobe is subdivided into bronchopulmonary segments.

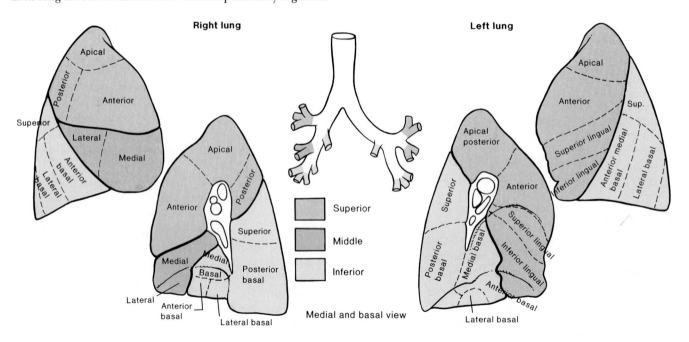

Right lung

Apical

Posterior

Anterior

Superior

Lateral

Medial

Anterior basal

Lateral basal

Apical

Anterior

Posterior

Superior

Medial

Medial

Basal

Posterior basal

Lateral

Anterior basal

Lateral basal

Left lung

Apical

Anterior

Sup.

Superior lingual

Inferior lingual

Anterior medial basal

Lateral basal

Apical posterior

Superior

Anterior

Posterior basal

Medial basal

Superior lingual

Inferior lingual

Anterior basal

Lateral basal

Superior

Middle

Inferior

Medial and basal view

434   Chapter 13

Each lobe is supplied by a secondary bronchus of the bronchial tree. It also has connections to blood and lymphatic vessels, and is enclosed by connective tissues. A lobe is divided by connective tissue into **bronchopulmonary segments** (figure 13.24). Each segment is supplied by a tertiary bronchus. There are ten segments in the right lung and eight in the left. Each segment is further subdivided into **lobules,** and each of these units contains terminal bronchioles, together with their alveolar ducts, alveolar sacs, alveoli, nerves, and associated blood and lymphatic vessels. Thus, the substance of a lung includes air passages, alveoli, blood vessels, connective tissues, lymphatic vessels, and nerves. Chart 13.2 summarizes the characteristics of the major parts of the respiratory system.

1. Where are the lungs located?
2. What is the function of the serous fluid within the pleural cavity?
3. How does the structure of the right lung differ from that of the left lung?
4. What kinds of structures make up a lung?

The Alveoli and the Respiratory Membrane

While other parts of the respiratory system move air in and out of the air passages, the alveoli carry on the vital process of exchanging gases between the air and the blood.

The Alveoli

The **alveoli** are microscopic air sacs clustered at the distal ends of the alveolar sacs. Each alveolus consists of a tiny space surrounded by a thin wall that separates it from adjacent alveoli. There are minute openings, called *alveolar pores,* in the walls of some alveoli, and although the function of these pores is not clear, they may permit air to pass from one alveolus to another (figure 13.25). This arrangement may provide alternate air pathways if the passages in some portions of the lung become obstructed.

Alveolar pores may also allow phagocytic cells, called alveolar macrophages, to move between adjacent alveoli (figure 13.26). These macrophages, which normally inhabit the alveoli, help keep the alveoli clean by engulfing various airborne agents, such as bacterial cells.

The Respiratory Membrane

The wall of an alveolus consists of an inner lining of simple squamous epithelium and a dense network of capillaries that are also lined with simple squamous cells. Thin basement membranes separate the layers of these flattened cells, and elastic and collagenous fibers in the spaces between them help support the wall. As figures 13.26 and 13.27 show, there are at least two thicknesses of epithelial cells and basement membranes between the air in an alveolus and the blood in a capillary. These layers make up the **respiratory membrane** (alveolar-capillary membrane), which is of vital importance because through this membrane gas exchange occurs between alveolar air and blood.

Part	Description	Function
Nose	Part of face centered above the mouth and below the space between the eyes	Nostrils provide entrance to nasal cavity; internal hairs begin to filter incoming air
Nasal cavity	Hollow space behind nose	Conducts air to pharynx; its mucous lining filters, warms, and moistens air
Sinuses	Hollow spaces lined with mucous membrane and located in various bones of the skull	Reduce weight of the skull; serve as resonant chambers
Pharynx	Chamber behind mouth cavity, and between nasal cavity and larynx	Passageway for air moving from nasal cavity to larynx, and for food moving from mouth cavity to esophagus
Larynx	Enlargement at the top of the trachea	Passageway for air; prevents foreign objects from entering trachea; houses vocal cords
Trachea	Flexible tube that connects larynx with bronchial tree	Passageway for air; its mucous lining continues to filter air
Bronchial tree	Branched tubes that lead from the trachea to the alveoli	Conducts air from the trachea to the alveoli; its mucous lining continues to filter air
Lungs	Soft, cone-shaped organs that occupy a large portion of the thoracic cavity	Contain the air passages, alveoli, blood vessels, connective tissues, lymphatic vessels, and nerves of the lower respiratory tract

Chart 13.2 Parts of the respiratory system

FIGURE 13.25
Alveolar pores (arrow) allow air to pass from one alveolus to another.

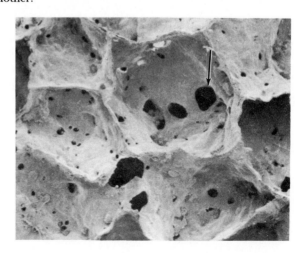

FIGURE 13.26
The respiratory membrane consists of the walls of the alveolus and the capillary.

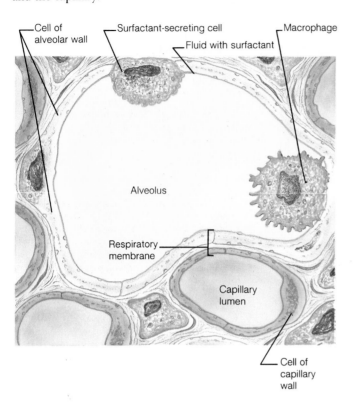

FIGURE 13.27
Electron micrograph of a capillary between two alveoli. Note the small space between the alveolar wall and the capillary wall. (AS = alveolar space; RBC = red blood cell; BM = basement membrane; IS = interstitial connective tissue; EN = epithelial nucleus.)

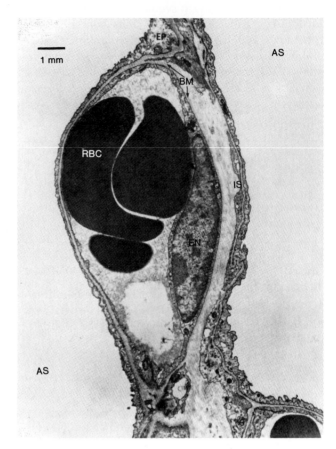

The squamous cells of the alveoli are continually replaced and have a life span of about three weeks. However, if these cells are severely damaged, they may be replaced by fibrous connective tissue.

The respiratory membrane is normally about 0.5 μm thick, and efficient gas exchange depends upon this thin membrane. Any condition that increases the thickness of this membrane, decreases gas exchange. For example, with the bacterial disease tuberculosis, lung tissue may be destroyed and replaced by fibrous tissue. This can result in a thickening of the respiratory membrane and may restrict gas exchange.

Breathing Mechanism

Breathing, or *pulmonary ventilation,* is the movement of air from outside the body into the bronchial tree and alveoli, followed by a reversal of this air movement. The actions responsible for these air movements are termed **inspiration** (inhalation) and **expiration** (exhalation).

Inspiration

Atmospheric pressure due to the weight of the air is the force that causes air to move into the lungs. At sea level, this pressure is sufficient to support a column of mercury about 760 millimeters high in a tube. Thus, normal air pressure is equal to 760 millimeters of mercury (Hg).

Air pressure is exerted on all surfaces in contact with the air, and because people breathe air, the inside surfaces of their lungs are also subjected to pressure. Therefore, the pressures on the inside of the lungs and alveoli, and on the outside of the thoracic wall are about the same (figure 13.28).

The *diaphragm* is located just below the lungs. It consists of an anterior group of skeletal muscle fibers (costal fibers), which originate from the ribs and sternum, and a posterior group (crural fibers), which originate from the vertebrae. Both groups of muscle fibers are inserted on a tendinous central portion of the diaphragm.

FIGURE 13.28
When the lungs are at rest, the pressure on the inside of the lungs is equal to the pressure on the outside of the thorax.

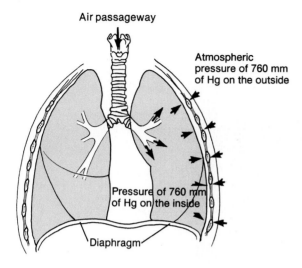

Air passageway

Atmospheric pressure of 760 mm of Hg on the outside

Pressure of 760 mm of Hg on the inside

Diaphragm

Chart 13.3 Major events in inspiration

1. Nerve impulses travel on phrenic nerves to muscle fibers in the diaphragm, causing them to contract.
2. As the dome-shaped diaphragm moves downward, the size of the thoracic cavity increases.
3. At the same time, the external intercostal muscles may contract, raising the ribs and causing the size of the thoracic cavity to increase still more.
4. As the size of the thoracic cavity increases, the pressure in the lungs decreases.
5. Atmospheric pressure, which is relatively greater on the outside, forces air into the respiratory tract through the air passages.
6. The lungs inflate.

During normal inspiration, muscle fibers in the dome-shaped diaphragm are stimulated to contract by impulses carried on the phrenic nerves. As this happens, the diaphragm moves downward, the size of the thoracic cavity is enlarged, and the pressure in the lungs is reduced about 1 millimeter Hg below that of atmospheric pressure. In response to this pressure, air is forced into the airways by atmospheric pressure.

While the diaphragm is contracting and moving downward, the *external intercostal muscles* between the ribs and certain thoracic muscles may be stimulated to contract. This action raises the ribs and elevates the sternum, so that the size of the thoracic cavity increases even more. As a result, the pressure inside is further reduced, and more air is forced into the airways by the greater atmospheric pressure. (See figure 8.13.)

The expansion of the lungs is aided by the fact that the parietal pleura, on the inner wall of the thoracic cavity, and the visceral pleura, attached to the surface of the lungs, are separated by only a thin film of serous fluid. *Surface tension* holds the moist surfaces of the pleural membranes tightly together. Consequently, when the thoracic wall is moved upward and outward by the action of the intercostal muscles, the parietal pleura is moved too, and the visceral pleura follows it. This expands the lungs in all directions. The steps in inspiration are summarized in chart 13.3.

The attraction between adjacent moist membranes is sufficient to cause the collapse of the tiny air sacs, which also have moist surfaces. However, certain alveolar cells (type II alveolar cells) secrete a substance called **surfactant** that reduces surface tension and decreases this tendency to collapse.

Sometimes the lungs of a newborn fail to produce enough surfactant, and the newborn's breathing mechanism is unable to overcome the force of surface tension. Consequently, the lungs cannot be ventilated, and the newborn is likely to die of suffocation. This condition is called *respiratory distress syndrome* and it is the primary cause of respiratory difficulty in immature newborns and in babies born to mothers with diabetes mellitus.

If a person needs to take a deeper than normal breath, the diaphragm and external intercostal muscles may be contracted to an even greater extent. Additional muscles, such as the pectoralis minors and sternocleidomastoids, can also be used to pull the thoracic cage further upward and outward, enlarging the thoracic cavity and decreasing the internal pressure still more (figure 13.29).

The ease with which the lungs can be expanded as a result of pressure changes occurring during breathing is called *compliance* (distensibility). In a normal lung, compliance decreases as lung volume increases, because an inflated lung is more difficult to expand than a deflated one. Conditions that tend to obstruct air passages, destroy lung tissue, or impede lung expansion in other ways also decrease compliance.

FIGURE 13.29

(a) Shape of the thorax at the end of normal inspiration. (b) Shape of the thorax at the end of maximal inspiration, aided by contraction of the sternocleidomastoid and pectoralis minor muscles.

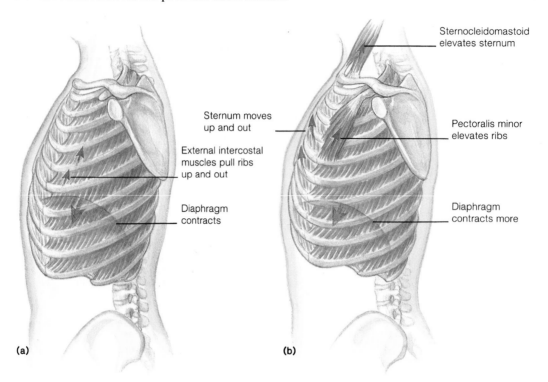

Sternocleidomastoid elevates sternum

Sternum moves up and out

External intercostal muscles pull ribs up and out

Diaphragm contracts

Pectoralis minor elevates ribs

Diaphragm contracts more

(a)

(b)

Expiration

The forces responsible for normal expiration come from *elastic recoil* of tissues and from surface tension. For example, the lungs and thoracic wall contain a considerable amount of elastic tissue, and as the lungs expand during inspiration, these tissues are stretched. When the diaphragm lowers, the abdominal organs beneath it are compressed. As the diaphragm and the external intercostal muscles relax following inspiration, the elastic tissues cause the lungs and thoracic cage to recoil, and they return to their original shapes. Similarly, elastic tissues within the abdominal organs cause them to spring back into their previous shapes, pushing the diaphragm upward. At the same time, the surface tension that develops between the moist surfaces of the alveolar linings tends to cause alveoli to decrease in diameter. Each of these factors tends to increase the pressure within the alveoli about 1 millimeter Hg above atmospheric pressure, so that the air inside the lungs is forced out through the respiratory passages. Thus, normal expiration is a passive process.

The recoil of the elastic fibers within the lung tissues tends to reduce the pressure in the pleural cavity. Consequently, the pressure between the pleural membranes (intrapleural pressure) is usually about 4 millimeters Hg less than atmospheric pressure.

Because the visceral and parietal pleural membranes are held together by surface tension, no actual space normally exists in the pleural cavity between them. However, if the thoracic wall is punctured, atmospheric air may enter the pleural cavity and create a real space between the membranes. This condition is called *pneumothorax,* and when it occurs, the lung on the affected side may collapse because of the lung's elasticity.

Pneumothorax may be treated by passing a tube (chest tube) through the thoracic wall into the pleural cavity and applying suction to the tube. In response to the suction, negative pressure is reestablished within the cavity, and the collapsed lung expands rapidly.

FIGURE 13.30

(*a*) Normal expiration is due to elastic recoil of the thoracic wall and abdominal organs; (*b*) maximal expiration is aided by contraction of the abdominal wall and posterior internal intercostal muscles.

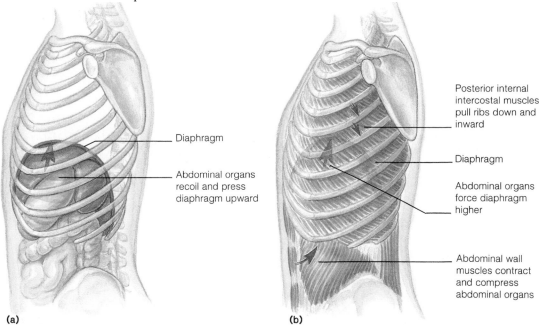

(a)

(b)

Diaphragm

Abdominal organs recoil and press diaphragm upward

Posterior internal intercostal muscles pull ribs down and inward

Diaphragm

Abdominal organs force diaphragm higher

Abdominal wall muscles contract and compress abdominal organs

If a person needs to exhale more air than normal, the posterior *internal intercostal muscles* can be contracted. These muscles pull the ribs and sternum downward and inward, increasing the pressure in the lungs. Also, the *abdominal wall muscles,* including the external and internal obliques, the transversus abdominis, and the rectus abdominis, can be used to squeeze the abdominal organs inward. Thus, the abdominal wall muscles can cause the pressure in the abdominal cavity to increase and force the diaphragm still higher against the lungs (figure 13.30). As a result of these actions, additional air may be squeezed out of the lungs. Chart 13.4 summarizes the steps in expiration.

Chart 13.4 Major events in expiration

1. The diaphragm and external respiratory muscles relax.
2. Elastic tissues of the lungs, thoracic cage, and abdominal organs, which were stretched during inspiration, suddenly recoil and surface tension causes alveolar walls to collapse.
3. Tissues recoiling around the lungs cause the pressure in the lungs to increase.
4. Air is pushed out of the lungs and into the air passages.

Nonrespiratory Air Movements

Air movements that occur in addition to breathing are called *nonrespiratory movements.* They are used to clear air passages, as in coughing and sneezing, or to express emotional feelings, as in laughing and crying. Other nonrespiratory air movements include yawning and hiccuping.

The most sensitive areas of the air passages are in the larynx and in regions near the branches of the major bronchi. The distal portions of the bronchioles (respiratory bronchioles), alveolar ducts, and alveoli lack a nerve supply. Consequently, before any material in these parts can trigger a cough reflex, it must be moved into the larger passages of the respiratory tract.

1. Describe the events in inspiration.
2. How does surface tension aid expansion of the lungs during inspiration?
3. What forces are responsible for normal expiration?

Some Respiratory Disorders

Although respiratory disorders are caused by a variety of factors, some are characterized by decreased ventilation. This group includes paralysis of various breathing muscles, bronchial asthma, emphysema, and lung cancer.

Paralysis of breathing muscles is sometimes caused by injuries to the respiratory center or to spinal nerve tracts that transmit motor impulses. Paralysis may also be the result of disease, such as *poliomyelitis,* which affects parts of the central nervous system and injures motor neurons. The consequences of such paralysis depend on the muscles affected. Sometimes, by increasing their responses, other muscles are able to compensate for functional losses of a paralyzed muscle. If unaffected muscles are unable to ventilate the lungs adequately, a person must be provided with some type of mechanical breathing device in order to survive.

Bronchial asthma is a condition commonly caused by an *allergic reaction* to foreign substances in the respiratory tract. Typically, the foreign substance is a plant pollen that enters with inhaled air. As a result of this reaction, the walls of the small bronchioles swell, the cells lining the respiratory tubes secrete abnormally large amounts of thick mucus, and the smooth muscles in these tubes contract. These muscles cause the bronchioles to constrict, reducing the diameters of the air passages. As these changes occur, the person finds it increasingly difficult to breathe and produces a characteristic wheezing sound, as air moves through narrowed passages.

An asthmatic person usually finds it harder to force air out of the lungs than to bring it in. This is because inspiration involves powerful breathing muscles, and as they contract, the lungs expand. This expansion helps open the air passages. Expiration, on the other hand, is usually a passive process due to elastic recoil of stretched tissues. Also, it causes compression of the tissues and decreases the diameters of the bronchioles, adding to the problem of moving air through the narrowed air passages.

Emphysema is a progressive, degenerative disease characterized by the destruction of many alveolar walls. As a result of this destruction, clusters of small air sacs merge to form larger chambers, so that the total surface area of the respiratory membrane decreases. At the same time, the alveolar walls tend to lose their elasticity and the capillary networks associated with the alveoli become less abundant (figure 13.31).

FIGURE 13.31
(*a*) As emphysema develops, the alveoli tend to merge, (*b*) forming larger chambers (×80).

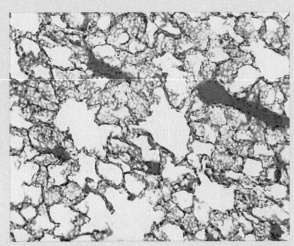
(a)

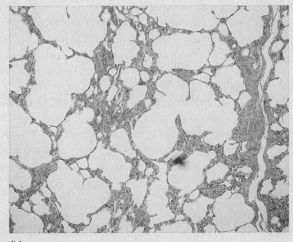
(b)

Because of the loss of tissue elasticity, the person with emphysema finds it increasingly difficult to force air out of the lungs. As was mentioned, normal expiration involves the passive elastic recoil of inflated tissues; in emphysema, abnormal muscular efforts are required to produce this movement.

The cause of emphysema is not clear, but some investigators believe it develops in response to prolonged exposure to respiratory irritants, such as those in tobacco smoke and polluted air. Emphysema is becoming one of the more common respiratory disorders among older persons, although it is not limited to this group.

Lung cancer, like other cancers, involves an uncontrolled growth of abnormal cells. These cells develop in and around the normal tissues and deprive them of nutrients. In effect, the cancer cells cause the death of normal cells by crowding them out.

Cancerous growths in the lungs often result from cancer cells that spread (metastasize) from other parts of the body, such as the breasts, alimentary tract, liver, or kidneys.

Primary pulmonary cancer, which begins in the lungs, is the most common form of cancer in males today. It is also becoming increasingly common among females and is rapidly replacing breast cancer as the leading cause of death from cancer among women. Primary pulmonary cancer may arise from epithelial cells, connective tissue cells, or various blood cells. The most common form arises from epithelium and is called *bronchogenic carcinoma,* which means it originates from the cells that line the tubes of the bronchial tree. This type of cancer seems to occur in response to excessive irritation such as that produced by prolonged exposure to tobacco smoke (figure 13.32).

Once lung cancer cells have appeared, they are likely to produce masses that obstruct air passages and reduce the amount of alveolar surface available for gas exchange. Furthermore, bronchogenic carcinoma is likely to spread to other tissues relatively quickly and establish secondary cancers. Common sites of such secondary cancers include the lymph nodes, liver, bones, the brain, and kidneys.

Lung cancer is often difficult to control. It is treated by surgical removal of the diseased portions of the lungs, exposure to ionizing radiation, and the use of drugs (chemotherapy). Despite these treatments, the survival rate among lung cancer victims remains extremely low.

FIGURE 13.32

Lung cancer usually starts in the lining (epithelium) of the bronchus. (*a*) The normal lining shows (*4*) columnar cells with (*2*) hairlike cilia, (*3*) goblet cells that secrete (*1*) mucus, and (*5*) basal cells from which new columnar cells arise. (*6*) A basement membrane separates the epithelial cells from (*7*) the underlying connective tissue. (*b*) In the first stage of lung cancer, the basal cells divide repeatedly. The goblet cells secrete excessive mucus, and the cilia function less efficiently in moving the heavy mucus secretion. (*c*) With the continued multiplication of basal cells, the columnar and goblet cells are displaced. The basal cells penetrate the basement membrane and invade the deeper connective tissue.

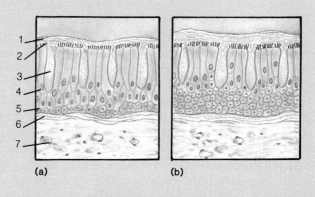

(a)   (b)

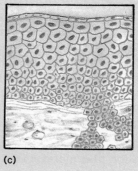

(c)

Control of Breathing

Although respiratory muscles can be controlled voluntarily, normal breathing is a rhythmic, involuntary act that continues when a person is unconscious.

The Respiratory Center

Breathing is controlled by a poorly defined group of neurons in the brain stem called the **respiratory center.** This center periodically initiates impulses that travel on spinal nerves to various breathing muscles, causing inspiration and expiration. The center is also able to adjust the rate and depth of breathing. As a result, cellular needs for a supply of oxygen and the removal of carbon dioxide are met, even during periods of strenuous physical exercise.

Components of the respiratory center are widely scattered throughout the pons and medulla oblongata. However, two areas of the center are of special interest: the rhythmicity area of the medulla and the pneumotaxic area of the pons, shown in figure 13.33.

The **medullary rhythmicity area** includes two groups of neurons that extend throughout the length of the medulla oblongata. They are called the dorsal and ventral respiratory groups.

The *dorsal respiratory group* is responsible for the basic rhythm of breathing. Neurons of this group emit bursts of impulses that signal the diaphragm and other inspiratory muscles to contract. The impulses last for about two seconds, then cease abruptly. The breathing muscles that contract in response to the impulses cause the volume of air entering the lungs to increase steadily. The neurons remain inactive while expiration occurs passively, then they emit another burst of inspiratory impulses so that the inspiration-expiration cycle is repeated.

The *ventral respiratory group* is quiescent during normal breathing. However, when there is need for more forceful breathing, neurons in this group generate impulses that increase inspiratory movement. Other neurons in the group activate muscles associated with forceful expiration as well. (See figure 13.33.)

Neurons in the **pneumotaxic area** transmit impulses to the dorsal respiratory group continuously and regulate the duration of inspiratory impulses originating from the dorsal group. In this way, the pneumotaxic neurons control the rate of breathing.

The respiratory center is located in the pons and the medulla oblongata.

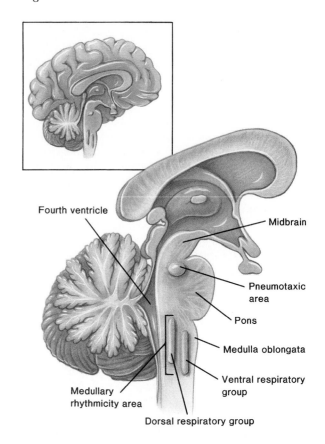

Fourth ventricle

Midbrain

Pneumotaxic area

Pons

Medulla oblongata

Ventral respiratory group

Medullary rhythmicity area

Dorsal respiratory group

Receptors and Nerve Pathways

Receptors associated with sensory pathways conduct nerve impulses to the respiratory center and may alter its activities. For example, chemoreceptors are located in structures called *carotid* and *aortic bodies,* which are found in certain large arteries (carotid arteries and aorta). (See figure 13.34.) When these receptors are stimulated, impulses are sent to the respiratory center, and the breathing rate is increased. *Stretch receptors* are found in the visceral pleura, bronchioles, and alveoli. When these receptors are activated, sensory impulses travel via the vagus nerves to the pneumotaxic area and the duration of respiratory movements is reduced. (See figure 13.35.)

FIGURE 13.34

Carotid and aortic bodies transmit impulses to the respiratory center.

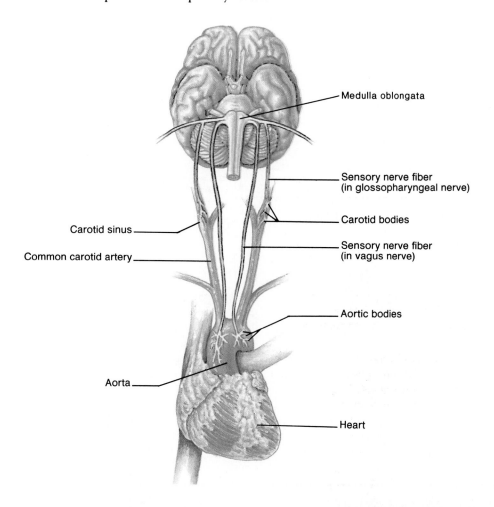

Medulla oblongata

Sensory nerve fiber
(in glossopharyngeal nerve)

Carotid bodies

Carotid sinus

Sensory nerve fiber
(in vagus nerve)

Common carotid artery

Aortic bodies

Aorta

Heart

Exercise is accompanied by an increase in breathing rate. The mechanism that seems to be responsible for most of the increase involves the cerebral cortex and proprioceptors associated with muscles and joints. (See chapter 10.) Specifically, the cortex seems to transmit stimulating impulses to the respiratory center whenever it signals skeletal muscles to contract. At the same time, muscular movements stimulate proprioceptors, and a joint reflex is triggered. In this reflex, sensory impulses are transmitted from the proprioceptors to the respiratory center, and the breathing rate increases.

1. Where is the respiratory center located?
2. Describe how the respiratory center maintains a normal breathing pattern.
3. Explain how the breathing pattern may be changed.

FIGURE 13.35
In the process of inspiration, motor impulses travel from the respiratory center to the diaphragm and external intercostal muscles, which contract and cause the lungs to expand.

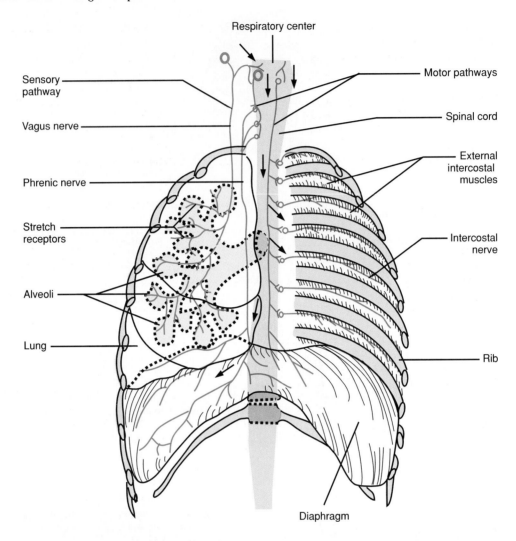

Clinical Terms Related to the Respiratory System

apnea (ap-ne′ah)   temporary absence of breathing.

atelectasis (at″e-lek′tah-sis)   the collapse of a lung or some portion of it.

bronchiolectasis (brong″ke-o-lek′tah-sis)   chronic dilation of the bronchioles.

bronchitis (brong-ki′tis)   inflammation of the bronchial lining.

Cheyne-Stokes respiration (chān stōks res″pi-ra′shun)   irregular breathing characterized by a series of shallow breaths that increase in depth and rate, followed by breaths that decrease in depth and rate.

dyspnea (disp′ne-ah)   difficulty in breathing.

eupnea (up-ne′ah)   normal breathing.

hyperpnea (hi″perp-ne′ah)   increased depth and rate of breathing.

lobar pneumonia (lo′ber nu-mo′ne-ah)   pneumonia that affects an entire lobe of a lung.

pleurisy (ploo′ri-se)   inflammation of the pleural membranes.

pneumoconiosis (nu″mo-ko″ne-o′sis)   a condition characterized by the accumulation of particles from the environment in the lungs, and the reaction of the tissues to their presence.

pneumothorax (nu″mo-tho′raks)   entrance of air into the space between the pleural membranes, followed by collapse of the lung.

rhinitis (ri-ni′tis)   inflammation of the nasal cavity lining.

sinusitis (si″nŭ-si′tis)   inflammation of the sinus cavity lining.

tracheostomy (tra″ke-ost′o-me)   an incision in the trachea for exploration or the removal of a foreign object.

Chapter Summary

Introduction (page 421)

The respiratory system includes the passages that transport air to and from the lungs, and the air sacs of the lungs in which gas exchanges occur. Respiration is the entire process by which gases are exchanged between the atmosphere and the body cells.

Organs of the Respiratory System (page 421)

The respiratory system includes the nose, nasal cavity, sinuses, pharynx, larynx, trachea, bronchial tree, and lungs.

1. The nose
   a. The nose is supported by bone and cartilage.
   b. Nostrils provide entrances for air.
2. The nasal cavity
   a. The nasal cavity is a space behind the nose.
   b. It is divided medially by the nasal septum.
   c. Nasal conchae divide the cavity into passageways and help increase surface area of mucous membranes.
   d. Mucous membranes filter, warm, and moisten incoming air.
   e. Particles trapped in the mucus are carried to the pharynx by ciliary action and are swallowed.
3. The sinuses
   a. Sinuses are spaces in the bones of the skull that open into the nasal cavity.
   b. They are lined with mucous membrane that is continuous with the lining of the nasal cavity.
4. The pharynx
   a. The pharynx is located behind the mouth, and between the nasal cavity and the larynx.
   b. It functions as a common passage for air and food.
   c. It aids in creating vocal sounds.
5. The larynx
   a. The larynx is an enlargement at the top of the trachea.
   b. It serves as a passageway for air and helps prevent foreign objects from entering the trachea.
   c. It is composed of muscles and cartilages, of which some are single and some are paired.
   d. It contains the vocal cords, which produce sounds by vibrating as air passes over them.
      (1) The pitch of a sound is related to the tension on the cords.
      (2) The intensity of a sound is related to the force of the air passing over the cords.
   e. The glottis and epiglottis help prevent food and liquid from entering the trachea.
6. The trachea
   a. The trachea extends into the thoracic cavity in front of the esophagus.
   b. It divides into right and left bronchi.
   c. The mucous lining continues to filter incoming air.
   d. The wall is supported by cartilaginous rings.
7. The bronchial tree
   a. The bronchial tree consists of branched air passages that lead from the trachea to the air sacs.
   b. The branches of the bronchial tree include primary bronchi, lobar bronchi, tertiary or segmental bronchi, bronchioles, terminal bronchioles, respiratory bronchioles, alveolar ducts, alveolar sacs, and alveoli.
   c. Structure of the respiratory tubes
      (1) As tubes branch, the amount of cartilage in the walls decreases and the muscular layer becomes more prominent.
      (2) Elastic fibers in the walls aid the breathing mechanism.
      (3) The epithelial lining changes from pseudostratified and ciliated to cuboidal and simple squamous.
   d. Functions of the respiratory tubes include distribution of air and exchange of gases between the alveolar air and the blood.
8. The lungs
   a. The left and right lungs are separated by the mediastinum and enclosed by the diaphragm and the thoracic cage.
   b. The visceral pleura is attached to the surface of the lungs; parietal pleura lines the thoracic cavity.
   c. The right lung has three lobes, and the left lung has two.
   d. A lobe is divided into bronchopulmonary segments.
   e. Each lobe is composed of lobules that contain alveoli, blood vessels, and supporting tissues.

The Alveoli and the Respiratory Membrane (page 435)

Alveoli carry on gas exchanges between the air and the blood.

1. The alveoli
   a. The alveoli are tiny air sacs clustered at the distal ends of the alveolar ducts.
   b. Some alveoli have openings into adjacent air sacs that provide alternate pathways for air when passages are obstructed.
2. The respiratory membrane
   a. The respiratory membrane consists of the alveolar and capillary walls.
   b. Gas exchanges take place through these walls.

Breathing Mechanism (page 436)

Inspiration and expiration movements are accompanied by changes in the size of the thoracic cavity.

1. Inspiration
   a. The pressure in the lungs is reduced when the diaphragm moves downward, and the thoracic cage moves upward and outward.
   b. Air is forced into the lungs by atmospheric pressure.
   c. Expansion of the lungs is aided by surface tension that holds the pleural membranes together.
   d. Surfactant reduces surface tension within the alveoli.
2. Expiration
   a. The forces of expiration come from the elastic recoil of tissues and surface tension within the alveoli.
   b. Expiration can be aided by thoracic and abdominal wall muscles that pull the thoracic cage downward and inward, and compress the abdominal organs.
3. Nonrespiratory air movements
   a. Nonrespiratory air movements are movements that occur in addition to breathing.
   b. They include coughing, sneezing, laughing, crying, hiccuping, and yawning.

Control of Breathing (page 442)

Normal breathing is rhythmic and involuntary, although the respiratory muscles can be controlled voluntarily.

1. The respiratory center
   a. The respiratory center is located in the brain stem, and includes parts of the medulla oblongata and pons.
   b. The medullary rhythmicity area includes two groups of neurons.
      (1) The dorsal respiratory group is responsible for the basic rhythm of breathing.
      (2) The ventral respiratory group increases inspiratory and expiratory movements during forceful breathing.
   c. The pneumotaxic area regulates the rate of breathing.
2. Receptors and nerve pathways
   Chemoreceptors and stretch receptors send sensory impulses to the respiratory center and alter its activity.

Clinical Application of Knowledge

1. If the upper respiratory passages are bypassed with a tracheostomy, how might the air entering the trachea be different from air normally passing through this canal? What problems may this create for the patient?
2. In certain respiratory disorders, such as emphysema, the amount of elastic tissue in the lungs may be lost. How might this alter breathing?
3. As a result of continued and prolonged irritation by tobacco smoke, the pseudostratified ciliated columnar epithelium that forms the inner lining of the upper respiratory tubes may be replaced by stratified squamous epithelium. What might be the consequences of this tissue change?
4. How might a collapsed lung change the appearance of a chest X ray? (See figure 6.44.)
5. A patient with bronchiogenic carcinoma has surgery, and the superior and middle lobes of the right lung are removed. How would you explain to the patient that the remaining lobe of the right lung will continue to function?

Review Activities

1. Describe the general functions of the respiratory system.
2. Explain how the nose and nasal cavity function in filtering incoming air.
3. Name and describe the locations of the major sinuses, and explain how a sinus headache may occur.
4. Distinguish between the pharynx and the larynx.
5. Name and describe the locations and functions of the cartilages of the larynx.
6. Distinguish between the false vocal cords and the true vocal cords.
7. Compare the structure of the trachea with the structure of the branches of the bronchial tree.
8. List the successive branches of the bronchial tree from the primary bronchi to the alveoli.
9. Describe how the structure of the respiratory tube changes as the branches become finer.
10. Explain the functions of the respiratory tubes.
11. Distinguish between visceral pleura and parietal pleura.
12. Name and describe the locations of the lobes of the lungs.
13. Define *respiratory membrane* and explain its function.
14. Explain how normal inspiration and forced inspiration are accomplished.
15. Define *surface tension* and explain how it aids the breathing mechanism.
16. Define *compliance*.
17. Explain how normal expiration and forced expiration are accomplished.
18. Describe the location of the respiratory center and name its major components.
19. Describe how the basic rhythm of breathing is controlled.
20. Explain the function of the pneumotaxic area of the respiratory center.
21. Describe the function of the chemoreceptors in the carotid and aortic bodies.

CHAPTER 14

The Cardiovascular System

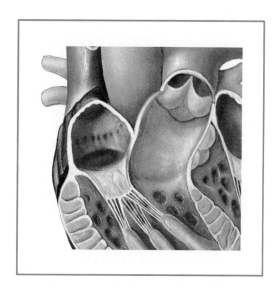

The plasma and cells of the blood carry substances that are necessary for the survival of all body cells. Waste substances from these body cells must be removed from the tissue fluid surrounding them. Blood, circulating in blood vessels, provides the medium that exchanges these necessary materials for waste from the tissue fluid. (See chapter 4.)

The *cardiovascular system* includes the heart and blood vessels. It moves blood between the body cells and organs of the integumentary, digestive, respiratory, and urinary systems, which communicate with the external environment. In performing this function, the heart acts as a pump that forces blood through the blood vessels. The blood vessels, in turn, form a closed system of ducts that transports blood and allows exchanges of gases, nutrients, and wastes between the blood and the body cells.

Chapter Outline

Introduction

Structure of the Heart
Size and Location of the Heart
Coverings of the Heart
Wall of the Heart
Heart Chambers and Valves
Skeleton of the Heart
Path of Blood through the Heart
Blood Vessels to the Heart

Actions of the Heart
The Cardiac Cycle
Cardiac Muscle Fibers
Cardiac Conduction System
Regulation of the Cardiac Cycle

Blood Vessels
Arteries and Arterioles
Capillaries
Venules and Veins

Paths of Circulation
The Pulmonary Circuit
The Systemic Circuit

The Arterial System
Principal Branches of the Aorta
Arteries to the Neck, Head, and
Brain
Arteries to the Shoulder and Arm
Arteries to the Thoracic and
Abdominal Walls
Arteries to the Pelvis and Leg

The Venous System
Characteristics of Venous Pathways
Veins from the Head, Neck, and
Brain
Veins from the Arm and Shoulder
Veins from the Abdominal and
Thoracic Walls
Veins from the Abdominal Viscera
Veins from the Leg and Pelvis

Clinical Terms Related to the
Cardiovascular System

Chapter Objectives

After you have studied this chapter, you should be able to

1. Name the organs of the cardiovascular system and discuss their functions.

2. Name and describe the location of the major parts of the heart and discuss the function of each part.

3. Trace the pathway of blood through the heart and the vessels of the coronary circulation.

4. Discuss the cardiac cycle and briefly explain how it is controlled.

5. Compare the structures and functions of the major types of blood vessels.

6. Compare the pulmonary and systemic circuits of the cardiovascular system.

7. Identify and locate the major arteries and veins of the pulmonary and systemic circuits.

8. Complete the review activities at the end of this chapter. Note that the items are worded in the form of specific learning objectives. You may want to refer to them before reading the chapter.

Aids to Understanding Words

angio-, a vessel: *angio*gram—an X-ray film of blood vessels.

cardia-, heart: peri*cardium*—a membrane that surrounds the heart.

diastol-, dilation: *diastole*—the portion of the cardiac cycle that occurs when the heart is relaxed (thus dilated).

myo-, muscle: *myo*cardium—the muscle tissue within the wall of the heart.

occlude, to close: *occlu*sion—an obstruction that may occur in a blood vessel.

papill-, nipple: *papill*ary muscle—a small mound of muscle within a chamber of the heart.

phleb-, vein: *phleb*itis—an inflammation of a vein.

scler-, hard: *scler*osis—condition in which a blood vessel wall loses its elasticity and becomes hard.

syn-, together: *syn*cytium—a mass of merging cells that act together.

systol-, contraction: *systole*—the portion of the cardiac cycle that occurs when the heart is contracting.

vas-, vessel: *vasa vaso*rum—small blood vessels found in the walls of larger blood vessels.

Introduction

A functional cardiovascular system is vital for survival, because without circulation, tissues lack a supply of oxygen and nutrients, and waste substances accumulate. Under such conditions, cells soon begin to undergo irreversible changes that quickly lead to the death of the organism. The general pattern of the cardiovascular system is shown in figure 14.1.

Structure of the Heart

The heart is a hollow, cone-shaped, muscular pump located within the mediastinum of the thorax and resting upon the diaphragm. (See reference plate 69.)

Size and Location of the Heart

Although its size varies with body size, the heart of an average adult is generally about 12 centimeters long and 9 centimeters wide. The heart is located in the mediastinum, and is bordered laterally by the lungs, posteriorly by the vertebral column, and anteriorly by the sternum (figure 14.2). Its *base*, which is attached to several large blood vessels, lies beneath the second rib. Its distal end extends downward and to the left, terminating as a bluntly pointed *apex* at the level of the fifth intercostal space. For this reason, it is possible to sense the *apical heartbeat* by feeling or listening to the chest wall between the fifth and sixth ribs, about 7.5 centimeters to the left of the midline. (See figure 6.44 for an X ray showing the position of the heart.)

Coverings of the Heart

The heart and the proximal ends of the large blood vessels to which it is attached are enclosed by a double-layered **parietal pericardium** (pericardial sac). The outer layer of this loose-fitting sac is the tough *fibrous pericardium* and the inner layer is the *serous pericardium*. At the base of the heart the serous pericardium turns back on itself to form the *visceral pericardium* (epicardium). This thin serous membrane forms the thin, outer layer of the heart wall.

The parietal pericardium is a tough, protective sac composed largely of white fibrous connective tissue and a serous membrane. It is attached to the central portion of the diaphragm, the back of the sternum, the vertebral column, and the large blood vessels emerging from the heart. (See figure 14.3.) Between the parietal and visceral membranes is a potential space, the *pericardial cavity*, that contains a small amount of serous fluid. This fluid reduces friction between the pericardial membranes as the heart moves within them (figure 14.4).

FIGURE 14.1

The cardiovascular system functions to transport blood between the body cells and organs that communicate with the external environment.

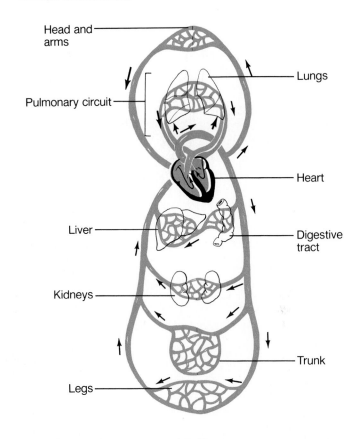

FIGURE 14.2

The heart is located behind the sternum, where it lies upon the diaphragm.

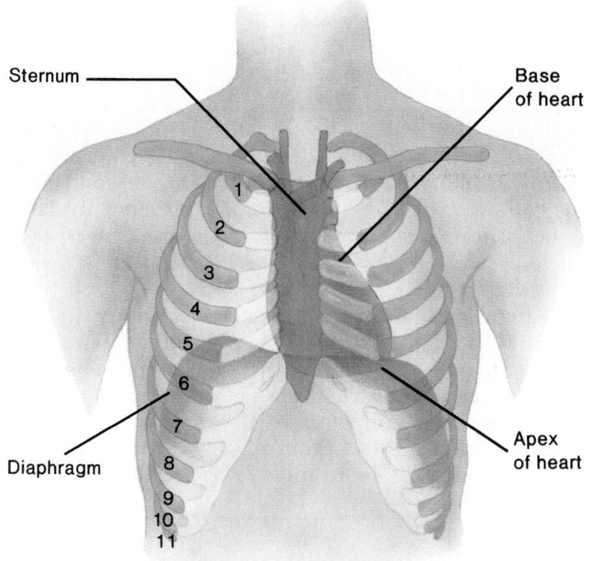

FIGURE 14.3
The heart is within the mediastinum and is enclosed by a layered pericardium.

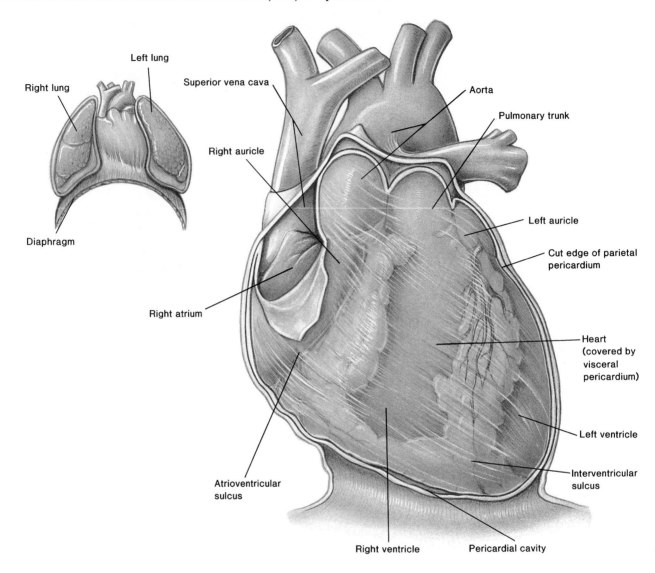

Left lung

Right lung

Superior vena cava

Aorta

Pulmonary trunk

Right auricle

Left auricle

Cut edge of parietal pericardium

Diaphragm

Right atrium

Heart (covered by visceral pericardium)

Left ventricle

Interventricular sulcus

Atrioventricular sulcus

Right ventricle

Pericardial cavity

If the pericardium becomes inflamed due to a bacterial or viral infection, the condition is called *pericarditis*. As a result of this inflammation, the layers of the pericardium sometimes become stuck together by adhesions, and this may cause considerable pain and interfere with heart movements.

Sometimes, as a result of disease or injury, fluid accumulates rapidly in the pericardial cavity. This condition, called *acute cardiac tamponade*, can be life threatening, because increasing pressure within the pericardial cavity may compress the heart and interfere with the flow of blood into its chambers. An early symptom of acute cardiac tamponade may be a visible engorgement of veins in the neck.

1. Where is the heart located?
2. Where would you listen to hear the apical heartbeat?
3. Distinguish between the visceral pericardium and the parietal pericardium.
4. What is the function of the fluid in the pericardial cavity?

Wall of the Heart

The wall of the heart is composed of three distinct layers: an outer epicardium, a middle myocardium, and an inner endocardium (figure 14.4).

The **epicardium**, also called the visceral pericardium, provides a protective layer. This serous membrane consists

FIGURE 14.4

(a) The wall of the heart consists of three layers: endocardium, myocardium, and epicardium; (b) light micrograph of a portion of the heart wall.

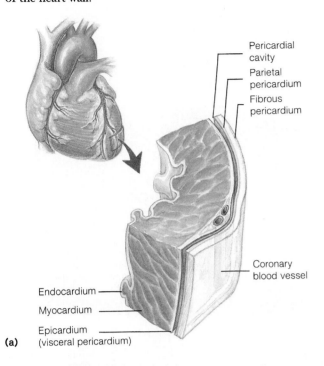

(a)

Pericardial cavity
Parietal pericardium
Fibrous pericardium
Coronary blood vessel
Endocardium
Myocardium
Epicardium (visceral pericardium)

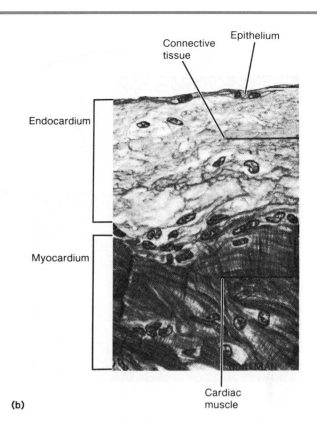

(b)

Connective tissue
Epithelium
Endocardium
Myocardium
Cardiac muscle

Chart 14.1 The wall of the heart

Layer	Composition	Function
Epicardium (visceral pericardium)	Serous membrane of connective tissue covered with epithelium and including blood capillaries, lymph capillaries, and nerve fibers	Forms a protective outer covering
Myocardium	Cardiac muscle tissue separated by connective tissues and including blood capillaries, lymph capillaries, and nerve fibers	Produces muscular contractions that force blood from the heart chambers
Endocardium	Membrane of epithelium and connective tissues, including elastic and collagenous fibers, blood vessels, and specialized muscle fibers	Forms a protective inner lining of the chambers and valves

of connective tissue covered by epithelium and includes blood capillaries, lymph capillaries, and nerve fibers. Its deeper portion often contains fat, particularly along the paths of larger blood vessels.

The middle layer, or **myocardium,** is relatively thick and consists largely of the cardiac muscle tissue responsible for forcing blood out of the heart chambers. The muscle fibers are arranged in planes separated by connective tissues that are richly supplied with blood capillaries, lymph capillaries, and nerve fibers.

The inner layer, or **endocardium,** consists of epithelium and connective tissue that contains many elastic and

collagenous fibers (figure 14.4). The connective tissue also contains blood vessels and some specialized cardiac muscle fibers, called *Purkinje fibers.* The function of these fibers is described in a subsequent section of this chapter.

The endocardium lines all of the heart chambers and covers structures, such as the heart valves, that project into them. This inner lining is also continuous with the inner linings of the blood vessels (endothelium) attached to the heart.

Chart 14.1 summarizes the characteristics of these three layers of the heart.

FIGURE 14.5

What features can you identify in (*a*) anterior view and (*b*) posterior view of the heart?

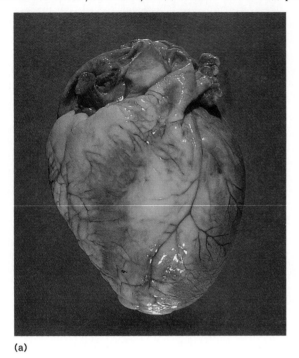

(a)

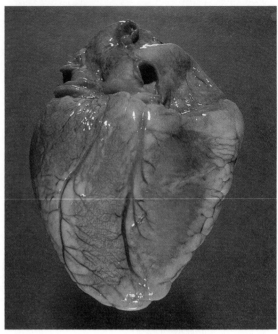

(b)

Endocarditis is an inflammation of the endocardium. This condition sometimes accompanies bacterial diseases, such as scarlet fever or syphilis, and may produce lasting effects by damaging the valves of the heart.

1. Describe the layers of the heart wall.
2. Name and locate the four chambers of the heart.
3. Name the orifices that occur between the upper and the lower chambers of the heart.
4. Name the structure that separates the right and left sides of the heart.

Heart Chambers and Valves

Internally, the heart is divided into four hollow chambers, two on the left and two on the right. The upper chambers, the **atria** (sing. *atrium*), have relatively thin walls and receive blood from veins. The lower chambers, the **ventricles,** force blood out of the heart into arteries. (Note: Veins are blood vessels that carry blood *toward* the heart; arteries carry blood away from the heart.)

The atrium and ventricle on the right side are separated from those on the left by a *septum*. The atrium on each side communicates with its corresponding ventricle through an opening called the **atrioventricular orifice,** which is guarded by an *atrioventricular valve* (A-V *valve*).

Grooves on the surface of the heart mark the divisions between its chambers, and they also contain major blood vessels that supply the heart tissues. The deepest of these grooves is the **atrioventricular** (coronary) **sulcus,** which encircles the heart between the atrial and ventricular portions. Two **interventricular** (anterior and posterior) **sulci** indicate the location of the interventricular septum that separates the right and left ventricles. Small, earlike projections called **auricles** extend outward from the atria (figures 14.3 and 14.5).

The right atrium receives blood from two large veins: the *superior vena cava* and the *inferior vena cava*. These veins return blood low in oxygen from various body parts. A smaller vein, the *coronary sinus,* also drains blood into the right atrium from the wall of the heart.

The atrioventricular orifice between the right atrium and the right ventricle is guarded by a large **tricuspid valve** composed of three leaflets or cusps, as its name implies. This valve permits blood to move from the right atrium into the right ventricle and prevents it from passing in the opposite direction. The cusps fold passively out of the way when the blood pressure is greater on the atrial side; when the pressure is greater on the ventricular side, they close passively (figures 14.6 and 14.7).

Strong, fibrous strings, called *chordae tendineae,* are attached to the cusps on the ventricular side. These strings originate from small mounds of muscle tissue, the **papillary muscles,** that project inward from the walls of the ventricle. When the tricuspid valve closes, the chordae tendineae and papillary muscles prevent the cusps from swinging back into the atrium.

FIGURE 14.6

A frontal section of the heart (*a*) showing the connection between the right ventricle and the pulmonary trunk, and (*b*) showing the connection between the left ventricle and the aorta.

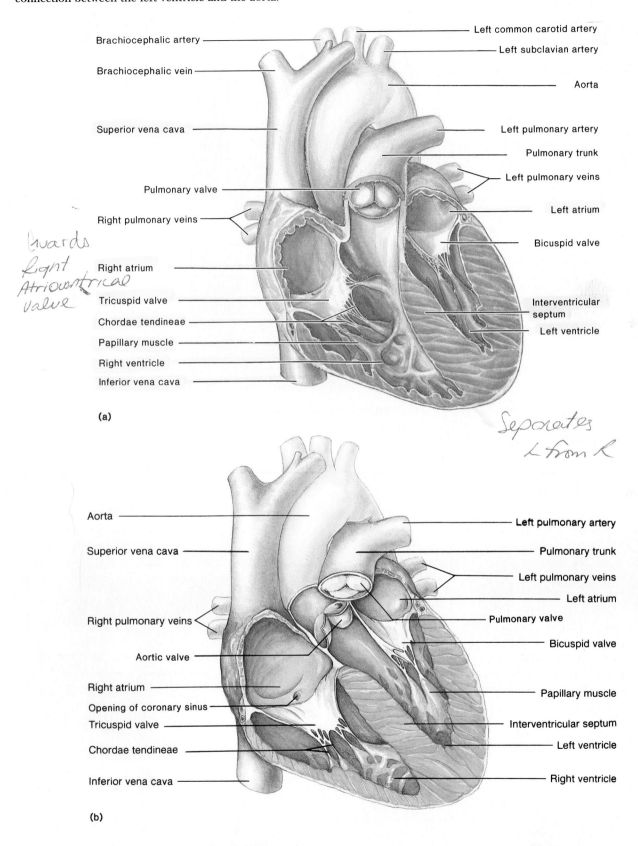

(a)

(b)

FIGURE 14.7
(*a*) A photograph of the right ventricle and tricuspid valve; (*b*) opening and closing of an atrioventricular valve.

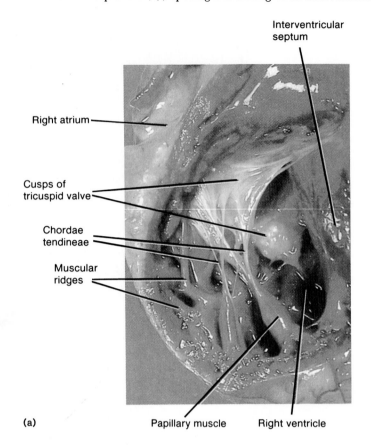

(a)

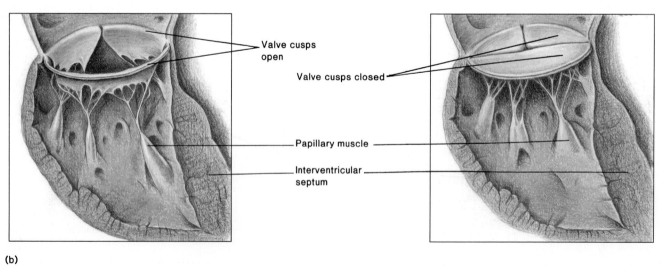

(b)

FIGURE 14.8

A transverse section through the ventricles. Note the difference in thickness of the ventricular walls.

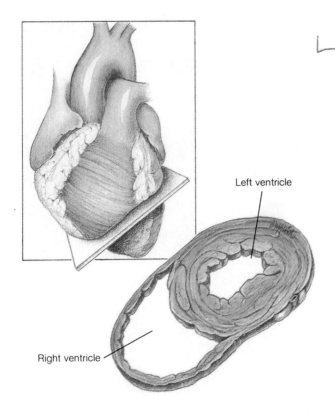

Left ventricle

Right ventricle

The right ventricle has a much thinner muscular wall than the left ventricle (figure 14.8). This right chamber pumps blood a fairly short distance to the lungs. The left ventricle, on the other hand, must force blood to all other parts of the body.

When the muscular wall of the right ventricle contracts, the blood inside its chamber is put under increasing pressure, and the tricuspid valve closes passively. As a result, the only exit is through the *pulmonary trunk,* which divides to form the left and right *pulmonary arteries.* At the base of this trunk is a **pulmonary valve** (pulmonary semi-lunar valve) that consists of three cusps, which are attached to the wall of the pulmonary trunk. This valve opens as the right ventricle contracts, and the cusps are passively pushed aside. However, when the ventricular muscles relax, the blood begins to back up in the pulmonary trunk. This causes the cusps to fill and extend into the middle of the pulmonary trunk, thus closing the valve. This action prevents a return blood flow into the ventricular chamber.

The left atrium receives blood from the lungs through four *pulmonary veins*—two from the right lung and two from the left. Blood passes from the left atrium into the left ventricle through the atrioventricular orifice, which is guarded by a valve. This valve consists of two leaflets, and is appropriately named the **bicuspid,** or **mitral, valve.** It prevents blood from flowing back into the left atrium from the ventricle. As with the tricuspid valve, the cusps of the bicuspid valve are prevented from swinging back into the left atrium by the papillary muscles and the chordae tendineae.

When the left ventricle contracts, the bicuspid valve closes passively, and the only exit for blood is through a large artery called the *aorta.* Its branches distribute blood to all parts of the body.

At the base of the aorta is an **aortic valve** (aortic semi-lunar valve) that consists of three cusps and is similar in structure and function to the pulmonary valve. (See figures 14.6 and 14.9.) It opens and allows blood to leave the left ventricle as it contracts. When the ventricular muscles relax, this valve closes and prevents blood from backing up into the ventricle. Chart 14.2 summarizes the locations and functions of the heart valves.

A heart disorder that affects up to 6% of the U.S. population is *mitral valve prolapse.* In this condition, one (or both) of the cusps of the bicuspid (mitral) valve is stretched so that it bulges into the left atrium during ventricular contraction. Although the valve continues to function adequately in most cases, sometimes blood regurgitates into the left atrium, causing some degree of disability. The cause of mitral valve prolapse is unknown.

Chart 14.2 Valves of the heart

Valve	Location	Function	Valve	Location	Function
Tricuspid valve	Right atrioventricular orifice	Prevents blood from moving from right ventricle into right atrium during ventricular contraction	Bicuspid (mitral) valve	Left atrioventricular orifice	Prevents blood from moving from left ventricle into left atrium during ventricular contraction
Pulmonary valve	Entrance to pulmonary trunk	Prevents blood from moving from pulmonary trunk into right ventricle during ventricular relaxation	Aortic valve	Entrance to aorta	Prevents blood from moving from aorta into left ventricle during ventricular relaxation

FIGURE 14.9

(a) A photograph of the aortic and pulmonary valves of the heart (superior view). Note the difference in thickness of the blood vessel walls; (b) these valves prevent blood from backing up into the ventricles.

(b) From *Human Physiology* by Elliott B. Mason. Copyright © 1983, Benjamin/Cummings Publishing Company, Menlo Park, Calif. Reprinted by permission.

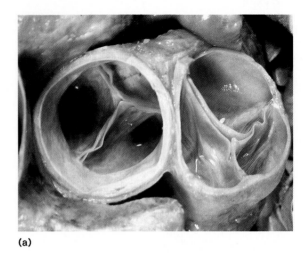

(a)

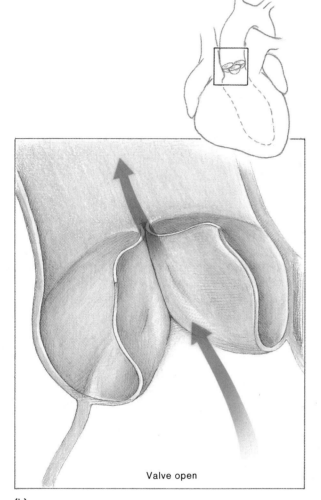

Valve open

Valve closed

(b)

1. Which blood vessels carry blood into the right atrium?
2. Where does the blood go after it leaves the right ventricle?
3. Which blood vessels carry blood into the left atrium?
4. What prevents blood from flowing back into the ventricles when they are relaxed?

Skeleton of the Heart

At their proximal ends, the pulmonary trunk and aorta are surrounded by rings of dense fibrous connective tissue. These rings are continuous with others that encircle the atrioventricular orifices. They provide firm attachments for the heart valves and for various muscle fibers. In addition, they prevent the outlets of the atria and ventricles from dilating during myocardial contraction. The fibrous rings together with other masses of dense fibrous tissue in the upper portion of the interventricular septum constitute the *skeleton of the heart* (figure 14.10).

Path of Blood through the Heart

Blood that is relatively low in oxygen and relatively high in carbon dioxide enters the right atrium through the venae cavae and the coronary sinus. As the right atrial wall contracts, blood passes through the right atrioventricular orifice and enters the chamber of the right ventricle (figure 14.11).

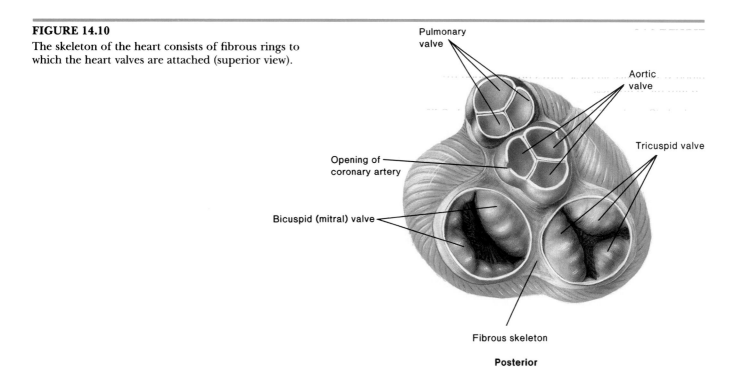

FIGURE 14.10
The skeleton of the heart consists of fibrous rings to which the heart valves are attached (superior view).

Pulmonary valve

Aortic valve

Tricuspid valve

Opening of coronary artery

Bicuspid (mitral) valve

Fibrous skeleton

Posterior

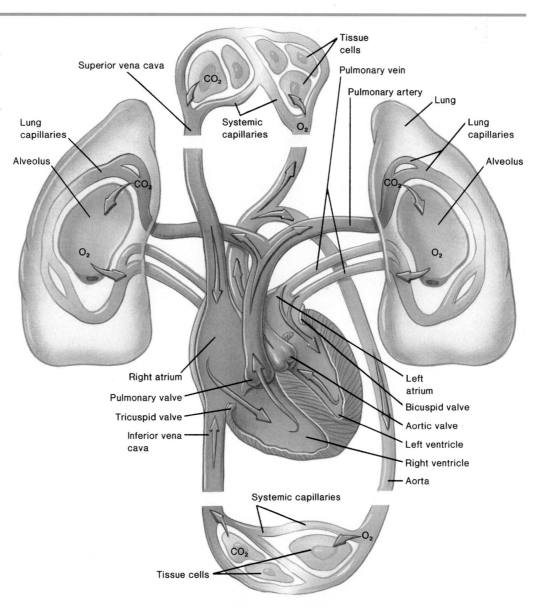

FIGURE 14.11
The right ventricle forces blood to the lungs, while the left ventricle forces blood to all other body parts. How does the composition of the blood in these two chambers differ?

Tissue cells

Superior vena cava

Pulmonary vein

Pulmonary artery

Lung

Lung capillaries

CO_2

Systemic capillaries

O_2

Alveolus

Lung capillaries

Alveolus

CO_2

CO_2

O_2

O_2

Right atrium

Left atrium

Pulmonary valve

Bicuspid valve

Tricuspid valve

Aortic valve

Inferior vena cava

Left ventricle

Right ventricle

Aorta

Systemic capillaries

O_2

CO_2

Tissue cells

FIGURE 14.12
The openings of the coronary arteries lie beyond the aortic semilunar valve.

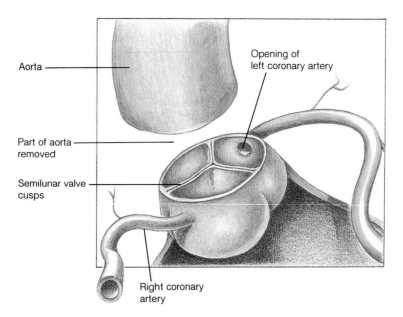

Aorta

Opening of
left coronary artery

Part of aorta
removed

Semilunar valve
cusps

Right coronary
artery

When the right ventricular wall contracts, the tricuspid valve closes the right atrioventricular orifice, and the blood moves into the pulmonary trunk and its branches (pulmonary circuit). From these vessels, blood enters the capillaries associated with the alveoli of the lungs. Gas exchanges occur between the blood in the capillaries and the air in the alveoli. The freshly oxygenated blood, now relatively low in carbon dioxide, returns to the heart through the pulmonary veins leading to the left atrium.

The left atrial wall contracts, and the blood moves through the left atrioventricular orifice and into the chamber of the left ventricle. When the left ventricular wall contracts, the bicuspid valve closes the left atrioventricular orifice, and the blood passes into the aorta and its branches (systemic circuit).

Blood Vessels to the Heart

Blood is supplied to the tissues of the heart by the first two branches of the aorta, called the **right** and **left coronary arteries.** Their openings lie just beyond the aortic semilunar valve (figures 14.10 and 14.12).

One branch of the left coronary artery, the *circumflex artery,* follows the atrioventricular sulcus between the left atrium and the left ventricle. Its branches supply blood to the walls of the left atrium and the left ventricle. Another branch of the left coronary artery, the *anterior interventricular artery* (left anterior descending artery), travels in the anterior interventricular sulcus, and its branches supply the walls of both ventricles.

The right coronary artery passes along the atrioventricular sulcus between the right atrium and the right ventricle. It gives off two major branches—a *posterior interventricular artery,* which travels along the posterior interventricular sulcus and supplies the walls of both ventricles, and a *marginal artery,* which passes along the lower border of the heart. Branches of the marginal artery supply the walls of the right atrium and the right ventricle (figures 14.13, 14.14, and 14.15).

If a branch of a coronary artery becomes abnormally constricted or obstructed, the myocardial cells it supplies may experience a blood oxygen deficiency called *ischemia.* As a result of ischemia, the person may experience a painful condition called *angina pectoris.* The discomfort usually occurs during physical activity, when the myocardial cells' need for oxygen exceeds the blood oxygen supply. However, the pain is commonly relieved by rest. Angina pectoris may also be triggered by an emotional disturbance. It may cause a sensation of heavy pressure, tightening, or squeezing in the chest. Although it is usually felt in the region behind the sternum or in the anterior portion of the upper thorax, the pain may radiate to other parts, including the neck, jaw, throat, arm, shoulder, elbow, back, or upper abdomen. Angina pectoris may be accompanied by profuse perspiration (diaphoresis), difficulty in breathing (dyspnea), nausea, or vomiting.

Sometimes a portion of the heart dies because a blood clot forms and completely obstructs a coronary artery or one of its branches (coronary thrombosis). This condition, called a *myocardial infarction* (more commonly called a heart attack), is one of the leading causes of death.

FIGURE 14.13

Blood vessels associated with the surface of the heart. (*a*) Anterior view; (*b*) posterior view.

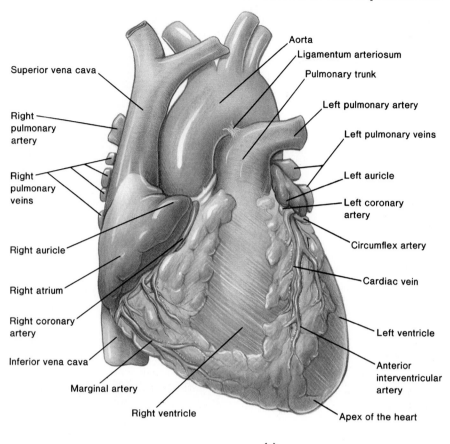

Aorta
Ligamentum arteriosum
Pulmonary trunk
Left pulmonary artery
Left pulmonary veins
Left auricle
Left coronary artery
Circumflex artery
Cardiac vein
Left ventricle
Anterior interventricular artery
Apex of the heart

Superior vena cava
Right pulmonary artery
Right pulmonary veins
Right auricle
Right atrium
Right coronary artery
Inferior vena cava
Marginal artery
Right ventricle

(a)

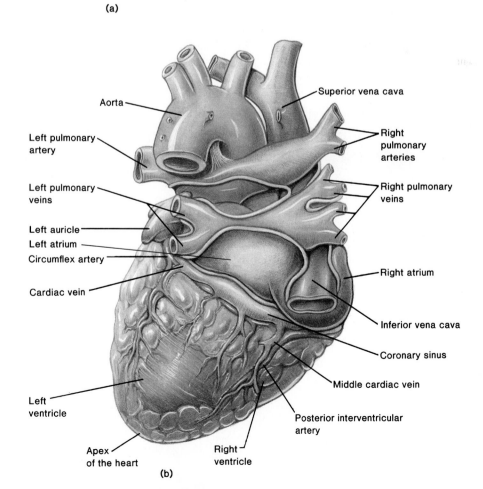

Aorta
Left pulmonary artery
Left pulmonary veins
Left auricle
Left atrium
Circumflex artery
Cardiac vein
Left ventricle

Superior vena cava
Right pulmonary arteries
Right pulmonary veins
Right atrium
Inferior vena cava
Coronary sinus
Middle cardiac vein
Posterior interventricular artery

Apex of the heart
Right ventricle

(b)

FIGURE 14.14

(*a*) Blood is supplied to heart tissues by branches of the coronary arteries; (*b*) blood is drained by branches of the cardiac veins.

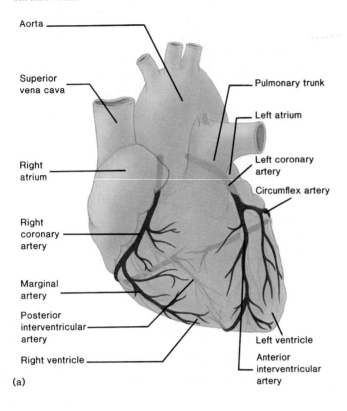

(a)

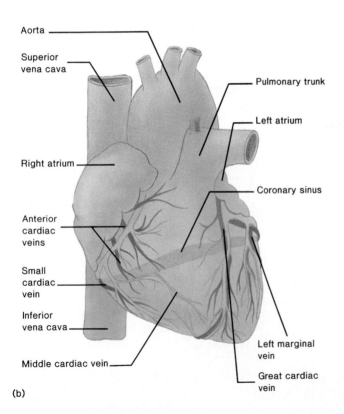

(b)

FIGURE 14.15

(*a*) A cast of the coronary arteries. These vessels supply blood to the heart. (*b*) An angiogram (X-ray film) of the coronary arteries. (The arrow indicates a blockage of the anterior interventricular artery.)

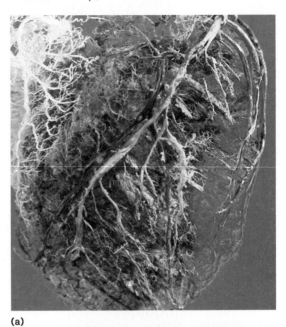

(a)

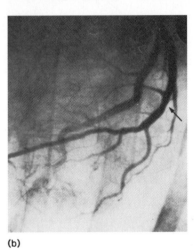

(b)

Because the heart must beat continually to supply blood to the body tissues, the myocardial cells require a constant supply of freshly oxygenated blood. The myocardium contains many capillaries fed by branches of the coronary arteries. The smaller branches of these arteries usually form interconnected networks, called *anastomoses,* that provide alternate pathways for blood.

In most body parts, blood flow in arteries reaches a peak during ventricular contraction. However, blood flow in the vessels of the myocardium is poorest during ventricular contraction. This is because the contracting muscle fibers of the myocardium compress nearby vessels, and this action interferes with blood flow. Also, the openings into the coronary arteries may be partially closed during ventricular contraction. Conversely, during ventricular relaxation, the myocardial vessels are no longer compressed and the orifices of the coronary arteries are open. Consequently, blood flow into the myocardium increases.

Blood that has passed through the capillaries of the myocardium is drained by branches of **cardiac veins,** whose paths roughly parallel those of the coronary arteries. As figure 14.14 shows, these veins join the **coronary sinus,** an enlarged vein on the posterior surface of the heart in the atrioventricular sulcus that empties into the right atrium.

In the *heart transplantation* procedure, the failing heart is removed except for the posterior walls of the right and left atria and their connections to the venae cavae and pulmonary veins. The donor heart is prepared similarly and is attached to the atrial cuffs remaining in the recipient's thorax. Finally, the recipient's aorta and pulmonary arteries are connected to those of the donor heart.

---

1. What structures make up the skeleton of the heart?
2. Review the path of blood through the heart.
3. What vessels supply blood to the myocardium?
4. How does blood return from the cardiac tissues to the right atrium?

Actions of the Heart

Although the previous discussion described the actions of the heart chambers separately, they do not function independently. Instead, their actions are regulated so that the atrial walls contract while the ventricular walls are relaxed, and ventricular walls contract while the atrial walls are relaxed. Such a series of events constitutes a complete heartbeat, or **cardiac cycle.** At the end of each cycle, the atria and the ventricles remain relaxed for a moment before a new cycle begins.

The Cardiac Cycle

When the atria are relaxed, blood flows into them from the large, attached veins. About 70% of the entering blood flows directly into the ventricles through the atrioventricular orifices before the atrial walls contract. Then, during atrial contraction (atrial systole), the remaining 30% of the blood is forced into the ventricles. This is followed by atrial relaxation (atrial diastole). (See figure 14.16.)

As the ventricles contract (ventricular systole), the A-V valves guarding the atrioventricular orifices close passively and begin to bulge back into the atria. At the same time, the papillary muscles contract, and by pulling on the chordae tendineae, they prevent the cusps of the A-V valves

---

FIGURE 14.16

(*a*) The ventricles fill with blood during ventricular diastole and (*b*) empty during ventricular systole.

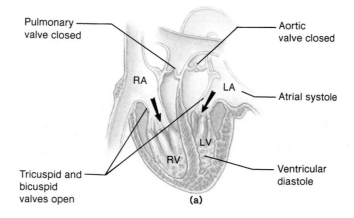

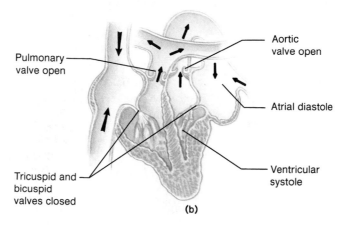

461

from bulging too far into the atria. During the ventricular contraction, the A-V valves remain closed. When the ventricles relax (ventricular diastole), the A-V valves open passively, and blood flows through them into the ventricles.

While the ventricles are contracting and the A-V valves are closed, the pulmonary and aortic valves open. Blood is ejected from the ventricles into the pulmonary trunk and aorta. When the ventricles are nearly empty, they relax. The pulmonary and aortic valves are closed by arterial blood flowing back toward the ventricles.

The sounds associated with a heartbeat can be heard with a stethoscope and are described as *lub-dup* sounds. These sounds are due to vibrations in heart tissues that are created as blood flow is suddenly speeded or slowed with the contraction and relaxation of heart chambers, and with the opening and closing of valves.

The first part of a heart sound (lub) occurs during the ventricular contraction, when the A-V valves are closing. The second part (dup) occurs during ventricular relaxation, when the semilunar valves are closing.

Heart sounds are of particular interest because they provide information concerning the condition of the heart valves. For example, an inflammation of the endocardium (endocarditis) may cause changes in the shapes of the valvular cusps (valvular stenosis). Then, when the cusps close, the closure may be incomplete, and some blood may leak back through the valve. If this happens, an abnormal sound called a *murmur* may be heard. The seriousness of a murmur depends on the amount of valvular damage. Fortunately for those who have serious problems, it may be possible to repair the damaged valves or to replace them by open heart surgery.

Using a stethoscope, it is possible to hear sounds associated with the aortic and pulmonary valves by listening from the second intercostal space on either side of the sternum. The *aortic sound* is heard on the right, and the *pulmonic sound* is heard on the left.

The sound associated with the bicuspid (mitral) valve can be heard from the fifth intercostal space at the nipple line on the left. The sound of the tricuspid valve can be heard at the tip of the sternum (figure 14.17).

Cardiac Muscle Fibers

As mentioned in chapter 5, cardiac muscle fibers are interconnected in branching networks that spread in all directions through the heart. (See figure 4.37.) When any portion of this net is stimulated, an impulse travels to all of its parts, and the whole structure contracts as a unit.

A mass of merging cells acting as a unit is called a **functional syncytium.** There are two such structures in the heart—one in the atrial walls and another in the ventricular walls. These masses of muscle fibers are separated from each other by portions of the heart's fibrous skeleton, except for a small area in the right atrial floor. In this region, the *atrial syncytium* and the *ventricular syncytium* are connected by fibers of the cardiac conduction system.

FIGURE 14.17
Thoracic regions where sounds of each heart valve are heard most easily.

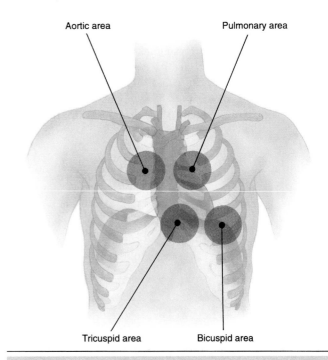

Aortic area

Pulmonary area

Tricuspid area

Bicuspid area

1. Describe the events of a cardiac cycle.
2. What causes heart sounds?
3. What is meant by a functional syncytium?
4. Where are the functional syncytia of the heart located?

Cardiac Conduction System

Throughout the heart there are clumps and strands of specialized cardiac muscle tissue whose fibers contain only a few myofibrils. Instead of contracting, these parts initiate and distribute impulses (cardiac impulses) throughout the myocardium. They comprise the **cardiac conduction system,** which coordinates the events of the cardiac cycle.

A key portion of this conduction system is called the **sinoatrial node** (S-A node). It consists of a small, elongated mass of specialized cardiac muscle tissue just beneath the epicardium. It is located in the posterior wall of the right atrium, below the opening of the superior vena cava, and its fibers are continuous with those of the *atrial syncytium.*

The membranes of the nodal cells are in contact with one another and have the ability to excite themselves. The S-A node initiates one impulse after another, seventy to eighty times a minute. Thus, it is responsible for the rhythmic contractions of the heart and is often called the **pacemaker.** As a cardiac impulse travels from the S-A node into the atrial syncytium, the right and left atria contract almost simultaneously. Instead of passing directly into the

FIGURE 14.18

The cardiac conduction system. What is the function of this system?

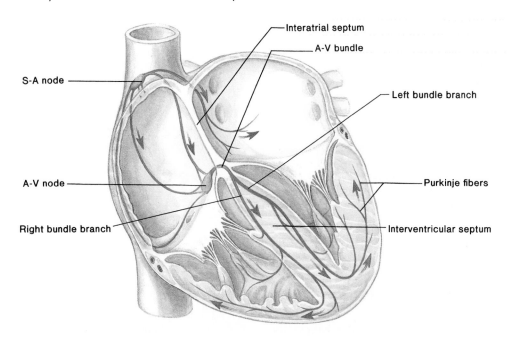

ventricular syncytium, which is separated from the atrial syncytium by the fibrous skeleton of the heart, the cardiac impulse passes along fibers of the conduction system (junctional fibers). These conducting fibers lead to a mass of specialized muscle tissue called the **atrioventricular node** (A-V node). This node, located in the floor of the right atrium near the interatrial septum and just beneath the endocardium, provides the only normal conduction pathway between the atrial and ventricular syncytia.

In about 50–55% of humans, a branch of the right coronary artery supplies blood to the S-A nodal tissue. In perhaps 40–45%, the blood is supplied by a branch of the left coronary artery, and in the remaining 8–10%, branches of both the right and left coronary arteries contribute to the nodal blood supply.

In most persons, a branch of the right coronary artery supplies the tissue of the A-V node; only rarely does the left coronary artery supply this node.

Once the cardiac impulse reaches the other side of the A-V node, it passes into a group of large fibers that make up the **A-V bundle** (bundle of His) and moves rapidly through them. The A-V bundle enters the upper part of the interventricular septum and divides into right and left **bundle branches** that lie just beneath the endocardium. About halfway down the septum, the branches give rise to enlarged **Purkinje fibers.**

The base of the aorta, which contains the aortic valves, is enlarged and protrudes somewhat into the interatrial septum close to the A-V bundle. Consequently, inflammatory conditions, such as bacterial endocarditis, involving the aortic valves (aortic valvulitis) may also affect the A-V bundle.

If a portion of the bundle is damaged, it may no longer conduct impulses normally. As a result, cardiac impulses may reach the two ventricles at different times, causing them to fail to contract together. This condition is called a *bundle branch block.*

The Purkinje fibers spread from the interventricular septum into the papillary muscles that project inward from the ventricular walls, and they continue downward to the apex of the heart. There they curve around the tips of the ventricles and pass upward over the lateral walls of these chambers. Along the way, the Purkinje fibers give off many small branches that become continuous with cardiac muscle fibers. These parts of the conduction system are shown in figure 14.18.

The muscle fibers in the ventricular walls are arranged in irregular whorls, so that when they are stimulated by impulses on Purkinje fibers, the ventricular walls contract with a twisting motion (figure 14.19). This action squeezes or wrings the blood out of the ventricular chambers and forces it into the arteries.

1. What kinds of tissues make up the cardiac conduction system?
2. Identify the parts of the cardiac conduction system.

FIGURE 14.19
The muscle fibers within the ventricular walls are arranged in patterns of whorls. The fibers of groups (*a*) and (*b*) surround both ventricles.

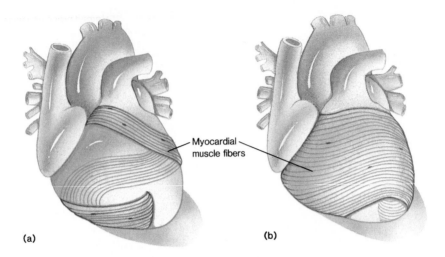

(a)   (b)

Regulation of the Cardiac Cycle

Since the S-A node normally controls the heart rate, changes in this rate often involve factors that affect the pacemaker. These include motor impulses carried on parasympathetic and sympathetic nerve fibers. (See figures 9.59 and 9.60.)

The parasympathetic fibers that supply the heart arise from neurons in the medulla oblongata and comprise parts of the *vagus nerves*. Most of these fibers branch to the S-A and A-V nodes. Impulses from these fibers decrease activity in the nodes; thus, the rate of the heartbeat decreases.

Sympathetic fibers reach the heart by means of the *acceleratory nerves*, whose branches join the S-A and A-V nodes as well as other areas of the atrial and ventricular myocardium. Impulses from these fibers cause an increase in the rate and the force of myocardial contractions.

A normal balance between the inhibitory effects of the parasympathetic fibers and the excitatory effects of the sympathetic fibers is maintained by the *cardiac center* of the medulla oblongata. In this region of the brain, masses of neurons function as *cardioinhibitor* and *cardioaccelerator reflex centers*. These centers receive sensory impulses from various parts of the circulatory system and relay motor impulses to the heart in response.

For example, receptors that are sensitive to being stretched are located in certain regions of the aorta (aortic sinus and aortic arch) and the carotid arteries (carotid sinuses). These receptors, called *pressoreceptors* (baroreceptors), can detect changes in blood pressure. For example, if the pressure rises, the receptors are stretched, and they signal the cardioinhibitor center in the medulla. In response, the medulla sends *parasympathetic motor impulses* to the heart, causing the heart rate and force of contraction to decrease (figure 14.20).

1. What nerves supply parasympathetic fibers to the heart? Sympathetic fibers?
2. How do parasympathetic and sympathetic impulses help control heart rate?
3. Where are pressoreceptors located?

Blood Vessels

The blood vessels are organs of the cardiovascular system that form a closed circuit of tubes carrying blood from the heart to the body cells and back again. These vessels include arteries, arterioles, capillaries, venules, and veins. The arteries and arterioles conduct blood away from the ventricles of the heart and lead to the capillaries. The capillaries function to exchange substances between the blood and the body cells, and the venules and veins return blood from the capillaries to the atria.

Arteries and Arterioles

Arteries are strong, elastic vessels adapted for carrying blood away from the heart under relatively high pressure. These vessels subdivide into progressively thinner tubes and eventually give rise to fine branches called **arterioles.**

The wall of an artery consists of three distinct layers, or *tunics*, shown in figure 14.21. The innermost layer (tunica intima) is composed of a layer of simple squamous epithelium, called *endothelium*, resting on a connective tissue membrane rich in elastic and collagenous fibers. The endothelial lining provides a smooth surface that allows blood cells and platelets to flow through without being damaged.

FIGURE 14.20

The cardiac center receives sensory impulses from pressoreceptors and regulates the activities of the S-A and A-V nodes by means of autonomic nerves.

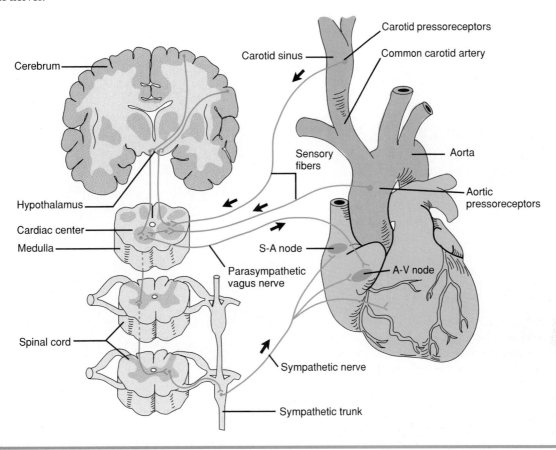

FIGURE 14.21

(a) The wall of an artery and (b) the wall of a vein.

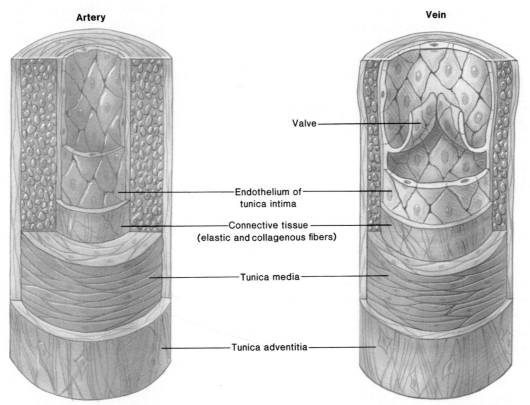

(a)

(b)

FIGURE 14.22

(a) Light micrograph of a portion of an elastic artery (×400) and (b) a muscular artery (×100).

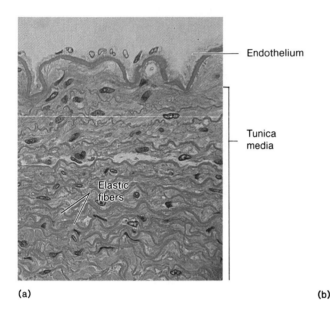

Endothelium

Tunica media

Elastic fibers

(a)

Tunica intima

Tunica media

Tunica adventitia

(b)

The middle layer (tunica media) makes up the bulk of the arterial wall. It includes smooth muscle fibers that encircle the tube, and elastic connective tissue. The large arteries, such as the aorta, are called *elastic arteries*. These vessels contain many elastic fibers as well as smooth muscle cells in the middle layer. This gives the vessels a tough elasticity, allowing them to stretch to accommodate the sudden increase in blood volume that accompanies each ventricular contraction. Intermediate size arteries are called *muscular arteries*. These vessels contain smooth muscle cells but few elastic fibers in the middle layer (figure 14.22).

The outer layer (tunica adventitia) is relatively thin and consists chiefly of connective tissue with irregularly arranged elastic and collagenous fibers. This layer attaches the artery to the surrounding tissues. It also contains minute vessels (vasa vasorum) that give rise to capillaries and provide blood to the more external cells of the artery wall.

Arterioles, which are microscopic continuations of arteries, give off branches called *metarterioles* that, in turn, join capillaries. Although the walls of the larger arterioles have three layers similar to those of arteries, these walls become thinner and thinner as the arterioles approach the capillaries. The wall of a very small arteriole consists only of an endothelial lining and some smooth muscle fibers, surrounded by a small amount of connective tissue (figures 14.23 and 14.24).

FIGURE 14.23

Small arterioles have some smooth muscle fibers in their walls; capillaries lack these fibers.

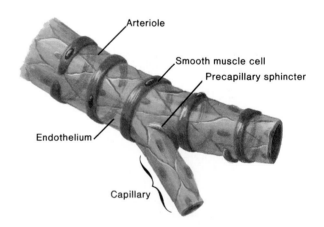

Arteriole

Smooth muscle cell

Precapillary sphincter

Endothelium

Capillary

The smooth muscles in the walls of arteries and arterioles are innervated by sympathetic branches of the autonomic nervous system. Impulses on these *vasomotor fibers* cause the smooth muscles to contract, thus reducing the diameter of the vessel. This action is called **vasoconstriction.** If such vasomotor impulses are inhibited, the muscle fibers relax and the diameter of the vessel increases. In this case, the artery is said to undergo **vasodilation.** Changes in the diameters of arteries greatly influence the flow and pressure of the blood (figure 14.25).

466   Chapter 14

FIGURE 14.24

(*a*) Scanning electron micrograph of an arteriole cross section (×3,900). (*b*) Light micrograph of an arteriole cross section.
(*a*) From R. G. Kessel and R. H. Kardon, *Tissues and Organs: A Text Atlas of Scanning Electron Microscopy*, © 1979, W. H. Freeman & Co.

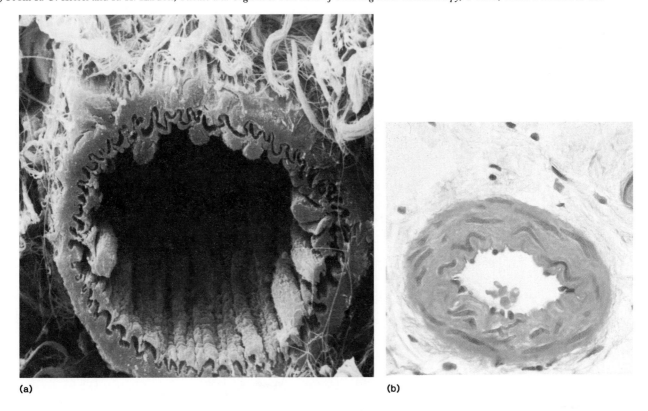

(a)　　　　　　　　　　　　　　(b)

FIGURE 14.25

(*a*) Relaxation of the smooth muscle in the arteriole wall produces vasodilation, while (*b*) contraction of the smooth muscle causes vasoconstriction.

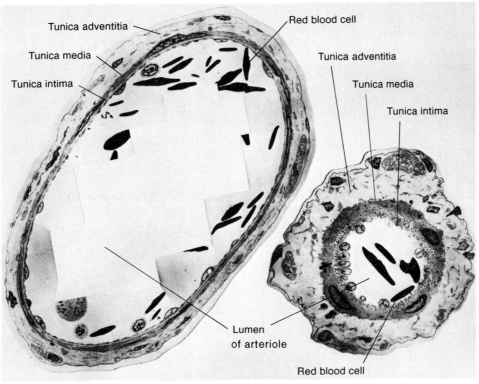

(a)　　　　　　　　　　　　　　(b)

FIGURE 14.26

(*a*) Some metarterioles provide arteriovenous shunts by connecting arterioles directly to venules. (*b*) Light micrograph of circulation in the retina of the human eye.

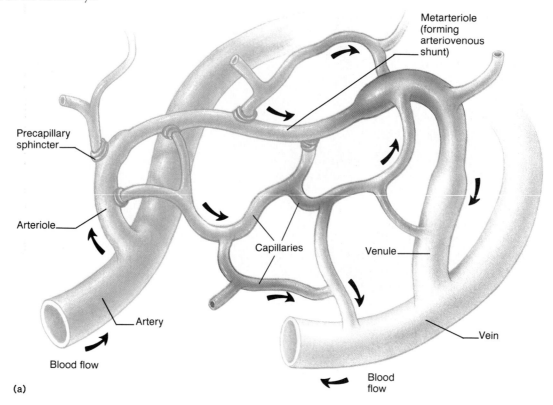

(a)

The arteriole and metarteriole walls are adapted for vasoconstriction and vasodilation in that their muscle fibers respond to impulses from the autonomic nervous system by contracting or relaxing. Thus, these vessels help control the flow of blood into the capillaries.

The vasomotor center of the medulla oblongata continually sends sympathetic impulses to the smooth muscles in the arteriole walls. As a result, these muscles are kept in a state of partial contraction. The vasomotor center can increase its outflow of sympathetic impulses, producing further vasoconstriction. When the pressoreceptors in the aortic arch and carotid sinuses signal the vasomotor center, the sympathetic outflow to the arteriole walls is inhibited. As a result, the vessels undergo vasodilation.

Sometimes metarterioles are connected directly to venules, and the blood entering them can bypass the capillaries. These connections between arteriole and venous pathways, shown in figure 14.26, are called *arteriovenous shunts*.

1. Describe the wall of an artery.
2. What is the function of the smooth muscle in the arterial wall?
3. How is the structure of an arteriole different from that of an artery?
4. How does the vasomotor center control the diameter of arterioles?

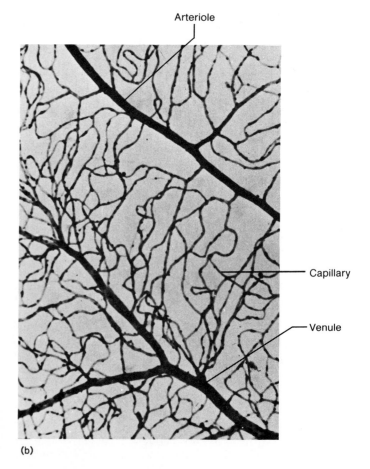

(b)

Capillaries

Capillaries are the smallest blood vessels. They form the connections between the smallest arterioles and the smallest venules. Capillaries are essentially extensions of the inner linings of these larger vessels, in that their walls consist of endothelium—a single layer of squamous epithelial cells and a basement membrane (figure 14.23). These thin walls form the semipermeable membranes through which substances in the blood are exchanged for substances in the tissue fluid surrounding body cells.

Capillary Permeability

The openings or pores in the capillary walls are usually thin slits occurring where two adjacent endothelial cells, or two parts of one cell overlap. The sizes of these pores, and consequently the permeability of the capillary wall, vary from tissue to tissue. For example, the pores are relatively small in the capillaries of smooth muscle, skeletal muscle, cardiac muscle, connective tissue and skin. These capillaries are called *continuous capillaries*. Larger pores in capillaries associated with the kidneys, endocrine glands, and the lining of the small intestine are called *fenestrated capillaries*. In these capillaries, there are also pores within the endothelial cells. Among the capillaries with the largest openings are those of the liver, spleen, and red bone marrow. These capillaries are called *sinusoids*. The pores in the walls of sinusoids commonly allow large molecules and even intact cells to pass through as they enter or leave the vessels (figures 14.27, 14.28, and 14.29).

In the brain, the endothelial cells of the capillary walls are more tightly fused by continuous tight junctions than are those in other body regions. Also, processes of astrocytes (see chapter 9) surround the capillaries (figure 14.30). Consequently, some substances that readily leave capillaries in other tissues enter brain tissues only slightly or not at all. This resistance to movement of some substances is called the *blood-brain barrier*. It is of particular interest because it prevents certain drugs from entering the brain tissues or cerebrospinal fluid in sufficient amounts to effectively treat certain diseases. The capillaries of the pituitary gland, pineal gland, and some portions of the hypothalamus are an exception, since they lack a blood-brain barrier. This allows these parts to respond to changes in the chemical composition of plasma.

Arrangement of Capillaries

The density of capillaries within tissues varies directly with the tissues' needs. Thus, muscle and nerve tissues, which use relatively large quantities of oxygen and nutrients, are richly supplied with capillaries, while cartilaginous tissues, the epidermis, and the cornea, which use fewer nutrients, lack capillaries.

The patterns of capillary arrangement also differ in various body parts. For example, some capillaries pass directly from arterioles to venules, but others lead to highly branched networks. Such arrangements make it possible for blood to follow different pathways through a tissue and meet the varying demands of its cells.

FIGURE 14.27

Types of capillary walls.

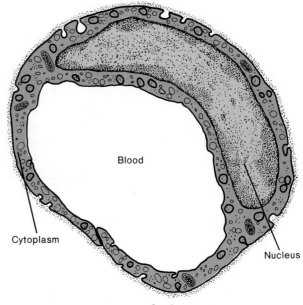

Continuous

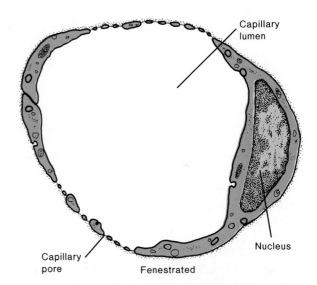

Fenestrated

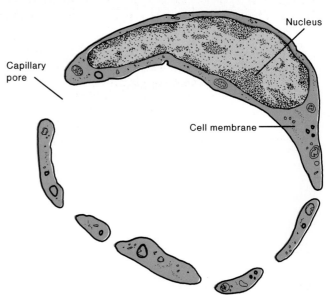

Sinusoid

FIGURE 14.28

(a) Transmission electron micrograph of a capillary cross section. Note the narrow opening at the cell junction through which substances are exchanged between the blood and tissue fluid. The lumen of the capillary is occupied by a red blood cell. (b) Highly magnified view of an endothelial junction.

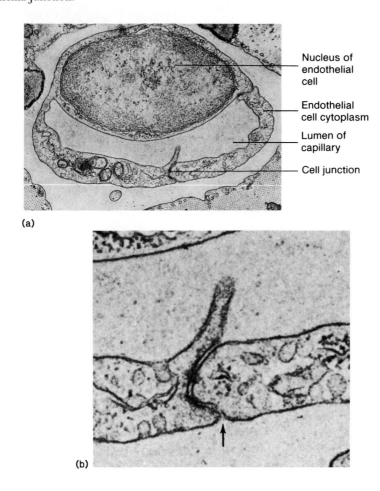

Nucleus of
endothelial
cell

Endothelial
cell cytoplasm

Lumen of
capillary

Cell junction

(a)

(b)

FIGURE 14.29

Leukocytes can squeeze between the cells of a capillary wall and enter the tissue space outside the blood system.

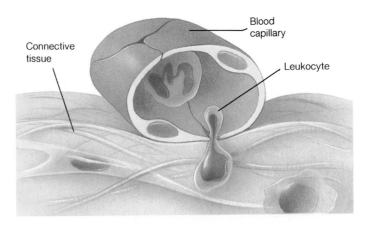

Connective
tissue

Blood
capillary

Leukocyte

FIGURE 14.30

(*a*) Astrocyte processes surround capillaries within the brain and aid in the formation of the blood-brain barrier; (*b*) light micrograph of a brain capillary and astrocytes (×250).

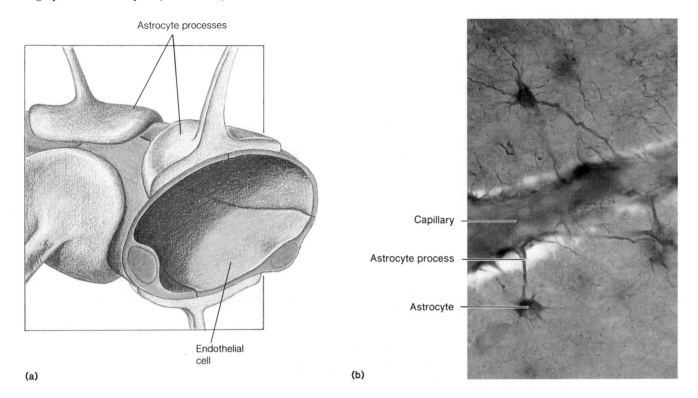

(a)

(b)

Regulation of Capillary Blood Flow

The distribution of blood in the various capillary pathways is regulated mainly by smooth muscles that encircle the capillary entrances. As figure 14.26 shows, these muscles form *precapillary sphincters* that may close a capillary by contracting or open it by relaxing.

---

1. Describe the wall of a capillary.
2. What is the function of a capillary?
3. How is blood flow into capillaries controlled?

Venules and Veins

Venules are the microscopic vessels that continue from the capillaries and merge to form **veins.** The veins, which carry blood back to the atria, follow pathways that roughly parallel those of the arteries.

The walls of veins are similar to those of arteries in that they are composed of three distinct layers. However,

the middle layer of the venous wall is poorly developed. Consequently, veins have thinner walls and contain less smooth muscle and less elastic tissue than arteries (figures 14.31 and 14.32).

Many veins, particularly those in the arms and legs, contain flaplike *valves* that project inward from their linings. These valves, shown in figure 14.33, are usually composed of two leaflets that close if the blood begins to back up in a vein. In other words, the valves aid in returning blood to the heart, since the valves open as long as the flow is toward the heart, but close if it is in the opposite direction.

When skeletal muscles contract, they thicken and press on nearby vessels, squeezing the blood inside. The flaplike semilunar valves in veins offer little resistance to blood flowing toward the heart. Consequently, as skeletal muscles exert pressure on veins with valves, some blood is moved from one valve section to another. This massaging action of contracting skeletal muscles helps push blood through the venous system toward the heart. (See figure 14.34.)

FIGURE 14.31

Note the structural differences in the cross sections of (*a*) an artery (×100) and (*b*) a vein (×160). (*c*) Scanning electron micrograph of a medium-sized artery (MA) and a medium-sized vein (MV) (×305).

(*c*) From R. G. Kessel and R. H. Kardon, *Tissues and Organs: A Text Atlas of Scanning Electron Microscopy*, © 1979, W. H. Freeman & Co.

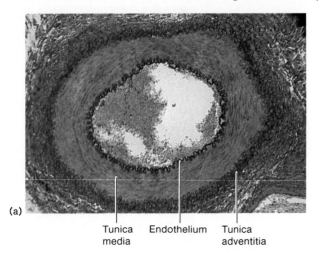

(a)

Tunica   Endothelium   Tunica
media   adventitia

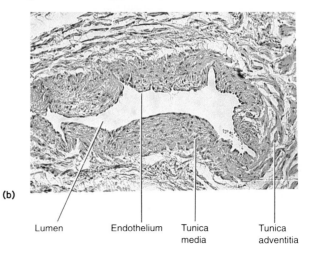

(b)

Lumen   Endothelium   Tunica   Tunica
media   adventitia

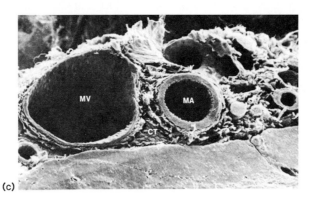

(c)

FIGURE 14.32

Light micrograph of a venule cross section (×250).

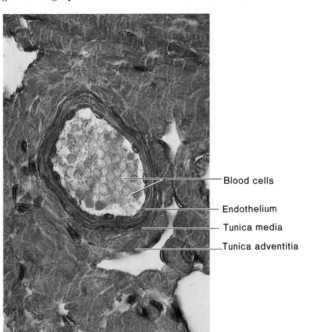

Blood cells

Endothelium

Tunica media

Tunica adventitia

FIGURE 14.33

Venous valves (*a*) allow blood to move toward the heart, but (*b*) prevent blood from moving away from the heart.

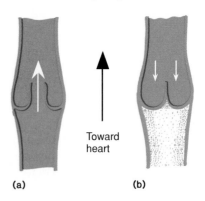

(a)   Toward   (b)

Toward
heart

FIGURE 14.34

The massaging action of skeletal muscles helps move blood through the venous system toward the heart.

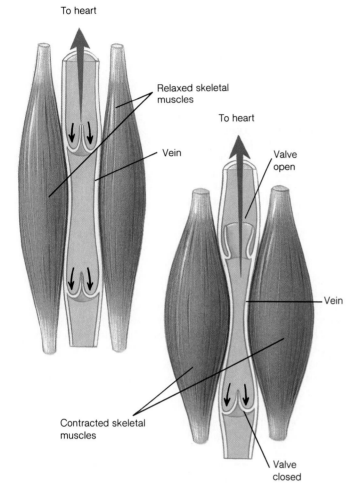

FIGURE 14.35

Most of the blood volume is contained within the veins and venules.

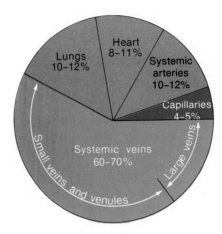

In addition to providing pathways for blood returning to the heart, the veins function as blood reservoirs that can be drawn on in times of need. For example, if a blood loss occurs, the muscular walls of veins are stimulated reflexly by sympathetic nerve impulses. The resulting venous constrictions ensure a nearly normal blood flow even when as much as 25% of the blood volume has been lost. Figure 14.35 illustrates the relative volumes of blood in the veins and other blood vessels. The characteristics of the blood vessels are summarized in chart 14.3.

1. How does the structure of a vein differ from that of an artery?
2. What are the functions of veins and venules?
3. What is the function of the venous valves?
4. How do skeletal muscles affect venous blood flow?

Chart 14.3 Characteristics of blood vessels

Vessel	Type of wall	Function
Artery	Thick, strong wall with three layers—an endothelial lining, a middle layer of smooth muscle and elastic tissue, and an outer layer of connective tissue	Carries blood from the heart to arterioles
Arteriole	Thinner wall than an artery, but with three layers; smaller arterioles have an endothelial lining, some smooth muscle tissue, and a small amount of connective tissue	Connects an artery to a capillary; helps control the blood flow into a capillary by undergoing vasoconstriction or vasodilation
Capillary	Single layer of squamous epithelium	Provides a semipermeable membrane through which nutrients, gases, and wastes are exchanged between the blood and tissue cells; connects an arteriole to a venule
Venule	Thinner wall, less smooth muscle and elastic tissue than an arteriole	Connects a capillary to a vein
Vein	Thinner wall than an artery, but with similar layers; the middle layer more poorly developed; some with flaplike valves	Carries blood from a venule to the heart; valves prevent a back flow of blood; serves as blood reservoir

Blood Vessel Disorders

It is estimated that nearly half of all deaths in the United States are due to the arterial disease called **atherosclerosis.** This condition is characterized by an accumulation of soft masses of fatty materials, particularly cholesterol, on the inside of the arterial wall. Such deposits are called *plaque,* and as they develop, they protrude into the lumens of the vessels and interfere with the blood flow (figure 14.36). Furthermore, plaque often creates a surface that can initiate the formation of a blood clot. As a result, persons with atherosclerosis may develop clots that cause blood deficiency (*ischemia*) or tissue death (*necrosis*) downstream from the obstruction.

Atherosclerosis is often associated with excessive use of saturated fats in the diet, elevated blood pressure, cigarette smoking, obesity, and lack of physical exercise. Emotional and genetic factors also may increase the susceptibility to atherosclerosis.

As individuals age, degenerative changes usually occur in the walls of their arteries. For example, there is a gradual loss of elastic and muscle tissue, and an increase in the fibrous connective tissue in the arterial walls. This condition, called **arteriosclerosis,** results in the arterial walls becoming hardened, or *sclerotic.* As this occurs, there is danger that a sclerotic vessel will rupture under the force of blood pressure. The walls of arteries affected by atherosclerosis often undergo accelerated arteriosclerotic changes.

Sometimes the wall of an artery is so weakened by the effects of disease that blood pressure causes a region of the artery to become dilated, forming a pulsating sac. This condition, called an **aneurysm,** tends to continue increasing in size. If the resulting sac develops by a longitudinal splitting of the middle layer of the arterial wall, it is called a *dissecting aneurysm.* An aneurysm may cause symptoms by pressing on nearby organs, or it may rupture and produce a great loss of blood.

Although most aneurysms seem to be caused by arteriosclerosis, they may also occur as a consequence of trauma, high blood pressure, infections, or congenital defects in blood vessels. Common sites of aneurysms include the thoracic and abdominal aorta, and the arterial circle.

Phlebitis, or inflammation of a vein, is a relatively common disorder. Although it may occur in association with an injury or infection, or as an aftermath of surgery, it sometimes develops for an unknown reason. If such an inflammation is restricted to a superficial vein, the blood flow may be rechanneled through other vessels. If it occurs in a deep vein, however, the consequences can be quite serious, particularly if the blood within the affected vessel clots and blocks the normal circulation. This condition is called *thrombophlebitis.*

Varicose veins are distinguished by the presence of abnormal and irregular dilations in superficial veins, particularly those in the lower legs. This condition is usually associated with prolonged, increased back pressure within the affected vessels due to the force of gravity, as occurs when a person stands. The problem can also be aggravated when venous blood flow is obstructed by crossing the legs or by sitting in a chair so that its edge presses against the popliteal area behind the knee.

Excessive back pressure causes the veins to stretch and their diameters to increase. Because the valves within these vessels do not change size, they soon lose their abilities to block the backward flow of blood, and blood tends to accumulate in the enlarged regions.

Increased venous pressure is also accompanied by rising pressure within the venules and capillaries that supply the veins. Consequently, tissues in affected regions typically become swollen and painful.

Although some people seem to inherit a weakness in their venous valves, *varicose veins* are most common in persons who stand or sit for prolonged periods. Pregnancy and obesity also seem to favor the development of this condition. The discomfort associated with varicose veins can sometimes be relieved by elevating the legs or by putting on support hosiery before arising in the morning, thus preventing the vessel dilation that occurs upon standing. Occasionally, surgical removal of the affected veins may be necessary.

FIGURE 14.36

As atherosclerosis develops, masses of fatty materials accumulate beneath the inner linings of certain arteries and arterioles, and protrude into their lumens. (*a*) Normal arteriole; (*b*), (*c*), and (*d*) accumulation of plaque on the inner wall of the arteriole.

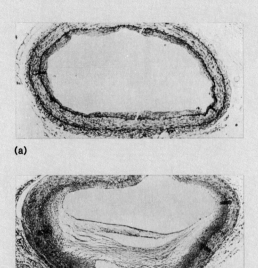

(a)

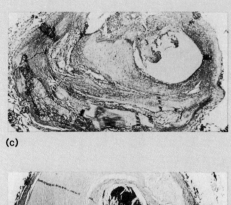

(c)

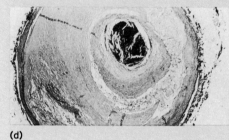

(b)

(d)

FIGURE 14.37
Sites where arterial pulse is most easily detected. (*a.* stands for artery.)

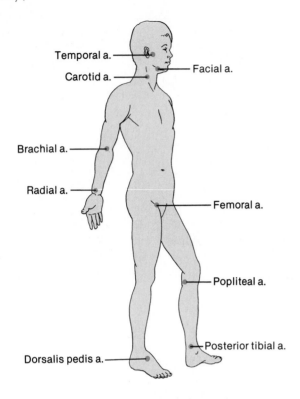

FIGURE 14.38

The pulmonary circuit consists of the vessels that carry blood between the heart and the lungs; all other vessels are included in the systemic circuit.

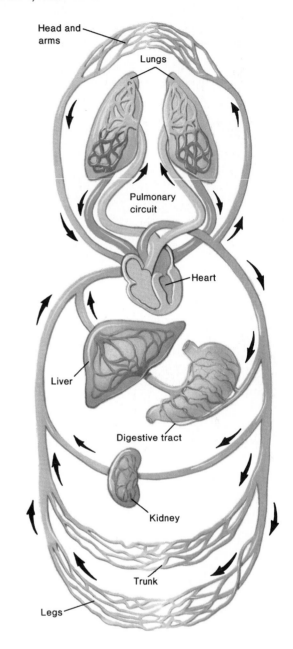

Blood pressure is the force exerted by the blood against the inner walls of blood vessels. Although such a force occurs throughout the vascular system, the term is most commonly used to refer to systemic arterial pressure.

Arterial blood pressure rises and falls in a pattern corresponding to the phases of the cardiac cycle.

The surge of blood entering the arterial system during a ventricular contraction causes the elastic walls of the arteries to stretch, but the pressure drops almost immediately as the contraction is completed, and the arterial walls recoil. This alternate expanding and recoiling of an arterial wall can be felt as a *pulse* in an artery that runs close to the surface. Figure 14.37 shows several sites where a pulse can be detected. The radial artery, for example, courses near the surface at the wrist and is commonly used to sense a person's radial pulse.

The pulse rate is equal to the rate at which the left ventricle is contracting, and for this reason it can be used to determine the heart rate. A pulse also can reveal something about blood pressure, because an elevated pressure produces a pulse that feels full, while a low pressure produces a pulse that is easily compressed.

Paths of Circulation

The blood vessels of the cardiovascular system can be divided into two major pathways—a pulmonary circuit and a systemic circuit. The **pulmonary circuit** consists of those vessels that carry blood from the heart to the lungs and back to the heart. The **systemic circuit** is responsible for carrying blood from the heart to all other parts of the body and back again (figure 14.38).

The circulatory pathways described in the following sections are those of an adult. The fetal pathways, which are somewhat different, are described in chapter 18.

FIGURE 14.39
Blood is carried to the lungs through branches of the pulmonary arteries and returns to the heart through pulmonary veins.

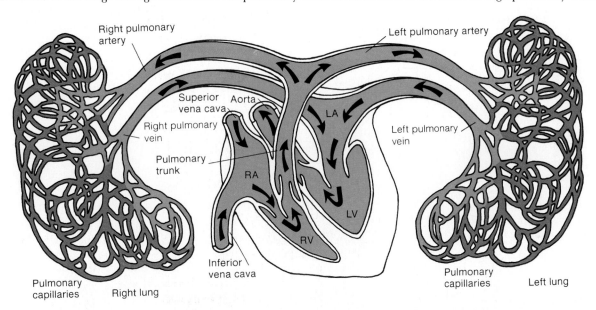

The Pulmonary Circuit

Blood enters the pulmonary circuit as it leaves the right ventricle through the **pulmonary trunk.** The pulmonary trunk extends upward and posteriorly from the heart, and about 5 centimeters above its origin, it divides into *right* and *left pulmonary arteries.* These branches penetrate the right and left lungs respectively. Within the lungs, they divide into *lobar branches* (three on the right side and two on the left) that accompany the main divisions of the bronchi into the lobes of the lungs. After repeated divisions, the lobar branches give rise to arterioles that continue into the capillary networks associated with the walls of the alveoli (figure 14.39).

The blood in the arteries and arterioles of the pulmonary circuit has a relatively low concentration of oxygen and a relatively high concentration of carbon dioxide. As explained in chapter 13, gas exchanges occur between the blood and the air as the blood moves through the *pulmonary capillaries.*

As a result of the gas exchanges occurring between the blood and the alveolar air, blood entering the venules of the pulmonary circuit is rich in oxygen and low in carbon dioxide. These venules merge to form small veins, which, in turn, converge to form still larger ones. Four *pulmonary veins*—two from each lung—return blood to the left atrium, and this completes the vascular loop of the pulmonary circuit.

The right pulmonary artery is normally somewhat larger and longer than the left. There is little normal variation in these arteries. Although there are usually four pulmonary veins, occasionally this number may vary. There may be three pulmonary veins from the right or left lungs. In some cases, the two vessels from the left lung may join to form one pulmonary vein.

The Systemic Circuit

The freshly oxygenated blood received by the left atrium is forced into the systemic circuit by the contraction of the left ventricle. This circuit includes the aorta and its branches leading to all body tissues, as well as the companion system of veins that returns blood to the right atrium.

1. Distinguish between the pulmonary and systemic circuits.
2. Trace a drop of blood through the pulmonary circuit from the right ventricle.

The Arterial System

The **aorta** is the largest artery in the body. It extends upward from the left ventricle, arches over the heart to the left, and descends just in front of the vertebral column. Figure 14.40 shows the aorta and its main branches.

FIGURE 14.40

The principal branches of the aorta.

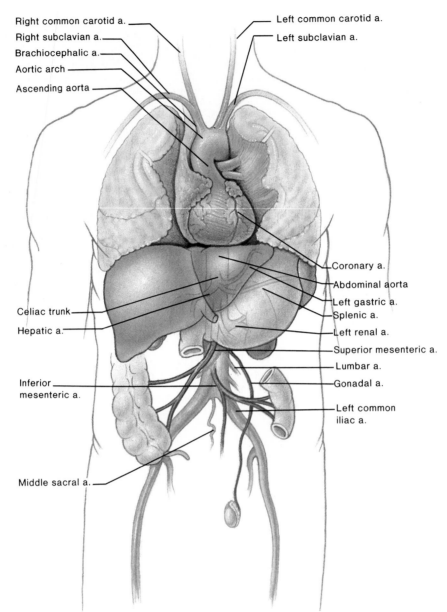

Right common carotid a.
Right subclavian a.
Brachiocephalic a.
Aortic arch
Ascending aorta

Left common carotid a.
Left subclavian a.

Coronary a.
Abdominal aorta
Left gastric a.
Splenic a.
Left renal a.
Superior mesenteric a.
Lumbar a.
Gonadal a.
Left common iliac a.

Celiac trunk
Hepatic a.

Inferior mesenteric a.

Middle sacral a.

Principal Branches of the Aorta

The first portion of the aorta is called the *ascending aorta.* Located at its base are the three cusps of the aortic semilunar valve, and opposite each cusp is a swelling in the aortic wall called an **aortic sinus.** The right and left *coronary arteries* spring from two of these sinuses. Blood flow into these arteries is intermittent and is driven by the elastic recoil of the aortic wall following a contraction of the left ventricle.

Several small structures called **aortic bodies** occur within the epithelial lining of the aortic sinuses. These bodies contain pressoreceptors that control blood pressure, and chemoreceptors that are sensitive to the blood concentrations of oxygen and carbon dioxide.

Three major arteries originate from the *arch of the aorta* (aortic arch). They are the brachiocephalic (innominate) artery, the left common carotid artery, and the left subclavian artery.

The **brachiocephalic** (brak″e-o-se-fal′ik) **artery** supplies blood to the tissues of the right arm and head, as its name suggests. It is the first branch from the aortic arch, and rises upward through the mediastinum to a point near the junction of the sternum and the right clavicle. There it divides, giving rise to the right **common carotid** (kah-rot′id) **artery,** which carries blood to the right side of the neck and head, and the right **subclavian** (sub-kla′ve-an) **artery,** which leads into the right arm. Branches of the subclavian artery also supply blood to parts of the shoulder, neck, and head.

FIGURE 14.41

(*a*) Abdominal aorta and its major branches; (*b*) angiogram (X-ray film) of the branches of the abdominal aorta.

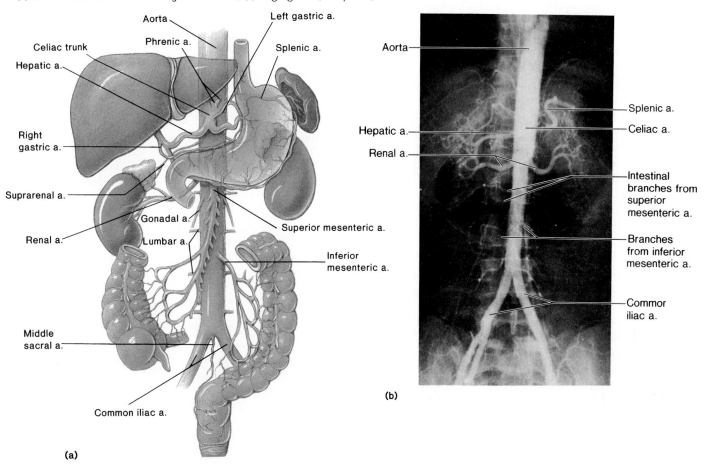

(a)

(b)

The *left common carotid artery* and the *left subclavian artery* are respectively the second and third branches of the aortic arch. They supply blood to regions on the left side of the body corresponding to those supplied by their counterparts on the right. (See figure 14.40 and reference plate 71.)

There are many normal variations of the first three branches of the aorta. For example, the first three arteries may branch from the ascending aorta. Also, these vessels may arise closer together or farther apart than normal.

Another common variation occurs when only the brachiocephalic and left subclavian arteries branch from the aorta. In this case, the left common carotid artery branches from the brachiocephalic artery. There also may be four major branches from the aorta if the left vertebral artery comes directly from the aortic arch.

Although the upper part of the *descending aorta* is positioned to the left of the midline, it gradually moves medially and finally lies directly in front of the vertebral column at the level of the twelfth thoracic vertebra.

The portion of the descending aorta above the diaphragm is known as the **thoracic** (tho-ras′ik) **aorta,** and it gives off numerous small branches to the thoracic wall and the thoracic visceral organs. These branches, the *bronchial, pericardial,* and *esophageal arteries,* supply blood to the structures for which they were named. Other branches become *mediastinal arteries,* supplying various tissues within the mediastinum, and *posterior intercostal arteries* that pass into the thoracic wall.

Below the diaphragm, the descending aorta becomes the **abdominal aorta,** and it gives off branches to the abdominal wall and various abdominal visceral organs (figure 14.41). These branches include the following:

1. **Celiac** (se′le-ak) **trunk.** This single vessel gives rise to the left *gastric, splenic,* and *hepatic arteries,* which supply upper portions of the digestive tube, the spleen, and the liver, respectively. (Note: The hepatic artery supplies the liver with about one-third of its blood flow, and this blood is oxygen-rich. The remaining two-thirds of the liver's blood flow arrives by means of the portal vein and is oxygen-poor.)

2. **Phrenic** (fren'ik) **arteries.** These paired arteries supply blood to the diaphragm.

3. **Superior mesenteric** (mes"en-ter'ik) **artery.** The superior mesenteric is a large unpaired artery that branches to many parts of the intestinal tract, including the jejunum, ileum, cecum, ascending colon, and transverse colon.

4. **Suprarenal arteries.** This pair of vessels supplies blood to the adrenal glands.

5. **Renal** (re'nal) **arteries.** The renal arteries pass laterally from the aorta into the kidneys. Each artery then divides into several lobar branches within the kidney tissues.

6. **Gonadal** (go'nad-al) **arteries.** In a female, paired *ovarian arteries* arise from the aorta and pass into the pelvis to supply the ovaries. In a male, *spermatic arteries* originate in similar locations. They course downward and pass through the body wall by way of the *inguinal canal* to supply the testes.

7. **Inferior mesenteric artery.** Branches of this single artery lead to the descending colon, the sigmoid colon, and the rectum.

8. **Lumbar arteries.** Three or four pairs of lumbar arteries arise from the posterior surface of the aorta in the region of the lumbar vertebrae. These arteries supply various muscles of the skin and the posterior abdominal wall.

9. **Middle sacral** (sa'kral) **artery.** This small, single vessel descends medially from the aorta along the anterior surfaces of the lower lumbar vertebrae. It carries blood to the sacrum and coccyx.

The descending aorta terminates near the brim of the pelvis, where it divides into right and left common iliac arteries. Branches from these vessels supply blood to lower regions of the abdominal wall, the pelvic organs, and the lower extremities.

Chart 14.4 summarizes these main branches of the aorta.

Arteries to the Neck, Head, and Brain

Blood is supplied to parts within the neck, head, and brain through branches of the subclavian and common carotid arteries (figure 14.42). The main divisions of the subclavian artery to these regions are the vertebral, thyrocervical, and costocervical arteries. The common carotid artery communicates to these parts by means of the internal and external carotid arteries.

The **vertebral** (ver'te-bral) **arteries** arise from the subclavian arteries in the base of the neck, near the tips of the lungs. They pass upward through the foramina of the transverse processes of the cervical vertebrae and enter the skull by way of the foramen magnum. Along their paths, these vessels supply blood to vertebrae, and to the ligaments and muscles associated with them.

Chart 14.4 Aorta and its principal branches		
Portion of aorta	**Major branch**	**General regions or organs supplied**
Ascending aorta	Right and left coronary arteries	Heart
Arch of aorta	Brachiocephalic artery	Right arm, right side of head
	Left common carotid artery	Left side of head
	Left subclavian artery	Left arm
Descending aorta		
Thoracic aorta	Bronchial artery	Bronchi
	Pericardial artery	Pericardium
	Esophageal artery	Esophagus
	Mediastinal artery	Mediastinum
	Posterior intercostal artery	Thoracic wall
Abdominal aorta	Celiac trunk	Organs of upper digestive system
	Phrenic artery	Diaphragm
	Superior mesenteric artery	Portions of small and large intestines
	Suprarenal artery	Adrenal gland
	Renal artery	Kidney
	Gonadal artery	Ovary or testis
	Inferior mesenteric artery	Lower portions of large intestine
	Lumbar artery	Posterior abdominal wall
	Middle sacral artery	Sacrum and coccyx
	Common iliac artery	Lower abdominal wall, pelvic organs, and leg

Within the cranial cavity, the vertebral arteries unite to form a single *basilar artery*. This vessel passes along the ventral brain stem and gives rise to branches leading to the pons, midbrain, and cerebellum. The basilar artery terminates by dividing into two *posterior cerebral arteries* that supply portions of the occipital and temporal lobes of the cerebrum. The posterior cerebral arteries also help form the **arterial circle** (*circle of Willis*) at the base of the brain. This circle creates a connection between the vertebral artery and internal carotid artery systems (figure 14.43). The union of these systems may provide alternate pathways through which blood can reach brain tissues in the event of an arterial occlusion, or blockage.

As many as 60% of all individuals show some variation in the arterial circle. In some, a vessel may be narrower on one side than the other. In other cases, one or more of the posterior cerebral or communicating arteries may be absent. One or more of these vessels may split and form two branches. Knowledge of the number and sizes of the vessels in the arterial circle is important in any surgery involving the vessels that supply the circle.

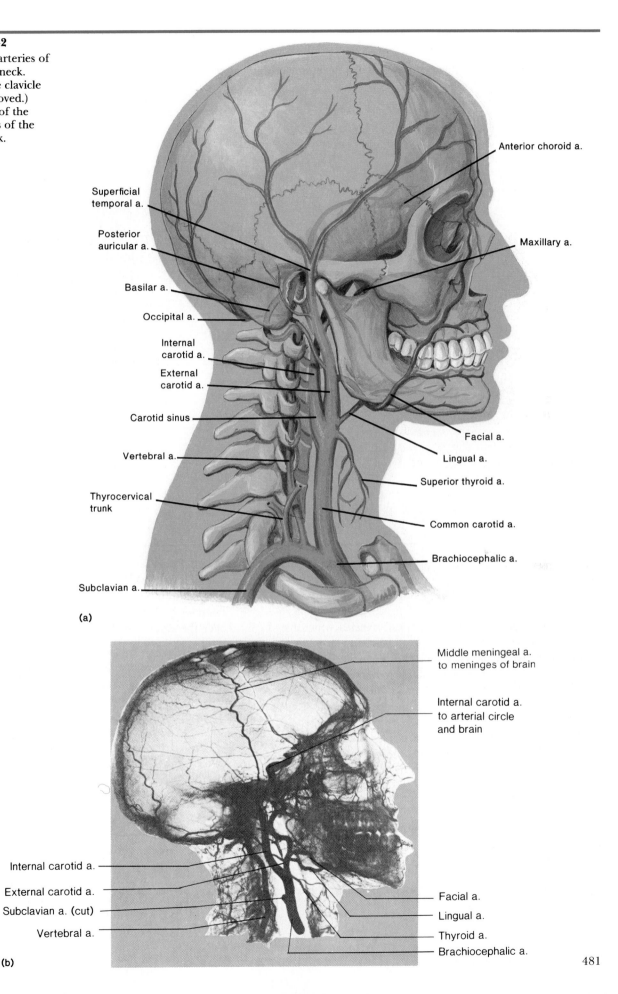

FIGURE 14.42
(*a*) The main arteries of the head and neck. (Note that the clavicle has been removed.)
(*b*) X-ray film of the major arteries of the head and neck.

(a)

Anterior choroid a.

Superficial temporal a.

Maxillary a.

Posterior auricular a.

Basilar a.

Occipital a.

Internal carotid a.

External carotid a.

Carotid sinus

Facial a.

Lingual a.

Vertebral a.

Superior thyroid a.

Thyrocervical trunk

Common carotid a.

Brachiocephalic a.

Subclavian a.

(b)

Middle meningeal a. to meninges of brain

Internal carotid a. to arterial circle and brain

Internal carotid a.

External carotid a.

Subclavian a. (cut)

Vertebral a.

Facial a.

Lingual a.

Thyroid a.

Brachiocephalic a.

481

FIGURE 14.43

The arterial circle is formed by the anterior cerebral arteries, which are connected by the anterior communicating artery, and the posterior cerebral arteries, which are connected to the internal carotid arteries by the posterior communicating arteries. (*aa.* stands for arteries.)

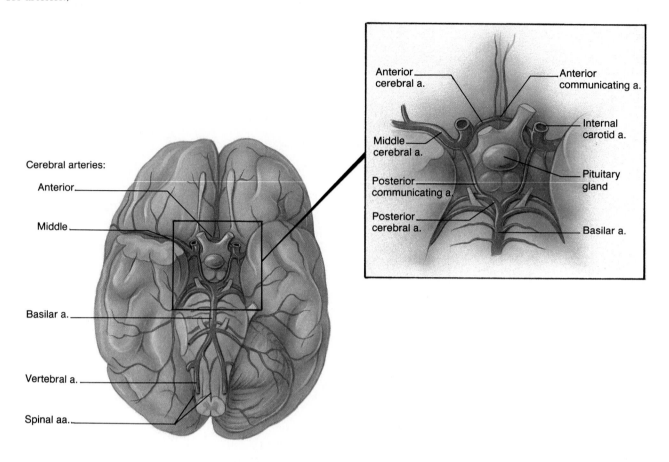

Cerebral arteries:
Anterior
Middle
Basilar a.
Vertebral a.
Spinal aa.

Anterior cerebral a.
Anterior communicating a.
Middle cerebral a.
Internal carotid a.
Posterior communicating a.
Pituitary gland
Posterior cerebral a.
Basilar a.

The **thyrocervical** (thi″ro-ser′vi-kal) **trunks** are short vessels that give off branches to the thyroid glands, parathyroid glands, larynx, trachea, esophagus, and pharynx, as well as to various muscles in the neck, shoulder, and back.

The **costocervical** (kos″to-ser′vi-kal) **arteries,** which are the third vessels to branch from the subclavians, carry blood to muscles in the neck, back, and thoracic wall.

The *left* and *right common carotid arteries* ascend deeply within the neck on either side. At the level of the upper laryngeal border, they divide to form the internal and external carotid arteries.

The **external carotid artery** courses upward on the side of the head, giving off branches to various structures in the neck, face, jaw, scalp, and base of the skull. The main vessels that originate from this artery include the following:

1. *Superior thyroid artery* to the hyoid bone, larynx, and thyroid gland.
2. *Lingual artery* to the tongue, muscles of the tongue, and salivary glands beneath the tongue.
3. *Facial artery* to the pharynx, palate, chin, lips, and nose.

4. *Occipital artery* to the scalp on the back of the skull, the meninges, the mastoid process, and various muscles in the neck.
5. *Posterior auricular artery* to the ear and the scalp over the ear.

The external carotid artery terminates by dividing into *maxillary* and *superficial temporal arteries.* The maxillary artery supplies blood to the teeth, gums, jaws, cheeks, nasal cavity, eyelids, and meninges. The temporal artery extends to the parotid salivary gland, and to various surface regions of the face and scalp.

The **internal carotid artery** follows a deep course upward along the pharynx to the base of the skull. Entering the cranial cavity, it provides the major blood supply to the brain. Its major branches include the following:

1. *Ophthalmic artery* to the eyeball, and to various muscles and accessory organs within the orbit.
2. *Posterior communicating artery* that forms part of the arterial circle.
3. *Anterior choroid artery* to the choroid plexus within the lateral ventricle of the brain and to a variety of nerve structures within the brain.

The internal carotid artery terminates by dividing into *anterior* and *middle cerebral arteries.* The middle cerebral artery passes through the lateral sulcus and supplies the lateral surface of the cerebrum, including the primary motor and sensory areas of the face and arms, the optic radiations, and the speech area (see chapter 9). The anterior cerebral artery extends anteriorly between the cerebral hemispheres and supplies the medial surface of the brain.

Near the base of each internal carotid artery is an enlargement called a **carotid sinus.** Like the aortic sinuses, these structures contain pressoreceptors that function in the reflex control of blood pressure. A number of small epithelial masses, called **carotid bodies,** also occur in the wall of the carotid sinus. These bodies are very vascular and contain chemoreceptors, which, along with the chemoreceptors of the aortic bodies, regulate various circulatory and respiratory actions.

> If a cerebral artery becomes occluded, the person may have a stroke, as brain tissue beyond the obstruction becomes ischemic. For example, if a branch of the middle cerebral artery is occluded, the symptoms may include varying degrees of paralysis or sensory loss in the face or arm, or various visual or speech disorders.

Arteries to the Shoulder and Arm

The subclavian artery, after giving off branches to the neck, continues into the upper arm (figure 14.44). It passes between the clavicle and the first rib, and becomes the axillary artery.

The **axillary artery** supplies branches to structures in the axilla and the chest wall, including the skin of the shoulder, part of the mammary gland, the upper end of the humerus, the shoulder joint, and various muscles in the back, shoulder, and chest. As this vessel leaves the axilla, it becomes the brachial artery.

The **brachial artery** courses along the humerus to the elbow. It gives rise to a *deep brachial artery* that curves posteriorly around the humerus and supplies the triceps muscle. Shorter branches pass into the muscles on the anterior side of the upper arm, while others descend on each side to the elbow and interconnect with arteries in the forearm. The resulting arterial network allows blood to reach the lower arm even if a portion of the distal brachial artery becomes obstructed.

Within the elbow, the brachial artery divides into an ulnar artery and a radial artery. The **ulnar** (ul'nar) **artery** leads downward on the ulnar side of the forearm to the wrist. Some of its branches join the anastomosis (an interconnected group of vessels) around the elbow joint, while others supply blood to flexor and extensor muscles in the lower arm.

FIGURE 14.44
The main arteries of the shoulder and arm.

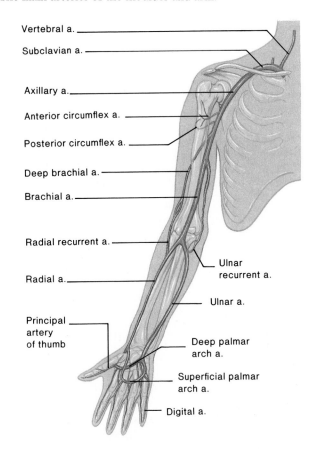

The **radial** (ra'de-al) **artery,** a continuation of the brachial artery, travels along the radial side of the forearm to the wrist. As it nears the wrist, it comes close to the surface and provides a convenient vessel for taking the pulse (radial pulse). Various branches of the radial artery join the anastomosis of the elbow and supply lateral muscles of the forearm.

At the wrist, branches of the ulnar and radial arteries join to form an interconnecting network of vessels. Arteries arising from this network supply blood to structures in the wrist, hand, and fingers.

Arteries to the Thoracic and Abdominal Walls

Blood reaches the thoracic wall through several vessels, including branches from the subclavian artery and the thoracic aorta (figure 14.45).

The subclavian artery contributes to this supply through a branch called the **internal thoracic artery.** This vessel originates in the base of the neck, and passes downward on the pleura and behind the cartilages of the upper six ribs. It gives off two *anterior intercostal arteries* to each of the upper six intercostal spaces; these two arteries supply the intercostal muscles, other intercostal tissues, and the mammary glands.

FIGURE 14.45
Arteries that supply the thoracic wall. (*m.* stands for muscle.)

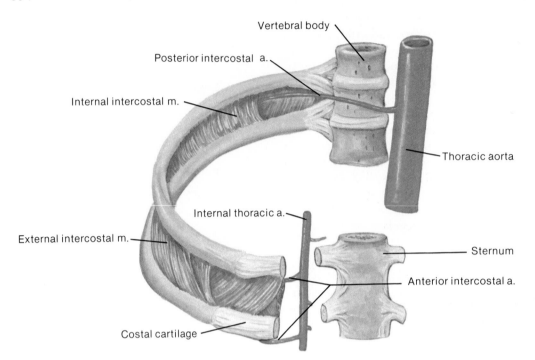

Posterior intercostal arteries arise from the thoracic aorta and enter the intercostal spaces between the third through the eleventh ribs. These arteries give off branches that supply the intercostal muscles, the vertebrae, the spinal cord, and various deep muscles of the back.

The blood supply to the anterior abdominal wall is provided primarily by branches of the *internal thoracic* and *external iliac arteries.* Structures in the posterior and lateral abdominal wall are supplied by paired vessels originating from the abdominal aorta, including the *phrenic* and *lumbar arteries* mentioned previously.

Arteries to the Pelvis and Leg

The abdominal aorta divides to form the **common iliac arteries** at the level of the pelvic brim, and these vessels provide blood to the pelvic organs, gluteal region, and legs.

Each common iliac artery descends a short distance and divides into an internal (hypogastric) branch and an external branch. The **internal iliac artery** gives off numerous branches to various pelvic muscles and visceral structures, as well as to the gluteal muscles and the external genitalia. Important branches of this vessel are shown in figure 14.46. They include the following:

1. *Iliolumbar artery* to the ilium and muscles of the back.
2. *Superior* and *inferior gluteal arteries* to the gluteal muscles, pelvic muscles, and skin of the buttocks.

3. *Internal pudendal artery* to muscles in the distal portion of the alimentary canal, the external genitalia, and the hip joint.
4. *Superior* and *inferior vesical arteries* to the urinary bladder. In males, these vessels also supply the seminal vesicles and the prostate gland.
5. *Middle* and *inferior rectal arteries* to the rectum.
6. *Uterine artery* to the uterus and vagina in females.

The **external iliac artery** provides the main blood supply to the legs (figure 14.47). It passes downward along the brim of the pelvis and gives off two large branches—an *inferior epigastric artery* and a *deep circumflex iliac artery.* These vessels supply muscles and skin in the lower abdominal wall (figure 14.46).

Midway between the symphysis pubis and the anterior superior iliac spine of the ilium, the external iliac artery passes beneath the inguinal ligament and becomes the femoral artery.

The femoral artery, vein, and nerve lie within an area called the *femoral triangle* (figure 14.48). This area is bounded by the sartorius and adductor longus muscles and the inguinal ligament. Since the femoral artery is near the body surface, a pulse can be felt within the femoral triangle. Also, pressure may be applied in the region of the pulse to stop bleeding from any point distal to the femoral triangle.

FIGURE 14.46
Arteries that supply the pelvic region.

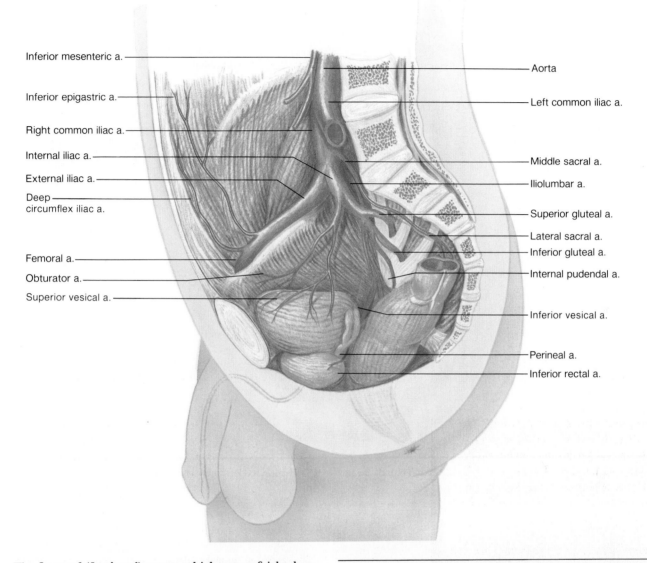

Inferior mesenteric a.
Inferior epigastric a.
Right common iliac a.
Internal iliac a.
External iliac a.
Deep circumflex iliac a.
Femoral a.
Obturator a.
Superior vesical a.

Aorta
Left common iliac a.
Middle sacral a.
Iliolumbar a.
Superior gluteal a.
Lateral sacral a.
Inferior gluteal a.
Internal pudendal a.
Inferior vesical a.
Perineal a.
Inferior rectal a.

The **femoral** (fem'or-al) **artery,** which passes fairly close to the anterior surface of the upper thigh, gives off many branches to muscles and superficial tissues of the thigh. These branches also supply the skin of the groin and the lower abdominal wall. Important subdivisions of the femoral artery include the following:

1. *Superficial circumflex iliac artery* to the lymph nodes and skin of the groin.
2. *Superficial epigastric artery* to the skin of the lower abdominal wall.
3. *Superficial* and *deep external pudendal arteries* to the skin of the lower abdomen and external genitalia.
4. *Profunda femoris artery* (the largest branch of the femoral artery) to the hip joint and various muscles of the thigh.
5. *Deep genicular artery* to distal ends of thigh muscles and to an anastomosis around the knee joint.

Two branches of the profunda femoris artery, the lateral and medial circumflex femoris arteries, supply blood to the head and neck of the femur. A fracture at the neck of the femur, which may occur in a person suffering from osteoporosis, may damage one of the circumflex femoris arteries and decrease the blood supply to the bone. This may delay healing of the bone.

As the femoral artery reaches the proximal border of the space behind the knee (popliteal fossa), it becomes the **popliteal** (pop-lit'e-al) **artery.** Branches of this artery supply blood to the knee joint and certain muscles in the thigh and calf. Also, many branches of the popliteal artery join the anastomosis of the knee and help provide alternate pathways for blood in the case of arterial obstructions. At the lower border of the popliteal fossa, the popliteal artery divides into the anterior and posterior tibial arteries.

FIGURE 14.47

(a) Main branches of the external iliac artery; (b) angiogram of the femoral artery.

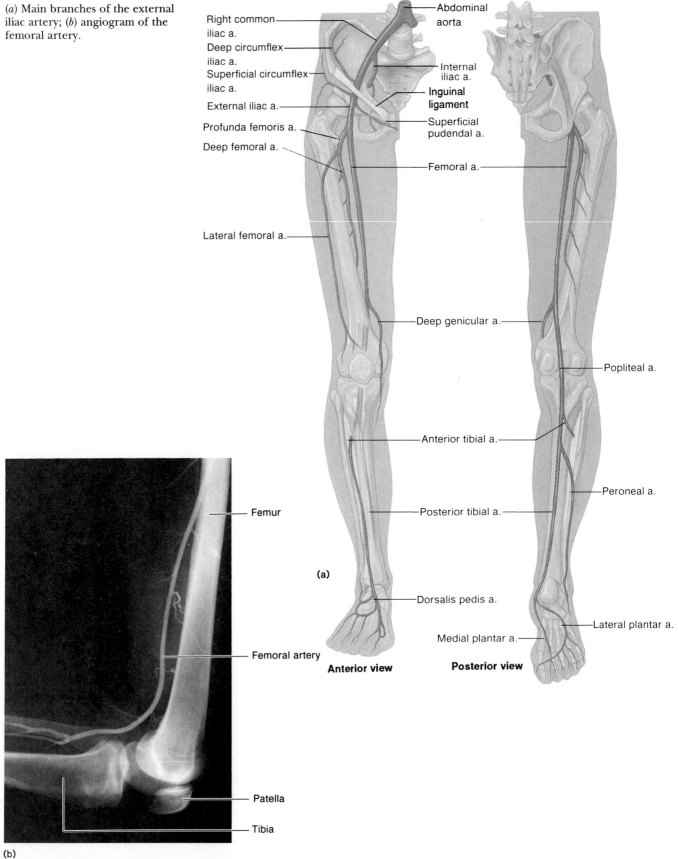

Right common iliac a.
Deep circumflex iliac a.
Superficial circumflex iliac a.
External iliac a.
Profunda femoris a.
Deep femoral a.
Lateral femoral a.

Abdominal aorta
Internal iliac a.
Inguinal ligament
Superficial pudendal a.
Femoral a.

Deep genicular a.
Popliteal a.
Anterior tibial a.
Peroneal a.
Posterior tibial a.
Dorsalis pedis a.
Lateral plantar a.
Medial plantar a.

Anterior view   **Posterior view**

(a)

Femur
Femoral artery
Patella
Tibia

(b)

FIGURE 14.48

The femoral artery, vein, and nerve lie within an area called the femoral triangle.

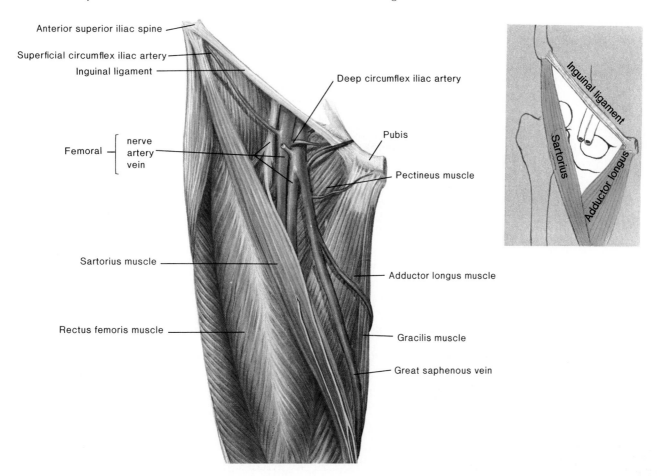

- Anterior superior iliac spine
- Superficial circumflex iliac artery
- Inguinal ligament
- Deep circumflex iliac artery
- Pubis
- Femoral — nerve / artery / vein
- Pectineus muscle
- Sartorius muscle
- Adductor longus muscle
- Rectus femoris muscle
- Gracilis muscle
- Great saphenous vein
- Inguinal ligament
- Sartorius
- Adductor longus

The **anterior tibial** (tib′e-al) **artery** passes downward between the tibia and the fibula, giving off branches to the skin and muscles in anterior and lateral regions of the lower leg. It also communicates with the anastomosis of the knee and with a network of arteries around the ankle. This vessel continues into the foot as the *dorsalis pedis artery,* which supplies blood to the foot and toes.

The **posterior tibial artery,** the larger of the two popliteal branches, descends beneath the calf muscles, giving off branches to skin, muscles, and other tissues of the lower leg along the way. Some of these vessels join the anastomoses of the knee and ankle. As it passes between the medial malleolus and the heel, the posterior tibial artery divides into the *medial* and *lateral plantar arteries.* Branches from these arteries supply blood to tissues of the heel, foot, and toes.

The largest branch of the posterior tibial artery is the *peroneal artery,* which travels downward along the fibula and contributes to the anastomosis of the ankle.

Following foot or leg surgery, healthcare professionals must palpate the pulses in the legs to check for adequate circulation, which is important since poor blood flow may lead to tissue death. The pulses are usually palpated from distal toward proximal locations. (See figure 14.37.) The dorsalis pedis arteries are absent in 10%–15% of the population. Consequently, these individuals will not have a pedal pulse. However, when circulation is adequate the posterior tibial pulse is always present.

Individuals suffering from arteriosclerosis may have arteries that are so hardened that a pulse cannot be palpated. In such cases, the healthcare professional may use a noninvasive instrument called a *Doppler device.* This instrument uses ultrasound to sense the velocity of blood. Thus, it can indicate that blood is flowing through a vessel even though a pulse cannot be palpated.

The major vessels of the arterial system are shown in figure 14.49.

FIGURE 14.49
Major vessels of the arterial system.

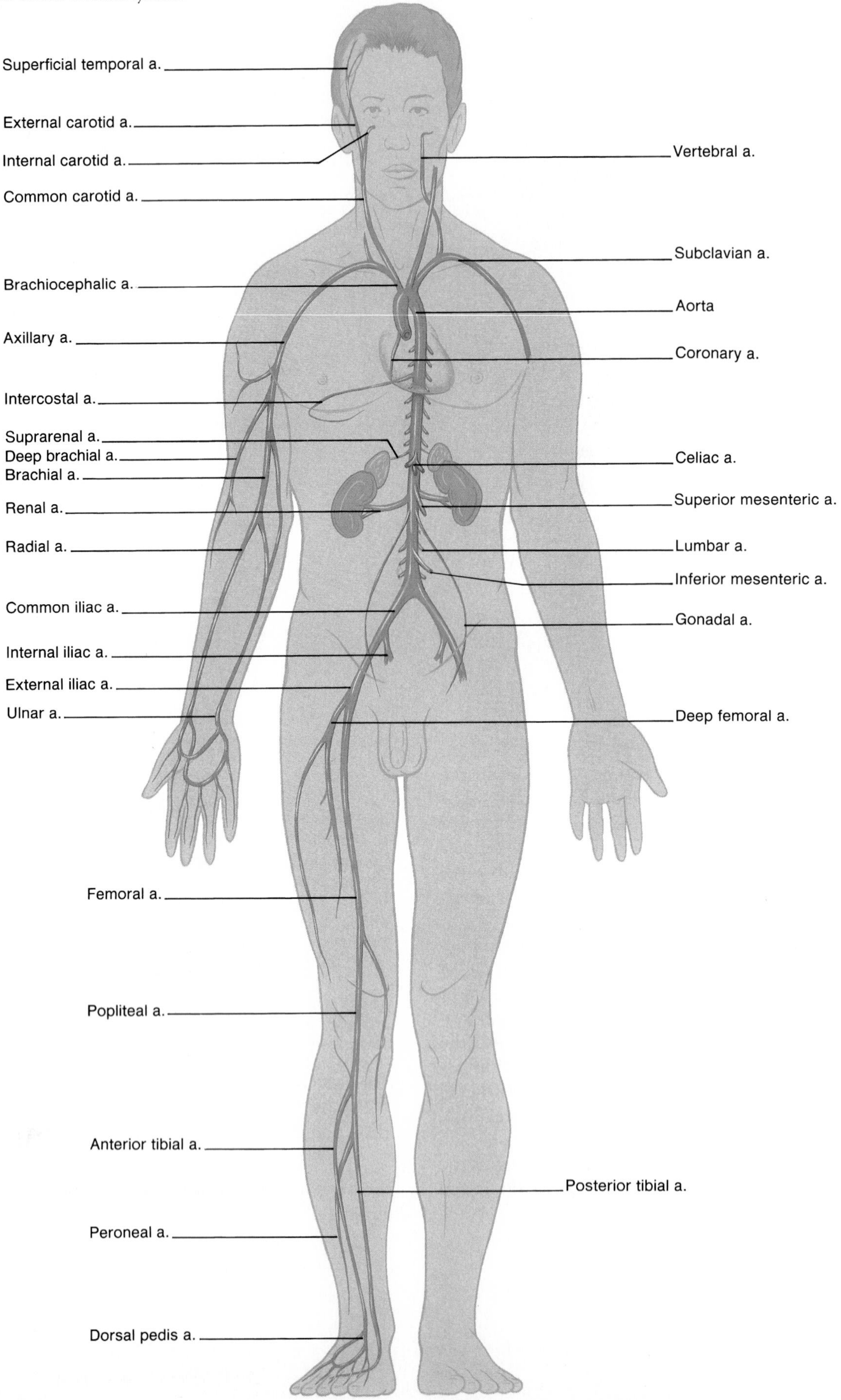

Superficial temporal a.

External carotid a.

Internal carotid a.

Common carotid a.

Brachiocephalic a.

Axillary a.

Intercostal a.

Suprarenal a.

Deep brachial a.

Brachial a.

Renal a.

Radial a.

Common iliac a.

Internal iliac a.

External iliac a.

Ulnar a.

Femoral a.

Popliteal a.

Anterior tibial a.

Peroneal a.

Dorsal pedis a.

Vertebral a.

Subclavian a.

Aorta

Coronary a.

Celiac a.

Superior mesenteric a.

Lumbar a.

Inferior mesenteric a.

Gonadal a.

Deep femoral a.

Posterior tibial a.

The Venous System

Venous circulation is responsible for returning blood to the heart after exchanges of gases, nutrients, and wastes have occurred between the blood and the body cells.

Characteristics of Venous Pathways

The vessels of the venous system begin with the merging of capillaries into venules, venules into small veins, and small veins into larger ones. Unlike arterial pathways, however, those of the venous system are difficult to follow. This is because the vessels are commonly interconnected in irregular networks, so that many unnamed tributaries may join to form a relatively large vein.

The larger, deep veins typically parallel the courses taken by arteries, and these veins often have the same names as their companions in the arterial system. Thus, with some exceptions, the name of a major artery also provides the name of the vein next to it. For example, the renal vein parallels the renal artery, the femoral vein accompanies the femoral artery, and so forth. The superficial veins are located in the fascia beneath the skin (figures 8.27 and 14.48).

The veins that carry blood from the lungs and myocardium back to the heart have already been described. The veins from all other parts of the body converge into two major pathways that lead to the right atrium. They are the *superior* and *inferior venae cavae.*

Veins from the Head, Neck, and Brain

Blood from the face, scalp, and superficial regions of the neck is drained by the **external jugular** (jug'u-lar) **veins.** These vessels descend on either side of the neck, passing over the sternocleidomastoid muscles and beneath the platysma. They empty into the **right** and **left subclavian veins** in the base of the neck (figure 14.50).

The **internal jugular veins,** which are somewhat larger than the external jugular veins, arise from numerous veins and venous sinuses of the brain, and from deep veins in various parts of the face and neck. They pass downward through the neck beside the common carotid arteries and also join the subclavian veins. These unions of the internal jugular and subclavian veins form large **brachiocephalic** (innominate) **veins** on each side. These vessels then merge in the mediastinum and give rise to the **superior vena cava,** which enters the right atrium.

FIGURE 14.50

The main veins of the head and neck. (Note that the clavicle has been removed.) (*v.* stands for vein.)

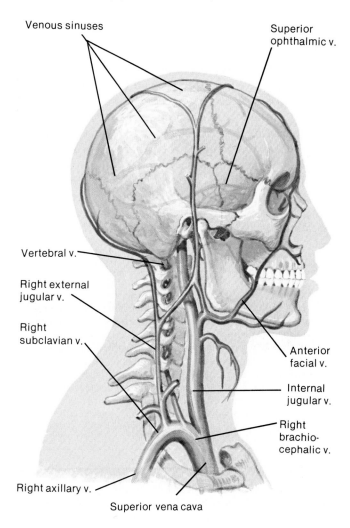

Venous sinuses

Superior ophthalmic v.

Vertebral v.

Right external jugular v.

Right subclavian v.

Anterior facial v.

Internal jugular v.

Right brachio-cephalic v.

Right axillary v.

Superior vena cava

The superior vena cava sometimes becomes compressed by the growth of a lung cancer, the enlargement of a lymph node, or an aortic aneurysm. This condition may interfere with return of blood from the upper body to the heart. It is characterized by pain, shortness of breath, distension of veins draining into the superior vena cava, and swelling of tissues in the face, head, and arms. In severe cases, compression of the superior vena cava results in restricted blood flow to the brain, and the person's life is threatened.

Veins from the Arm and Shoulder

The arm is drained by a set of deep veins and a set of superficial ones. The deep veins generally parallel the arteries in each region and are given similar names, such as *radial vein, ulnar vein, brachial vein,* and *axillary vein.* The superficial veins are interconnected in complex networks just beneath the skin. They also communicate with the deep vessels of the arm, providing many alternate pathways through which blood can leave the tissues (figure 14.51).

The main vessels of the superficial network are the basilic and cephalic veins. They arise from anastomoses in the hand and wrist on the ulnar and radial sides, respectively.

The **basilic vein** passes along the back of the forearm on the ulnar side for a distance and then curves forward to the anterior surface below the elbow. It continues ascending on the medial side until it reaches the middle of the upper arm. There it penetrates the tissues deeply and joins the **brachial vein.** As the basilic and brachial veins merge, they form the **axillary vein.**

The **cephalic vein** courses upward on the lateral side of the arm from the hand to the shoulder. In the shoulder, it pierces the tissues and empties into the axillary vein. Beyond the axilla, the axillary vein becomes the *subclavian vein.*

When the shoulder is depressed, the midclavicular line can be used to locate the position of the subclavian vein. (See figure 14.51.) This site is used when inserting a needle and intravenous catheter (a small, hollow tube). The catheter is threaded into the superior vena cava and a concentrated nutrient solution may be infused through it. The nutrients are diluted by the large volume of blood in the superior vena cava. The peripheral veins used for other intravenous infusions cannot be used with such concentrated solutions because the veins may be damaged by them.

In the bend of the elbow, a *median cubital vein* ascends from the cephalic vein on the lateral side of the arm to the basilic vein on the medial side. This vein is often used as a site for *venipuncture,* when it is necessary to remove a sample of blood for examination or to add certain fluids to the blood.

Veins from the Abdominal and Thoracic Walls

The abdominal and thoracic walls are drained mainly by tributaries of the brachiocephalic and azygos veins. For example, the *brachiocephalic vein* receives blood from the *internal thoracic vein,* which generally drains the tissues supplied by the internal thoracic artery. Some *intercostal veins* also empty into the brachiocephalic vein (figure 14.52).

The **azygos** (az′i-gos) **vein** originates in the dorsal abdominal wall and ascends through the mediastinum on the right side of the vertebral column to join the superior vena cava. It drains most of the muscular tissue in the abdominal and thoracic walls.

Tributaries of the azygos vein include the *posterior intercostal veins* on the right side, which drain the intercostal spaces, and the *superior* and *inferior hemiazygos veins,* which receive blood from the posterior intercostal veins on the

FIGURE 14.51
The main veins of the arm and shoulder.

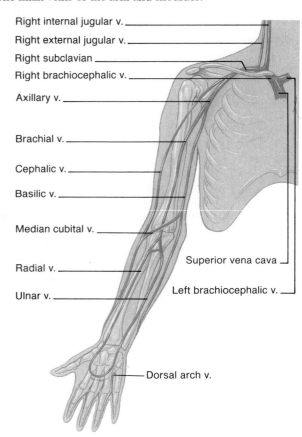

Right internal jugular v.
Right external jugular v.
Right subclavian
Right brachiocephalic v.
Axillary v.
Brachial v.
Cephalic v.
Basilic v.
Median cubital v.
Radial v.
Ulnar v.
Superior vena cava
Left brachiocephalic v.
Dorsal arch v.

left. The right and left *ascending lumbar veins,* with tributaries that include vessels from the lumbar and sacral regions, also connect to the azygos system.

Veins from the Abdominal Viscera

Although veins usually carry blood directly to the atria of the heart, those that drain the abdominal viscera are exceptions (figure 14.53). They originate in the capillary networks of the stomach, intestines, pancreas, and spleen, and carry blood from these organs through a **portal** (por′tal) **vein** to the liver. There the blood enters capillary-like **hepatic sinusoids** (he-pat′ik si′nu-soids). This unique venous pathway is called the **hepatic portal system.** (See figure 14.54.)

The tributaries of the portal vein include the following vessels:

1. *Right* and *left gastric veins* from the stomach.
2. *Superior mesenteric vein* from the small intestine, ascending colon, and transverse colon.
3. *Splenic vein* from a convergence of several veins draining the spleen, pancreas, and a portion of the stomach. Its largest tributary, the *inferior mesenteric vein,* brings blood upward from the descending colon, sigmoid colon, and rectum.

FIGURE 14.52

Veins that drain the thoracic wall.

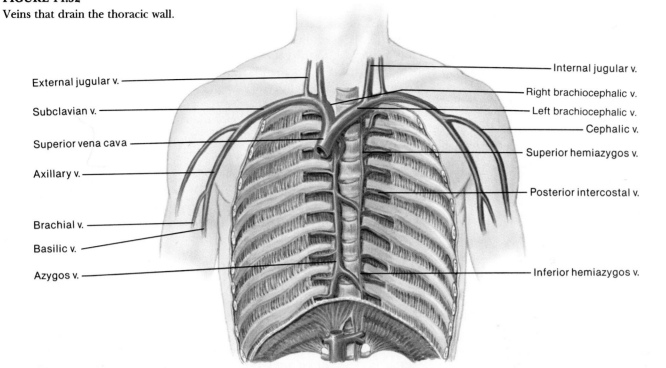

External jugular v.

Subclavian v.

Superior vena cava

Axillary v.

Brachial v.

Basilic v.

Azygos v.

Internal jugular v.

Right brachiocephalic v.

Left brachiocephalic v.

Cephalic v.

Superior hemiazygos v.

Posterior intercostal v.

Inferior hemiazygos v.

FIGURE 14.53

Veins that drain the abdominal viscera.

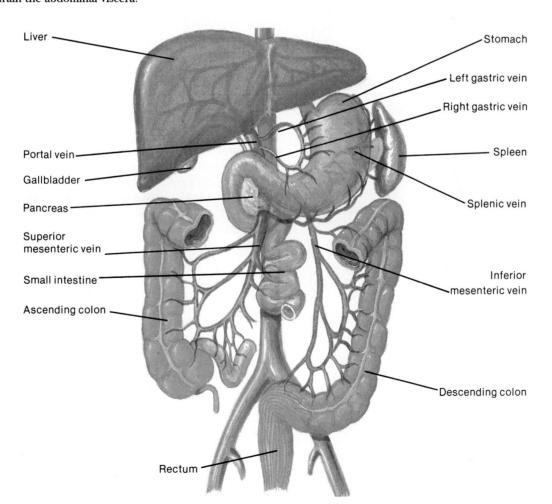

Liver

Portal vein

Gallbladder

Pancreas

Superior
mesenteric vein

Small intestine

Ascending colon

Rectum

Stomach

Left gastric vein

Right gastric vein

Spleen

Splenic vein

Inferior
mesenteric vein

Descending colon

About 80% of the blood flowing to the liver in the hepatic portal system comes from capillaries in the stomach and intestines, and is rich in nutrients. As discussed in chapter 12, the liver modifies and stores some nutrients and detoxifies harmful substances. The hepatic macrophages remove and destroy bacteria.

FIGURE 14.54
In this schematic drawing, the hepatic portal vein drains one set of capillaries and leads to another set.

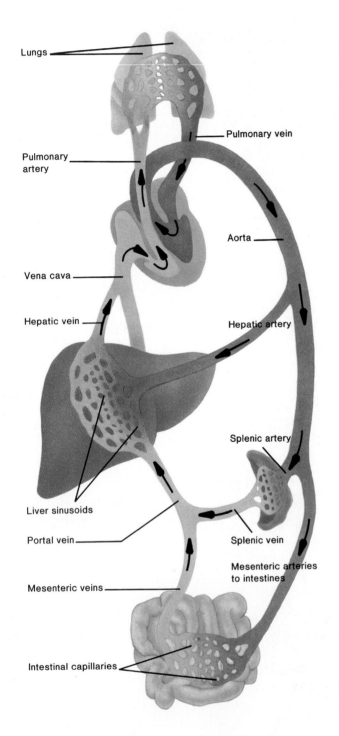

Lungs

Pulmonary artery

Pulmonary vein

Aorta

Vena cava

Hepatic vein

Hepatic artery

Liver sinusoids

Splenic artery

Portal vein

Splenic vein

Mesenteric veins

Mesenteric arteries to intestines

Intestinal capillaries

After passing through the hepatic sinusoids of the liver, blood in the hepatic portal system is carried through a series of merging vessels into **hepatic veins.** These veins empty into the *inferior vena cava,* and thus the blood is returned to the general circulation.

Other veins also empty into the inferior vena cava as it ascends through the abdomen. They include the *lumbar, gonadal, renal, suprarenal,* and *phrenic veins.* Generally, these vessels drain regions that are supplied by arteries with corresponding names.

Veins from the Leg and Pelvis

As in the arm, veins that drain blood from the leg can be divided into deep and superficial groups (figure 14.55). The deep veins of the lower leg, such as the *anterior* and *posterior tibial veins,* have names that correspond with the arteries they accompany. At the level of the knee, these vessels form a single trunk, the **popliteal vein.** This vein continues upward through the thigh as the **femoral vein,** which, in turn, becomes the **external iliac vein** just behind the inguinal ligament.

The superficial veins of the foot and leg interconnect to form a complex network beneath the skin. These vessels drain into two major trunks: the small and great saphenous veins.

The **small saphenous** (sah-fe′nus) **vein** begins in the lateral portion of the foot and passes upward behind the lateral malleolus. It ascends along the back of the calf, enters the popliteal fossa, and joins the *popliteal vein.*

The **great saphenous vein,** which is the longest vein in the body, originates on the medial side of the foot. It ascends in front of the medial malleolus and extends upward along the medial side of the leg. In the thigh just below the inguinal ligament, it penetrates deeply and joins the femoral vein. Near its termination, the great saphenous vein receives tributaries from a number of vessels that drain the upper thigh, groin, and lower abdominal wall.

In addition to communicating freely with each other, the saphenous veins communicate extensively with the deep veins of the leg. As a result, there are many pathways by which blood can be returned to the heart from the lower extremities.

When a person stands, the saphenous veins are subjected to increased blood pressure because of gravitational forces. When such pressure is prolonged, these veins are especially prone to developing abnormal dilations characteristic of varicose veins. The saphenous veins commonly serve as a source of blood vessel material for vascular bypass surgery.

In the pelvic region, blood is carried away from organs of the reproductive, urinary, and digestive systems by vessels leading to the **internal iliac vein.** This vein is formed

FIGURE 14.55
The main veins of the leg and pelvis.

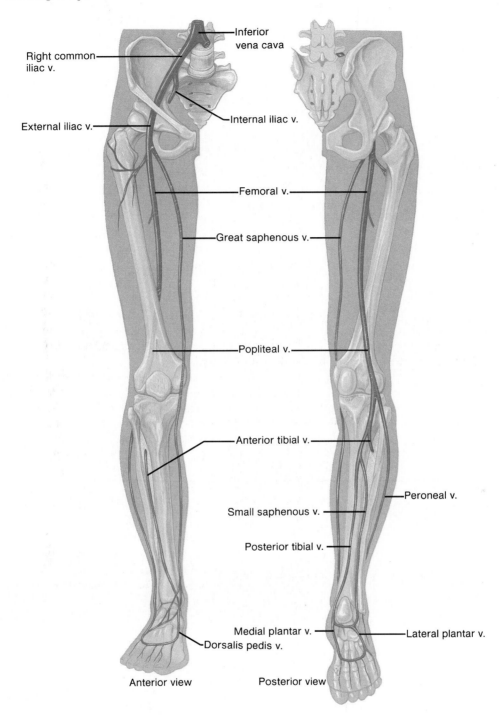

Right common iliac v.

External iliac v.

Inferior vena cava

Internal iliac v.

Femoral v.

Great saphenous v.

Popliteal v.

Anterior tibial v.

Peroneal v.

Small saphenous v.

Posterior tibial v.

Medial plantar v.

Dorsalis pedis v.

Lateral plantar v.

Anterior view

Posterior view

by tributaries corresponding to the branches of the internal iliac artery, such as the *gluteal, pudendal, vesical, rectal, uterine,* and *vaginal veins.* Typically, these veins have many interconnections and form complex networks (plexuses) in the regions of the rectum, urinary bladder, and prostate gland (in the male), or uterus and vagina (in the female).

The internal iliac veins originate deep within the pelvis and ascend to the pelvic brim. There they unite with the *right* and *left external iliac veins* to form the **common iliac veins.** These vessels, in turn, merge to produce the *inferior vena cava* at the level of the fifth lumbar vertebra.

Figure 14.56 shows the major vessels of the venous system.

FIGURE 14.56
Major vessels of the venous system.

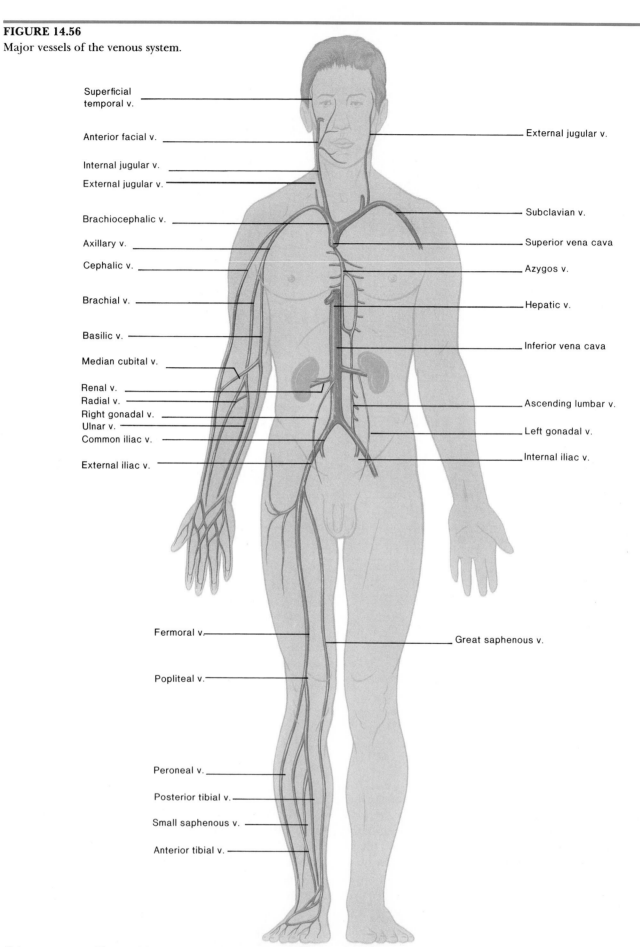

Superficial
temporal v.

Anterior facial v.

Internal jugular v.

External jugular v.

Brachiocephalic v.

Axillary v.

Cephalic v.

Brachial v.

Basilic v.

Median cubital v.

Renal v.

Radial v.

Right gonadal v.

Ulnar v.

Common iliac v.

External iliac v.

Fermoral v.

Popliteal v.

Peroneal v.

Posterior tibial v.

Small saphenous v.

Anterior tibial v.

External jugular v.

Subclavian v.

Superior vena cava

Azygos v.

Hepatic v.

Inferior vena cava

Ascending lumbar v.

Left gonadal v.

Internal iliac v.

Great saphenous v.

Clinical Terms Related to the Cardiovascular System

aneurysm (an'u-rizm)   a saclike swelling in the wall of a blood vessel, usually an artery.

angiospasm (an'je-o-spazm")   a muscular spasm in the wall of a blood vessel.

arteriography (ar"te-re-og'rah-fe)   injection of radiopaque solution into the vascular system for X-ray examination of arteries.

asystole (a-sis'to-le)   condition in which the myocardium fails to contract.

cardiac tamponade (kar'de-ak tam"po-nād')   compression of the heart by an accumulation of fluid within the pericardial cavity.

congestive heart failure (kon-jes'tiv hart fāl'yer)   condition in which the heart is unable to pump an adequate amount of blood to the body cells.

endarterectomy (en"dar-ter-ek'to-me)   removal of the inner wall of an artery to reduce an arterial occlusion.

palpitation (pal"pi-ta'shun)   awareness of a heartbeat that is unusually rapid, strong, or irregular.

pericardiectomy (per"i-kar"de-ek'to-me)   an excision of the pericardium.

phlebitis (flě-bi'tis)   inflammation of a vein, usually in the legs.

phlebotomy (flě-bot'o-me)   incision of a vein for the purpose of withdrawing blood.

sinus rhythm (si'nus rithm)   normal cardiac rhythm regulated by the S-A node.

valvotomy (val-vot'o-me)   an incision of a valve.

venography (ve-nog'rah-fe)   injection of radiopaque solution into the vascular system for X-ray examination of veins.

Chapter Summary

Introduction (page 449)
The cardiovascular system is vital for providing oxygen and nutrients to tissues and for removing wastes.

Structure of the Heart (page 449)
1. Size and location of the heart
   a. The heart is about 12 centimeters long and 9 centimeters wide.
   b. It is located within the mediastinum and rests on the diaphragm.
2. Coverings of the heart
   a. The heart is enclosed in a pericardium.
   b. The pericardial cavity is a potential space between the visceral and parietal membranes.
3. Wall of the heart
   The wall of the heart is composed of the epicardium, myocardium, and endocardium.

4. Heart chambers and valves
   a. The heart is divided into four chambers—two atria and two ventricles—that communicate through atrioventricular orifices on each side.
   b. Right chambers and valves
      (1) The right atrium receives blood from the venae cavae and coronary sinus.
      (2) The right atrioventricular orifice is guarded by the tricuspid valve.
      (3) The right ventricle pumps blood into the pulmonary trunk.
      (4) The base of the pulmonary trunk is guarded by a pulmonary valve.
   c. Left chambers and valves
      (1) The left atrium receives blood from the pulmonary veins.
      (2) The left atrioventricular orifice is guarded by the bicuspid valve.
      (3) The left ventricle pumps blood into the aorta.
      (4) The base of the aorta is guarded by an aortic valve.
5. Skeleton of the heart
   a. The skeleton of the heart consists of fibrous rings that enclose bases of the pulmonary artery, aorta, and atrioventricular orifices.
   b. The fibrous rings provide attachments for valves and muscle fibers, and prevent the orifices from dilating excessively during ventricular contractions.
6. Path of blood through the heart
   a. Blood that is relatively low in oxygen concentration and high in carbon dioxide concentration enters the right side of the heart from the venae cavae and is pumped into the pulmonary circulation.
   b. After blood is oxygenated in the lungs and some carbon dioxide is removed, it returns to the left side of the heart through the pulmonary veins.
   c. From the left ventricle, it moves into the aorta.
7. Blood vessels to the heart
   a. Blood is supplied through the coronary arteries.
   b. It is returned to the right atrium through the cardiac veins and coronary sinus.

Actions of the Heart (page 461)
1. The cardiac cycle
   Atria contract while ventricles relax; ventricles contract while atria relax.
2. Cardiac muscle fibers
   a. Fibers are interconnected to form a functional syncytium.
   b. If any part of the syncytium is stimulated, the whole structure contracts as a unit.
   c. Except for a small region in the floor of the right atrium, the atrial syncytium is separated from the ventricular syncytium by the fibrous skeleton.
3. Cardiac conduction system
   a. This system is composed of specialized muscle tissue and functions to initiate and conduct impulses through the myocardium.
   b. Impulses from the S-A node pass to the A-V node; impulses travel along the A-V bundle, bundle branches, and Purkinje fibers.

c. Muscle fibers in the ventricular walls are arranged in whorls that squeeze blood out of the ventricles when they contract.
4. Regulation of the cardiac cycle
S-A and A-V nodes are innervated by branches of sympathetic and parasympathetic nerve fibers.
   a. Parasympathetic impulses cause heart action to decrease; sympathetic impulses cause heart action to increase.
   b. Autonomic impulses are regulated by the cardiac center in the medulla oblongata.

Blood Vessels (page 464)
The blood vessels form a closed circuit of tubes that transport blood between the heart and body cells. The tubes include arteries, arterioles, capillaries, venules, and veins.
1. Arteries and arterioles
   a. Arteries are adapted to carry blood away from the heart.
   b. Arterioles are branches of arteries.
   c. Walls of arteries and arterioles consist of layers of endothelium, smooth muscle, and connective tissue.
      (1) Elastic arteries contain many elastic fibers in the middle tunic.
      (2) Muscular arteries have few elastic fibers.
   d. The smooth muscle cells are innervated by autonomic fibers that can stimulate vasoconstriction or vasodilation.
2. Capillaries
Capillaries form connections between arterioles and venules. The capillary wall consists of a single layer of cells that forms a semipermeable membrane.
   a. Capillary permeability
      (1) The openings in the capillary walls are thin slits between adjacent endothelial cells.
      (2) The sizes of the openings vary from tissue to tissue.
      (3) Endothelial cells of brain capillaries are tightly fused, forming a blood-brain barrier.
   b. Arrangement of capillaries
   Capillary density varies directly with tissue needs.
   c. Regulation of capillary blood flow
      (1) Capillary blood flow is regulated by precapillary sphincters.
      (2) Precapillary sphincters open when cells are low in oxygen and nutrients, and close when cellular needs are met.
3. Venules and veins
   a. Venules continue from capillaries and merge to form veins.
   b. Veins carry blood to the heart.
   c. Venous walls are similar to arterial walls, but are thinner and contain less muscle and elastic tissue.
   d. Many veins contain flaplike valves that prevent blood from backing up.

Paths of Circulation (page 476)
1. The pulmonary circuit
The pulmonary circuit is composed of vessels that carry blood from the right ventricle to the lungs, pulmonary capillaries, and vessels that lead back to the left atrium.
2. The systemic circuit
   a. The systemic circuit is composed of vessels that lead from the heart to the body cells and back to the heart.
   b. It includes the aorta and its branches, and the veins that return blood to the heart.

The Arterial System (page 477)
1. Principal branches of the aorta
   a. Branches of the ascending aorta include the right and left coronary arteries.
   b. Branches of the aortic arch include the brachiocephalic, left common carotid, and left subclavian arteries.
   c. Branches of the descending aorta include thoracic and abdominal groups.
   d. The descending aorta terminates by dividing into right and left common iliac arteries.
2. Arteries to the neck, head, and brain.
These include branches of the subclavian and common carotid arteries.
3. Arteries to the shoulder and arm
   a. The subclavian artery passes into the upper arm, and in various regions is called the axillary and brachial artery.
   b. Branches of the brachial artery include the ulnar and radial arteries.
4. Arteries to the thoracic and abdominal walls
   a. The thoracic wall is supplied by branches of the subclavian artery and thoracic aorta.
   b. The abdominal wall is supplied by branches of the abdominal aorta and other arteries.
5. Arteries to the pelvis and leg
The common iliac artery supplies the pelvic organs, gluteal region, and leg.

The Venous System (page 489)
1. Characteristics of venous pathways
   a. Veins are responsible for returning blood to the heart.
   b. Larger veins usually parallel the courses of major arteries.
   c. Superficial veins are found in the fascia under the skin.
2. Veins from the head, neck, and brain
   a. These regions are drained by the jugular veins.
   b. Jugular veins unite with subclavian veins to form the brachiocephalic veins.

3. Veins from the arm and shoulder
   a. The arm is drained by sets of superficial and deep veins.
   b. Major superficial veins are the basilic and cephalic veins.
   c. The median cubital vein in the bend of the elbow is often used as a site for venipuncture.
4. Veins from the abdominal and thoracic walls
   These are drained by tributaries of the brachiocephalic and azygos veins.
5. Veins from the abdominal viscera
   a. Blood from the abdominal viscera generally enters the hepatic portal system and is carried to the liver.
   b. Blood in the portal system is rich in nutrients.
   c. The liver modifies and stores nutrients.
   d. From the liver, the blood is carried by hepatic veins to the inferior vena cava.
6. Veins from the leg and pelvis
   a. These regions are drained by sets of deep and superficial veins.
   b. Deep veins include the tibial veins, and superficial veins include the saphenous veins.

Clinical Application of Knowledge

1. In a rare defect, an individual may lack a left coronary artery. How would such a person maintain blood flow to the myocardium on the left side of the heart?
2. Early investigators injected certain dyes into the blood vessels, but found that they failed to stain the brain tissue. How could this observation be explained?
3. If a patient develops a blood clot in the femoral vein of the left leg and a portion of the clot breaks loose, where is the blood flow likely to carry the clot? What symptoms is this condition likely to produce?
4. If a cardiologist inserted a catheter into a patient's right femoral artery, through which arteries would the tube have to pass in order to reach the entrance of the left coronary artery?
5. Cirrhosis of the liver is a disease commonly associated with alcoholism. In this condition, the blood flow through the hepatic blood vessels is often obstructed. As a result of such obstruction, the blood backs up, and the capillary pressure greatly increases in the organs drained by the hepatic portal system. What effects might this increasing capillary pressure produce, and which organs would be affected by it?
6. A bitter-tasting substance is injected into the cubital vein. Which vessels would the substance pass through before it could be sensed by the taste buds of the tongue?

Review Activities

1. Describe the general structure, function, and location of the heart.
2. Describe the pericardium.
3. Describe the layers of the cardiac wall.
4. Identify and describe the location of the chambers and valves of the heart.
5. Describe the skeleton of the heart and explain its function.
6. Trace the path of blood through the heart.
7. Trace the path of blood through the coronary circulation.
8. Describe a cardiac cycle.
9. Describe the arrangement of the cardiac muscle fibers.
10. Distinguish between the S-A node and A-V node.
11. Describe the parts of the cardiac conduction system and explain how it functions in controlling the cardiac cycle.
12. Discuss how the nervous system functions in the regulation of the cardiac cycle.
13. Distinguish between an artery and an arteriole.
14. Explain how vasoconstriction and vasodilation are controlled.
15. Describe the structure and function of a capillary.
16. Describe the structure and function of the blood-brain barrier.
17. Explain how the blood flow through a capillary is controlled.
18. Distinguish between a venule and a vein.
19. Explain how veins function as blood reservoirs.
20. Distinguish between the pulmonary and systemic circuits of the cardiovascular system.
21. Trace the path of blood through the pulmonary circuit.
22. Describe the aorta and name its principal branches.
23. On a diagram, locate and identify the major arteries that supply the abdominal visceral organs.
24. On a diagram, locate and identify the major arteries that supply parts in the head, neck, and brain.
25. On a diagram, locate and identify the major arteries that supply parts in the shoulder and arm.
26. On a diagram, locate and identify the major arteries that supply parts in the thoracic and abdominal walls.
27. On a diagram, locate and identify the major arteries that supply parts in the pelvis and leg.
28. What is the function of an anastomosis of arteries, such as that found in the elbow or knee?
29. Describe the relationship between the major venous pathways and the major arterial pathways.
30. On a diagram, locate and identify the major veins that drain parts in the head, neck, and brain.
31. On a diagram, locate and identify the major veins that drain parts in the arm and shoulder.
32. On a diagram, locate and identify the major veins that drain parts in the abdominal and thoracic walls.
33. On a diagram, locate and identify the major veins that drain parts of the abdominal viscera.
34. On a diagram, locate and identify the major veins that drain parts of the leg and pelvis.

C H A P T E R 15

The Lymphatic System

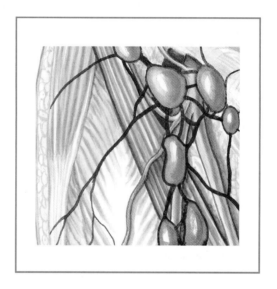

When substances are exchanged between the blood and tissue fluid, more fluid normally leaves the blood capillaries than returns to them. If the fluid remaining in the tissue spaces were allowed to accumulate, the pressure in tissues would increase. The lymphatic system prevents such an imbalance by providing pathways through which tissue fluid can be transported as lymph from the spaces to veins, where it becomes part of the blood.

The lymphatic system also helps defend the tissues against infections.

Chapter Outline

Introduction

Lymphatic Pathways
  Lymphatic Capillaries
  Lymphatic Vessels
  Lymphatic Trunks and Collecting
    Ducts

Tissue Fluid and Lymph
  Tissue Fluid and Lymph Formation
  Function of Lymph

Movement of Lymph
  Flow of Lymph
  Obstruction of Lymph Movement

Lymph Nodes
  Structure of a Lymph Node
  Locations of Lymph Nodes
  Functions of Lymph Nodes

Thymus and Spleen
  The Thymus
  The Spleen

Body Defenses Against Infection

Cells of Immunity
  Origin of Lymphocytes
  Functions of Lymphocytes

Clinical Terms Related to the Lymphatic
  System and Immunity

Chapter Objectives

After you have studied this chapter, you should be able to

1. Describe the general functions of the lymphatic system.

2. Describe the locations of the major lymphatic pathways.

3. Describe how tissue fluid and lymph are formed, and explain the function of lymph.

4. Explain how lymphatic circulation is maintained and the consequence of lymphatic obstruction.

5. Describe a lymph node and its major functions.

6. Describe the location of the major chains of lymph nodes.

7. Discuss the structures and functions of the thymus and spleen.

8. Explain how two major types of lymphocytes are formed.

9. Complete the review activities at the end of this chapter. Note that these items are worded in the form of specific learning objectives. You may want to refer to them before reading the chapter.

Aids to Understanding Words

edem-, a swelling: *edem* a—condition in which fluids accumulate in the tissues and cause them to swell.

immun-, free: *immun*ity—resistance to/ freedom from a specific disease.

inflamm-, setting on fire: *inflamm*ation—a condition characterized by localized redness, heat, swelling, and pain in the tissues.

lymph-, water: *lymph*atic vessel— vessel that transports the watery fluid called lymph.

nod-, knot: *nod*ule—a small mass of lymphocytes surrounded by connective tissue.

patho-, disease: *patho*gen—a disease-causing agent.

-phage, to eat: macro*phage*—a large cell that engulfs and destroys foreign cells.

reticulo-, net: *reticulo*endothelial tissue—groups of cells that form networks in the spleen and other lymphatic organs.

Introduction

The lymphatic system is closely associated with the cardio-vascular system because it includes a network of vessels that assist in circulating body fluids. These vessels transport excess fluid away from the interstitial spaces that exist between the cells in most tissues, and return it to the blood stream. The organs of the lymphatic system also help defend the body against invasion by disease-causing agents (figure 15.1).

Lymphatic Pathways

The lymphatic pathways begin as lymphatic capillaries. These tiny tubes merge to form larger lymphatic vessels, which, in turn, lead to collecting ducts that unite with veins in the thorax.

Lymphatic Capillaries

Lymphatic capillaries are microscopic, closed-end tubes. They extend into the interstitial spaces, forming complex networks that parallel the networks of blood capillaries (figure 15.2). The walls of the lymphatic capillaries, like those of blood capillaries, consist of a single layer of squamous epithelial cells. This thin wall makes it possible for tissue fluid (interstitial fluid) from the interstitial space to enter the lymphatic capillary. Once the fluid is inside a lymphatic capillary, it is called **lymph.**

The villi of the small intestine contain specialized lymphatic capillaries called *lacteals,* described in chapter 12. These vessels transport recently absorbed fats away from the digestive tract.

FIGURE 15.1

Lymphatic vessels transport fluid from interstitial spaces to the bloodstream.

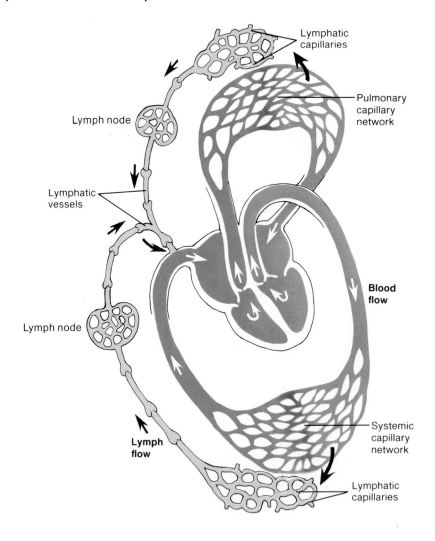

Lymphatic Vessels

Lymphatic vessels, which are formed by the merging of lymphatic capillaries, have walls similar to those of veins. That is, their walls are composed of three layers: an endothelial lining, a middle layer of smooth muscle and elastic fibers, and an outer layer of connective tissue. Also, like veins, the lymphatic vessels have flaplike *valves* that help prevent the backflow of lymph. Figure 15.3 shows one of these valves.

Typically, lymphatic vessels lead to specialized organs called **lymph nodes.** After leaving these structures, the vessels merge to form still larger lymphatic trunks.

Lymphatic Trunks and Collecting Ducts

The **lymphatic trunks** drain lymph from relatively large regions of the body, and are named for the regions they serve. For example, the *lumbar trunk* drains lymph from the legs, lower abdominal wall, and the pelvic organs; the

---

FIGURE 15.2

Lymph capillaries are microscopic closed-end tubes that begin in the interstitial spaces of most tissues.

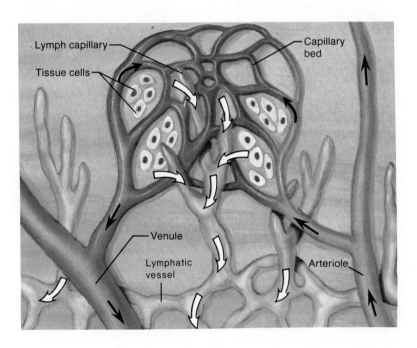

FIGURE 15.3

A light micrograph of the flaplike valve (arrow) within a lymphatic vessel (×25). What is the function of this valve?

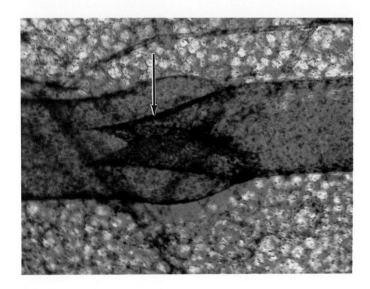

FIGURE 15.4

Lymphatic vessels merge into larger lymphatic trunks, which in turn drain into collecting ducts.

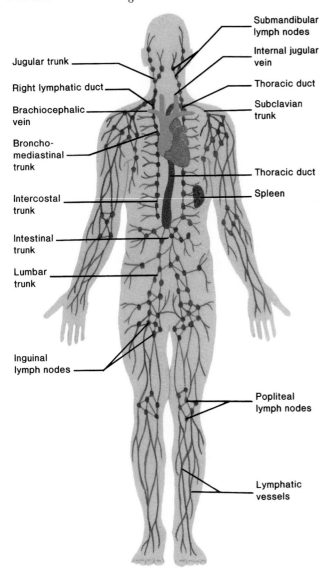

- Submandibular lymph nodes
- Internal jugular vein
- Jugular trunk
- Thoracic duct
- Right lymphatic duct
- Subclavian trunk
- Brachiocephalic vein
- Broncho-mediastinal trunk
- Thoracic duct
- Spleen
- Intercostal trunk
- Intestinal trunk
- Lumbar trunk
- Inguinal lymph nodes
- Popliteal lymph nodes
- Lymphatic vessels

FIGURE 15.5

A lymphangiogram (X-ray film) of the lymphatic vessels and lymph nodes of the pelvic region.

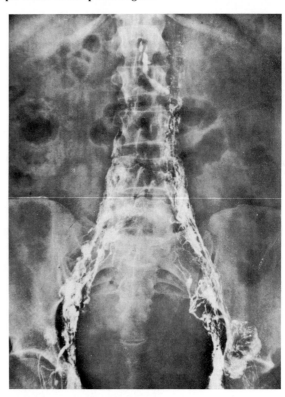

empties into the left subclavian vein near the junction of the left jugular vein. This duct drains lymph from the intestinal, lumbar, and intercostal trunks, as well as from the left subclavian, left jugular, and left bronchomediastinal trunks. Many individuals have an enlarged portion of the thoracic duct in the abdominal area, called the *cisterna chyli*.

> There is great variation in the junction between the thoracic duct and the circulatory system. In 35%–45% of individuals, the thoracic duct joins the internal jugular vein. In 10%–15% of individuals, the duct joins the subclavian vein. In approximately 35% of individuals, the thoracic duct terminates at the junction of the internal jugular and subclavian veins. In a small percentage of people, the thoracic duct joins the brachiocephalic vein.

The **right lymphatic duct** originates in the right thorax at the union of the right jugular, right subclavian, and right bronchomediastinal trunks. It empties into the right subclavian vein near the junction of the right jugular vein.

After leaving the two collecting ducts, lymph enters the venous system and becomes part of the plasma just before the blood returns to the right atrium.

To summarize, lymph from lower body regions, the left arm, and the left side of the head and neck enters the thoracic duct; lymph from the right side of the head and neck, the right arm, and right thorax enters the right lymphatic duct (figure 15.6). Chart 15.1 traces a typical lymphatic pathway.

intestinal trunk drains organs of the abdominal viscera; the *intercostal* and *bronchomediastinal trunks* receive lymph from portions of the thorax; the *subclavian trunk* drains the arm; and the *jugular trunk* drains portions of the neck and head. These lymphatic trunks then join one of two **collecting ducts**—the thoracic duct or the right lymphatic duct. Figure 15.4 shows the location of the major lymphatic trunks and collecting ducts, and figure 15.5 shows a lymphangiogram (or X-ray film) of some lymphatic vessels and lymph nodes.

The **thoracic duct** is the larger and longer of the two collecting ducts. It begins in the abdomen, passes upward through the diaphragm beside the aorta, ascends in front of the vertebral column through the mediastinum, and

FIGURE 15.6

(a) The right lymphatic duct drains lymph from the upper right side of the body, while the thoracic duct drains lymph from the rest of the body; (b) most of the lymph from the breast drains into the axillary area.

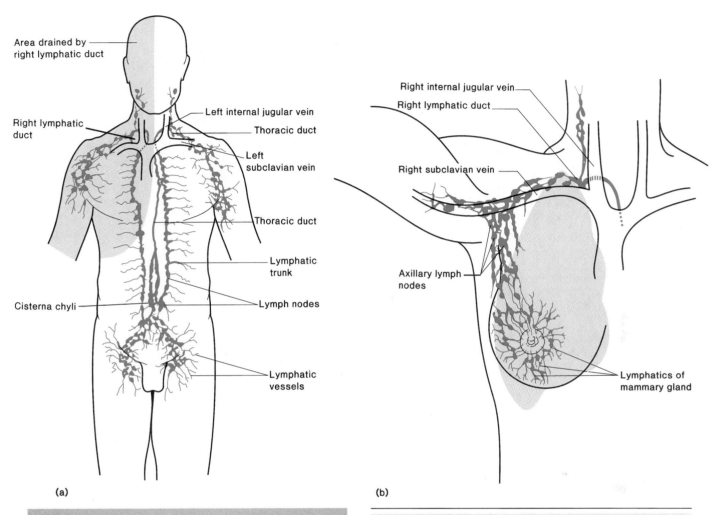

(a)

(b)

Chart 15.1 Typical lymphatic pathway

Tissue fluid
  leaves the interstitial space and becomes

Lymph
  as it enters the

Lymphatic capillary
  that merges with other capillaries to form the

Afferent lymphatic vessel
  that enters the

Lymph node
  where lymph is filtered and leaves via the

Efferent lymphatic vessel
  that merges with other vessels to form the

Lymphatic trunk
  that merges with other trunks and joins the

Collecting duct
  that empties into the

Subclavian vein
  where lymph is added to the blood.

The skin is richly supplied with lymphatic capillaries. Consequently, if the skin is broken, or if something is injected into it (such as venom from a stinging insect), foreign particles are likely to enter the lymphatic system relatively rapidly.

1. What is the general function of the lymphatic system?
2. Through what lymphatic vessels would lymph pass in traveling from a leg to the blood stream?

Tissue Fluid and Lymph

Lymph is essentially *tissue fluid* that has entered a lymphatic capillary. Thus, the formation of lymph is closely associated with the formation of tissue fluid.

Tissue Fluid and Lymph Formation

Tissue fluid originates from blood plasma. It is composed of water and dissolved substances that leave the blood capillaries.

Although tissue fluid contains various nutrients and gases found in plasma, it generally lacks large molecules. Some smaller molecules (proteins) do leak out of the blood capillaries and enter the tissue spaces. Usually, these smaller molecules are not reabsorbed when water and other dissolved substances move back into the venule ends of these capillaries.

As molecules accumulate in the tissue spaces, the volume of fluid in the interstitial spaces then increases, as does the pressure within the spaces. This increasing pressure is responsible for forcing some of the tissue fluid into the lymphatic capillaries, where it becomes lymph (figure 15.2).

Function of Lymph

Most of the protein molecules that leak out of the blood capillaries are carried away by lymph and are returned to the blood stream. At the same time, lymph transports various foreign particles, such as bacterial cells or viruses that have entered the tissue fluids, to lymph nodes.

Although these proteins and foreign particles cannot easily enter blood capillaries, the lymphatic capillaries are especially adapted to receive them. Specifically, the epithelial cells that form the walls of these vessels are arranged so that the edge of one cell overlaps the edge of an adjacent cell, but is not attached to it. This arrangement, shown in figure 15.7, creates flaplike valves in the lymphatic capillary wall, which are pushed inward when the pressure is greater on the outside of the lymphatic capillary, but close when the pressure is greater on the inside.

The epithelial cells of the lymphatic capillary wall are also attached to surrounding connective tissue cells by thin filaments, so that the lumen of a lymphatic capillary remains open even when the outside pressure is increased.

---

1. How would you explain the relationship between tissue fluid and lymph?
2. Describe the arrangement of epithelial cells in a lymph capillary.
3. What are the major functions of lymph?

Movement of Lymph

Although the entrance of lymph into the lymphatic capillaries is influenced by the pressure of tissue fluid, the movement of lymph through the lymphatic vessels is controlled largely by muscular activity.

FIGURE 15.7

Tissue fluid enters lymphatic capillaries through flaplike valves between adjacent epithelial cells.

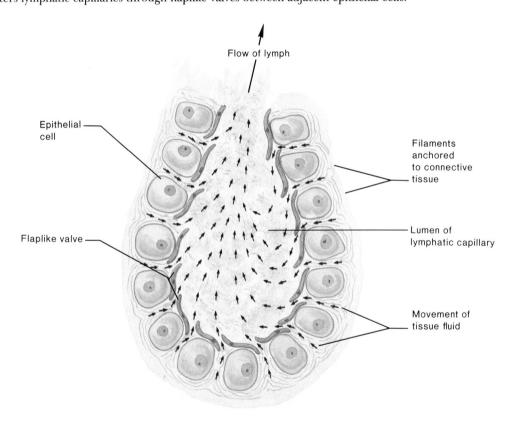

Flow of lymph

Epithelial cell

Flaplike valve

Filaments anchored to connective tissue

Lumen of lymphatic capillary

Movement of tissue fluid

Flow of Lymph

Lymph, like venous blood, may not flow readily through the lymphatic vessels without the aid of outside forces. These forces include contraction of skeletal muscles, pressure changes due to the action of breathing muscles, and contraction of smooth muscles in the walls of larger lymphatic vessels.

As *skeletal muscles* contract, they compress lymphatic vessels. This squeezing action causes the lymph inside the vessel to move, but because the lymphatic vessels contain valves that prevent backflow, the lymph can only move toward a collecting duct. Similarly, the smooth muscles in the walls of larger lymphatic vessels may contract and compress the lymph inside. This action also helps force the fluid onward.

Breathing muscles aid the circulation of lymph (as they do that of venous blood) by creating relatively low pressure in the thorax during inhalation. Lymph (and venous blood as well) is squeezed out of the abdominal vessels and forced into the thoracic vessels. Once again, backflow of lymph (and blood) is prevented by valves within the lymphatic (and blood) vessels.

Obstruction of Lymph Movement

The continuous movement of fluid from interstitial spaces into blood capillaries and lymphatic capillaries causes the volume of fluid in these spaces to remain stable. However, conditions sometimes occur that interfere with lymph movement, and tissue fluids accumulate in the spaces, causing *edema.*

For example, lymphatic vessels may be obstructed as a result of surgical procedures in which portions of the lymphatic system are removed. Because the affected pathways can no longer drain lymph from the tissues, proteins and fluid tend to accumulate in the tissue spaces.

> Because lymphatic vessels tend to carry particles away from tissues, these vessels may also transport cancer cells and promote their spread to other sites (metastasis). For this reason, the lymphatic tissues (lymph nodes) in the axillary regions are commonly biopsied during the surgical removal of cancerous breast tissue (mastectomy). When lymphatic tissue is removed during the procedure, lymphatic drainage from the arm and nearby tissues is sometimes obstructed, and these parts may become edematous following surgery.

1. What factors promote the flow of lymph?
2. What is the consequence of lymphatic obstruction?

Lymph Nodes

Lymph nodes (lymph glands) are structures located along the lymphatic pathways. They contain large numbers of *lymphocytes* and *macrophages* that are vital in the defense against invading microorganisms.

Structure of a Lymph Node

Lymph nodes vary in size and shape; however, they are usually less than 2.5 centimeters in length and are somewhat bean-shaped. A section of a typical lymph node is illustrated in figure 15.8.

FIGURE 15.8

(*a*) A section of a lymph node; (*b*) light micrograph of a lymph node (×2.5). What factors promote the flow of lymph through a node?

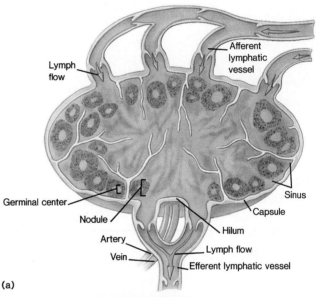

(a)

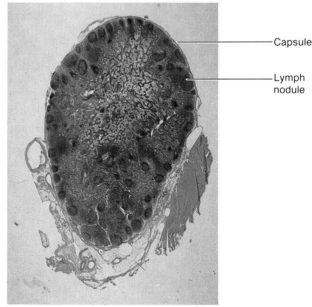

(b)

The Lymphatic System   505

FIGURE 15.9
Lymph enters and leaves a lymph node through lymphatic vessels.

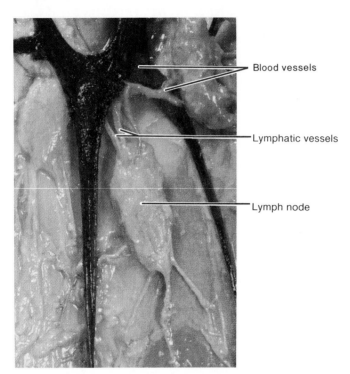

FIGURE 15.10
Major locations of lymph nodes.

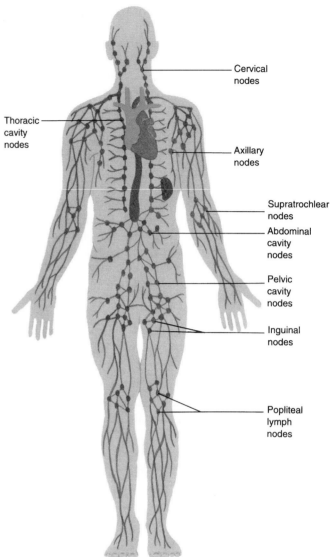

The indented region of a bean-shaped node is called the **hilum,** and it is the portion through which blood vessels and nerves connect with the structure. The lymphatic vessels leading to a node (afferent vessels) enter separately at various points on its convex surface, but the lymphatic vessels leaving the node (efferent vessels) exit from the hilum.

Each lymph node is enclosed by a capsule of white fibrous connective tissue. This tissue also extends into the node and partially subdivides it into compartments containing dense masses of lymphocytes and macrophages. These masses, called **nodules,** represent the structural units of the node (figure 15.8).

Spaces within the node, called **lymph sinuses,** provide a complex network of chambers and channels through which lymph circulates as it passes through the node. Lymph enters a lymph node through an *afferent lymphatic vessel,* moves slowly through the lymph sinuses, and leaves through an *efferent lymphatic vessel* (figure 15.9).

Sometimes lymphatic vessels become inflamed due to a bacterial infection. When this happens in superficial lymphatic vessels, painful reddish streaks may appear beneath the skin—for example, in an arm or a leg. This condition is called *lymphangitis,* and it is usually followed by *lymphadenitis,* an inflammation of the lymph nodes. Affected nodes may become greatly enlarged and quite painful.

Nodules also occur singly or in groups associated with the mucous membranes of the respiratory and digestive tracts. The *tonsils* (described in chapter 12) are composed of partially encapsulated lymph nodules. Also, aggregations of nodules (Peyer's patches) are scattered throughout the mucosal lining of the ileum of the small intestine.

Locations of Lymph Nodes

Lymph nodes generally occur in groups or chains along the paths of the larger lymphatic vessels. Although they are widely distributed throughout the body, lymph nodes are absent in the tissues of the central nervous system. The major locations of lymph nodes (illustrated in figure 15.10) are as follows:

FIGURE 15.11
Locations of lymph nodes within the cervical region.

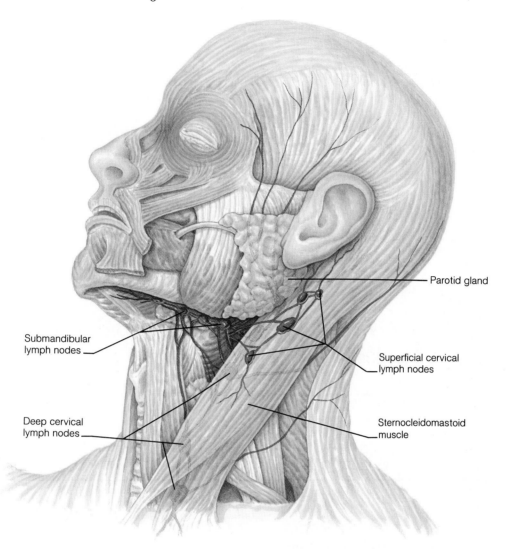

1. **Cervical region.** Nodes in the cervical region occur along the lower border of the mandible, in front of and behind the ears, and deep within the neck along the paths of the larger blood vessels. These nodes are associated with the lymphatic vessels that drain the skin of the scalp and face, as well as the tissues of the nasal cavity and pharynx (figure 15.11).

2. **Axillary region.** Nodes in the underarm region receive lymph from vessels that drain the arm, the wall of the thorax, most of the mammary glands (breasts), and the upper wall of the abdomen. (See figure 15.6.)

3. **Inguinal region.** Nodes in the inguinal region receive lymph from the legs, the external genitalia, and the lower abdominal wall (figure 15.12).

4. **Pelvic cavity.** Within the pelvic cavity, nodes occur primarily along the paths of the iliac blood vessels. They receive lymph from the lymphatic vessels of the pelvic viscera.

5. **Abdominal cavity.** Nodes within the abdominal cavity occur in chains along the main branches of the mesenteric arteries and the abdominal aorta. These nodes receive lymph from the abdominal viscera (figure 15.13).

6. **Thoracic cavity.** Nodes of the thoracic cavity occur within the mediastinum and along the trachea and bronchi. They receive lymph from the thoracic viscera and from the internal wall of the thorax (figure 15.14).

FIGURE 15.12
Locations of lymph nodes within the inguinal region.

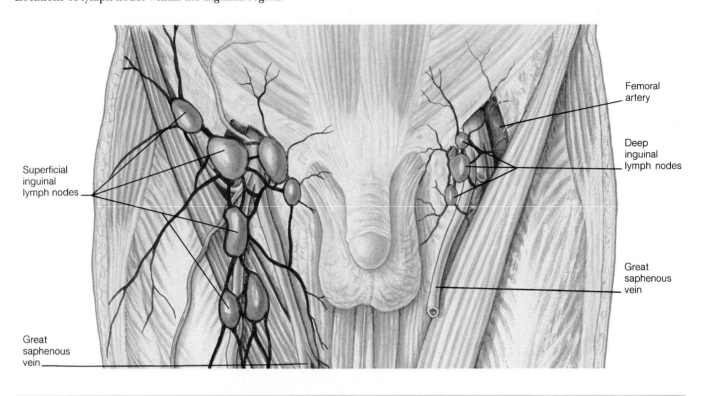

Femoral artery

Deep inguinal lymph nodes

Superficial inguinal lymph nodes

Great saphenous vein

Great saphenous vein

FIGURE 15.13
Lymph nodes within the pelvic and abdominal cavities.

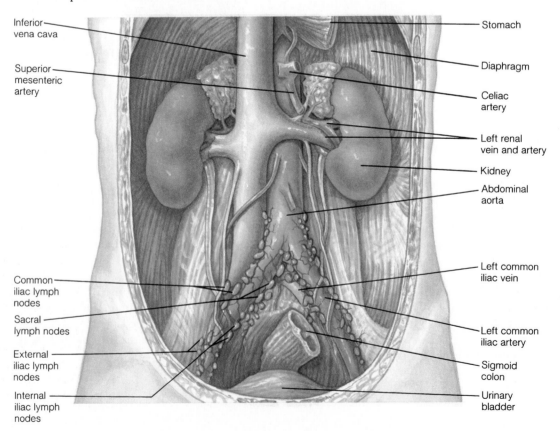

Inferior vena cava

Superior mesenteric artery

Common iliac lymph nodes

Sacral lymph nodes

External iliac lymph nodes

Internal iliac lymph nodes

Stomach

Diaphragm

Celiac artery

Left renal vein and artery

Kidney

Abdominal aorta

Left common iliac vein

Left common iliac artery

Sigmoid colon

Urinary bladder

FIGURE 15.14
Lymph nodes within the thoracic cavity.

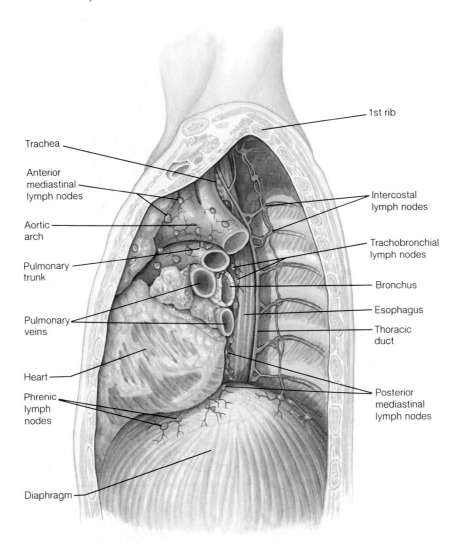

Trachea

Anterior
mediastinal
lymph nodes

Aortic
arch

Pulmonary
trunk

Pulmonary
veins

Heart

Phrenic
lymph
nodes

Diaphragm

1st rib

Intercostal
lymph nodes

Trachobronchial
lymph nodes

Bronchus

Esophagus

Thoracic
duct

Posterior
mediastinal
lymph nodes

The supratrochlear lymph nodes (cubital lymph nodes), located superficially on the medial side of the elbow, often become enlarged in children as a result of infections associated with numerous cuts and scrapes on the hands. Similarly, the popliteal lymph nodes, located in the popliteal fossa, may become inflamed following cuts on the feet.

Functions of Lymph Nodes

As mentioned previously, lymph nodes contain large numbers of *lymphocytes*. The lymph nodes, in fact, are centers for lymphocyte proliferation, although such cells proliferate in other tissues as well. Lymphocytes act against foreign particles, such as bacterial cells and viruses, that are carried to the lymph nodes by the lymphatic vessels.

The lymph nodes also contain *macrophages* that engulf and destroy foreign substances, damaged cells, and cellular debris. (See figure 4.11.)

FIGURE 15.15
The thymus gland is a bilobed organ located between the lungs and above the heart.

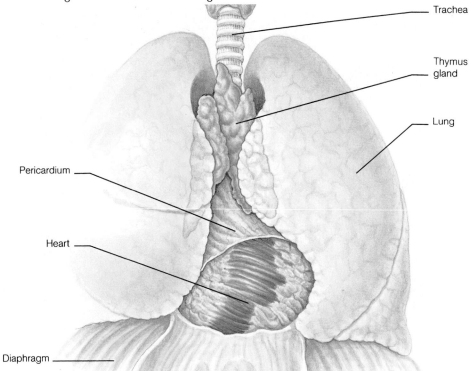

Trachea

Thymus gland

Lung

Pericardium

Heart

Diaphragm

Thus, the lymph nodes function as sites of proliferation for lymphocytes, which help defend the body against microorganisms, and the filtration of potentially harmful foreign particles and cellular debris from lymph before it is returned to the blood stream.

1. How would you distinguish between a lymph node and a lymph nodule?
2. In what body regions are lymph nodes most abundant?
3. What are the major functions of lymph nodes?

Thymus and Spleen

Two other lymphatic organs whose functions are closely related to those of the lymph nodes are the thymus and the spleen.

The Thymus

The **thymus** (thymus gland), shown in figure 15.15, is a soft, bilobed structure whose lobes are surrounded by connective tissue. It is located within the mediastinum, in front of the aortic arch and behind the upper part of the sternum, extending from the root of the neck to the pericardium. Although the thymus varies in size from person to person, it is usually relatively large during infancy and early childhood. After puberty it decreases in size, and in an adult it may be quite small. In an elderly person, the thymus is often largely replaced by fat and connective tissue.

The thymus is composed of lymphatic tissue that is subdivided into *lobules* by connective tissues extending inward from its surface (figure 15.16). Each lobule has an outer cortex and an inner medulla. The cortex contain large numbers of lymphocytes that developed from precursor cells originating in the bone marrow. The majority of these cells (thymocytes) remain inactive; however, some of them develop into T-lymphocytes, a group of cells that leaves the thymus and functions in providing immunity.

Epithelial cells within the thymus secrete a hormone called *thymosin*, which is thought to stimulate the maturation of the T-lymphocytes after they leave the thymus and migrate to other lymphatic tissues.

FIGURE 15.16

A cross section of the thymus gland (×10). Note how the organ is divided into lobules.

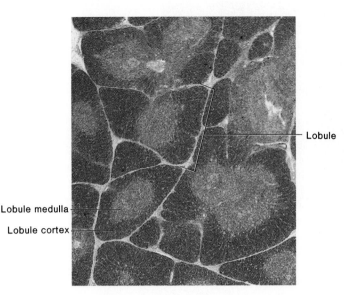

FIGURE 15.17

The spleen resembles a large lymph node.

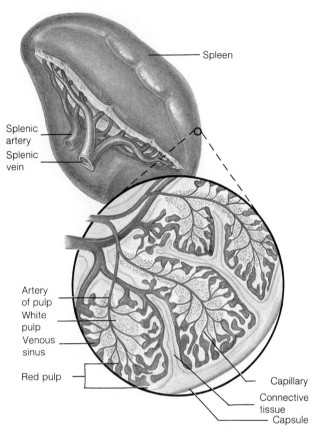

The Spleen

The **spleen** is the largest of the lymphatic organs. It is located in the upper-left portion of the abdominal cavity, just beneath the diaphragm and behind the stomach. (See reference plates 4, 5, and 6.)

The spleen resembles a large lymph node in some respects. For example, it is enclosed in connective tissue that extends inward from the surface and partially subdivides the organ into chambers, or *lobules*. It also has a *hilum* on one surface through which blood vessels enter. However, unlike the sinuses in a lymph node, the spaces (venous sinuses) within the chambers of the spleen are filled with *blood* instead of lymph.

Within the lobules of the spleen, the tissues are called *pulp* and are of two types: white pulp and red pulp. The *white pulp* is distributed throughout the spleen in tiny islands. This tissue is composed of nodules (splenic nodules), which are similar to those found in lymph nodes and contain large numbers of lymphocytes. The *red pulp*, which fills the remaining spaces of the lobules, surrounds the venous sinuses. This pulp contains relatively large numbers of red blood cells, which are responsible for its color, along with many lymphocytes and macrophages (figures 15.17, 15.18, and 15.19).

The blood capillaries within the red pulp are quite permeable. Red blood cells can squeeze through the pores in these capillary walls and enter the venous sinuses. The older, more fragile red blood cells may rupture as they make this passage and the resulting cellular debris is removed by macrophages located within the splenic sinuses.

The macrophages also engulf and destroy foreign particles, such as bacteria, that may be carried in the blood as it flows through the sinuses. Thus, the spleen filters blood much as the lymph nodes filter lymph.

The lymphocytes of the spleen, like those of the thymus, lymph nodes, and nodules, help defend the body against infections.

Chart 15.2 summarizes the characteristics of the major organs of the lymphatic system.

FIGURE 15.18
Photograph of a spleen.

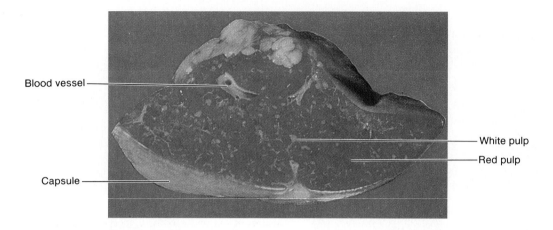

Blood vessel

White pulp
Red pulp

Capsule

FIGURE 15.19
Light micrograph of a portion of the spleen (×40).

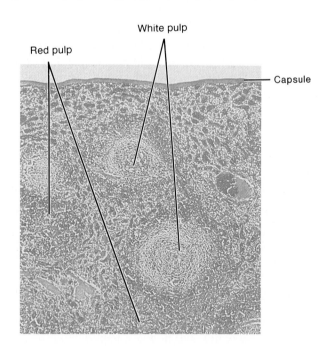

Red pulp

White pulp

Capsule

Chart 15.2 Major organs of the lymphatic system

Chart 15.2 Major organs of the lymphatic system

Organ	Location	Function
Lymph nodes	In groups or chains along the paths of larger lymphatic vessels	Center for lymphocyte proliferation; house T-lymphocytes and B-lymphocytes that are responsible for immunity; macrophages filter foreign particles and cellular debris from lymph
Thymus	Within the mediastinum behind the upper portion of the sternum	Houses lymphocytes; changes undifferentiated lymphocytes into T-lymphocytes
Spleen	In the upper-left portion of the abdominal cavity beneath the diaphragm and behind the stomach	Macrophages filter foreign particles, damaged red blood cells, and cellular debris from the blood; houses lymphocytes

During fetal development, pulp cells of the spleen produce blood cells, much as red bone marrow cells do in later life. As the time of birth approaches, this splenic function ceases. However, in certain diseases in which large numbers of red blood cells are destroyed, the splenic pulp cells may resume forming blood cells.

1. Why are the thymus and spleen considered organs of the lymphatic system?
2. What are the major functions of the thymus and the spleen?

Body Defenses Against Infection

An infection is a condition caused by the presence of a disease-causing agent. Such agents are termed **pathogens,** and they include viruses and microorganisms such as bacteria, fungi, and protozoans, as well as other parasitic forms of life.

The human body is equipped with a variety of defense mechanisms that help prevent the entrance of pathogens or act to destroy them if they do enter the tissues.

For example, the *skin* and the *mucous membranes* lining the tubes of the respiratory, digestive, urinary, and reproductive systems create mechanical barriers against the entrance of infectious agents. As long as these barriers remain unbroken, many pathogens are unable to penetrate them.

Some monocytes develop into *macrophages* (histiocytes), which become fixed in various tissues or attached to the inner walls of blood vessels and lymphatic vessels. These relatively nonmotile cells can divide and produce new macrophages, and are found in such organs as the lymph nodes, spleen, liver, and lungs. This diffuse group of cells constitutes the **reticuloendothelial tissue** or **reticuloendothelial system** (tissue macrophage system).

The name *reticuloendothelium* describes two characteristics of cells that make up this tissue. They are capable of forming fibrous networks, or *reticula,* and are often associated with the linings of blood vessels, the *endothelium.* The reticuloendothelial cells remove foreign particles from lymph and from blood.

The cells that line the vascular sinuses of the red bone marrow are also reticuloendothelial cells. Although these cells are especially concerned with the formation of red and white blood cells, they are also capable of engulfing particles.

1. What is a pathogen?
2. Which body structures form mechanical barriers to pathogens?
3. Define *reticuloendothelial tissue.*

Cells of Immunity

Immunity is resistance to specific foreign agents, such as pathogens, or to the toxins they release. The cells that function in immune mechanisms include lymphocytes and macrophages.

Origin of Lymphocytes

Lymphocytes originate from bone marrow cells (stem cells), although later they proliferate and mature in various lymphatic tissues.

Before they become specialized, or *differentiated,* developing lymphocytes are released from the marrow and are carried away by the blood. About half of them reach the thymus gland, where they remain for a time. Within the thymus, these undifferentiated cells (thymocytes) undergo special processing, and thereafter they are called *T-lymphocytes,* or T-cells. Later, the T-cells are transported away from the thymus by the blood, where they comprise 70%–80% of the circulating lymphocytes. They reside in various organs of the lymphatic system and are particularly abundant in lymph nodes, the thoracic duct, and the white pulp of the spleen.

Lymphocytes that have been released from the bone marrow and do not reach the thymus gland, differentiate into *B-lymphocytes,* or B-cells. Before they can mature, however, it may be necessary for these B-cells to pass through lymphoid tissue in some presently unknown region of the body, where they are specially processed.

FIGURE 15.20
Bone marrow releases undifferentiated lymphocytes that, after processing, become T-lymphocytes and B-lymphocytes.

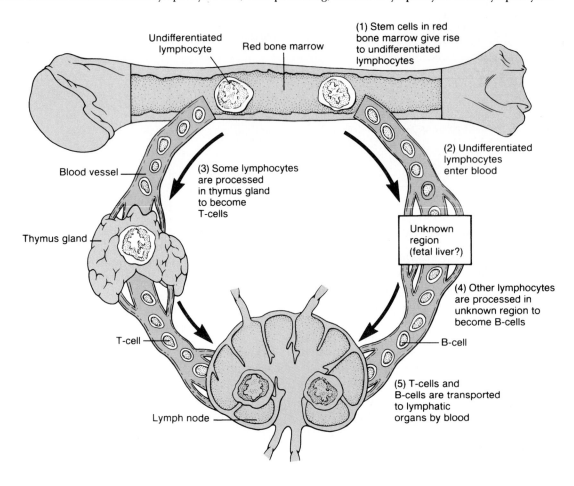

B-lymphocytes are distributed by the blood and constitute 20%–30% of the circulating lymphocytes. They settle in various lymphatic organs with the T-lymphocytes and are abundant in the lymph nodes, spleen, bone marrow, secretory glands, intestinal lining, and reticuloendothelial tissue (figures 15.20 and 15.21).

Functions of Lymphocytes

Prior to birth, body cells somehow make an inventory of the various chemicals present in the body. Subsequently, the substances that are present (self-substances) can be distinguished by the lymphocytes from foreign (nonself) substances. Such foreign substances, to which lymphocytes respond, are called **antigens.**

T-cells and B-cells respond to antigens in different ways. For example, some T-cells (cytotoxic T-cells) attach themselves to antigen-bearing cells, including certain bacterial cells, and interact with these cells directly—that is, with cell-to-cell contact.

FIGURE 15.21

Scanning electron micrograph of a human circulating lymphocyte (×36,000).

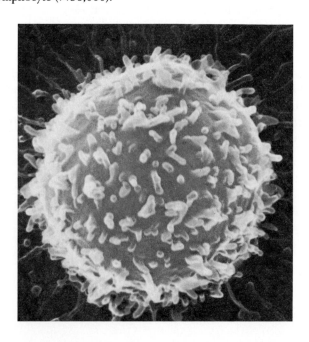

514   Chapter 15

Chart 15.3 A comparison of T-lymphocytes and B-lymphocytes

Characteristic	T-lymphocytes	B-lymphocytes
Origin of undifferentiated cell	Bone marrow	Bone marrow
Site of differentiation	Thymus gland	Region outside thymus gland
Primary locations	Lymphatic tissues, 70%–80% of circulating lymphocytes	Lymphatic tissues, 20%–30% of circulating lymphocytes

B-cells act indirectly against antigens by producing and secreting chemicals called *antibodies*. Antibodies are carried by the body fluids and react in various ways to destroy specific antigens or antigen-bearing particles.

Chart 15.3 compares T- and B-lymphocytes.

Acquired immune deficiency syndrome (AIDS) is a disease first recognized in 1981 whose incidence is roughly doubling each year. It is caused by a virus called human immunodeficiency virus (HIV-1). This virus infects certain T-cells, macrophages, B-cells, endothelial cells, and certain neuroglial cells.

When the virus infects cells, viral chromosomes are incorporated into the cellular chromosomes. Then, the virus may become dormant, failing to produce any noticeable effects for some time. During this latency period, which may last for several years, the person may show no symptoms of AIDS.

If the virus becomes active, it will induce the production of new viral particles that can infect other T-cells and kill them. As a consequence, the person's immune system is greatly impaired, and the group of symptoms that characterize AIDS develops. These symptoms include enlargement of lymph nodes, weight loss, and fever, as well as severe infections (following depression of the immune system) and the appearance of certain forms of cancer. The AIDS virus may also infect neuroglial cells, causing a loss of white matter and a variety of neurological problems. Some patients develop serious neurological dysfunctions without impairment of their immune systems.

1. Define immunity.
2. Explain the difference in origin between a T-lymphocyte and a B-lymphocyte.

Clinical Terms Related to the Lymphatic System and Immunity

asplenia (ah-sple′ne-ah)   the absence of a spleen.
lymphadenectomy (lim-fad″ĕ-nek′to-me)   surgical removal of lymph nodes.
lymphadenopathy (lim-fad″ĕ-nop′ah-the)   enlargement of the lymph nodes.
lymphadenotomy (lim-fad″ĕ-not′o-me)   an incision of a lymph node.
lymphoma (lim-fo′mah)   a tumor composed of lymphatic tissue.
lymphosarcoma (lim″fo-sar-ko′mah)   a cancer within the lymphatic tissue.
splenectomy (sple-nek′to-me)   surgical removal of the spleen.
splenitis (sple-ni′tis)   an inflammation of the spleen.
splenomegaly (sple″no-meg′ah-le)   an abnormal enlargement of the spleen.
splenotomy (sple-not′o-me)   incision of the spleen.
thymectomy (thi-mek′to-me)   surgical removal of the thymus gland.

Chapter Summary

Introduction (page 500)
The lymphatic system is closely associated with the cardiovascular system. It transports excess tissue fluid to the blood stream and helps defend the body against invasion by disease-causing microorganisms.

Lymphatic Pathways (page 500)
1. Lymphatic capillaries
   a. Lymphatic capillaries are microscopic, closed-end tubes that extend into interstitial spaces.
   b. They receive lymph through their thin walls.
   c. Lacteals are lymphatic capillaries in the villi of the small intestine.
2. Lymphatic vessels
   a. Lymphatic vessels are formed by the merging of lymphatic capillaries.
   b. They have walls similar to veins and possess valves that prevent backflow of lymph.
   c. They lead to lymph nodes and then merge into lymphatic trunks.
3. Lymphatic trunks and collecting ducts
   a. Lymphatic trunks drain lymph from relatively large body regions.
   b. Trunks lead to two collecting ducts within the thorax.
   c. Collecting ducts join the subclavian veins.

Tissue Fluid and Lymph (page 503)
1. Tissue fluid and lymph formation
   a. Tissue fluid originates from blood plasma, and includes water and dissolved substances that passed through the capillary wall.

b. It generally lacks large molecules, but some smaller protein molecules leak into interstitial spaces.
c. As proteins accumulate in tissue fluid, pressure increases also.
d. Increasing pressure within interstitial spaces forces some tissue fluid into lymphatic capillaries. This fluid becomes lymph.
2. Function of lymph
a. Lymph returns protein molecules to the blood stream.
b. It transports foreign particles to the lymph nodes.

Movement of Lymph (page 504)
1. Flow of lymph
a. Lymph may not flow readily without aid from external forces.
b. Forces that aid movement of lymph include squeezing action of skeletal muscles and low pressure in the thorax created by breathing movements.
2. Obstruction of lymph movement
a. Any condition that interferes with the flow of lymph results in edema.
b. Obstruction of lymphatic vessels due to surgery also results in edema.

Lymph Nodes (page 505)
1. Structure of a lymph node
a. Lymph nodes are usually bean-shaped, with blood vessels, nerves, and efferent lymphatic vessels attached to the indented region; afferent lymphatic vessels enter at points on the convex surface.
b. Lymph nodes are enclosed in connective tissue that extends into the nodes and divides them into nodules.
c. Nodules contain masses of lymphocytes and macrophages, and spaces through which lymph flows.
2. Locations of lymph nodes
a. Lymph nodes generally occur in groups or chains along the paths of larger lymphatic vessels.
b. They occur primarily in cervical, axillary, and inguinal regions, and within the pelvic, abdominal, and thoracic cavities.
3. Functions of lymph nodes
a. Lymph nodes are centers for proliferation of lymphocytes that act against foreign particles.
b. They contain macrophages that remove foreign particles from lymph.

Thymus and Spleen (page 510)
1. The thymus
a. The thymus is a soft, bilobed organ located within the mediastinum.
b. It tends to decrease in size after puberty.
c. It is composed of lymphatic tissue that is subdivided into lobules.
d. Lobules contain lymphocytes, most of which are inactive, that develop from precursor cells in bone marrow.
e. Some lymphocytes leave the thymus and become T-lymphocytes.
f. The thymus may secrete a hormone called thymosin, which stimulates lymphocytes that have migrated to other lymphatic tissues.
2. The spleen
a. The spleen is located in the upper-left portion of the abdominal cavity.
b. It resembles a large lymph node that is encapsulated and subdivided into lobules by connective tissue.
c. Spaces within lobules are filled with blood.
d. It contains numerous macrophages and lymphocytes that filter foreign particles and damaged red blood cells from the blood.

Body Defenses Against Infection (page 513)
Infection is caused by the presence of pathogens. The body is equipped with defenses against infection.

1. Mechanical barriers include skin and mucous membranes. They prevent the entrance of many pathogens as long as they remain unbroken.
2. Monocytes give rise to macrophages that remain fixed in tissues.
3. Cells associated with the linings of blood vessels in bone marrow, liver, spleen, and lymph nodes constitute the reticuloendothelial tissue.

Cells of Immunity (page 513)
1. Lymphocytes originate in bone marrow and are released into the blood before they become differentiated.
2. Some reach the thymus, where they become T-lymphocytes.
3. Others become B-lymphocytes after being processed in some unknown region of the body.
4. Both T- and B-lymphocytes tend to reside in organs of the lymphatic system.
5. Lymphocytes respond to antigens.
a. T-cells contact antigen-bearing cells.
b. B-cells produce antibodies that react to antigens.

Clinical Application of Knowledge

1. Based on your understanding of the functions of lymph nodes, how would you explain the fact that enlarged nodes are often removed for microscopic examination as an aid to diagnosing certain disease conditions?
2. Why is it true that an injection into the skin is, to a large extent, an injection into the lymphatic system?
3. Why is knowledge of lymph node locations and direction of lymph flow important in predicting the spread of cancer cells?
4. When a breast is removed surgically for the treatment of breast cancer, the lymph nodes in the nearby axillary region are sometimes excised also. Why is this procedure likely to be followed by swelling of the arm on the treated side?
5. If an infant was found to be lacking a thymus because of a developmental disorder, what could be predicted about the infants susceptibility to infections? Why?

Review Activities

1. Explain how the lymphatic system is related to the cardiovascular system.
2. Trace the general pathway of lymph from the interstitial spaces to the blood stream.
3. Identify and describe the location of the major lymphatic trunks and collecting ducts.
4. Distinguish between tissue fluid and lymph.
5. Describe the primary functions of lymph.
6. Explain how a lymphatic obstruction leads to edema.
7. Describe the structure of a lymph node and list its major functions.
8. Locate the major body regions occupied by lymph nodes.
9. Describe the structure and functions of the thymus gland.
10. Describe the structure and functions of the spleen.
11. Define *reticuloendothelial tissue* and explain its importance.
12. Review the origin and differentiation of T-lymphocytes and B-lymphocytes.

CHAPTER 16

The Urinary System

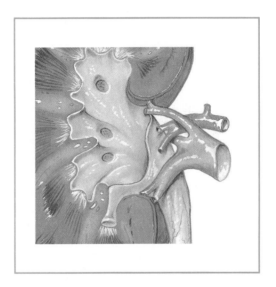

Body cells form a variety of wastes as by-products of body processes, and if these substances accumulate, their effects are likely to be toxic.

Body fluids, such as blood and lymph, carry wastes away from the tissues that produce them. The urinary system is composed of organs that remove wastes from the blood. The wastes are then carried outside the body through tubular organs.

Chapter Outline

Introduction

The Kidneys
    Location of the Kidneys
    Structure of a Kidney
    Functions of the Kidneys
    Renal Blood Vessels
    The Nephrons

Elimination of Urine
    The Ureters
    The Urinary Bladder
    Micturition
    The Urethra

Clinical Terms Related to the Urinary
System

Chapter Objectives

After you have studied this chapter, you
should be able to

1. Name the organs of the urinary
system and list their general
functions.

2. Describe the locations of the kidneys
and the structure of a kidney.

3. List the functions of the kidneys.

4. Trace the pathway of blood through
the major vessels within a kidney.

5. Describe a nephron and explain the
functions of its major parts.

6. Describe the structure of the ureters,
urinary bladder, and urethra.

7. Discuss the process of micturition
and explain how it is controlled.

8. Complete the review activities at the
end of this chapter. Note that the
items are worded in the form of
specific learning objectives. You may
want to refer to them before reading
the chapter.

Aids to Understanding Words

calyc-, a small cup: major *calyces*—
cuplike subdivisions of the renal
pelvis.

cort-, covering: renal *cortex*—shell of
tissue surrounding the inner region
of the kidney.

detrus-, to force away: *detrus*or
muscle—muscle within the bladder
wall that causes urine to be
expelled.

glom-, little ball: *glom*erulus—cluster of
capillaries within a renal corpuscle.

juxta-, near to: *juxta*medullary
nephron—a nephron located near
the renal medulla.

mict-, to pass urine: *mict*urition—
process of expelling urine from the
bladder.

nephr-, pertaining to the kidney:
*nephr*on—functional unit of a
kidney.

papill-, nipple: renal *papill*ae—small
elevations that project into a renal
calyx.

ren-, kidney: *ren*al cortex—outer region
of the kidney.

trigon-, a triangular shape: *trigone*—
triangular area on the internal floor
of the bladder.

Introduction

The urinary system consists of the following parts: a pair of glandular *kidneys,* which remove substances from the blood, form urine, and help regulate various body processes; a pair of tubular *ureters,* which transport urine away from the kidneys; a saclike *urinary bladder,* which serves as a urine reservoir; and a tubular *urethra,* which conveys urine to the outside of the body. These organs are shown in figures 16.1 and 16.2.

The Kidneys

A **kidney** is a reddish brown, bean-shaped organ with a smooth surface. It is about 12 centimeters long, 6 centimeters wide, and 3 centimeters thick in an adult, and is enclosed in a tough, fibrous *renal capsule.*

Location of the Kidneys

The kidneys lie on either side of the vertebral column in depressions high on the posterior wall of the abdominal cavity.

Although the positions of the kidneys may vary slightly with changes in posture and with breathing movements, their upper and lower borders are generally at the levels of the twelfth thoracic and third lumbar vertebrae, respectively. The left kidney is usually about 1.5 to 2 centimeters higher than the right one.

The kidneys are positioned *retroperitoneally,* which means they are behind the parietal peritoneum and against the deep muscles of the back. They are held in position by connective tissue (renal fascia) and the masses of adipose tissue (renal fat) that surround them. (See figures 16.3 and 16.4.)

Structure of a Kidney

The lateral surface of each kidney is convex, but its medial side is deeply concave. The resulting medial depression leads into a hollow chamber called the **renal sinus.** The entrance to this sinus is termed the *hilum,* and through it passes various blood vessels, nerves, lymphatic vessels, and the ureter (figure 16.1).

FIGURE 16.1

The urinary system includes the kidneys, ureters, urinary bladder, and urethra. What are the general functions of this system?

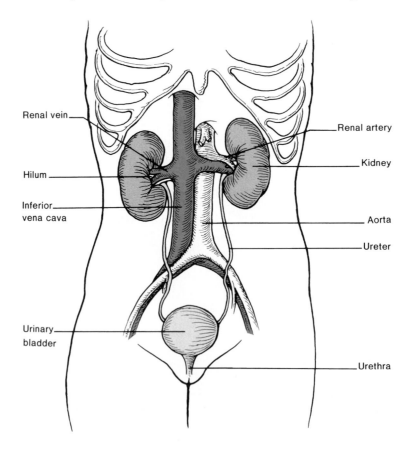

FIGURE 16.2

What features of the urinary system do you recognize in this artificially colored X-ray film?

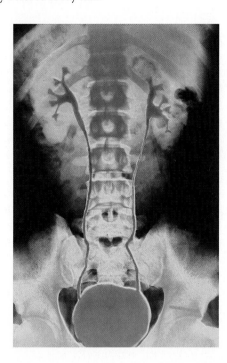

FIGURE 16.4

Sagittal section of a kidney.

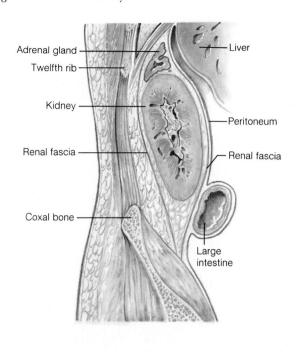

FIGURE 16.3

The kidneys are behind the parietal peritoneum and are surrounded and supported by adipose tissue.

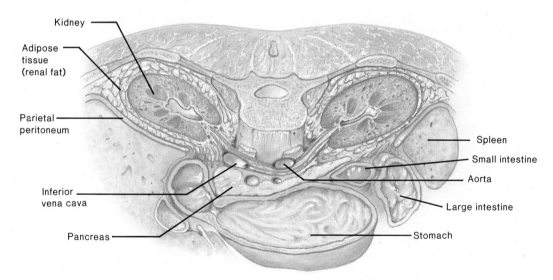

The superior end of the ureter is expanded to form a funnel-shaped sac called the **renal pelvis,** which is located inside the renal sinus. The pelvis is subdivided into two or three tubes called *major calyces* (sing. *calyx*), and they, in turn, are subdivided into 8–14 *minor calyces* (figure 16.5).

A series of small elevations project into the renal sinus from its wall. These projections are called *renal papillae,* and each of them is pierced by tiny openings that lead into a minor calyx.

The substance of the kidney includes two distinct regions: an inner medulla and an outer cortex. The **renal medulla** is composed of conical masses of tissue called *renal pyramids,* whose bases are directed toward the lateral surface of the kidney, and whose apexes form the renal papillae. The tissue of the medulla appears striated due to the presence of microscopic tubules leading from the cortex to the renal papillae.

FIGURE 16.5

(*a*) Longitudinal section of a kidney; (*b*) a renal pyramid containing nephrons; (*c*) a single nephron.

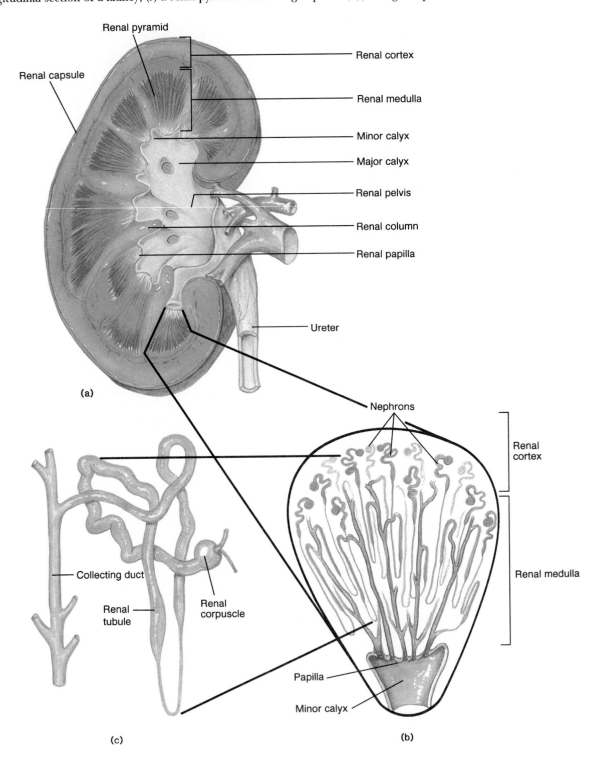

Renal pyramid

Renal cortex

Renal capsule

Renal medulla

Minor calyx

Major calyx

Renal pelvis

Renal column

Renal papilla

Ureter

(a)

Nephrons

Renal cortex

Collecting duct

Renal tubule

Renal corpuscle

Renal medulla

Papilla

Minor calyx

(c)

(b)

The **renal cortex,** which appears somewhat granular, forms a shell around the medulla. Its tissue dips into the medulla between adjacent renal pyramids, forming *renal columns.* The granular appearance of the cortex is due to the random arrangement of tiny tubules associated with **nephrons,** the functional units of the kidney.

During the development of a human kidney, several pyramidal masses, or lobes, fuse to form the final structure. Consequently, lobulation is evident on the surface of a fetal kidney, and this condition sometimes persists into adulthood.

Functions of the Kidneys

The kidneys remove wastes from the blood and excrete them to the outside. They also carry on important regulatory activities.

The kidneys help regulate the volume and composition of body fluids. These functions involve complex mechanisms leading to the formation of urine.

---

1. Where are the kidneys located?
2. Describe the structure of a kidney.
3. Name the functional unit of a kidney.
4. What are the general functions of the kidneys?

Renal Blood Vessels

Blood is supplied to the kidneys by **renal arteries** that arise from the abdominal aorta (figure 16.6). These arteries transport a relatively large volume of blood.

A renal artery enters a kidney through the hilum and gives off several branches, called the *interlobar arteries,* that pass between the renal pyramids. At the junction between the medulla and the cortex, the interlobar arteries branch to form a series of incomplete arches, the *arciform arteries* (arcuate arteries), which, in turn, give rise to *interlobular arteries.* Lateral branches of the interlobular arteries, called **afferent arterioles,** lead to the nephrons.

Venous blood is returned through a series of vessels that correspond generally to the arterial pathways. For example, the venous blood passes through interlobular, arciform, interlobar, and renal veins. The **renal vein** then joins the inferior vena cava as it courses through the abdominal cavity. (Branches of the renal arteries and veins are shown in figures 16.7, 16.8, and 16.9.)

Patients with end-stage renal disease are sometimes treated with a *kidney transplant.* In this surgical procedure, a kidney from a living donor or a cadaver whose tissues are similar to those of the recipient, is placed in the depression on the medial surface of the right or left ilium (iliac fossa). The renal artery and vein of the donor kidney are connected to the recipient's iliac artery and vein respectively, and the kidney's ureter is attached to the dome of the recipient's urinary bladder.

FIGURE 16.6

Blood vessels associated with the kidneys and adrenal glands.

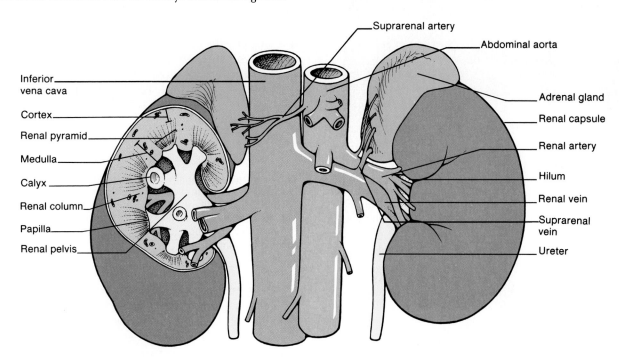

FIGURE 16.7
Main branches of the renal artery and vein.

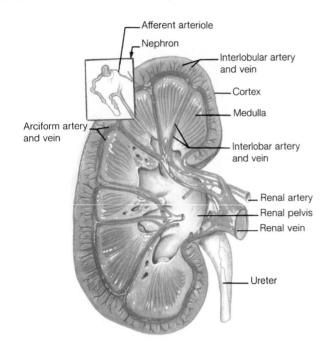

FIGURE 16.8
A cast of the ureter, renal pelvis, and branches of the renal artery.

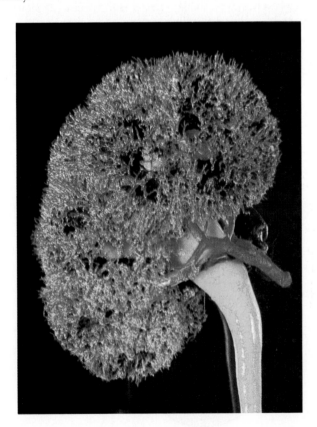

FIGURE 16.9
A scanning electron micrograph of a cast of the renal blood vessels associated with the glomeruli (×260).
R. G. Kessel and R. H. Kardon, *Tissues and Organs: A Text Atlas of Scanning Electron Microscopy,* © 1979, W. H. Freeman & Co.

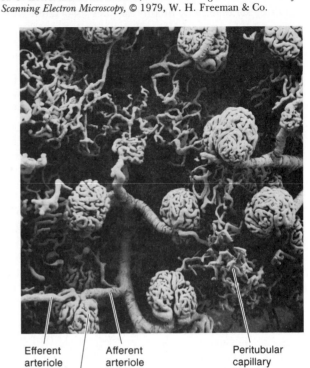

The Nephrons

Structure and Function of a Nephron

A kidney contains about one million nephrons, each consisting of a **renal corpuscle** and a **renal tubule** (figures 16.5 and 16.10).

A renal corpuscle (malpighian corpuscle) is composed of a tangled cluster of blood capillaries called a **glomerulus,** which is surrounded by a thin-walled, saclike structure called the **glomerular** (Bowman's) **capsule,** (figure 16.11). The glomerulus filters fluid from the blood. This fluid, called filtrate, then moves into the glomerular capsule.

> The glomerular capillaries are more permeable than the capillaries in most other tissues due to the presence of numerous tiny openings (fenestrae) in their walls. These capillaries provide a large surface area to filter blood plasma. This surface area is estimated to be about 2 square meters—approximately equal to the surface area of an adult's skin.

The glomerular capsule is an expansion at the closed end of a renal tubule. It is composed of two layers of squamous epithelial cells: a visceral layer that closely covers the glomerulus, and an outer parietal layer that is continuous with the visceral layer and with the wall of the renal tubule.

FIGURE 16.10

Structure of a nephron and the blood vessels associated with it. (The arrows indicate the direction of blood flow.)

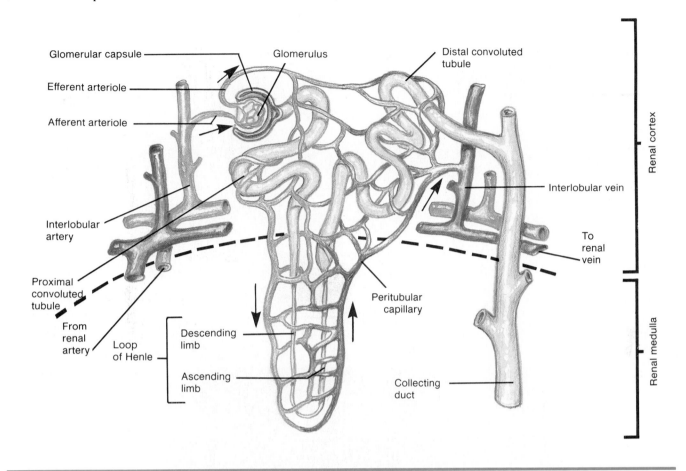

FIGURE 16.11

A scanning electron micrograph of a glomerulus surrounded by a glomerular capsule.

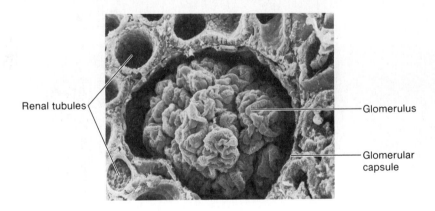

FIGURE 16.12

(a) Podocytes form the visceral layer of the glomerular capsule and surround the glomerular capillaries. (b) Scanning electron micrograph of a glomerulus (×8,000). Note the slit pores between the pedicels.

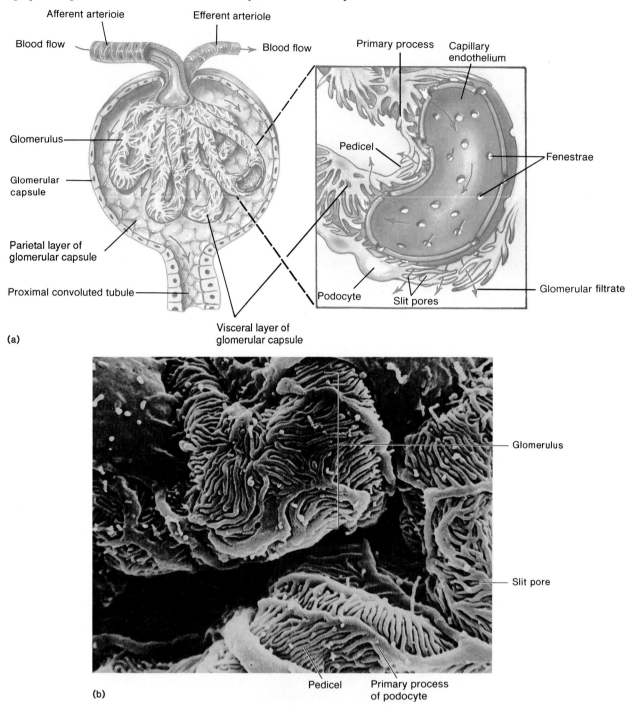

(a)

(b)

The cells of the parietal layer are typical squamous epithelial cells; however, those of the visceral layer are highly modified epithelial cells called *podocytes*. Each podocyte has several primary processes extending from its cell body, and these processes, in turn, bear numerous secondary processes, or *pedicels*. The pedicels of each cell interdigitate with those of adjacent podocytes, and the clefts between them form a complicated system of *slit pores*. (See figures 16.12 and 16.13.) Filtrate from the glomerulus moves through the slit pores.

The renal tubule carries filtrate away from the glomerular capsule. Each renal tubule is lined with a single layer of epithelial cells.

The first portion of the renal tubule becomes highly coiled and is named the *proximal convoluted tubule*. The cuboidal epithelial cells in this portion have numerous microscopic projections called *microvilli* that form a "brush border" on their free surfaces. These tiny extensions greatly increase the surface area exposed to glomerular

FIGURE 16.13

(a) A transmission electron micrograph and (b) a drawing of a glomerular capillary and podocytes. Substances are filtered through the capillary pores, the basement membrane, and the slit pores between the pedicels (arrows in part b).

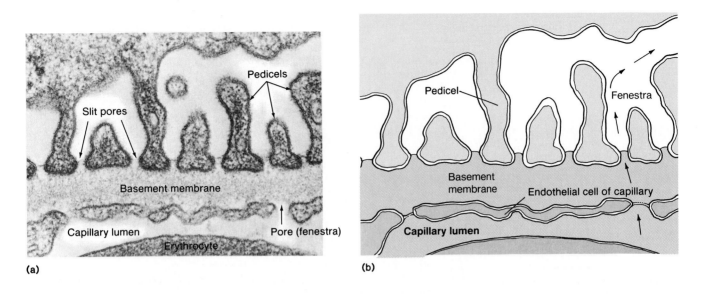

(a)

(b)

FIGURE 16.14

Cross sections of a renal tubule.

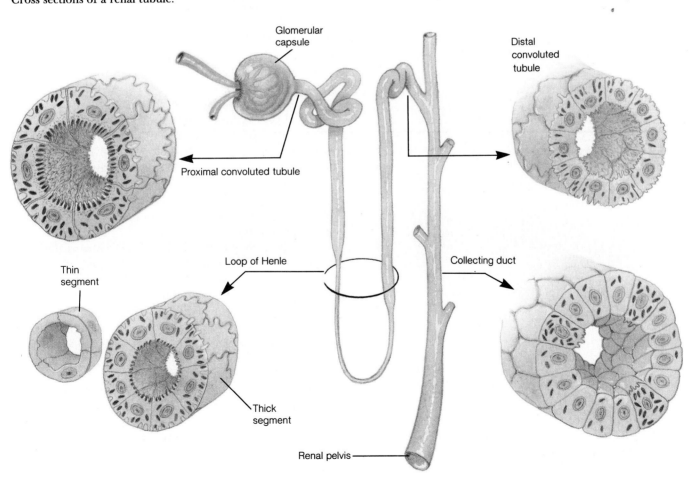

FIGURE 16.15
(*a*) Cells of the proximal convoluted tubule have many microvilli that enhance the reabsorption of substances; (*b*) a transmission electron micrograph of the proximal convoluted tubule, showing the microvilli (Mv) and mitochondria (M).

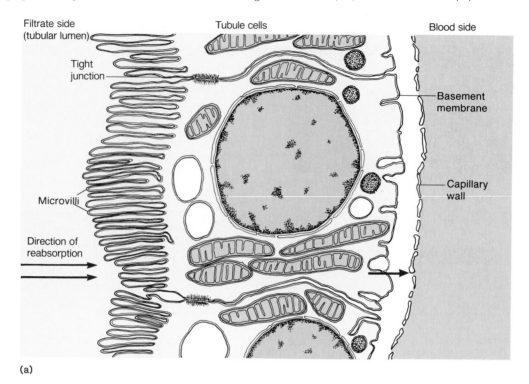

(a)

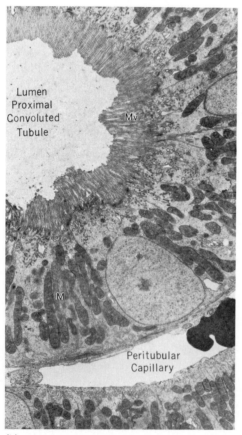

(b)

filtrate (figures 16.14 and 16.15). This enhances the reabsorption of substances through the epithelium and into the surrounding blood vessels.

The proximal convoluted tubule dips toward the renal pelvis to become the *descending limb of the loop of Henle*. The tubule then curves back toward its renal corpuscle and forms the *ascending limb of the loop of Henle*. The epithelium of the descending limb (thin segment) is composed of flattened cuboidal epithelial cells that lack microvilli (figure 16.16). The ascending limb (thick segment) is lined with cuboidal epithelium. Reabsorption of water and certain salts occurs in the loop of Henle.

The ascending limb returns to the region of the renal corpuscle, where it becomes highly coiled again and is then called the *distal convoluted tubule*. This distal portion is shorter than the proximal tubule, and its convolutions are less complex. This segment is also lined with cuboidal epithelial cells, but they possess few microvilli. Certain waste substances are secreted into the filtrate within the distal convoluted tubule.

Several distal convoluted tubules merge in the renal cortex to form a *collecting duct,* which, in turn, passes into the renal medulla, becoming larger and larger as it is joined by other collecting ducts. The resulting tube (papillary duct) empties into a minor calyx through an opening in a renal papilla. The parts of a nephron are shown in figures 16.14 and 16.17, and its functions are summarized in chart 16.1.

FIGURE 16.16

Light micrograph of cross sections of renal tubules (×250).

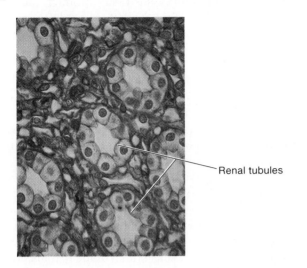

Renal tubules

Chart 16.1 Functions of nephron parts	
Part	**Function**
Renal Corpuscle	
Glomerulus	Filtration of water and dissolved substances from plasma
Glomerular capsule	Receives glomerular filtrate
Renal Tubule	
Proximal convoluted tubule	Reabsorption of many dissolved substances and water
Descending limb of the loop of Henle	Reabsorption of water
Ascending limb of the loop of Henle	Reabsorption of certain salts
Distal convoluted tubule	Reabsorption of dissolved substances and water
	Active secretion of certain substances

FIGURE 16.17

(*a*) Light micrograph of the human renal cortex (about ×150).
(*b*) Light micrograph of the renal medulla.

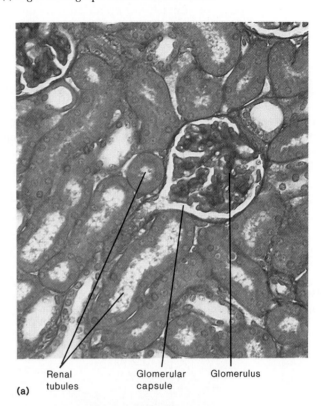

Renal
tubules   Glomerular   Glomerulus
               capsule

(a)

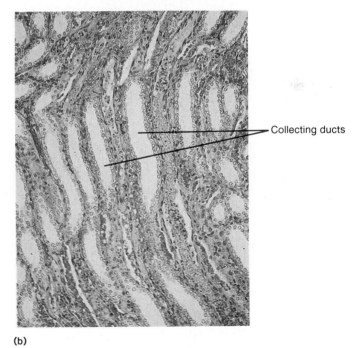

Collecting ducts

(b)

The Urinary System   529

Juxtaglomerular Apparatus

Near its beginning, the distal convoluted tubule passes between the afferent and efferent arterioles, and contacts them. At the point of contact, the epithelial cells of the distal tubule are quite narrow and densely packed. These cells comprise a structure called the *macula densa.*

Close by, in the walls of the arterioles near their attachments to the glomerulus, are some large smooth muscle cells. They are called *juxtaglomerular cells,* and together with the cells of the macula densa, they constitute the **juxtaglomerular apparatus** (complex). This structure plays an important role in regulating the flow of blood through various renal vessels (figure 16.18).

Cortical and Juxtamedullary Nephrons

Most nephrons have corpuscles located in the renal cortex near the surface of the kidney. These are called *cortical nephrons,* and have relatively short loops of Henle that usually do not reach the renal medulla.

Another group, called *juxtamedullary nephrons,* have corpuscles close to the renal medulla, and their loops of Henle extend deep into the medulla. Although they represent only about 20% of the total, these nephrons play an important role in regulating the volume of urine produced (figure 16.19).

Blood Supply of a Nephron

The cluster of capillaries that forms a glomerulus arises from an **afferent arteriole.** After passing through the capillary of the glomerulus, blood enters an **efferent arteriole** (rather than a venule) whose diameter is somewhat less than that of the afferent vessel.

The efferent arteriole branches into a complex, freely interconnecting network of capillaries that surrounds the various portions of the renal tubule. This network is called the **peritubular capillary system** (figures 16.10 and 16.19).

Special branches of this system, which receive blood primarily from the efferent arterioles of the juxtamedullary

FIGURE 16.18

The juxtaglomerular apparatus consists of the macula densa and the juxtaglomerular cells.

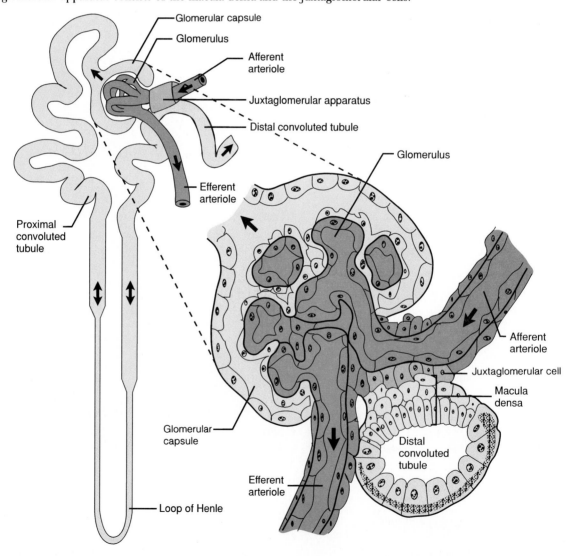

Glomerulonephritis

Nephritis refers to an inflammation of the kidney; *glomerulonephritis* refers to an inflammation affecting the glomeruli. This latter condition may occur in acute or chronic forms, and can lead to renal failure.

Acute glomerulonephritis (AGN) usually results from an abnormal immune reaction that develops one to three weeks following a certain type of bacterial infection (beta-hemolytic streptococci). As a rule, the infectious condition occurs in some other part of the body and does not affect the kidneys directly. Instead, the presence of bacteria triggers an immune reaction. As a consequence of this reaction, the glomerular capillaries may be blocked by bacteria and white blood cells.

Most patients eventually regain normal kidney function; however, in severe cases the renal functions may fail completely, and without treatment, the person is likely to die within a week or so.

Chronic glomerulonephritis is a progressive disease in which increasing numbers of nephrons are slowly damaged until finally the kidneys are unable to perform their usual functions. This condition is usually associated with certain diseases other than streptococcal infections and involves tissue changes in which the glomerular membranes are slowly replaced by fibrous tissue. As this happens, the functions of the nephrons are permanently lost, and eventually the kidneys may fail.

FIGURE 16.19

(*a*) Cortical nephrons are close to the surface of a kidney; juxtamedullary nephrons are near the renal medulla. (*b*) Enlarged view of a cortical nephron. (The arrows indicate the direction of blood flow.)

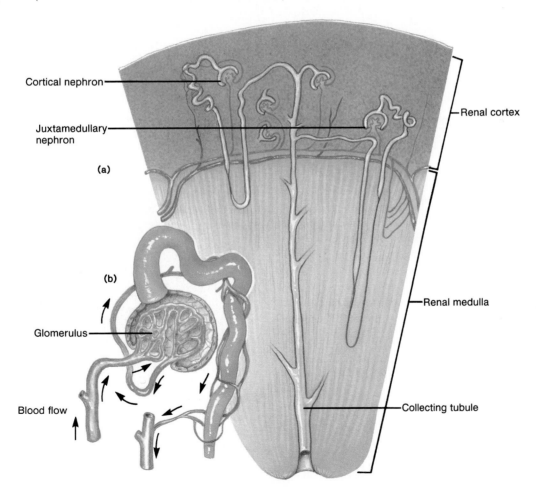

The Urinary System   531

FIGURE 16.20

The capillary loop of the vasa recta is closely associated with the loop of Henle of a juxtamedullary nephron.

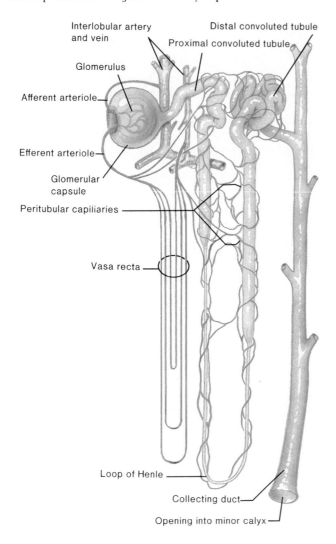

Elimination of Urine

After being formed by nephrons, urine passes from the collecting ducts through openings in the renal papillae and enters the minor and major calyces of the kidney. From there, it passes through the renal pelvis and is conveyed by a ureter to the urinary bladder. It is excreted to the outside of the body by means of the urethra.

The Ureters

Each **ureter** is a tubular organ about 25 centimeters long, which begins as the funnel-shaped renal pelvis. It extends downward behind the parietal peritoneum and runs parallel to the vertebral column. Within the pelvic cavity, it courses forward medially to join the urinary bladder from underneath.

The wall of a ureter is composed of three layers. The inner layer, or *mucous coat,* includes several thicknesses of epithelial cells and is continuous with the linings of the renal tubules and the urinary bladder. The middle layer, or *muscular coat,* consists largely of smooth muscle fibers arranged in circular and longitudinal bundles. The outer layer, or *fibrous coat,* is composed of connective tissue (figure 16.21).

> Because the linings of the ureters and the urinary bladder are continuous, infectious agents such as bacteria may ascend from the bladder into the ureters. An inflammation of the bladder, called *cystitis,* occurs more commonly in women than in men because the female urethral pathway is shorter. An inflammation of the ureter is called *ureteritis.*

Although the ureter is simply a tube leading from the kidney to the urinary bladder, its muscular wall helps move urine. Muscular peristaltic waves originating in the renal pelvis force urine along the length of the ureter. These waves are initiated by the presence of urine in the renal pelvis.

The opening through which the urine enters the urinary bladder is covered by a flaplike fold of mucous membrane. This fold acts as a valve, allowing urine to move inward from the ureter but preventing it from backing up.

If a ureter becomes obstructed, as when a small kidney stone (renal calculus) is present in its lumen, strong peristaltic waves are initiated in the proximal portion of the tube. Such waves may help move the stone into the bladder. At the same time, the presence of a stone usually stimulates a sympathetic reflex (ureterorenal reflex) that results in constriction of the renal arterioles and reduces the production of urine in the kidney on the affected side.

nephrons, form capillary loops called *vasa recta.* These loops dip into the renal medulla and are closely associated with the loops of the juxtamedullary nephrons.

The vessels of the peritubular capillary network and the vasa recta absorb substances from the nephron. After flowing through the vasa recta, blood is returned to the renal cortex, where it joins blood from other branches of the peritubular capillary system and enters the venous system of the kidney (figure 16.20).

1. Describe the system of vessels that supplies blood to a kidney.
2. Name the parts of a nephron.
3. What parts comprise the juxtaglomerular apparatus?
4. Distinguish between a cortical nephron and a juxtamedullary nephron.
5. Describe the blood supply of a nephron.

FIGURE 16.21

Cross section of a ureter (×160).

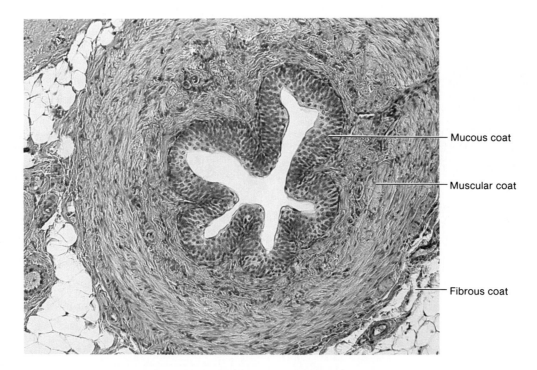

Mucous coat

Muscular coat

Fibrous coat

Kidney stones, which are usu-
ally composed of calcium oxalate, calcium phosphate, uric
acid, or magnesium phosphate, sometimes form in the renal
pelvis. If such a stone passes into a ureter, it may produce
severe pain. This pain commonly begins in the region of the
kidney and tends to radiate into the abdomen, pelvis, and legs.
The pain may also be accompanied by nausea and vomiting.

1. Describe the structure of a ureter.
2. How is urine moved from the renal pelvis?
3. What prevents urine from backing up from the urinary
   bladder into the ureters?
4. How does an obstruction in a ureter affect urine
   production?

The Urinary Bladder

The **urinary bladder** is a hollow, distensible, muscular
organ. It is located within the pelvic cavity, behind the
symphysis pubis and beneath the parietal peritoneum
(figure 16.22). In a male, it lies against the rectum posteriorly, and in a female it contacts the anterior walls of the
uterus and vagina.

Although the bladder is somewhat spherical, its shape
is altered by the pressures of surrounding organs. When
it is empty, the inner wall of the bladder is thrown into
many folds, but as it fills with urine, the wall becomes
smoother. At the same time, the superior surface of the
bladder expands upward into a dome.

FIGURE 16.22

The urinary bladder is located within the pelvic cavity and
behind the symphysis pubis. In a male, it lies against the
rectum.

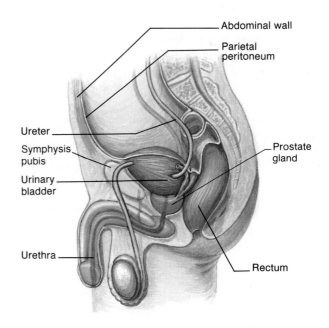

Abdominal wall

Parietal
peritoneum

Ureter

Symphysis
pubis

Urinary
bladder

Prostate
gland

Urethra

Rectum

When it is greatly distended, the bladder pushes above
the pubic crest and into the region between the abdominal
wall and the parietal peritoneum. The dome can reach the
level of the umbilicus and press against the coils of the small
intestine.

FIGURE 16.23

(*a*) Frontal section of the male urinary bladder; (*b*) posterior view of the urinary bladder; (*c*) light micrograph of the wall of a human urinary bladder.

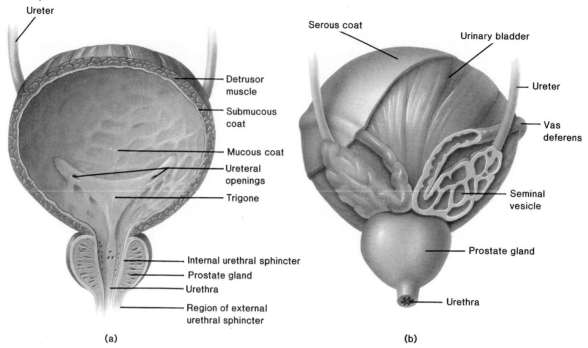

(a)

(b)

The internal floor of the bladder includes a triangular area called the *trigone*, which has an opening at each of its three angles (figure 16.23). Posteriorly, at the base of the trigone, the openings are those of the ureters. Anteriorly, at the apex of the trigone, there is a short, funnel-shaped extension called the neck of the bladder. This part contains the opening to the urethra. The trigone generally remains in a fixed position even though the rest of the bladder changes shape during distension and contraction, thus preventing a reflux of urine into the ureters.

The wall of the urinary bladder consists of four layers. The inner layer, or *mucous coat,* includes several thicknesses of transitional epithelial cells, similar to those lining the ureters and the upper portion of the urethra. The thickness of this tissue changes as the bladder expands and contracts. Thus, during distension the tissue appears to be only two or three cells thick, but during contraction it appears to be five or six cells thick (see figure 4.7).

The second layer of the wall is the *submucous coat.* It consists of connective tissue and contains many elastic fibers.

The third layer of the bladder wall, or *muscular coat,* is composed primarily of coarse bundles of smooth muscle fibers. These bundles are interlaced in all directions and at all depths, and together they comprise the **detrusor muscle.** The portion of the detrusor muscle that sur-

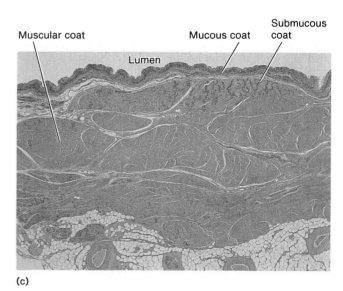

(c)

rounds the neck of the bladder forms the internal urethral sphincter. This muscle is supplied with parasympathetic nerve fibers that function in the micturition reflex.

The outer layer of the bladder wall, or *serous coat,* consists of the parietal peritoneum. This layer occurs only on the upper surface of the bladder. Elsewhere, the outer coat is composed of fibrous connective tissue.

Micturition

Micturition (urination) is the process by which urine is expelled from the urinary bladder. It involves the contraction of the detrusor muscle and may be aided by contractions of muscles in the abdominal wall and pelvic floor, and by fixation of the thoracic wall and diaphragm. Micturition also involves the relaxation of the *external urethral sphincter*. This muscle, which is part of the urogenital diaphragm, surrounds the urethra about 3 centimeters from the bladder and is composed of voluntary skeletal muscle tissue.

The need to urinate is usually stimulated by distension of the bladder wall as it fills with urine. As the wall expands, stretch receptors are stimulated, and the micturition reflex is triggered.

The *micturition reflex center* is located in the sacral segments of the spinal cord. When it is signalled by sensory impulses from the stretch receptors, *parasympathetic* motor impulses travel out to the detrusor muscle, which undergoes rhythmic contractions in response. This action is accompanied by a sensation of urgency.

Although the urinary bladder may hold as much as 600 milliliters of urine, the desire to urinate usually is experienced when it contains about 150 milliliters. Then, as the volume of urine increases to 300 milliliters or more, the sensation of fullness becomes increasingly uncomfortable.

However, because the external urethral sphincter is composed of skeletal muscle, it can be consciously controlled. It ordinarily remains contracted until a decision is made to urinate. This control is aided by nerve centers in the brain stem and cerebral cortex that are able to partially inhibit the micturition reflex. When a person decides to urinate, the external urethral sphincter is allowed to relax, and the micturition reflex is no longer inhibited. Nerve centers within the pons and the hypothalamus may function to make the micturition reflex more effective. Consequently, the detrusor muscle contracts, and urine is excreted to the outside through the urethra. Within a few moments, the neurons of the micturition reflex seem to fatigue, the detrusor muscle relaxes, and the bladder begins to fill with urine again.

The Urethra

The **urethra** is a tube that conveys urine from the urinary bladder to the outside of the body. Its wall is lined with mucous membrane and contains a relatively thick layer of smooth muscle tissue, whose fibers are generally directed longitudinally. It also contains numerous mucous glands, called *urethral glands,* that secrete mucus into the urethral canal.

In a female, the urethra is about 4 centimeters long. It passes forward from the bladder, courses below the symphysis pubis, and empties between the labia minora. Its opening, the external urethral meatus, is located anterior to the vaginal opening and about 2.5 centimeters posterior to the clitoris.

In a male, the urethra, which functions both as a urinary canal and a passageway for cells and secretions from various reproductive organs, can be divided into three sections: the prostatic urethra, the membranous urethra, and the penile urethra (figure 16.24).

The *prostatic urethra* is about 2.5 centimeters long and passes from the urinary bladder through the *prostate gland,* which is located just below the bladder. Ducts from various reproductive structures join the urethra in this region.

The *membranous urethra* is about 2 centimeters long. It begins just distal to the prostate gland, passes through the urogenital diaphragm, and is surrounded by the fibers of the external urethral sphincter muscle.

The *penile urethra* is about 15 centimeters long and passes through the corpus spongiosum of the penis, where it is surrounded by erectile tissue. It is lined with transitional epithelium (figure 16.25). This portion of the urethra terminates as the *external urethral orifice* at the tip of the penis.

FIGURE 16.24

(a) Longitudinal section of the male urinary bladder and urethra; (b) longitudinal section of the female urinary bladder and urethra.

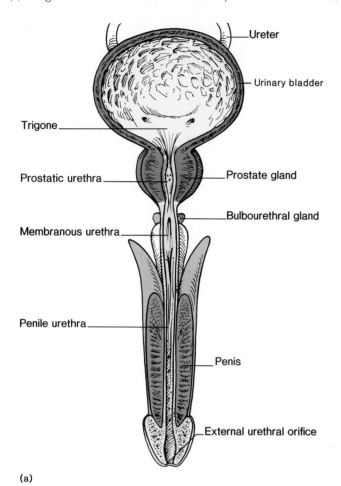

- Ureter
- Urinary bladder
- Trigone
- Prostatic urethra
- Prostate gland
- Bulbourethral gland
- Membranous urethra
- Penile urethra
- Penis
- External urethral orifice

(a)

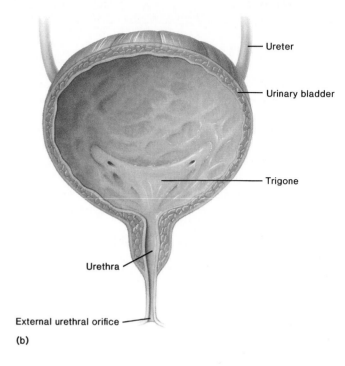

- Ureter
- Urinary bladder
- Trigone
- Urethra
- External urethral orifice

(b)

FIGURE 16.25

Cross section through the urethra (×10).

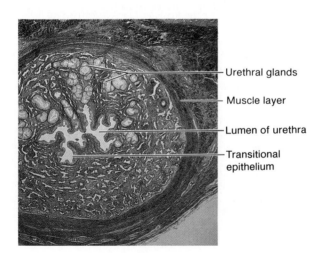

- Urethral glands
- Muscle layer
- Lumen of urethra
- Transitional epithelium

Clinical Terms Related to the Urinary System

anuria (ah-nu're-ah)   an absence of urine due to kidney failure or to an obstruction in a urinary pathway.

cystectomy (sis-tek'to-me)   surgical removal of the urinary bladder.

cystoscope (sis'to-skōp)   instrument used for visual examination of the interior of the urinary bladder.

cystotomy (sis-tot'o-me)   an incision of the wall of the urinary bladder.

nephrectomy (ně-frek'to-me)   surgical removal of a kidney.

nephrolithiasis (nef''ro-li-thi'ah-sis)   presence of a stone or stones in the kidney.

nephroptosis (něf''rop-to'sis)   a movable or displaced kidney.

pyelolithotomy (pi''ě-lo-li-thot'o-me)   removal of a stone from the renal pelvis.

pyelonephritis (pi''ě-lo-ně-fri'tis)   inflammation of the renal pelvis.

pyelotomy (pi''ě-lot'o-me)   incision into the renal pelvis.

ureteritis (u-re''ter-i'tis)   inflammation of the ureter.

urethritis (u''re-thri'tis)   inflammation of the urethra.

Chapter Summary

Introduction (page 520)
The urinary system consists of the kidneys, ureters, urinary bladder, and urethra.

The Kidneys (page 520)
1. Location of the kidneys
   a. The kidneys are on either side of the vertebral column, high on the posterior wall of the abdominal cavity.
   b. They are positioned behind the parietal peritoneum, and held in place by adipose and connective tissue.
2. Structure of a kidney
   a. A kidney contains a hollow renal sinus.
   b. The ureter expands into the renal pelvis, which, in turn, is divided into major and minor calyces.
   c. Renal papillae project into the renal sinus.
   d. Kidney tissue is divided into a renal medulla and a renal cortex.
3. Functions of the kidneys
   a. Kidneys remove wastes from the blood and excrete them to the outside.
   b. They also help regulate the volume and composition of the body fluids.
4. Renal blood vessels
   a. Arterial blood flows through the renal artery, interlobar arteries, arciform arteries, interlobular arteries, and afferent arterioles.
   b. Venous blood returns through a series of vessels that correspond to those of the arterial pathways.
5. The nephrons
   a. Structure of the nephron
      (1) The nephron is the functional unit of the kidney.
      (2) It consists of a renal corpuscle and a renal tubule.
         (a) The corpuscle consists of a glomerulus and a glomerular capsule.
         (b) Portions of the renal tubule include the proximal convoluted tubule, the loop of Henle (ascending and descending limbs), the distal convoluted tubule, and the collecting duct.
         (c) The renal tubule is lined with a single layer of epithelial tissue.
      (3) The collecting duct empties into the minor calyx of the renal pelvis.
   b. Juxtaglomerular apparatus
      (1) The juxtaglomerular apparatus is located at the point of contact between the distal convoluted tubule and the afferent and efferent arterioles.
      (2) It consists of the macula densa and the juxtaglomerular cells.
   c. Cortical and juxtamedullary nephrons
      (1) Cortical nephrons are the most numerous and have corpuscles near the surface of the kidney.
      (2) Juxtamedullary nephrons have corpuscles near the medulla.
   d. Blood supply of a nephron
      (1) The glomerular capillary receives blood from the afferent arteriole and passes it to the efferent arteriole.
      (2) The efferent arteriole gives rise to the peritubular capillary system that surrounds the renal tubule.
      (3) Capillary loops, called vasa recta, dip down into the medulla.

Elimination of Urine (page 532)
1. The ureters
   a. Each ureter is a tubular organ that extends from the kidney to the urinary bladder.
   b. Its wall has mucous, muscular, and fibrous layers.
   c. Peristaltic waves in the ureter force urine to the bladder.
   d. An obstruction in the ureter stimulates strong peristaltic waves and a reflex that causes the kidney to decrease urine production.
2. The urinary bladder
   a. The urinary bladder is a distensible organ that stores urine and forces it into the urethra.
   b. The openings for the ureters and urethra are located at the three angles of the trigone in the floor of the urinary bladder.
   c. Muscle fibers in the wall form the detrusor muscle.
3. Micturition
   a. Micturition is the process by which urine is expelled.
   b. It involves contraction of the detrusor muscle and relaxation of the external urethral sphincter.
   c. Micturition reflex
      (1) Stretch receptors in the bladder wall are stimulated by distension.
      (2) The micturition reflex center in the sacral spinal cord sends parasympathetic motor impulses to the detrusor muscle.
      (3) Urination can be controlled by means of the voluntary external urethral sphincter and nerve centers in the brain that inhibit the micturition reflex.
      (4) When the decision to urinate is made, the external urethral sphincter is allowed to relax and nerve centers in the brain act to facilitate the micturition reflex.
4. The urethra
   a. The urethra conveys urine from the bladder to the outside.
   b. In females, it empties between the labia minora.
   c. In males, it conveys products of reproductive organs as well as urine.
      (1) There are three portions of the male urethra: prostatic, membranous, and penile.
      (2) The urethra empties at the tip of the penis.

Clinical Application of Knowledge

1. Why would you expect a person with a history of developing kidney stones to be placed on a low calcium diet?

2. How might a female's urinary bladder be affected during pregnancy, when the uterus increases in size?

3. The antibiotic penicillin is excreted by the kidneys into the urine. If a physician prescribed oral penicillin therapy for a patient with an infection of the urinary bladder, how would you describe for the patient the route by which the drug would reach the bladder?

4. Urinary bladder infections are more common in women than in men. How might this observation be related to the anatomy of the female and male urethras?

Review Activities

1. Name the organs of the urinary system and list their general functions.

2. Describe the external and internal structure of a kidney.

3. List the functions of the kidneys.

4. Name the vessels through which blood passes as it travels from the renal artery to the renal vein.

5. Distinguish between a renal corpuscle and a renal tubule.

6. Name the parts through which fluid passes as it travels from the glomerulus to the collecting duct.

7. Describe the location and structure of the juxtaglomerular apparatus.

8. Explain how the epithelial cells of the proximal convoluted tubule are adapted for reabsorption.

9. Distinguish between cortical and juxtamedullary nephrons.

10. Describe the structure and function of a ureter.

11. Explain how the muscular wall of the ureter aids in moving urine.

12. Discuss what happens if a ureter becomes obstructed.

13. Describe the structure and location of the urinary bladder.

14. Define *detrusor muscle*.

15. Describe the micturition reflex.

16. Explain how the micturition reflex can be voluntarily controlled.

17. Compare the male and female urethras.

UNIT 5
The Human Life Cycle

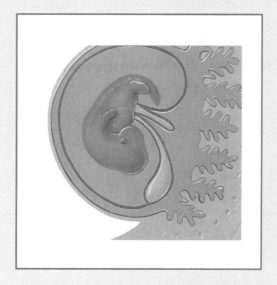

The chapters of unit 5 are concerned with the reproduction, growth, and development of the human organism. They describe how the organs of the male and female reproductive systems produce an embryo and how this offspring grows and develops.

CHAPTER 17

The Reproductive Systems

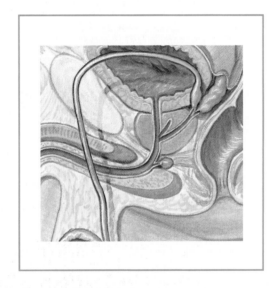

The male and female reproductive systems are specialized to produce offspring. These systems are unique in that their functions are not necessary for the survival of each individual. Instead, their functions are vital to the continuation of the human species.

Organs of the male and female reproductive systems are adapted to produce sex cells, sustain these cells, and transport them to a location where fertilization may occur. In addition, specialized organs of the female system are adapted to support the life of an offspring that may develop from a fertilized egg and transport this offspring to the outside of the female's body.

Chapter Objectives

After you have studied this chapter, you should be able to

1. State the general functions of the male reproductive system.

2. Name the parts of the male reproductive system and describe the general functions of each part.

3. Describe the structure of a testis and explain how sperm cells are formed.

4. Trace the path followed by sperm cells from their site of formation to the outside.

5. Describe the structure of the penis.

6. State the general functions of the female reproductive system.

7. Name the parts of the female reproductive system and describe the general functions of each part.

8. Describe the structure of an ovary, and explain how egg cells and follicles are formed.

9. Review the structure and function of the mammary glands.

10. Complete the review activities at the end of this chapter. Note that the items are worded in the form of specific learning objectives. You may want to refer to them before reading the chapter.

Aids to Understanding Words

crur-, lower part: *crura*—diverging parts at the base of the penis by which it is attached to the pelvic arch.

fimb-, a fringe: *fimb*riae—irregular extensions on the margin of the infundibulum of the uterine tube.

follic-, small bag: *follic*le—ovarian structure that contains an egg cell.

genesis, origin: spermato*genesis*—process by which sperm cells are formed.

gubern-, to guide: *gubern*aculum—fibromuscular cord that guides the descent of a testis.

labi-, lip: *labi*a minora—flattened, longitudinal folds that extend along the margins of the vestibule.

mons, mountain: *mons* pubis—rounded elevation of fatty tissue overlying the symphysis pubis in a female.

puber-, adult: *puber*ty—time when a person becomes able to function

Introduction

Organs of the male and female reproductive systems are concerned with the creation of offspring, and each organ is adapted to perform specialized tasks. For example, some produce sex cells, while others sustain these cells or transport them from one location to another. Still other parts produce and secrete hormones, which regulate the formation of sex cells and play roles in the development and maintenance of male and female sexual characteristics.

Organs of the Male Reproductive System

Organs of the male reproductive system are specialized to produce and maintain male sex cells (sperm cells), to transport these cells together with various supporting fluids to the female reproductive tract, and to produce and secrete male sex hormones.

The *primary sex organs* (gonads) of the male reproductive system are the two *testes* in which sperm cells (spermatozoa) and the male sex hormones are formed. The other structures of the male reproductive system are termed *accessory sex organs* (secondary sex organs), and they include two groups: the internal reproductive organs and the external reproductive organs (figure 17.1).

The Testes

The **testes** are ovoid structures about 5 centimeters in length and 3 centimeters in diameter. Each testis is suspended by a spermatic cord and is contained within the cavity of the saclike *scrotum.*

Descent of the Testes

In a male fetus, the testes originate from masses of tissue located behind the parietal peritoneum, near the developing kidneys. Usually about a month or two before birth, these organs descend to regions in the lower abdominal cavity and pass through the abdominal wall into the scrotum.

The descent of the testes is stimulated by the male sex hormone *testosterone,* which is secreted by the developing testes. The actual movement of these organs seems to be aided by a fibromuscular cord called the **gubernaculum.** This cord is attached to the developing testis and extends into the inguinal region of the abdominal cavity. It passes through the abdominal wall and is fastened to the skin on the outside. As the testis descends, apparently guided by the gubernaculum, it passes through the **inguinal canal** of the abdominal wall and enters the scrotum, where it remains anchored by the gubernaculum. Each testis carries with it a developing *vas deferens,* and various blood vessels

and nerves. These structures later form parts of the spermatic cord, which suspends the testis in the scrotum (figure 17.2).

If the testes fail to descend into the scrotum, they will not produce sperm cells. In fact, in this condition, called *cryptorchidism,* the cells that normally produce sperm cells degenerate, and the male is sterile. This failure to produce sperm cells is apparently caused by the unfavorable temperature of the abdominal cavity, which is a few degrees higher than the scrotal temperature.

During the descent of a testis, a pouch of peritoneum, called the *vaginal process,* moves through the inguinal canal and into the scrotum. In about one-quarter of males, this process remains more or less open. Such an opening provides a potential passageway through which a loop of intestine may be forced, by excessive abdominal pressure, producing a condition called an *indirect inguinal hernia.* If the protruding intestinal loop is so tightly constricted within the inguinal canal that its blood supply is interrupted, the condition is called a *strangulated hernia.* Without prompt treatment, the strangulated tissues may die.

---

1. What are the primary sex organs of the male reproductive system?
2. Describe the descent of the testes.
3. What happens if the testes fail to descend into the scrotum?

Structure of the Testes

A testis is enclosed by a tough, white, fibrous capsule called the *tunica albuginea.* Along its posterior border, the connective tissue thickens and extends into the organ, forming a mass called the *mediastinum testis.* From this structure, thin dividers of connective tissue, called septa, pass into the testis and subdivide it into about 250 *lobules.*

A lobule contains one to four highly coiled, convoluted **seminiferous tubules,** each of which is approximately 70 centimeters long when uncoiled. These tubules course posteriorly and unite to form a complex network of channels called the *rete testis.* The rete testis is located within the mediastinum testis and gives rise to several ducts that join a tube called the **epididymis.** The epididymis, in turn, is coiled on the outer surface of the testis.

The seminiferous tubules are lined with a specialized stratified epithelium that includes the *spermatogenic cells,* which give rise to the sperm cells. Other specialized cells, called *interstitial cells* (cells of Leydig), are located in the spaces between the seminiferous tubules. They produce and secrete male sex hormones (figures 17.3 and 17.4).

FIGURE 17.1

(a) Sagittal view of male reproductive organs; (b) posterior view.

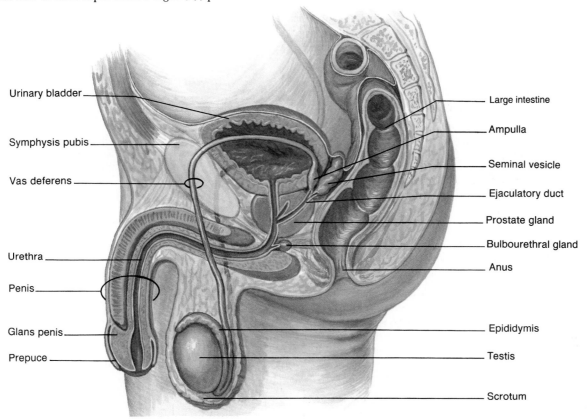

Urinary bladder

Symphysis pubis

Vas deferens

Urethra

Penis

Glans penis

Prepuce

Large intestine

Ampulla

Seminal vesicle

Ejaculatory duct

Prostate gland

Bulbourethral gland

Anus

Epididymis

Testis

Scrotum

(a)

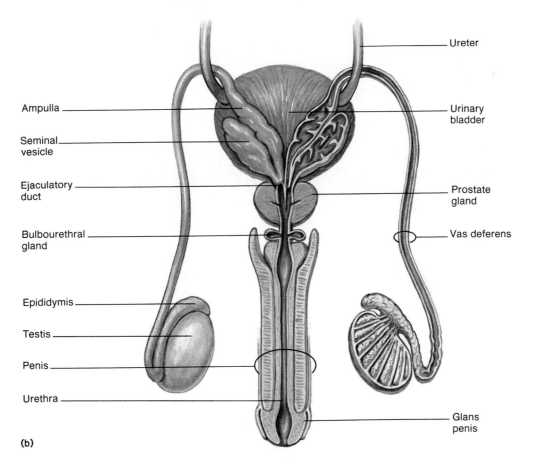

Ampulla

Seminal vesicle

Ejaculatory duct

Bulbourethral gland

Epididymis

Testis

Penis

Urethra

Ureter

Urinary bladder

Prostate gland

Vas deferens

Glans penis

(b)

FIGURE 17.2

During fetal development (*a-c*), each testis descends through an inguinal canal and enters the scrotum. What is the function of the gubernaculum when this occurs?

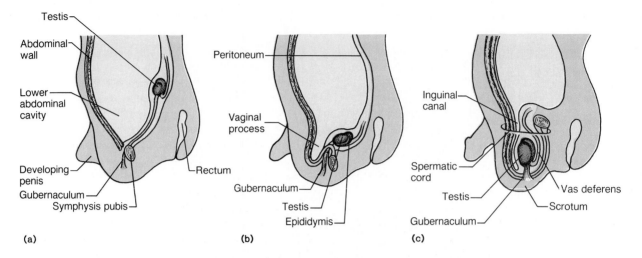

(a)   (b)   (c)

FIGURE 17.3

(*a*) Sagittal section of a testis; (*b*) enlarged cross section of a seminiferous tubule.

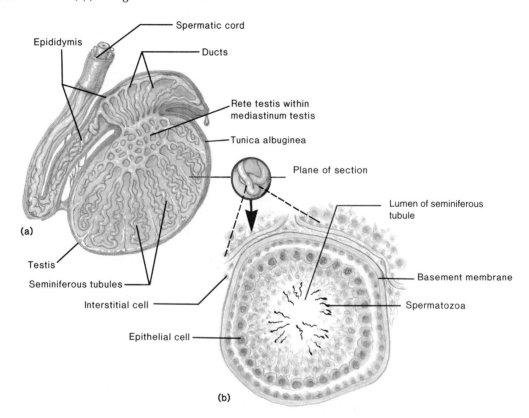

FIGURE 17.4
Scanning electron micrograph of cross sections of human
seminiferous tubules (about ×100).
R. G. Kessel and R. H. Kardon, *Tissues and Organs: A Text Atlas of
Scanning Electron Microscopy,* © 1979, W. H. Freeman & Co.

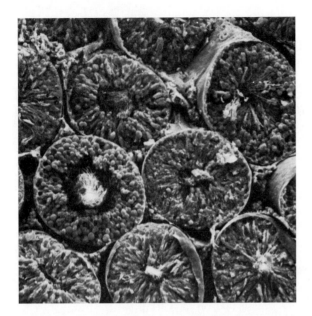

The epithelial cells of the sem-
iniferous tubules sometimes give rise to testicular cancer, one
of the more common types of cancer occurring in young men.
In most cases, the first sign of this condition is a painless enlargement of a testis, or the development of a scrotal mass
that seems to be attached to a testis. When testicular cancer
is suspected, a tissue sample is usually removed (biopsied) and
examined microscopically. If cancer cells are present, the affected testis is surgically removed (orchiectomy). Depending
upon the type of cancerous tissue present and the extent of
the disease, a patient may be treated with radiation or with
chemotherapy employing one or more drugs. As a result of
such treatment, the cure rate for testicular cancer is high.

1. Describe the structure of a testis.
2. Where are the sperm cells produced within the testes?
3. What cells produce male sex hormones?

Formation of Sperm Cells

The epithelium of the seminiferous tubules includes two
types of cells: supporting cells (Sertoli's cells) and spermatogenic cells. The *supporting cells* are tall, columnar cells
that extend the full thickness of the epithelium from its
base to the lumen of the seminiferous tubule. Numerous,
thin processes project from these cells, filling the spaces
between nearby spermatogenic cells. They support,
nourish, and regulate the *spermatogenic cells,* which give rise
to sperm cells (spermatozoa).

In a young male, all the spermatogenic cells are undifferentiated and are called *spermatogonia.* Each of these
cells contains 46 chromosomes in its nucleus, which is the
usual number for human cells. (See figure 17.5.)

During early adolescence, certain hormones stimulate
spermatogonia to become active. Some of them undergo
mitosis, giving rise to new spermatogonia and providing a
reserve supply of these undifferentiated cells. Others enlarge and become *primary spermatocytes,* which then divide
by a special type of cell division called **meiosis.**

Meiosis

The sex cells of each individual carry unique combinations
of inherited information. This uniqueness results from the
process of meiosis.

Meiosis occurs during spermatogenesis and oogenesis,
and as a result of it, the chromosome numbers of the resulting sex cells are reduced by one-half. This process involves two successive divisions: a first and second meiotic
division. In the *first meiotic division,* the homologous chromosomes of the parent cell are separated, and the chromosome number is reduced in the newly formed cells.
(Chromosomes that carry similar information are called
homologous.) During the *second meiotic division,* the chromatids separate and the result is the formation of sex cells
(figure 17.5).

Like mitosis, described in chapter 3, meiosis is a continuous process without marked interruptions between
steps. However, for convenience, the process can be divided into stages as follows:

1. **First meiotic prophase.** During this stage, the
   individual chromosomes appear as thin threads
   within the nucleus. The threads become shorter
   and thicker; the nucleoli disappear; the nuclear
   envelope fades away; and the spindle fibers become
   organized (figure 17.6).

   Throughout this stage, the individual
   chromosomes, which were replicated during the
   interphase prior to meiosis, are composed of two
   identical chromatids. Each pair of chromatids is
   held together by a central region called the
   centromere (kinetochore).

   As the prophase continues, homologous
   chromosomes approach each other, lie side by side,
   and become tightly intertwined. This process of
   pairing is called *synapsis.* During synapsis, the
   chromatids of the homologous chromosomes
   contact one another at various points. In fact, the
   chromatids may break in one or more places and
   exchange parts, forming chromatids with new
   combinations of information. This process of
   exchanging genetic information is called **crossing
   over.**

FIGURE 17.5

Spermatogenesis is a meiotic process that involves two successive divisions. (Note: only 4 of 46 chromosomes in the primary spermatocyte are shown.)

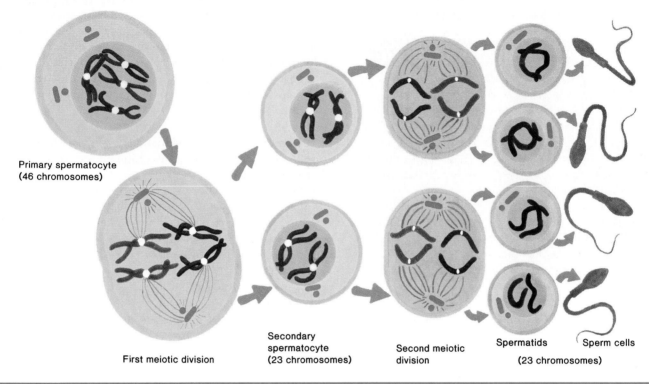

Primary spermatocyte
(46 chromosomes)

First meiotic division

Secondary
spermatocyte
(23 chromosomes)

Second meiotic
division

Spermatids   Sperm cells

(23 chromosomes)

FIGURE 17.6

Stages in the first meiotic division.

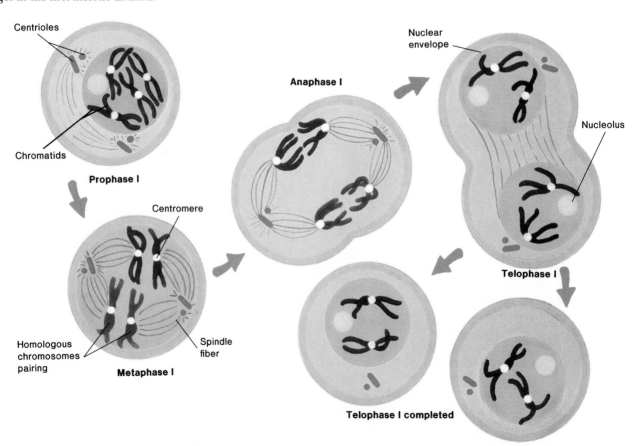

Centrioles

Chromatids

Prophase I

Centromere

Homologous
chromosomes
pairing

Metaphase I

Spindle
fiber

Anaphase I

Nuclear
envelope

Nucleolus

Telophase I

Telophase I completed

2. **First meiotic metaphase.** During the first metaphase, shown in figure 17.6, the synaptic pairs of chromosomes become lined up about midway between the poles of the developing spindle. Each pair (two chromosomes consisting of four chromatids) becomes associated with a spindle fiber.

3. **First meiotic anaphase.** During the first meiotic anaphase the centromeres do not separate (figure 17.6), and as a result, the homologous chromosomes become separated, and the chromatids of each chromosome move together to one end of the spindle. Thus, each new cell receives only one member of a homologous pair of chromosomes, and the chromosome number is thereby reduced by one-half.

4. **First meiotic telophase.** In meiotic telophase the parent cell divides into two cells (figure 17.6). Also during this phase, nuclear envelopes appear around the chromosome sets, the nucleoli reappear, and the spindle fibers disappear.

The first meiotic telophase is followed by a short *interphase* and the beginning of the second meiotic division. This division is essentially the same as mitosis, and it can also be divided into *prophase, metaphase, anaphase,* and *telophase.* These stages are shown in figure 17.7.

During the **second meiotic prophase,** the chromosomes reappear. They are still composed of pairs of chromatids, and the chromatids are held together by centromeres. Near the end of this phase, the chromosomes move into positions midway between the poles of the developing spindle.

In the **second meiotic metaphase,** the double-stranded chromosomes become attached to spindle fibers, and during the **second meiotic anaphase,** the centromeres separate so that the chromatids are free to move to opposite poles of the spindle. As a result of the **second meiotic telophase,** each cell divides into two new cells, and new nuclei are organized around the sets of single-stranded chromosomes.

---

1. Identify the two types of cells found in the epithelium of seminiferous tubules.
2. Describe the major events that occur during meiosis.

FIGURE 17.7

Stages in the second meiotic division.

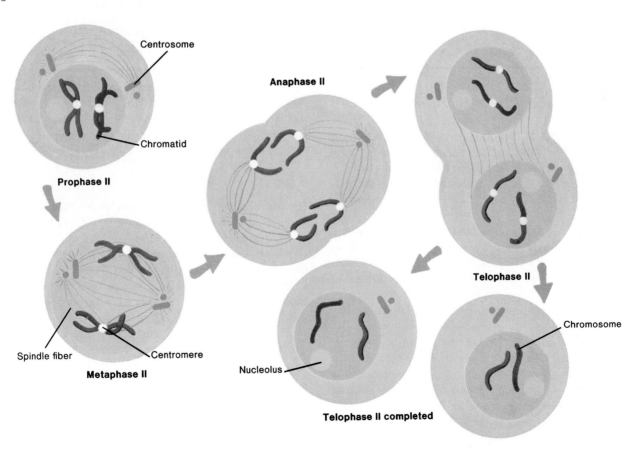

The Reproductive Systems   547

FIGURE 17.8

(a) Light micrograph of seminiferous tubules (×200); (b) spermatogonia give rise to primary spermatocytes by mitosis; the spermatocytes, in turn, give rise to sperm cells by meiosis.

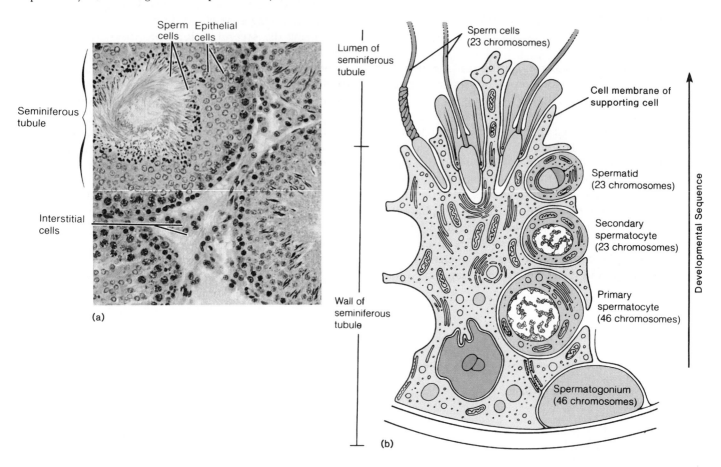

Spermatogenesis

In the course of meiosis, the primary spermatocytes each divide to form two *secondary spermatocytes.* Each of these cells, in turn, divides to form two *spermatids,* which mature into sperm cells. Consequently, for each primary spermatocyte that undergoes meiosis, four sperm cells with 23 chromosomes in each of their nuclei are formed. This process of producing sperm cells is called **spermatogenesis** (figure 17.8).

The spermatogonia are located near the base of the germinal epithelium. As spermatogenesis occurs, cells in more advanced stages are pushed along the sides of supporting cells toward the lumen of the seminiferous tubule.

Near the base of the epithelium, membranous processes from adjacent supporting cells are fused by specialized junctions (occluding junctions) into complexes that divide the tissue into two layers. The spermatogonia are located on one side of this barrier, and the cells in more advanced stages are on the other side. This membranous complex seems to help maintain a favorable environment for the development of sperm cells.

Spermatogenesis occurs continually throughout the reproductive life of a male. The resulting sperm cells collect in the lumen of each seminiferous tubule. They then pass through the rete testis to the epididymis, where they remain for a time to mature.

Structure of a Sperm Cell

A mature sperm cell is a tiny, tadpole-shaped structure about 60 micrometers long. It consists of a flattened head, a cylindrical body, and an elongated tail.

As spermatocytes mature into sperm cells, portions of the cytoplasm, containing various organelles, pinch off. Consequently, the *head* of a sperm cell, which is oval in outline, is composed primarily of a nucleus and contains the 23 chromosomes in highly compacted form. It has a small part at its anterior end called the *acrosome,* which contains lysosomal substances that aid the sperm cell in penetrating an egg cell at the time of fertilization (figure 17.9).

FIGURE 17.9

(a) The head of the sperm develops largely from the nucleus of the formative cell; (b) parts of a mature sperm cell.

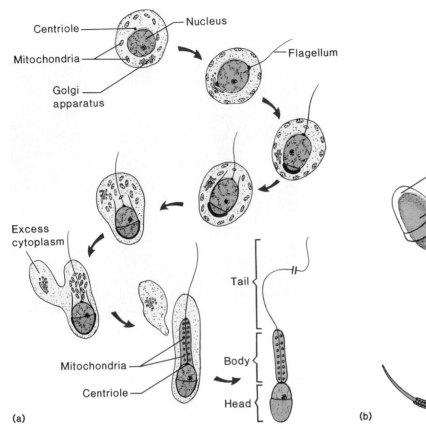

(a)

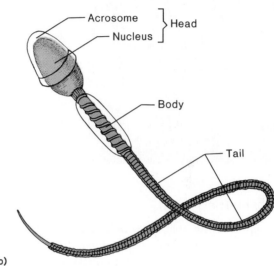

(b)

The *body* of the sperm cell contains a central, filamentous core and a large number of mitochondria arranged in a spiral. The *tail* consists of several longitudinal fibrils enclosed in an extension of the cell membrane. The scanning electron micrograph in figure 17.10 shows a few mature sperm cells.

1. Explain the function of supporting cells in the germinal epithelium.
2. Describe the process of spermatogenesis.
3. Describe the structure of a sperm cell.

Male Internal Accessory Organs

The *internal accessory organs* of the male reproductive system include the epididymides, vasa deferentia, ejaculatory ducts, and urethra, as well as the seminal vesicles, prostate gland, and bulbourethral glands.

FIGURE 17.10

Scanning electron micrograph of human sperm cells (×4,000).

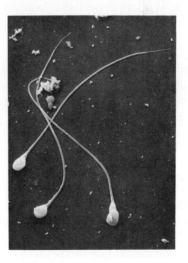

FIGURE 17.11
Cross section of a human epididymis (×50).

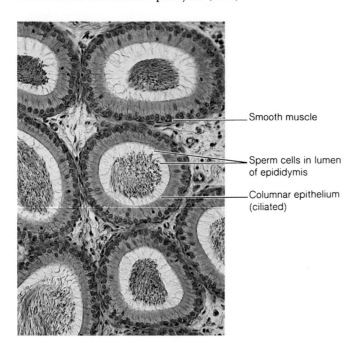

Smooth muscle

Sperm cells in lumen
of epididymis

Columnar epithelium
(ciliated)

FIGURE 17.12
Scanning electron micrograph of cross section of the vas
deferens (×70).
R. G. Kessel and R. H. Kardon, *Tissues and Organs: A Text Atlas of
Scanning Electron Microscopy,* © 1979, W. H. Freeman & Co.

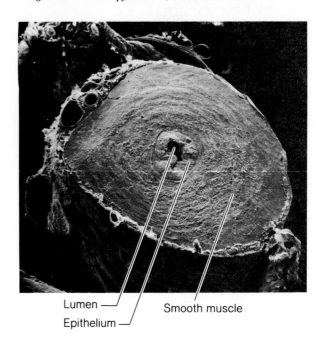

Lumen

Smooth muscle

Epithelium

The Epididymis

Each **epididymis** (pl. *epididymides*) is a tightly coiled,
threadlike tube about 6 meters long (figures 17.1 and
17.11). This tube is connected to ducts within a testis. It
emerges from the top of the testis, descends along its posterior surface, then courses upward to become the *vas
deferens.*

The inner lining of the epididymis is composed of
pseudostratified columnar cells that bear nonmotile cilia.
These cells are thought to secrete nutrients that help sustain the lives of the stored sperm cells and promote their
maturation.

When immature sperm cells reach the epididymis, they
are nonmobile. However, as they travel through the epididymis as a result of rhythmic peristaltic contractions they
undergo *maturation.* Following this aging process, the
sperm cells are able to move independently and fertilize
egg cells.

The Vas Deferens

Each **vas deferens** (pl. *vasa deferentia*), also called *ductus
deferens,* is a muscular tube about 45 centimeters long. It
begins at the lower end of the epididymis and passes
upward along the medial side of a testis to become part of
the spermatic cord. It passes through the inguinal canal,
enters the abdominal cavity outside of the parietal peritoneum, and courses over the pelvic brim. From there, it
extends backward and medially into the pelvic cavity, where
it ends behind the urinary bladder.

FIGURE 17.13
A light micrograph of the vas deferens (×250).

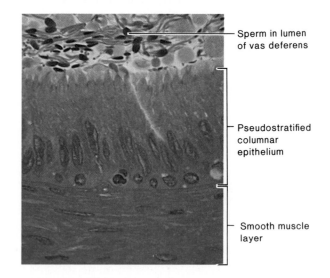

Sperm in lumen
of vas deferens

Pseudostratified
columnar
epithelium

Smooth muscle
layer

Near its termination, the vas deferens becomes dilated
into a portion called the *ampulla.* Just outside the prostate
gland, the tube becomes slender again and unites with the
duct of a seminal vesicle. The fusion of these two ducts
forms an **ejaculatory duct,** which passes through the substance of the prostate gland and empties into the urethra
through a slitlike opening (figures 17.1, 17.12, and 17.13).

FIGURE 17.14

A light micrograph of a seminal vesicle.

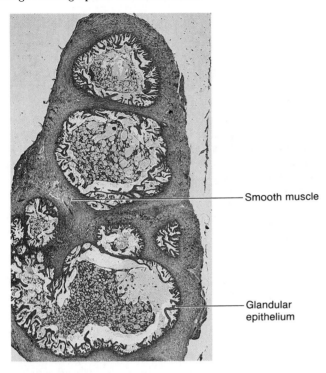

Smooth muscle

Glandular epithelium

The Seminal Vesicle

A **seminal vesicle** is a convoluted, saclike structure about 5 centimeters long that is attached to the vas deferens near the base of the urinary bladder.

The glandular tissue lining the inner wall of the seminal vesicle secretes a fluid that provides nutrients and enhances the movement of sperm. Contraction of the smooth muscle within the wall of the seminal vesicle empties its contents into the ejaculatory duct (figure 17.14).

---

1. Describe the structure of the epididymis.
2. Trace the path of the vas deferens.
3. What is the function of a seminal vesicle?

The Prostate Gland

The **prostate gland** is a chestnut-shaped structure about 4 centimeters across and 3 centimeters thick surrounding the beginning of the urethra, just below the urinary bladder. It is enclosed by connective tissue and is composed of many branched tubular glands. These glands are separated by septa of connective tissue and smooth muscle that extend inward from the capsule. Their ducts open into the urethra (figure 17.15).

The prostate gland secretes a thin, milky fluid that helps sustain sperm cells entering the female reproductive tract. The prostate gland releases its secretions into the urethra as a result of smooth muscle contractions in its capsular wall. This increases the volume of the semen.

FIGURE 17.15

A light micrograph of the prostate gland.

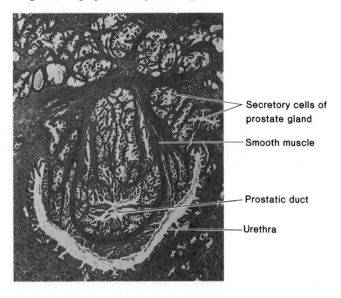

Secretory cells of prostate gland

Smooth muscle

Prostatic duct

Urethra

Although the prostate gland is relatively small in male children, it begins to grow in early adolescence and reaches its adult size a few years later. As a rule, its size remains unchanged between age 20 and 50 years. In older males the prostate gland usually enlarges. This tends to squeeze the urethra and interfere with urine excretion.

The treatment for an enlarged prostate gland is usually surgical. If the obstruction is slight, the procedure may be performed through the urethral canal and is called a *transurethral prostatic resection.*

The prostate gland is a common site of cancer in older males. Such cancers are usually stimulated to grow more rapidly by the male sex hormone testosterone, and are inhibited by the female sex hormone estrogen. Consequently, treatment for this type of cancer may involve removing the testes (the main source of testosterone), administering drugs that block the action of testosterone, or administering estrogen. Although such treatment usually does not stop the cancer, it may slow its development.

The Bulbourethral Glands

The **bulbourethral glands** (Cowper's glands) are two small structures about the size of peas that are located below the prostate gland lateral to the membranous urethra and enclosed by fibers of the external urethral sphincter muscle (figure 17.1).

These glands are composed of numerous tubes whose epithelial linings secrete a mucuslike fluid. This fluid is released in response to sexual stimulation and provides a small quantity of lubricating fluid to the end of the penis. Most of the lubricating fluid secreted in preparation for intercourse, however, is provided by female reproductive organs.

Male Infertility

In a male, infertility is lack of ability to induce fertilization of an egg cell. This condition can result from a variety of disorders. For example, if the testes fail to descend into the scrotum, the higher temperature of the abdominal cavity prevents the formation of sperm cells by causing cells in the seminiferous tubules to degenerate. Similarly, certain diseases, such as mumps, may cause inflammation of the testes (orchitis) and produce infertility by destroying cells of the seminiferous tubules.

Other males are infertile because of a deficiency of sperm cells in their seminal fluid. Normally, a milliliter of this fluid contains about 120 million sperm cells, and although the esti-

mates of the number of cells necessary for fertility vary, 20 million sperm cells per milliliter in a release of 3 to 5 milliliters is often cited as the minimum for fertility.

Even though a single sperm cell is needed to fertilize an egg cell, many sperm must be present at the time. This is because many sperm cells are necessary to remove the layers of cells that normally surround an egg cell, thus exposing the egg cell for fertilization.

Still other males seem to be infertile because of the quality of the sperm cells they produce. In such cases, the sperm cells may have poor motility, or they may have abnormal shapes related to the presence of defective chromosomes.

Semen

The fluid conveyed by the urethra to the outside during ejaculation is called **semen**. It consists of sperm cells from the testes and secretions of the seminal vesicles, prostate gland, and bulbourethral glands. It has a milky appearance, and contains a variety of nutrients and substances that enhance sperm cell survival and movement through the female reproductive tract.

The volume of seminal fluid released varies from 2 to 6 milliliters, and the average number of sperm cells present in the fluid is about 120 million per milliliter.

Sperm cells remain immobile while they are in the ducts of the testis and epididymis, but become activated as they are mixed with the secretions of accessory glands.

Although sperm cells are able to live for many weeks in the ducts of the male reproductive tract, they tend to survive for only a day or two after being expelled to the outside even when they are maintained at body temperature. However, they can be stored and kept viable for years, if frozen at a temperature below −100° C.

1. Where is the prostate gland located?
2. What is the function of the secretion of the prostate gland?
3. What is the function of the bulbourethral glands?
4. Which structures produce semen?

Male External Reproductive Organs

The male external reproductive organs are the scrotum, which encloses the testes, and the penis, through which the urethra passes.

The Scrotum

The **scrotum** is a pouch of skin and subcutaneous tissue that hangs from the lower abdominal region behind the penis.

Although its subcutaneous tissue lacks fat, the scrotal wall contains a layer of smooth muscle fibers that constitute the *dartos muscle*. When these muscle fibers are contracted, the scrotal skin becomes wrinkled and is held close to the testes; when the fibers are relaxed, the scrotum hangs more loosely.

The scrotum is subdivided into chambers by a medial septum, and each chamber is occupied by a testis. Each chamber also contains a serous membrane that provides a covering for the front and sides of the testis, and the epididymis. This covering helps ensure that the testis will move smoothly within the scrotum (figure 17.1).

The Penis

The **penis** is a cylindrical organ that conveys urine and semen through the urethra to the outside. It is also specialized to become enlarged and stiffened by a process called erection, so that it can be inserted into the female vagina during sexual intercourse.

FIGURE 17.16

(a) Interior structure of the penis; (b) cross section of the penis.

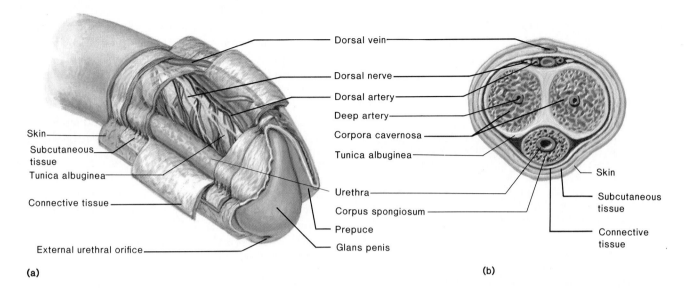

Dorsal vein

Dorsal nerve

Dorsal artery

Deep artery

Corpora cavernosa

Tunica albuginea

Skin

Subcutaneous tissue

Tunica albuginea

Connective tissue

Skin

Subcutaneous tissue

Connective tissue

Urethra

Corpus spongiosum

Prepuce

Glans penis

External urethral orifice

(a)

(b)

The *body*, or shaft, of the penis is composed of three columns of erectile tissue, which include a pair of dorsally located *corpora cavernosa* and a single *corpus spongiosum* below. The penis is enclosed by skin, a thin layer of subcutaneous tissue, and a layer of connective tissue. In addition, each column is surrounded by a tough capsule of white fibrous connective tissue called a *tunica albuginea* (figure 17.16).

The corpus spongiosum, through which the urethra extends, is enlarged at its distal end to form a sensitive, cone-shaped **glans penis.** This glans covers the ends of the corpora cavernosa and bears the urethral opening—the *external urethral orifice.* The skin of the glans is very thin and hairless. A loose fold of skin called the *prepuce* (foreskin) begins just behind the glans and extends forward to cover it as a sheath. The prepuce is sometimes removed by a surgical procedure called *circumcision.*

At the *root* of the penis, the columns of erectile tissue become separated. The corpora cavernosa diverge laterally in the perineum and are firmly attached to the medial surfaces of the pubic arch by connective tissue. These diverging parts form the *crura* of the penis. The single corpus spongiosum is enlarged between the crura as the *bulb* of the penis, which is attached to membranes of the perineum.

The functions of the male reproductive organs are summarized in chart 17.1.

1. Describe the structure of the penis.
2. What is circumcision?
3. How is the penis attached to the perineum?

Chart 17.1 Functions of the male reproductive organs

Organ	Function
Testes	
Seminiferous tubules	Production of sperm cells
Interstitial cells	Production and secretion of male sex hormones
Epididymis	Storage and maturation of sperm cells; conveys sperm cells to the vas deferens
Vas deferens	Conveys sperm cells to ejaculatory duct
Seminal vesicle	Secretes fluid containing nutrients
Prostate gland	Secretes fluid that enhances survival of sperm cells
Bulbourethral gland	Secretes fluid that lubricates end of penis
Scrotum	Encloses and protects testes
Penis	Conveys urine and semen to outside of body; inserted into vagina during sexual intercourse; glans penis is richly supplied with sensory nerve endings associated with feelings of pleasure during sexual stimulation

During puberty, testosterone, a male sex hormone, stimulates the enlargement of the testes and various accessory organs of the reproductive system, and causes the development of the male secondary sexual characteristics. (Note: The primary male sexual characteristic is the presence of testes.) These secondary sexual characteristics are associated with the adult male body, and they include the following:

1. Increased growth of body hair, particularly on the face, chest, axillary region, and pubic region, but sometimes accompanied by decreased growth of hair on the scalp.
2. Enlargement of the larynx and thickening of the vocal folds, accompanied by the development of a lower-pitched voice.
3. Thickening of the skin.
4. Increased muscular growth accompanied by the development of broader shoulders and a relatively narrow waist.
5. Thickening and strengthening of the bones.

Testosterone causes bones to thicken and strengthen by promoting the deposition of calcium in osseous tissues. Because of this, testosterone is sometimes used to treat elderly persons suffering from osteoporosis, a condition in which the bones thin due to excessive bone resorption.

Organs of the Female Reproductive System

The organs of the female reproductive system are specialized to produce and maintain female sex cells, or egg cells, transport these cells to the site of fertilization, provide a favorable environment for a developing offspring, move the offspring to the outside, and produce female sex hormones.

The *primary sex organs* (gonads) of this system are the ovaries, which produce the female sex cells and sex hormones. The other parts of the reproductive system comprise the internal and external *accessory organs*.

The Ovaries

The **ovaries** are solid, ovoid structures measuring about 3.5 centimeters in length, 2 centimeters in width, and 1 centimeter in thickness. They are located, one on each side, in a shallow depression (ovarian fossa) in the lateral wall of the pelvic cavity (figure 17.17).

Attachments of the Ovaries

Each ovary is attached to several ligaments that help hold it in position. The largest of these, formed by a fold of peritoneum, is called the *broad ligament*. It is also attached to the uterine tubes and the uterus.

FIGURE 17.17
Organs of the female reproductive system.

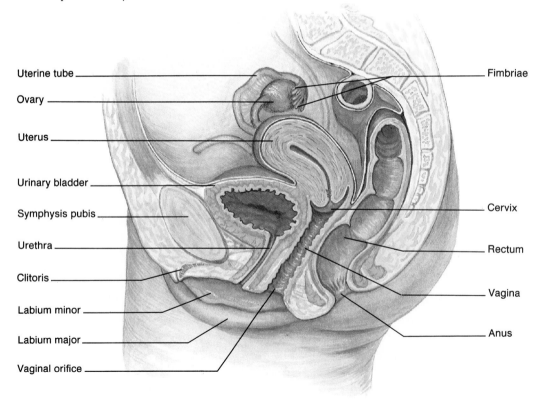

At its upper end, the ovary is held by a small fold of peritoneum, called the *suspensory ligament,* that contains the ovarian blood vessels and nerves. At its lower end, it is attached to the uterus by a rounded, cordlike thickening of the broad ligament called the *ovarian ligament* (figures 17.18 and 17.25).

Descent of the Ovaries

Like the testes in a male fetus, the ovaries in a female fetus originate from masses of tissue behind the parietal peritoneum, near the developing kidneys. During development, these structures descend to locations just below the pelvic brim, where they remain attached to the lateral pelvic wall.

Structure of the Ovaries

The tissues of an ovary can be subdivided into two rather indistinct regions: an inner *medulla* and an outer *cortex.*

The ovarian medulla is largely composed of loose connective tissue, and contains numerous blood vessels, lymphatic vessels, and nerve fibers. The ovarian cortex is composed of more compact tissue and has a somewhat granular appearance due to the presence of tiny masses of cells called *ovarian follicles.*

The free surface of the ovary is covered by a layer of cuboidal cells called the **germinal epithelium.** Just beneath this epithelium is a layer of dense connective tissue called *tunica albuginea.*

---

1. What are the primary sex organs of the female?
2. Describe the descent of the ovary.
3. Describe the structure of an ovary.

Primordial Follicles

During prenatal development (before birth), small groups of cells in the outer region of the ovarian cortex form several million **primordial follicles.** Each of these structures consists of a single, large cell, called a *primary oocyte,* which is closely surrounded by a layer of flattened epithelial cells called *follicular cells.*

Early in development, the primary oocytes begin to undergo meiosis, but the process soon halts and is not continued until puberty. Once the primordial follicles have appeared, no new ones are formed. Instead, the number of oocytes in the ovary steadily declines, as many of the oocytes degenerate. Of the several million oocytes formed originally, only a million or so remain at the time of birth, and perhaps 400,000 are present at puberty. Of these, probably fewer than 400–500 will be released from the ovary during the reproductive life of a person.

FIGURE 17.18

The ovaries are located on each side, against the lateral walls of the pelvic cavity.

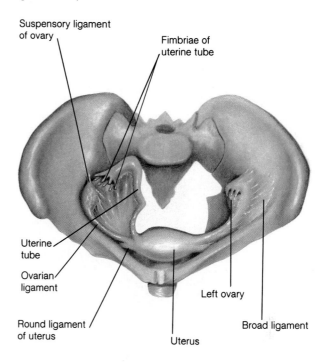

Oogenesis

Beginning at puberty, some of the primary oocytes are stimulated to continue meiosis, and as in the case of sperm cells, the resulting cells have one-half as many chromosomes (23) in their nuclei as the parent cells.

When a primary oocyte divides, the division of the cellular cytoplasm is very unequal. One of the resulting cells, called a *secondary oocyte,* is quite large, and the other, called the *first polar body,* is very small.

The large secondary oocyte represents a future *egg cell* (ovum) in that it can be fertilized by uniting with a sperm cell. If this happens, the oocyte divides unequally to produce a tiny *second polar body* and a relatively large fertilized egg cell, or **zygote.** (See figures 17.19 and 17.20.)

Thus, the result of this process, called **oogenesis,** is one secondary oocyte, or future egg cell, and one polar body. After being fertilized, the secondary oocyte divides to produce a second polar body and a zygote that can give rise to an embryo. The polar bodies have no further function, and they soon degenerate.

---

1. How does the timing of egg cell production differ from that of sperm cell production?
2. Describe the major events of oogenesis.

FIGURE 17.19

During the process of oogenesis, a single egg cell (secondary oocyte) results from the meiosis of a primary oocyte. If the egg cell is fertilized, it forms a second polar body and becomes a zygote.

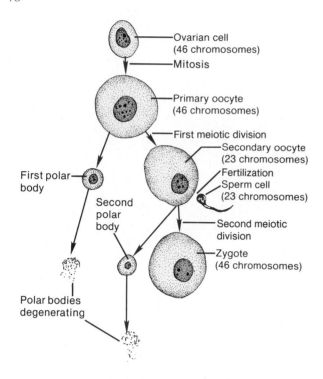

Ovarian cell (46 chromosomes)
Mitosis
Primary oocyte (46 chromosomes)
First meiotic division
Secondary oocyte (23 chromosomes)
Fertilization
Sperm cell (23 chromosomes)
Second meiotic division
Zygote (46 chromosomes)
First polar body
Second polar body
Polar bodies degenerating

FIGURE 17.20

(a) Light micrograph of a primary oocyte during metaphase I of meiosis. The arrow indicates the chromosomes. (b) A secondary oocyte and a polar body (arrow).

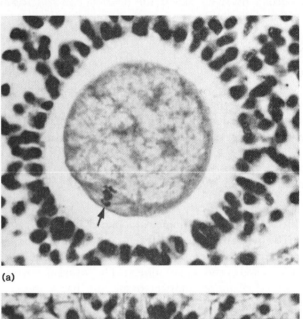

(a)

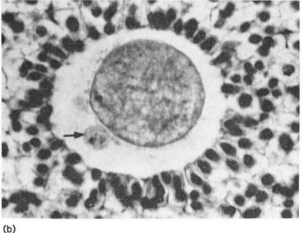

(b)

Maturation of a Follicle

At *puberty*, the ovaries begin to enlarge. At the same time, some of the primordial follicles begin to undergo maturation, becoming primary follicles (figure 17.21).

During this maturation process, the oocyte of a follicle enlarges, and the surrounding follicular cells proliferate by mitosis, giving rise to a stratified epithelium composed of cells called *granulosa cells*. A noncellular layer, called the *zona pellucida*, gradually separates the oocyte from the granulosa cells, and at this stage, the structure is called a *primary follicle*.

Meanwhile, the ovarian cells outside the follicle become organized into two cellular layers—an *inner vascular layer* (theca interna), composed largely of loose connective tissue and blood vessels, and an *outer fibrous layer* (theca externa), composed of tightly packed connective tissue cells.

The follicular cells continue to proliferate, and when there are six to twelve layers of cells, several irregular, fluid-filled spaces appear among them. These spaces soon join together to form a single cavity (antrum), and the oocyte is pressed to one side of the follicle. At this stage, the follicle has a diameter of about 0.2 millimeters and is called a *secondary follicle*. (See figure 17.22.)

Ten to fourteen days after the process begins, the follicle reaches maturity. The mature follicle (preovulatory, or Graafian, follicle) is about 10 millimeters or more across, and its fluid-filled cavity bulges outward on the surface of the ovary, like a blister. The oocyte within the mature follicle is a large, spherical cell, surrounded by a relatively thick, extracellular coat (zona pellucida), to which a mantle of follicular cells (corona radiata) is attached. Processes from these follicular cells extend through the zona pellicuda and may supply the oocyte with nutrients.

Although as many as twenty primary follicles may begin the process of maturation at any one time, usually only one follicle reaches full development, and the others degenerate.

FIGURE 17.21

(*a*) Light micrograph of the surface of a mammalian ovary (×50). (*b*) Structure of a secondary follicle.

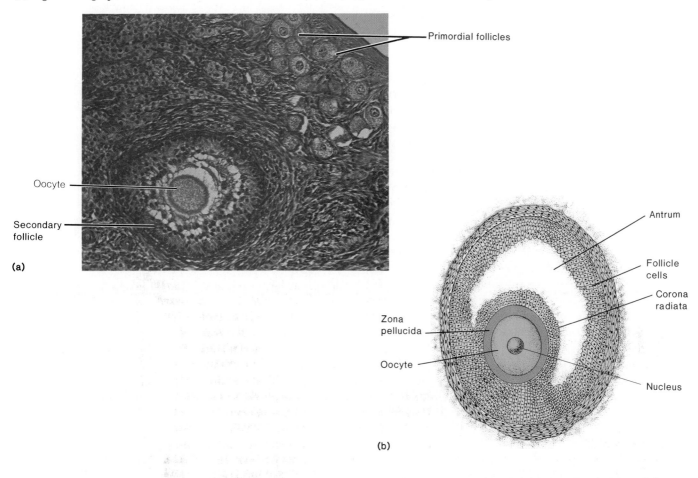

Primordial follicles

Oocyte

Secondary follicle

(a)

Antrum

Follicle cells

Corona radiata

Zona pellucida

Oocyte

Nucleus

(b)

FIGURE 17.22

(*a*) What features can you identify in this light micrograph of a maturing follicle (×250)? (*b*) Scanning electron micrograph of a maturing human follicle.

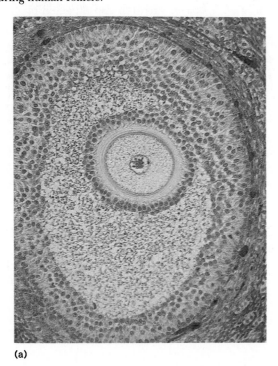

(a)

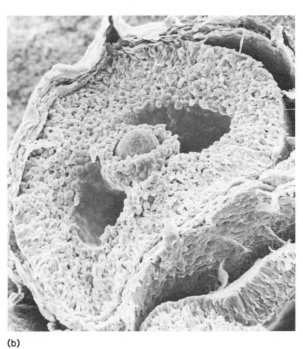

(b)

Ovulation

As a follicle matures, its primary oocyte undergoes oogenesis, giving rise to a secondary oocyte and a first polar body. These cells are released from the follicle by the process called ovulation.

Ovulation is stimulated by hormones from the anterior pituitary gland, which apparently cause the mature follicle to swell rapidly and its wall to weaken. Eventually, the wall ruptures and the follicular fluid, accompanied by the oocyte, oozes outward from the surface of the ovary. The expulsion of a mammalian oocyte is shown in figure 17.23.

Following ovulation, the remnants of the follicle in the ovary undergo rapid changes. The space occupied by the follicular fluid fills with blood, and the follicular cells enlarge greatly to form a new glandular structure within the ovary, called the **corpus luteum.**

After ovulation, the oocyte and one or two layers of follicular cells surrounding it are usually propelled to the opening of a nearby uterine tube. If the oocyte is not fertilized by union with a sperm cell within a relatively short time, it will degenerate. The maturation of a follicle and the release of an oocyte are illustrated in figure 17.24.

1. What causes a primary follicle to mature?
2. What changes occur in a follicle and its oocyte during maturation?
3. What happens to an egg cell following ovulation?

Female Internal Accessory Organs

The internal accessory organs of the female reproductive system include a pair of uterine tubes, a uterus, and a vagina.

The Uterine Tubes

The **uterine tubes** (fallopian tubes, or oviducts) are suspended by portions of the broad ligament, and have openings into the peritoneal cavity near the ovaries. Each tube, which is about 10 centimeters long and 0.7 centimeters in diameter, passes medially to the uterus, penetrates its wall, and opens into the uterine cavity.

Near each ovary, a uterine tube expands to form a funnel-shaped *infundibulum,* which partially encircles the ovary medially. On its margin, the infundibulum bears a number of irregular, branched extensions called *fimbriae* (figure 17.25). Although the infundibulum generally does not touch the ovary, one of the larger extensions (ovarian fimbria) is connected directly to it.

The wall of a uterine tube consists of an inner mucosal layer, a middle muscular layer, and an outer covering of peritoneum. The mucosal layer is drawn into numerous

FIGURE 17.23
Light micrograph of a follicle during ovulation.

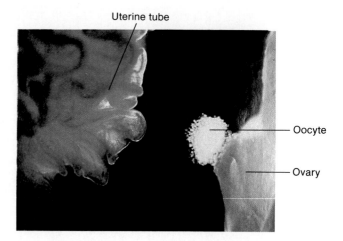

longitudinal folds and is lined with simple columnar epithelial cells, some of which are *ciliated* (figures 17.26 and 17.27). The epithelium secretes mucus, and the cilia beat toward the uterus. These actions help draw the egg cell and expelled follicular fluid into the infundibulum following ovulation.

Ciliary action also aids the transport of the egg cell down the uterine tube, and peristaltic contractions of the tube's muscular layer help force the egg along.

The Uterus

The **uterus** is a hollow, muscular organ, shaped somewhat like an inverted pear. It receives the embryo that results from a fertilized egg cell, and sustains its life during development.

The *broad ligament,* which is also attached to the ovaries and uterine tubes, extends from the lateral walls of the uterus to the pelvic walls and floor, creating a septum across the pelvic cavity (figure 17.25). A fibrous sheet along the sides of the lower uterus and vagina form the *cardinal ligament,* which provides a deep continuation of this septum. Also, a flattened band of tissue within the broad ligament, called the *round ligament,* connects the upper end of the uterus to the pelvic wall (figures 17.18 and 17.25).

Although the size of the uterus changes greatly during pregnancy, in its nonpregnant, adult state it is about 7 centimeters long, 5 centimeters wide (at its broadest point), and 2.5 centimeters in diameter. The uterus is located medially within the anterior portion of the pelvic cavity, above the vagina, and is usually bent forward over the urinary bladder.

The upper two-thirds, or *body* of the uterus has a dome-shaped top and is joined by the uterine tubes that enter its wall at its broadest part.

FIGURE 17.24

(*a*) As a follicle matures, the egg cell enlarges and becomes surrounded by a mantle of follicular cells and fluid. Eventually, the mature follicle ruptures and the egg cell is released; (*b*) light micrograph of a mammalian (monkey) ovary (×42).

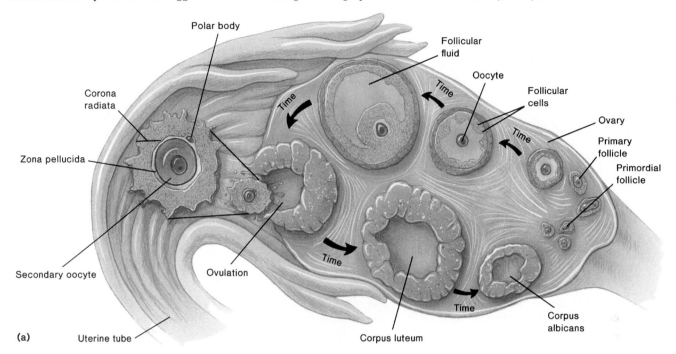

(a)

Polar body

Follicular fluid

Oocyte

Follicular cells

Corona radiata

Ovary

Primary follicle

Primordial follicle

Zona pellucida

Time

Time

Time

Secondary oocyte

Ovulation

Time

Corpus albicans

Uterine tube

Corpus luteum

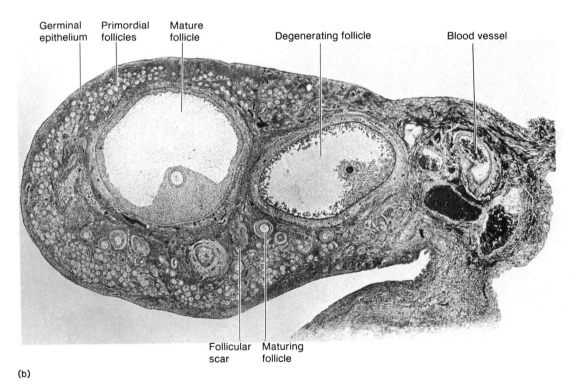

(b)

Germinal epithelium

Primordial follicles

Mature follicle

Degenerating follicle

Blood vessel

Follicular scar

Maturing follicle

FIGURE 17.25

The funnel-shaped infundibulum of the uterine tube partially encircles the ovary. What factors aid the movement of an egg cell into the infundibulum following ovulation?

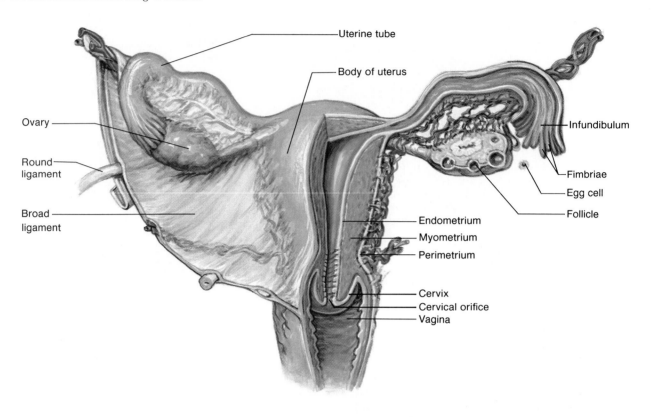

Uterine tube

Body of uterus

Ovary

Round ligament

Broad ligament

Infundibulum

Fimbriae

Egg cell

Follicle

Endometrium

Myometrium

Perimetrium

Cervix

Cervical orifice

Vagina

FIGURE 17.26

Scanning electron micrograph of the ciliated cells that line the uterine tube (×650).

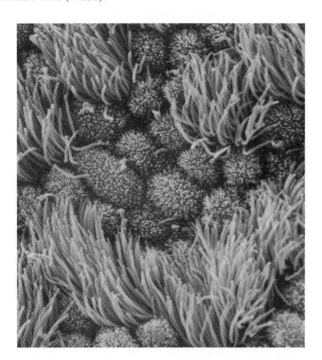

FIGURE 17.27

Light micrograph of the uterine tube.

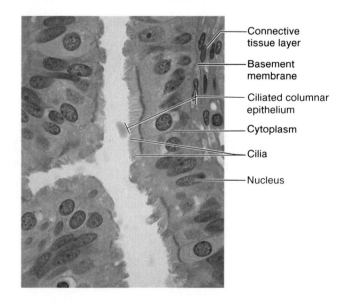

Connective tissue layer

Basement membrane

Ciliated columnar epithelium

Cytoplasm

Cilia

Nucleus

The lower one-third of the uterus is called the **cervix.** This tubular part extends downward into the upper portion of the vagina. The cervix surrounds the opening called the *cervical orifice* (ostium uteri), through which the uterus is connected with the vagina.

Cancer developing within the tissues of the uterine cervix can usually be detected by means of a relatively simple and painless procedure called the *Pap* (Papanicolaou) *smear test*. This technique involves scraping a tiny sample of cervical tissue, smearing the sample on a glass slide, staining it, and examining it for the presence of abnormal cells.

Because this test can reveal certain types of cervical cancers in the early stages of development, when they may be cured completely, the American Cancer Society recommends that women between 20 and 65 years of age have a Pap test every three years.

The uterine wall is relatively thick and is composed of three layers: the endometrium, the myometrium, and the perimetrium. (See figure 17.28.) The **endometrium** is the inner mucosal layer lining the uterine cavity. This lining is covered with columnar epithelium and contains numerous tubular glands. The **myometrium,** a very thick, muscular layer, consists largely of bundles of smooth muscle fibers arranged in longitudinal, circular, and spiral patterns, interlaced with connective tissues. During the monthly female reproductive cycle and during pregnancy, the endometrium and myometrium undergo extensive changes (figure 17.29). The **perimetrium** consists of an outer serosal layer that covers the body of the uterus and part of the cervix.

FIGURE 17.28

Light micrograph of the uterine wall (×10).

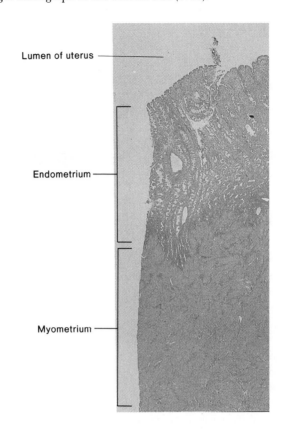

FIGURE 17.29

During the female reproductive cycle, the endometrium thickens and becomes more vascular. At the end of the cycle, the thickened lining disintegrates and sloughs away.

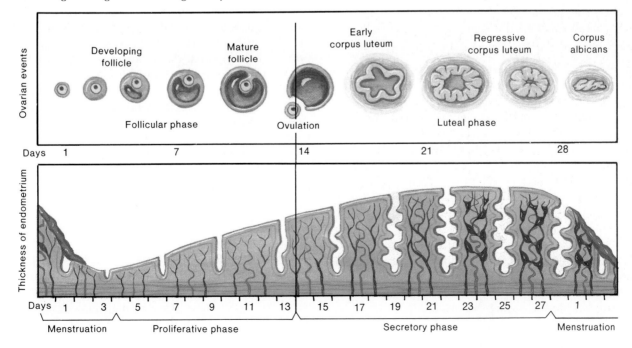

FIGURE 17.30

The vagina is lined with stratified squamous epithelium (×50).

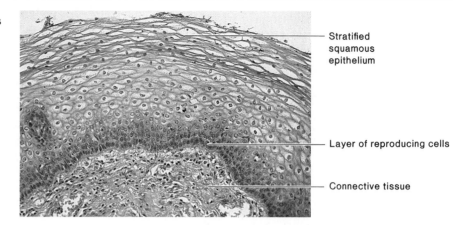

Stratified squamous epithelium

Layer of reproducing cells

Connective tissue

The Vagina

The **vagina** is a fibromuscular tube, about 9 centimeters in length, extending from the uterus to the outside. It conveys uterine secretions, receives the erect penis during sexual intercourse, and transports the offspring during the birth process.

The vagina extends upward and back into the pelvic cavity. It is posterior to the urinary bladder and urethra, anterior to the rectum, and is attached to these parts by connective tissues. The upper one-fourth of the vagina is separated from the rectum by a pouch (rectouterine pouch). The tubular vagina also surrounds the end of the cervix, and the recesses that occur between the vaginal wall and the cervix are termed *fornices* (sing. fornix) (figure 17.25).

The fornices are clinically important since they are relatively thin-walled and allow the internal abdominal organs to be palpated during a physical examination. Also, the posterior fornix, which is somewhat longer than the others, provides a surgical access to the peritoneal cavity through the vagina.

The *vaginal orifice* is partially closed by a thin membrane of connective tissue and stratified squamous epithelium called the **hymen.** A central opening of varying size allows uterine and vaginal secretions to pass to the outside.

The vaginal wall consists of three layers. The inner *mucosal layer* consists of stratified squamous epithelium and is drawn into numerous longitudinal and transverse ridges (vaginal rugae). This layer is devoid of mucous glands; therefore, the mucus found in the lumen of the vagina comes from glands of the cervix (figure 17.30).

The middle *muscular layer* consists mainly of smooth muscle fibers arranged in longitudinal and circular patterns. At the lower end of the vagina is a thin band of striated muscle. This band helps close the vaginal opening; however, a voluntary muscle (bulbospongiosus) is primarily responsible for closing this orifice.

The outer *fibrous layer* consists of dense fibrous connective tissue interlaced with elastic fibers, and it attaches the vagina to surrounding organs.

1. How is an egg cell moved along a uterine tube?
2. Describe the structure of the uterus.
3. What is the function of the uterus?
4. Describe the structure of the vagina.

Female External Reproductive Organs

The external accessory organs of the female reproductive system include the labia majora, the labia minora, the clitoris, and the vestibular glands. As a group, these structures, which surround the openings of the urethra and vagina, compose the **vulva.** They are shown in figure 17.31.

The Labia Majora

The **labia majora** (sing. labium majus) enclose and protect the other external reproductive organs. They correspond to the scrotum of the male and are composed primarily of rounded folds of adipose tissue and a thin layer of smooth muscle covered by skin. On the outside this skin includes numerous hairs, sweat glands, and sebaceous glands, while on the inside it is thinner and hairless.

The labia majora lie closely together and are separated longitudinally by a cleft (pudendal cleft) that includes the urethral and vaginal openings. At their anterior ends, the labia merge to form a medial, rounded elevation of fatty tissue called the *mons pubis,* which overlies the symphysis pubis. At their posterior ends, the labia are somewhat tapered, and they merge into the perineum near the anus.

The Labia Minora

The **labia minora** (sing. labium minus) are flattened longitudinal folds located within the cleft between the labia majora. These folds extend along either side of the vestibule. They are composed of connective tissue that is richly supplied with blood vessels, causing a pinkish appearance. This tissue is covered with stratified squamous epithelium.

FIGURE 17.31

Female external reproductive organs and vestibular bulbs.

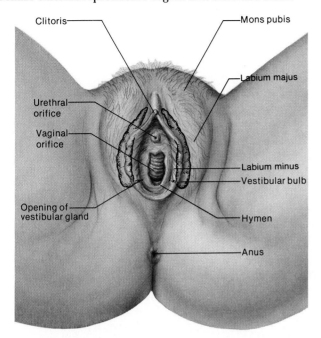

Clitoris

Mons pubis

Urethral orifice

Labium majus

Vaginal orifice

Labium minus

Vestibular bulb

Opening of vestibular gland

Hymen

Anus

Chart 17.2 Functions of the female reproductive organs

Organ	Function
Ovary	Production of egg cells and female sex hormones
Uterine tube	Conveys egg cell toward uterus; site of fertilization; conveys developing embryo to uterus
Uterus	Protects and sustains life of embryo during pregnancy
Vagina	Conveys uterine secretions to outside of body; receives erect penis during sexual intercourse; transports fetus during birth process
Labia majora	Enclose and protect other external reproductive organs
Labia minora	Form margins of vestibule; protect openings of vagina and urethra
Clitoris	Glans is richly supplied with sensory nerve endings
Vestibule	Space between labia minora that includes vaginal and urethral openings
Vestibular glands	Secrete fluid that moistens and lubricates vestibule

Posteriorly, the labia minora merge with the labia majora, while anteriorly they converge to form a hoodlike covering around the clitoris.

The Clitoris

The **clitoris** is a small projection at the anterior end of the vulva between the labia minora. Although most of it is embedded in surrounding tissues, it is usually about 2 centimeters long and 0.5 centimeters in diameter. The clitoris corresponds to the male penis and has a similar structure. More specifically, it is composed of two columns of erectile tissue called *corpora cavernosa*. These columns are separated by a septum and are surrounded by a covering of dense fibrous connective tissue.

At the root of the clitoris, the corpora cavernosa diverge to form *crura*, which, in turn, are attached to the sides of the pubic arch. At its anterior end, a small mass of erectile tissue forms a **glans**, which is richly supplied with sensory nerve fibers.

The Vestibule

The **vestibule** of the vulva is the space enclosed by the labia minora. The vagina opens into the posterior portion of the vestibule, and the urethra opens in the midline, just anterior to the vagina and about 2.5 centimeters posterior to the glans of the clitoris.

A pair of **vestibular glands** (Bartholin's glands), which correspond to the male bulbourethral glands, lie one on either side of the vaginal opening. Their ducts open into the vestibule near the lateral margins of the vaginal orifice.

Beneath the mucosa of the vestibule on either side is a mass of vascular erectile tissue. These structures, shown in figure 17.31, are called *vestibular bulbs*. They are separated from each other by the vagina and the urethra, and they extend forward from the level of the vaginal opening to the clitoris.

The various functions of the female reproductive organs are summarized in chart 17.2.

1. What is the male counterpart of the labia majora? Of the clitoris?
2. What structures are located within the vestibule?

The primary source of estrogen (in a nonpregnant female) is the ovaries. At puberty, these organs secrete increasing amounts of the hormone. The estrogen stimulates enlargement of various accessory reproductive organs, including the vagina, uterus, uterine tubes, ovaries, and the external structures. Estrogen also is responsible for the development and maintenance of female secondary sexual characteristics, which include:

1. Development of the breasts and the ductile system of the mammary glands within the breasts.
2. Increased deposition of adipose tissue in the subcutaneous layer generally, and particularly in the breasts, thighs, and buttocks.
3. Increased vascularization of the skin.

Certain other changes that occur in females at puberty seem to be related to *androgen* (testosterone) concentrations. For example, increased growth of hair in the pubic and axillary regions seems to be due to the presence of androgen secreted by the adrenal cortices. Conversely, the development of the female skeletal configuration, which includes narrow shoulders and broad hips, seems to be related to a lack of androgen.

The Reproductive Systems 563

Female Infertility

It is estimated that about 60% of infertile marriages are the result of female disorders. Some of the more common of these disorders involves decreased secretion of certain hormones followed by failure of the female to ovulate (anovulation).

Another cause of female infertility is *endometriosis,* in which tissue resembling the inner lining of the uterus (endometrium) is present abnormally in the abdominal cavity. Some investigators believe that small pieces of the endometrium may move up through the uterine tubes and become implanted in the abdominal cavity. In any case, once this tissue is present in the cavity, it undergoes changes similar to those of the uterine lining during the reproductive cycle. However, when the tissue begins to break down at the end of the cycle, it cannot be expelled to the outside. Instead, its products remain in the abdominal cavity where they may irritate its lining (peritoneum) and cause considerable abdominal pain. These products also tend to stimulate the formation of fibrous tissue (fibrosis), which, in turn, may encase the ovary, preventing ovulation mechanically or may obstruct the uterine tubes.

Still other women become infertile as a result of infections, such as gonorrhea, which may cause the uterine tubes to become inflamed and obstructed, or may stimulate the production of viscous mucus that can plug the cervix and prevent the entrance of sperm cells.

The Mammary Glands

The **mammary glands** are accessory organs of the female reproductive system that are specialized to secrete milk following pregnancy.

Location of the Glands

The mammary glands are located in the subcutaneous tissue of the anterior thorax within hemispherical elevations called *breasts.* The breasts overlie the *pectoralis major* muscles and extend from the second to the sixth ribs and from the sternum to the axillae.

A *nipple* is located near the tip of each breast at about the level of the fourth intercostal space, and it is surrounded by a circular area of pigmented skin called the *areola* (figure 17.32).

Structure of the Glands

A mammary gland is composed of fifteen to twenty irregularly shaped lobes. Each lobe contains glands (alveolar glands), and a duct (lactiferous duct) that leads to the nipple and opens to the outside. The lobes are separated by dense connective and adipose tissues. These tissues also support the glands and attach them to the fascia of the underlying pectoral muscles. Other connective tissue, which forms dense strands called *suspensory ligaments,* extends inward from the dermis of the breast to the fascia, helping to support the weight of the breast.

Breast cancer, one of the more common types of cancer in women, usually begins as a small, painless lump that may be a tumor. Since an early diagnosis of such a tumor is of prime importance in successful treatment, the American Cancer Society recommends that women beyond the age of 20 examine their breasts each month, paying particular attention to the upper, outer portions. The examination should be made just after menstruation when the breasts are usually soft, and any lump that is discovered should be checked immediately by a physician.

It is also recommended that after age 35 women have their breasts examined at regular intervals with *mammography*—a breast cancer detection technique that makes use of relatively low-dosage X ray (figure 17.33).

More specifically, the American Cancer Society recommends that women between the ages of 35 and 40 have a baseline mammogram; those between the ages of 40 and 49 have a mammogram every one to two years; and those over 50 years of age have a mammogram yearly. It has been determined that a breast cancer can be detected on a *mammogram* (an X-ray film of the breast) perhaps two years before the growing tumor could be felt.

Whenever a questionable lump is detected by physical examination or mammography, a biopsy should be performed so that the tissue can be observed microscopically. As a rule, such a microscopic examination is necessary before breast cancer can be diagnosed with certainty.

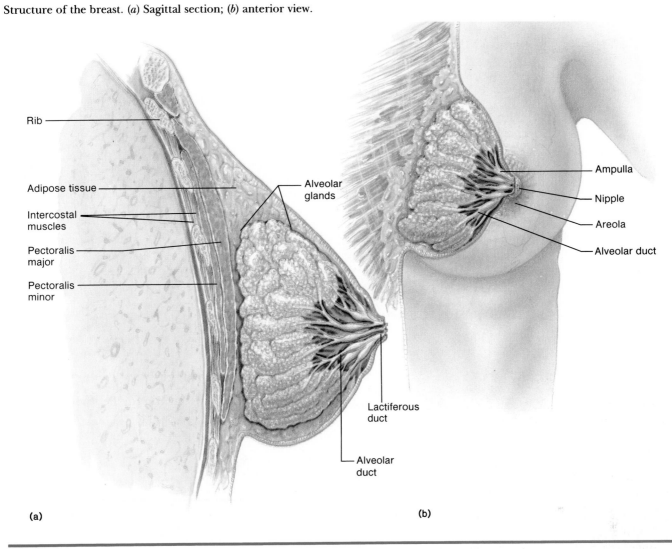

(a)

(b)

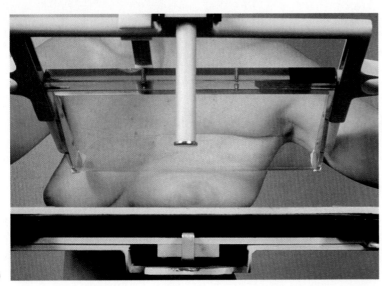

(a)

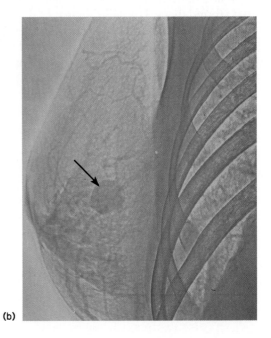

(b)

FIGURE 17.34

(a) Light micrograph of an inactive (nonpregnant) mammary gland; (b) light micrograph of an active (lactating) mammary gland.

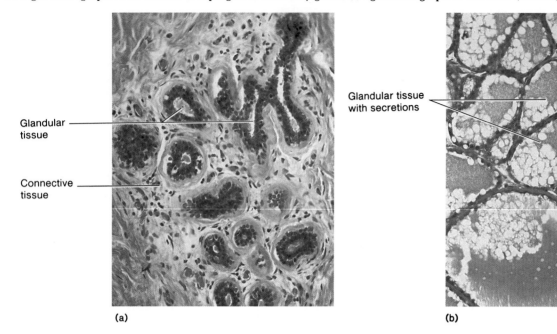

Glandular tissue

Connective tissue

Glandular tissue with secretions

(a)

(b)

Development of the Breasts

The mammary glands of male and female children are similar. As children reach *puberty,* the male glands fail to develop, while ovarian hormones stimulate the female glands to develop. As a result, the alveolar glands and ducts enlarge, and fat is deposited so that the breasts become surrounded by adipose tissue, except for the region of the areola.

During pregnancy, further development of the mammary glands is stimulated. The ductile systems grow and become branched, and have large quantities of fat deposited around them. The development of the alveolar glands at the ends of the ducts also occurs. As a result, the breasts may double in size. At the same time, fatty tissue is largely replaced by glandular tissue, and the mammary glands become capable of secreting milk. These changes are promoted by the presence of certain female sex hormones (figure 17.34).

Production and Secretion of Milk

Following childbirth, the mammary glands are stimulated to secrete large quantities of milk. This does not occur until 2 or 3 days following birth, and in the meantime, the glands secrete a few milliliters of a fluid called *colostrum* each day. Although colostrum contains some of the nutrients found in milk, it lacks fat.

The milk produced does not flow readily through the ductile system of the mammary gland, but must be actively

FIGURE 17.35

Milk is ejected from an alveolar gland by the action of myoepithelial cells.

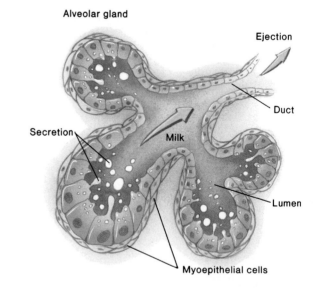

Alveolar gland

Ejection

Duct

Secretion

Milk

Lumen

Myoepithelial cells

ejected by contraction of specialized *myoepithelial cells* surrounding the alveolar glands. The contraction of these cells and the consequent ejection of milk through the ducts result from a reflex action (figure 17.35).

This reflex is elicited when the breast is suckled, or the nipple or areola is otherwise mechanically stimulated. The myoepithelial cells then contract. Consequently, milk is ejected into a suckling infant's mouth in about 30 seconds.

Sensory impulses triggered by mechanical stimulation of the nipples also signal the continued secretion of a hormone that stimulates milk production. If milk is not removed regularly, however, within about one week the mammary glands lose their capacity to produce milk.

1. Describe the structure of a mammary gland.
2. How does pregnancy affect the mammary glands?
3. How is milk stimulated to flow into the ductile system of a mammary gland?

Clinical Terms Related to the Reproductive Systems

conization (ko″nĭ-za′shun)   the surgical removal of a cone of tissue from the cervix for examination.

curettage (ku″rĕ-tahzh′)   surgical procedure in which the cervix is dilated and the endometrium of the uterus is scraped (commonly called a D and C).

endometriosis (en″do-mĕ″tre-o′sis)   a condition in which tissue resembling the endometrium of the uterine lining is present and growing in the abdominal cavity.

endometritis (en″do-mĕ-tri′tis)   inflammation of the uterine lining.

epididymitis (ep″ĭ-did″ĭ-mi′tis)   inflammation of the epididymis.

hysterectomy (his″tĕ-rek′to-me)   the surgical removal of the uterus.

mastitis (mas″ti′tis)   inflammation of a mammary gland.

oophorectomy (o″of-o-rek′to-me)   surgical removal of an ovary.

oophoritis (o″of-o-ri′tis)   inflammation of an ovary.

orchiectomy (or″ke-ĕk′to-me)   surgical removal of a testis.

orchitis (or-ki′tis)   inflammation of a testis.

prostatectomy (pros″tah-tek′to-me)   surgical removal of a portion or all of the prostate gland.

prostatitis (pros″tah-ti′tis)   inflammation of the prostate gland.

salpingectomy (sal″pin-jek′to-me)   surgical removal of a uterine tube.

vaginitis (vaj″ĭ-ni′tis)   inflammation of the vaginal lining.

Chapter Summary

Introduction (page 542)
Reproductive organs are specialized to produce and maintain sex cells, transport these cells, and produce hormones.

Organs of the Male Reproductive System (page 542)
Primary sex organs are the testes, which produce sperm cells and male sex hormones. Accessory organs include internal and external reproductive organs.

The Testes (page 542)
1. Descent of the testes
   a. Testes originate behind the parietal peritoneum near the level of the developing kidneys.
   b. The gubernaculum guides the descent of testes into the lower abdominal cavity and through the inguinal canal.
   c. Undescended testes fail to produce sperm cells because of the relatively high abdominal temperature.
2. Structure of the testes
   a. The testes are composed of lobules separated by connective tissue and filled with seminiferous tubules.
   b. Seminiferous tubules unite to form the rete testis that joins the epididymis.
   c. Seminiferous tubules are lined with germinal epithelium that produces sperm cells.
   d. Interstitial cells that produce male sex hormones occur between the seminiferous tubules.
3. Formation of sperm cells
   a. Meiosis includes two successive divisions.
      (1) In the first meiotic division, homologous chromosomes of the parent cell are separated and the chromosome number is reduced by one-half.
      (2) In the second meiotic division, the chromosomes act as they do in mitosis.
   b. Epithelium consists of supporting cells and spermatogenic cells.
   c. Sperm cells are produced from spermatogonia by the process of spermatogenesis.
      (1) The number of chromosomes in sperm cells is reduced by one-half (46 to 23) by meiosis.
      (2) Spermatogenesis produces four sperm cells from each primary spermatocyte.
   d. Membranous processes of adjacent supporting cells form a barrier within the epithelium that separates early and advanced stages of spermatogenesis.
4. Structure of a sperm cell
   a. A sperm head contains a nucleus with 23 chromosomes.
   b. A sperm body contains many mitochondria.
   c. A sperm tail propels the cell.

Male Internal Accessory Organs (page 549)
1. The epididymis
   a. The epididymis is a tightly coiled tube on the outside of the testis that leads into the vas deferens.
   b. It stores immature sperm cells as they mature.
2. The vas deferens
   a. The vas deferens is a muscular tube that forms part of the spermatic cord.
   b. It passes through the inguinal canal, enters the abdominal cavity, courses medially into the pelvic cavity, and ends behind the urinary bladder.
   c. It fuses with the duct from the seminal vesicle to form the ejaculatory duct.
3. The seminal vesicle
   a. The seminal vesicle is a saclike structure attached to the vas deferens.
   b. This secretion is emptied into the ejaculatory duct.
4. The prostate gland
   a. This gland surrounds the urethra just below the urinary bladder.

b. It secretes thin, milky fluid.

c. It may enlarge in older males and interfere with urination.

5. The bulbourethral glands

    a. These are two small structures beneath the prostate gland.

    b. They secrete fluid that serves as a lubricant for the penis in preparation for sexual intercourse.

6. Semen

    a. Semen is composed of sperm cells and secretions of seminal vesicles, the prostate gland, and bulbourethral glands.

    b. This fluid contains nutrients and activates sperm cells.

Male External Reproductive Organs (page 552)

1. The scrotum

    a. The scrotum is a pouch of skin and subcutaneous tissue that encloses the testes.

    b. The dartos muscle in the scrotal wall causes the skin of the scrotum to be held close to the testes or to hang loosely.

2. The penis

    a. The penis conveys urine and seminal fluid.

    b. It is specialized to become erect for insertion into the vagina during sexual intercourse.

    c. The body of the penis is composed of three columns of erectile tissue surrounded by connective tissue.

    d. The root of the penis is attached to the pelvic arch and membranes of the perineum.

Organs of the Female Reproductive System (page 554)

The primary sex organs of the female reproductive system are the ovaries, which produce female sex cells and sex hormones. Accessory organs include internal and external reproductive organs.

The Ovaries (page 554)

1. Attachments of the ovaries

    a. The ovaries are held in position by several ligaments.

    b. These ligaments include broad, suspensory, and ovarian ligaments.

2. Descent of the ovaries

    a. The ovaries descend from behind the parietal peritoneum near the developing kidneys.

    b. They are attached to the pelvic wall just below the pelvic brim.

3. Structure of the ovaries

    a. The ovaries are divided into a medulla and a cortex.

    b. The medulla is composed of connective tissue, blood vessels, lymphatic vessels, and nerves.

    c. The cortex contains ovarian follicles and is covered by germinal epithelium.

4. Primordial follicles

    a. During development, groups of cells in the ovarian cortex form millions of primordial follicles.

    b. Each primordial follicle contains a primary oocyte and several follicular cells.

    c. The primary oocyte begins to undergo meiosis, but the process is soon halted and is not continued until puberty.

    d. The number of oocytes steadily decreases throughout the life of a female.

5. Oogenesis

    a. Beginning at puberty, some oocytes are stimulated to continue meiosis.

    b. When a primary oocyte undergoes oogenesis, it gives rise to a secondary oocyte in which the original chromosome number is reduced by one-half (46 to 23).

    c. A secondary oocyte represents an egg cell and can be fertilized to produce a zygote.

6. Maturation of a follicle

    a. At puberty, primordial follicles become primary follicles.

    b. During maturation, the oocyte enlarges, the follicular cells multiply, and a fluid-filled cavity appears and produces a secondary follicle.

    c. Ovarian cells surrounding the follicle form two layers.

    d. Usually only one follicle reaches full development.

7. Ovulation

    a. Ovulation is the release of an oocyte from an ovary.

    b. The resulting oocyte is released when the follicle ruptures.

    c. After ovulation, the oocyte is drawn into the opening of the uterine tube.

Female Internal Accessory Organs (page 558)

1. The uterine tubes

    a. These tubes convey egg cells toward the uterus.

    b. The end of each tube is expanded and its margin bears irregular extensions.

    c. Movement of an egg cell into the opening is aided by ciliated cells that line the tube and by peristaltic contractions in the wall of the tube.

2. The uterus

    a. The uterus receives the embryo and sustains its life during development.

    b. The cervix of the uterus is partially enclosed by the vagina.

    c. The uterine wall includes the endometrium, myometrium, and perimetrium.

3. The vagina

    a. The vagina connects the uterus to the vestibule.

    b. It receives the erect penis, conveys uterine secretions to the outside, and transports the fetus during birth.

    c. The vaginal orifice is partially closed by a thin membrane, called the hymen.

    d. Its wall consists of a mucosal layer, muscular layer, and outer fibrous layer.

Female External Reproductive Organs (page 562)

1. The labia majora

    a. The labia majora are rounded folds of fatty tissue and skin that enclose and protect the other external reproductive parts.

    b. The upper ends form a rounded, fatty elevation over the symphysis pubis.

2. The labia minora

    a. The labia minora are flattened, longitudinal folds between the labia majora.

    b. They form the sides of the vestibule and anteriorly form the hoodlike covering of the clitoris.

3. The clitoris
   a. The clitoris is a small projection at the anterior end of the vulva.
   b. It is composed of two columns of erectile tissue.
   c. Its root is attached to the sides of the pubic arch.
4. The vestibule
   a. The vestibule is the space between the labia majora that encloses the vaginal and urethral openings.
   b. Vestibular glands secrete mucus into the vestibule during sexual stimulation.

The Mammary Glands (page 564)
1. Location of the glands
   a. The mammary glands are located in subcutaneous tissue of the anterior thorax within the breasts.
   b. The breasts extend between the second and sixth ribs, and from the sternum to the axillae.
2. Structure of the glands
   a. The mammary glands are composed of lobes that contain tubular glands.
   b. Lobes are separated by dense connective and adipose tissues.
   c. The mammary glands are connected to the nipple by ducts.
3. Development of the breasts
   a. Male breasts remain nonfunctional.
   b. A hormone stimulates female breast development.
      (1) Alveolar glands and ducts enlarge.
      (2) Fat is deposited around and within breasts.
   c. During pregnancy the breasts change.
      (1) The ductile system grows.
      (2) Alveolar glands develop.
4. Production and secretion of milk
   a. Following childbirth, the mammary glands begin to secrete milk.
   b. Reflex response to mechanical stimulation of the nipple causes milk to be ejected from the alveolar ducts.
   c. As long as milk is removed from glands, more milk is produced; if milk is not removed, production ceases.

Clinical Application of Knowledge

1. What changes, if any, might occur in the secondary sexual characteristics of an adult male following removal of one testis? Following removal of both testes? Following removal of the prostate gland?
2. What is the reason for using ultrasonography, instead of some other imaging techniques, when examining the uterus and uterine tubes?
3. A vasectomy is a surgical procedure in which each vas deferens is severed near the epididymis and the cut ends are tied. This prevents sperm from leaving the epididymis. Following vasectomy, will this person be able to produce semen? Explain your answer.
4. What effect would it have on a woman's secondary sexual characteristics if a single ovary were removed? What effect would it have if both ovaries were removed?

Review Activities

1. List the general functions of the male reproductive system.
2. Distinguish between the primary and accessory male reproductive organs.
3. Describe the descent of the testes.
4. Define *cryptorchidism*.
5. Describe the structure of a testis.
6. Explain the function of the supporting cells in the testis.
7. List the major steps in spermatogenesis.
8. Describe a sperm cell.
9. Describe the epididymis and explain its function.
10. Trace the path of the vas deferens from the epididymis to the ejaculatory duct.
11. On a diagram, locate the seminal vesicles.
12. On a diagram, locate the prostate gland and describe the function of its secretion.
13. On a diagram, locate the bulbourethral glands.
14. Define *semen*.
15. Describe the structure of the scrotum.
16. Describe the structure of the penis.
17. List the general functions of the female reproductive system.
18. Distinguish between the primary and accessory female reproductive organs.
19. Describe how the ovaries are held in position.
20. Describe the descent of the ovaries.
21. Describe the structure of an ovary.
22. Define *primordial follicle*.
23. List the major steps in oogenesis.
24. Describe how a follicle matures.
25. Define ovulation.
26. On a diagram, locate the uterine tubes and explain their function.
27. Describe the structure of the uterus.
28. Describe the structure of the vagina.
29. Distinguish between the labia majora and the labia minora.
30. On a diagram, locate the clitoris and describe its structure.
31. Define *vestibule*.
32. Describe the structure of a mammary gland.

C H A P T E R 1 8

Human Growth and Development

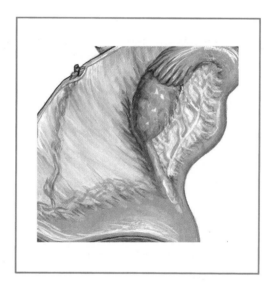

The products of the female and male reproductive systems are egg cells and sperm cells, respectively. When an egg cell and a sperm cell unite, a zygote is formed by the process of fertilization. Such a single-celled zygote is the first cell of an off-spring, and it is capable of giving rise to an adult of the subsequent generation. The processes by which this is accomplished are called *growth* and *development*.

Chapter Outline

Introduction

Pregnancy
    Transport of Sex Cells
    Fertilization

Prenatal Period
    Period of Cleavage
    Embryonic Stage
    Fetal Stage
    Fetal Circulation
    The Birth Process

Neonatal Period

Clinical Terms Related to Growth
    and Development

Chapter Objectives

After you have studied this chapter, you should be able to

1. Distinguish between growth and development.

2. Define pregnancy and describe the process of fertilization.

3. Describe the major events that occur during the period of cleavage.

4. Explain how the primary germ layers originate and list the structures produced by each layer.

5. Describe the formation and function of the placenta.

6. Define fetus and describe the major events that occur during the fetal stage of development.

7. Trace the general path of blood through the fetal circulatory system.

8. Describe the birth process.

9. Describe the major circulatory adjustments that occur in the newborn.

10. Complete the review activities at the end of this chapter. Note that the items are worded in the form of specific learning objectives. You may want to refer to them before reading the chapter.

Aids to Understanding Words

allant-, sausage-shaped: *allant*ois—tubelike structure that extends from the yolk sac into the connecting stalk of the embryo.

chorio-, skin: *chorio*n—outermost membrane that surrounds the fetus and other fetal membranes.

cleav-, to divide: *cleav*age—period of development characterized by a division of the zygote into smaller and smaller cells.

lacun-, a pool: *lacun*a—space between the chorionic villi that fills with maternal blood.

morul-, mulberry: *morul*a—embryonic structure consisting of a solid ball of about 16 cells, looking somewhat like a mulberry.

nat-, to be born: pre*nat*al—period of development before birth.

troph-, nourishment: *troph*oblast—cellular layer that surrounds the inner cell mass and helps nourish it.

umbil-, the navel: *umbil*ical cord—structure attached to the fetal navel (umbilicus) that connects the fetus to the placenta.

Introduction

Growth refers to an increase in size. In a human, growth usually reflects an increase in cell numbers as a result of *mitosis,* followed by enlargement of the newly formed cells and enlargement of the body.

Development, on the other hand, is the continuous process by which an individual changes from one life phase to another. These life phases include a **prenatal period,** which begins with the fertilization of an egg cell and ends at birth, and a **postnatal period,** which begins at birth and ends with death in old age (figure 18.1).

Pregnancy

Pregnancy is the condition characterized by the presence of a developing offspring within the uterus. It results from the union of an egg cell and a sperm cell—an event called **fertilization.**

Transport of Sex Cells

Ordinarily, before fertilization can occur, an egg cell (secondary oocyte) must be released by ovulation and enter a uterine tube.

During sexual intercourse, semen containing sperm cells is deposited in the vagina near the cervix. To reach the egg cell, the sperm cells must move upward through the uterus and uterine tube. This movement is aided by the lashing movements of the sperm tails and by muscular contractions within the walls of the uterus and uterine tube (figure 18.2).

The sperm transport mechanism is relatively inefficient, however, because even though as many as 300 million to 500 million sperm cells may be deposited in the vagina, only a few hundred of them ever reach an egg cell.

Studies indicate that an egg cell may survive for only 12 to 24 hours following ovulation, while sperm cells may live up to 72 hours within the female reproductive tract. Consequently, sexual intercourse probably must occur no more than 72 hours before ovulation or 24 hours following ovulation if fertilization is to take place.

Sperm cells are thought to reach the upper portions of the uterine tube within an hour following sexual intercourse. Although many sperm cells may reach an egg cell, only one will actually fertilize the egg (figure 18.3).

Fertilization

When a sperm cell reaches an egg cell, it moves through the follicular cells that adhere to the egg's surface (corona radiata) and binds to the *zona pellucida* surrounding the egg cell membrane. The sperm cell penetrates the zona with the aid of substances that the sperm cell secretes.

The sperm cell's plasma membrane fuses with that of the egg, and the sperm movement ceases. At the same time, the egg cell membrane becomes unresponsive to other sperm cells. The union of the egg and sperm cell membranes also triggers an action in some lysosome-like granules (cortical granules) that occur just beneath the egg cell membrane. These granules release substances that cause the zona pellucida to harden. This reduces the chance that other sperm cells will reach the egg and forms a protective layer around the newly formed, fertilized egg cell.

After the sperm cell has fused with the egg cell membrane, it passes through the membrane and enters the cytoplasm. During this process, the sperm cell loses its tail,

FIGURE 18.1

(a) Growth involves an increase in size; (b) development refers to the process of changing from one phase of life to another.

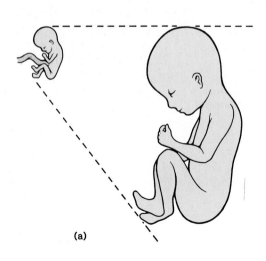

(a)

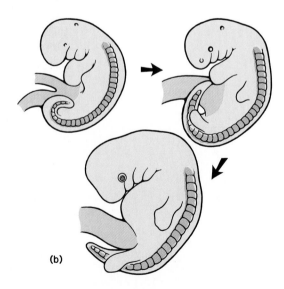

(b)

FIGURE 18.2

The paths of the egg and sperm cells through the female reproductive tract. What factors aid the movement of these cells?

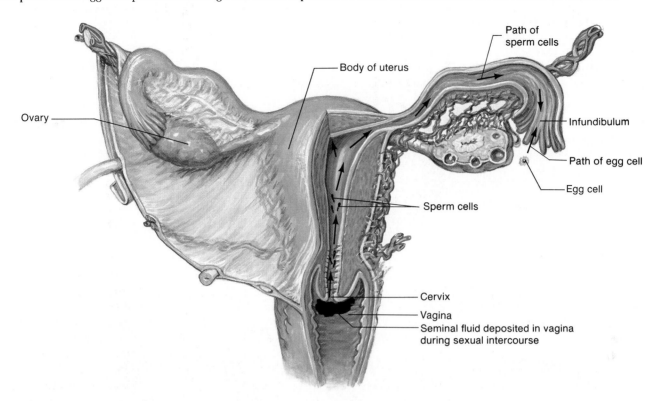

and its head swells to form a nucleus. As explained previously, the egg cell (secondary oocyte) then divides unequally to form a relatively large cell and a tiny second polar body, which is later expelled. The nucleus of the egg cell and that of the sperm cell come together in the center of the larger cell. Their nuclear envelopes disappear and their chromosomes combine, thus completing the process of **fertilization.** This process is diagrammed in figure 18.4.

Because the sperm cell and the egg cell each provide 23 chromosomes, the product of fertilization is a cell with 46 chromosomes—the usual number for a human cell. This cell is called a **zygote,** and is the first cell of the future offspring.

1. Where in the female reproductive system does fertilization normally take place?
2. List the events that occur during fertilization.

Prenatal Period

The prenatal period of development usually lasts for 40 weeks (ten lunar months) and can be divided into three stages: a period of cleavage, an embryonic stage, and a fetal stage.

FIGURE 18.3

Scanning electron micrograph of sperm cells on the surface of an egg cell (×1,200).

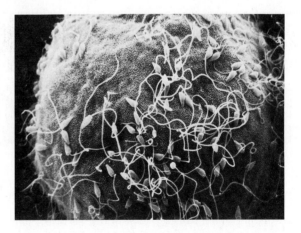

Period of Cleavage

Fertilization normally occurs within a uterine tube. About 30 hours after the *zygote* is formed, it undergoes *mitosis,* giving rise to two cells. These cells, in turn, divide to form four cells; they divide into eight cells; and so forth. With each subsequent division, the resulting cells are smaller and smaller. This distribution of the zygote's contents into

FIGURE 18.4

Steps in the fertilization process: (*1*) Sperm cell reaches corona radiata surrounding the egg cell. (*2*) Acrosome of sperm cell releases protein-digesting chemical. (*3* and *4*) Sperm cell penetrates zona pellucida surrounding egg cell. (*5*) Sperm cell's plasma membrane fuses with egg cell membrane.

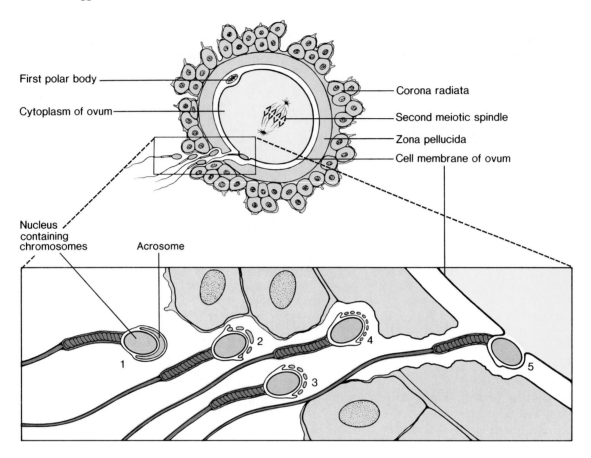

smaller and smaller cells is called *cleavage,* and the cells produced in this way are called *blastomeres* (figures 18.5 and 18.6).

It is usually not possible to determine the actual time of fertilization because reliable records concerning sexual activities are seldom available. However, the approximate time can be calculated by adding fourteen days to the date of the onset of the last menstruation. This time can then be used to calculate the fertilization age of an embryo. The expected time of birth can be estimated by adding 266 days to the fertilization date. Most fetuses are born within 10 to 15 days of this calculated time.

The tiny mass of cells formed by cleavage is moved through the uterine tube to the cavity of the uterus. This movement is aided by the action of cilia of the tubular epithelium and by weak peristaltic contractions of smooth muscles in the tubular wall. Secretions from the epithelial lining are thought to provide the developing organism with nutrients.

The trip to the uterus takes about three days. At the end of this time, the structure consists of a solid ball of about sixteen cells, called a *morula* (figure 18.7).

The morula enters the uterine cavity and remains unattached for about three days. During this time, the zona pellucida degenerates, and the morula develops a fluid-filled central cavity. Once this cavity appears, the morula becomes a hollow ball of cells called a **blastocyst** (figure 18.8).

Within the blastocyst, cells in one region group together to form an *inner cell mass* that eventually gives rise to the **embryo** proper—the body of the developing offspring. The cells forming the wall of the blastocyst make up the *trophoblast,* which forms structures that assist the embryo in its development.

FIGURE 18.5

During the period of cleavage, the cells divide by mitosis and become smaller and smaller.

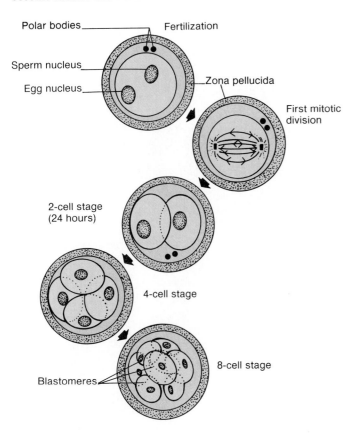

FIGURE 18.6

(a) A human egg cell surrounded by follicle cells. Note the sperm cells in the outer layer of the follicle. (b) The two-cell stage of development (×1,000).

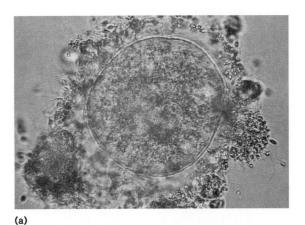

(a)

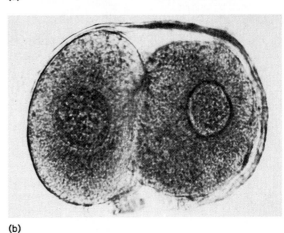

(b)

FIGURE 18.7

A human morula.

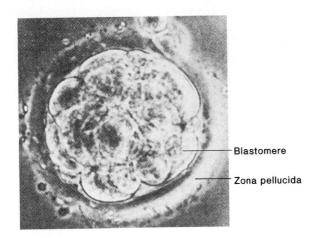

Sometimes two ovarian follicles release egg cells simultaneously, and if both are fertilized, the resulting zygotes can develop into fraternal (dizygotic) twins. Such twins are no more alike genetically than any brothers or sisters from the same parents. In other instances, twins develop from a single fertilized egg (monozygotic twins). This can happen if two inner cell masses form within a blastocyst and each produces an embryo. Twins of this type usually share a single placenta, and they are identical genetically. Thus, they are always the same sex and are very similar in appearance.

About the sixth day, the blastocyst begins to attach itself to the uterine lining. This attachment is apparently aided by a secretion that digests a portion of the endometrium. The blastocyst sinks slowly into the resulting depression, becoming completely buried in the uterine lining. At the same time, the endometrium lining is stimulated to thicken below the implanting blastocyst, and cells of the trophoblast begin to produce tiny, fingerlike processes (microvilli) that grow into the endometrium. This

FIGURE 18.8

(a) A morula consists of a solid ball of cells; (b) a blastocyst has a fluid-filled cavity.

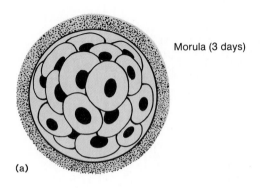

Morula (3 days)

(a)

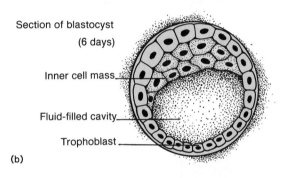

Section of blastocyst
(6 days)

Inner cell mass

Fluid-filled cavity

Trophoblast

(b)

FIGURE 18.9

(a) About the sixth day of development, the blastocyst contacts the uterine wall and (b) begins to become implanted within the wall.

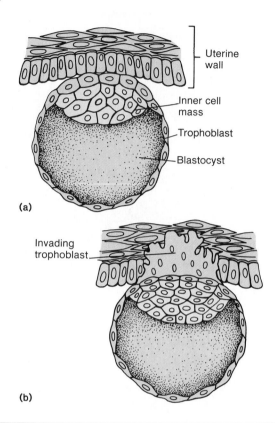

Uterine wall

Inner cell mass

Trophoblast

Blastocyst

(a)

Invading trophoblast

(b)

FIGURE 18.10

Light micrograph of a blastocyst in contact with the endothelium of the uterine wall (×300).

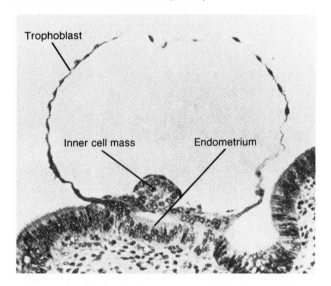

Trophoblast

Inner cell mass

Endometrium

process of **implantation** occurs near the end of the first week of development, and completes the period of cleavage (figures 18.9, 18.10, 18.11, and 18.12).

Figure 18.13 summarizes the events in early human development.

Occasionally, developing offspring may become implanted in tissues outside the uterus, including those of a uterine tube, ovary, cervix, or an organ in the abdominal cavity. The result is an *ectopic pregnancy.* Most commonly, this occurs within a uterine tube and is termed a *tubal pregnancy.*

In a tubal pregnancy, the tube usually ruptures as the embryo enlarges. This is accompanied by severe pain and heavy bleeding through the vagina. The treatment involves prompt surgical removal of the embryo and repair or removal of the damaged uterine tube.

Usually, the blastocyst becomes implanted in the upper posterior wall of the uterus. Sometimes, however, implantation occurs in the lower portion near the cervix, and as the placenta develops, it may partially or totally cover the opening of the cervix. This condition is called *placenta previa,* and it is likely to produce complications since any expansion of the cervix may damage placental tissues and cause bleeding.

1. Distinguish between growth and development.
2. What is a zygote?
3. What changes characterize the period of cleavage?
4. How does a blastocyst become attached to the endometrium of the uterus?
5. In what way does the endometrium respond to the activities of the blastocyst?

FIGURE 18.11

Light micrograph of a human embryo (arrow), undergoing implantation in the uterine wall.

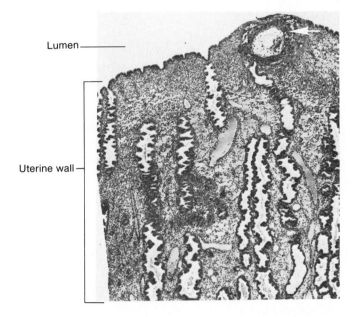

FIGURE 18.12

An embryo (arrow) appears as a red blister bulging out from the wall of this dissected uterus.

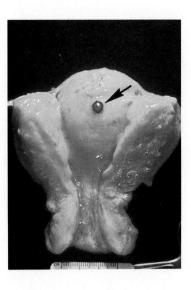

FIGURE 18.13

Stages in early human development.

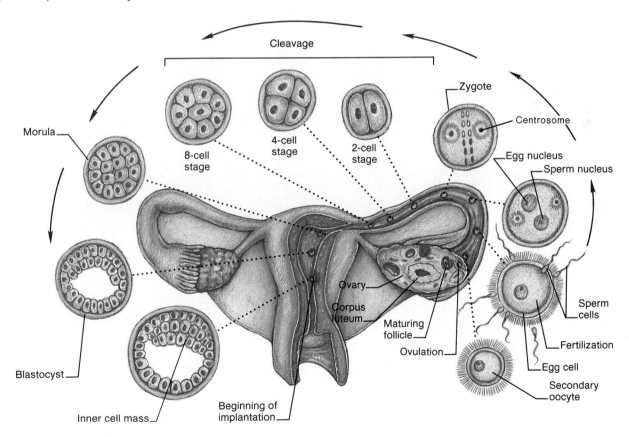

In Vitro Fertilization

A woman who is infertile because her uterine tubes are blocked may become pregnant by means of *in vitro fertilization.* In one such technique, oocytes are removed from the woman's ovary and mixed with sperm in a dish to achieve fertilization (*in vitro* means "in glass" and refers to the artificial environment of the fertilization dish). Later, the resulting embryos are transferred into the woman's uterus for development.

The in vitro fertilization procedure usually begins with the administration of some substance that will induce the development of ovarian follicles. The growth of the follicles can be monitored using ultrasonography, and when they have reached a certain diameter, the patient is given a hormone to induce ovulation.

Oocytes released from the ovary are harvested with the aid of a *laparoscope*—an optical instrument used to examine the abdominal interior. The oocytes are incubated at 37° C, and when mature, they are mixed in a dish with sperm that have been washed to remove various inhibitory factors.

Fertilized eggs are incubated in a special medium. After 50–60 hours, when the developing embryos have reached the 8- or 16-cell stage, normal ones are transferred through the woman's cervix and into her uterus with the aid of a specially designed catheter. She is then treated with a hormone to promote a favorable uterine environment for implantation of the embryos. As a result of this procedure, successful implantation occurs in about 20%–30% of the cases.

FIGURE 18.14
Early in the embryonic stage of development, the three primary germ layers are formed.

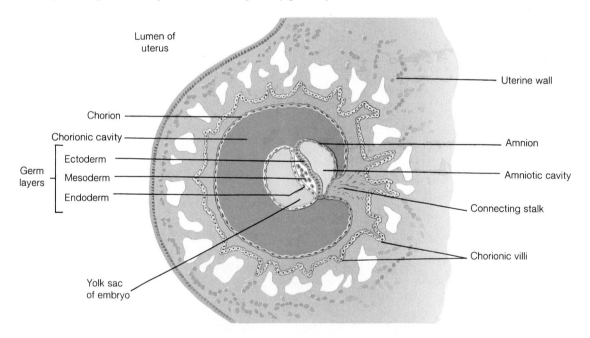

Embryonic Stage

The **embryonic stage** extends from the second week through the eighth week of development. It is characterized by the formation of the placenta, the development of the main internal organs, and the appearance of the major external body structures.

Early in this stage, the cells of the inner cell mass become organized into a flattened **embryonic disk** that consists of two distinct layers: an outer *ectoderm* and an inner *endoderm.* A short time later, a third layer of cells, the *mesoderm,* forms between the ectoderm and endoderm.

These three layers of cells are called the **primary germ layers,** and they are responsible for forming all of the body organs. (See figure 18.14.)

More specifically, *ectodermal cells* give rise to the nervous system, portions of special sensory organs, the epidermis, hair, nails, glands of the skin, and the linings of the mouth and anal canal. *Mesodermal cells* form all types of muscle tissue, bone tissue, bone marrow, blood, blood vessels, lymphatic vessels, various connective tissues, internal reproductive organs, kidneys, and the epithelial linings of the body cavities. *Endodermal cells* produce the epithelial linings of the digestive tract, respiratory tract, urinary bladder, and urethra (figure 18.15).

FIGURE 18.15

Each of the primary germ layers is responsible for the formation of a particular set of organs.

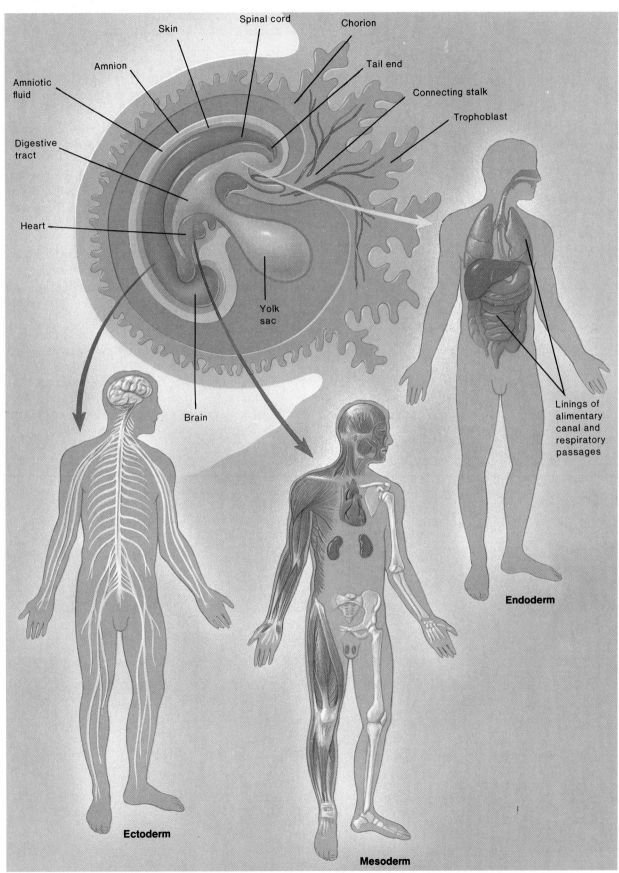

FIGURE 18.16

During the fourth week, (a) the flat embryonic disk becomes (b) a cylindrical structure.

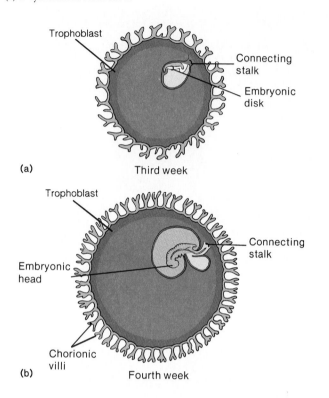

During the fourth week of development (figure 18.16), the flat embryonic disk is transformed into a cylindrical structure, which is attached to the developing placenta by a *connecting stalk* (body stalk). By this time, the head and jaws are appearing, the heart is beating and forcing blood through blood vessels, and tiny buds that will give rise to the arms and legs are forming (figure 18.17).

During the fifth through the seventh weeks, as shown in figures 18.18 and 18.19, the head grows rapidly and becomes rounded and erect. The face, which is developing eyes, nose, and mouth, becomes more humanlike. The arms and legs elongate, and fingers and toes appear (figure 18.20).

By the end of the seventh week, all the main internal organs have become established, and as these structures enlarge, they affect the shape of the body. Consequently, the body takes on a humanlike appearance.

Meanwhile, the embryo continues to become implanted within the uterus. As mentioned, early in this process slender projections grow out from the trophoblast into the surrounding endometrium. These extensions, which are called *chorionic villi,* become branched, and by the end of the fourth week they are well formed.

While the chorionic villi are developing, embryonic blood vessels form within them, which are continuous with those vessels passing through the connecting stalk to the body of the embryo. At the same time, irregular spaces called **lacunae** are eroded around and between the villi. These spaces become filled with maternal blood that escapes from eroded endometrial blood vessels.

FIGURE 18.17

(a) A human embryo at three weeks; (b) at 3.5 weeks. The brain and spinal cord are formed by longitudinal folds that develop in the ectoderm. (c) An embryo at about 29 days.

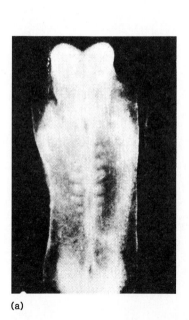

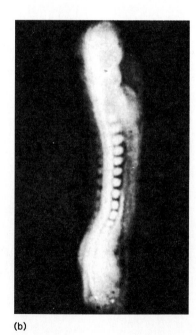

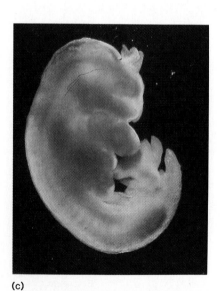

(a)   (b)   (c)

FIGURE 18.18

(*a*) Human embryo after about five weeks of development; (*b*) six-week-old human embryo.

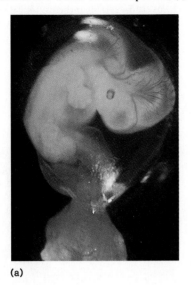

(a)

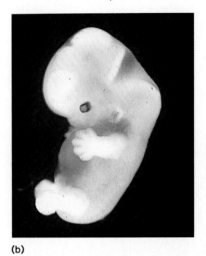

(b)

FIGURE 18.19

In the fifth through the seventh weeks of development, the embryonic body and face develop a humanlike appearance.

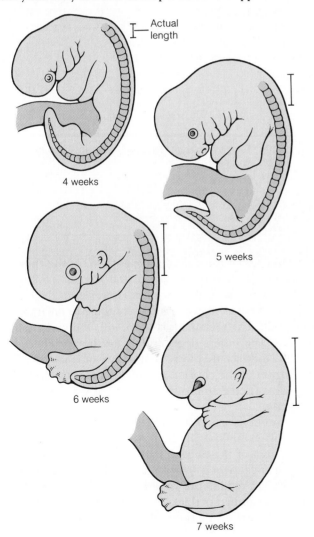

FIGURE 18.20

What structures can you identify in this photograph of a 7-week-old human embryo?

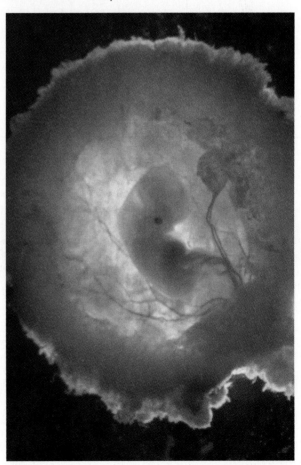

FIGURE 18.21

As illustrated in the section of a villus, the placental membrane consists of the epithelial wall of an embryonic capillary and the epithelial wall of a chorionic villus. What is the significance of this membrane?

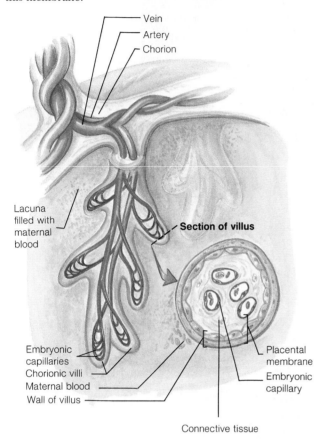

FIGURE 18.22

The placenta consists of an embryonic portion and a maternal portion. (Blue vessels indicate blood with a low oxygen content; red vessels indicate high oxygen content.)

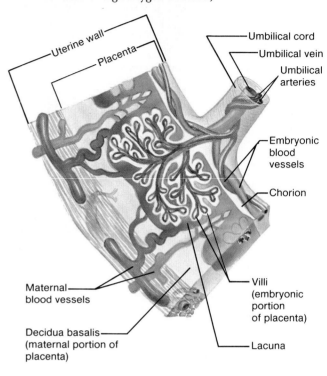

A thin membrane separates embryonic blood within the capillary of a chorionic villus from maternal blood in a lacuna. This membrane, called the **placental membrane,** is composed of the epithelium of the villus and the epithelium of the capillary (figure 18.21). Through this membrane, exchanges take place between the maternal blood and the embryonic blood. Oxygen and nutrients move from the maternal blood into the embryonic blood, and carbon dioxide and other wastes move from the embryonic blood into the maternal blood.

Factors that can cause congenital malformations by affecting an embryo during its period of rapid growth and development are called *teratogens.* Such agents include various drugs and certain microorganisms.

Because most drugs are able to pass freely through the placental membrane, substances ingested by the mother may affect the fetus. Thus, fetal drug addiction may occur following the mother's use of various addicting drugs such as heroin.

Similarly, depressant drugs administered to the mother during labor can produce effects within the fetus, such as depressing the activity of its respiratory system.

1. What major events occur during the embryonic stage of development?
2. What tissues and structures develop from ectoderm? From mesoderm? From endoderm?
3. Describe the structure and function of a chorionic villus.

Until about the end of the eighth week, the chorionic villi cover the entire surface of the former trophoblast, which is now called the **chorion.** However, as the embryo and the chorion surrounding it continue to enlarge, only those villi that remain in contact with the endometrium endure. The others degenerate, and the portions of the chorion to which they were attached become smooth. Thus, the region of the chorion still in contact with the uterine wall is restricted to a disk-shaped area that becomes the **placenta.**

The embryonic portion of the placenta is composed of the chorion and its villi; the maternal portion is composed of the area of the uterine wall (decidua basalis) to which the villi are attached. When it is fully formed, the placenta appears as a reddish brown disk, about 20 centimeters long and 2.5 centimeters thick. It usually weighs about 0.5 kilogram. Figure 18.22 shows the structure of the placenta.

FIGURE 18.23

(*a, b, c*) As the amnion develops, it surrounds the embryo, and (*d*) the umbilical cord is formed. What structures comprise this cord?

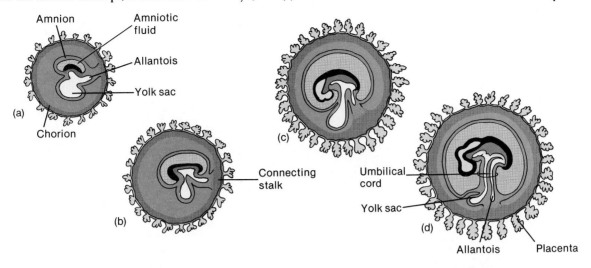

FIGURE 18.24

As the amniotic cavity enlarges, the amnion contacts the chorion, and the two membranes fuse to form the amniochorionic membrane.

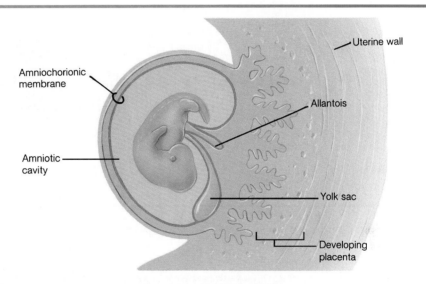

Usually the placenta is attached to the uterus near the upper posterior wall. However, it may be attached at any place on the uterine wall. The placement of the placenta may result in complications if it covers the opening to the cervix.

While the placenta is forming from the chorion, another membrane, called the **amnion,** develops around the embryo. This second membrane begins to appear during the second week. Its margin is attached around the edge of the embryonic disk, and fluid called **amniotic fluid** fills the space between them.

As the embryo is transformed into a cylindrical structure, the margins of the amnion are folded around it so that the embryo becomes enclosed by the amnion and surrounded by amniotic fluid. As this process continues, the amnion envelops the tissues on the underside of the embryo, by which it is attached to the chorion and the developing placenta. In this manner, as figure 18.23 illustrates, the **umbilical cord** is formed.

When the umbilical cord is fully developed, it is about 1 centimeter in diameter and about 55 centimeters in length. It begins at the umbilicus of the embryo and is inserted into the central region of the placenta. The cord contains three blood vessels—two *umbilical arteries* and one *umbilical vein*—through which blood passes between the embryo and the placenta (see figure 18.22).

The umbilical cord also suspends the embryo in the amniotic cavity, and the amniotic fluid provides a watery environment in which the embryo can grow freely without being compressed by surrounding tissues. The amniotic fluid also protects the embryo from being jarred by movements of the mother's body.

Eventually, the amniotic cavity becomes so enlarged that the membrane of the amnion contacts the thicker chorion around it, and the two membranes become fused into an *amniochorionic membrane* (figures 18.23, 18.24, and 18.25).

FIGURE 18.25

(a) The developing placenta as it appears during the seventh week of development; (b) photograph of an embryo attached to the placenta.

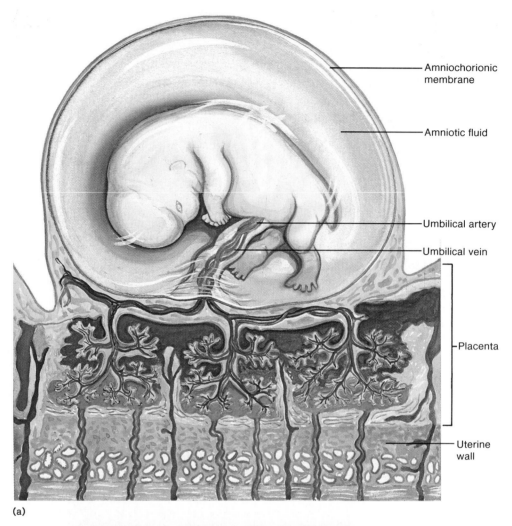

- Amniochorionic membrane
- Amniotic fluid
- Umbilical artery
- Umbilical vein
- Placenta
- Uterine wall

(a)

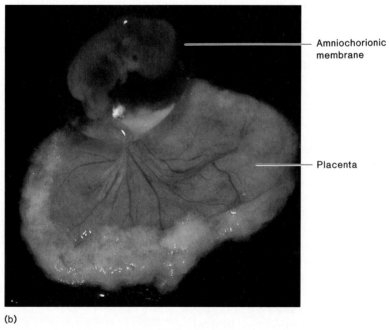

- Amniochorionic membrane
- Placenta

(b)

In addition to the amnion and chorion, two other embryonic membranes appear during development. They are the yolk sac and the allantois.

The **yolk sac** appears during the second week, and is attached to the underside of the embryonic disk (figures 18.23 and 18.24). It forms blood cells in the early stages of development and gives rise to the cells that later become sex cells. Portions of the yolk sac also enter into the formation of the embryonic digestive tube. Part of this membrane becomes incorporated into the umbilical cord, while the remainder lies in the cavity between the chorion and the amnion near the placenta.

The **allantois** forms during the third week as a tube extending from the early yolk sac into the connecting stalk of the embryo. It too forms blood cells and gives rise to the umbilical arteries and vein (figures 18.23 and 18.24).

The *embryonic stage* is completed at the end of the eighth week. It is the most critical period of development, for during this time the embryo becomes implanted within the uterine wall and all the essential external and internal body parts are formed. Any disturbances in the developmental processes occurring during the embryonic stage are likely to result in major malformations or malfunctions.

By the beginning of the eighth week, the embryo is usually 30 millimeters in length and weighs less than 5 grams. Although its body is quite unfinished, it is recognizable as a human being.

The eighth week of development occurs two weeks after a pregnant woman has missed her second menstrual period. Since these first few weeks are critical periods in development, it is important that a woman seek health care as soon as she thinks she may be pregnant.

---

1. Describe the development of the amnion.
2. What blood vessels are found in the umbilical cord?
3. What is the function of amniotic fluid?
4. What is the significance of the yolk sac?

Fetal Stage

The fetal stage begins at the end of the eighth week of development and lasts until the time of birth. During this period the offspring is called a **fetus,** and although the existing body structures continue to grow and mature, only a few new parts appear. The rate of growth is great, however, and body proportions change considerably. For example, at the beginning of the fetal stage, the head is disproportionately large and the legs are relatively short (figure 18.26).

FIGURE 18.26
During development, the body proportions change considerably.

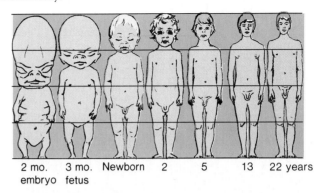

2 mo. 3 mo. Newborn 2   5   13   22 years
embryo fetus

During the third lunar month, growth in body length is accelerated, while the growth of the head slows. (Note: A lunar month equals 28 days.) The arms achieve the relative length they will maintain throughout development, and ossification centers appear in most of the bones. By the twelfth week, the external reproductive organs are distinguishable as male or female (figure 18.27).

In the fourth lunar month, the body grows very rapidly and reaches a length of 13 to 17 centimeters. The legs lengthen considerably, and the skeleton continues to ossify.

In the fifth lunar month, the rate of growth decreases somewhat. The legs achieve their final relative proportions, and the skeletal muscles become active so that the mother may feel fetal movements (quickening). Some hair appears on the head, and the skin becomes covered with fine, downy hair (lanugo). The skin is also coated with a cheesy mixture of sebum from the sebaceous glands and dead epidermal cells (vernix caseosa).

During the sixth lunar month, the body gains a substantial amount of weight. The eyebrows and eyelashes appear. The skin is quite wrinkled and translucent. It is also reddish, due to the presence of dermal blood vessels.

In the seventh lunar month, the skin becomes smoother as fat is deposited in the subcutaneous tissues. The eyelids, which fused together during the third month, reopen. At the end of this month, a fetus is about 37 centimeters in length.

If a fetus is born prematurely, its chance of surviving increases directly with its age and weight. One factor that affects the chance of survival is the development of the lungs. Thus, fetuses have increased chances of surviving if their lungs are sufficiently developed so that they have the thin respiratory membranes necessary for rapid exchange of oxygen and carbon dioxide, and if the lungs produce enough surfactant to reduce the alveolar surface tension (see chapter 13). A fetus weighing less than 700 grams at birth seldom survives, even when given intensive care.

FIGURE 18.27
(a) Human fetus after about 10 weeks of development (note the vessels of the placenta); (b) after 12 weeks of development.

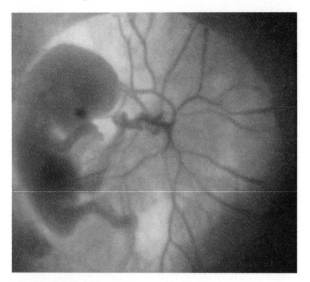

(a)

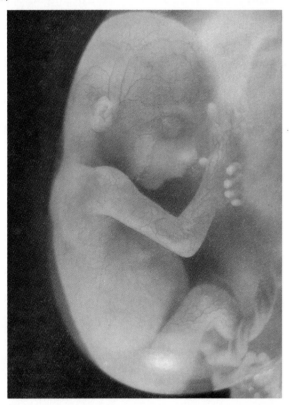

(b)

In the eighth lunar month, the fetal skin is still reddish and somewhat wrinkled. The testes of males descend from regions near the developing kidneys through the inguinal canals and into the scrotum.

During the ninth lunar month, the fetus reaches a length of about 47 centimeters. The skin is smooth, and the body appears chubby due to an accumulation of subcutaneous fat. The reddishness of the skin fades to pinkish

or bluish pink, even in fetuses of dark-skinned parents, because melanin is not produced until the skin is exposed to light.

At the end of the tenth lunar month, the fetus is said to be full term. It is about 50 centimeters long and weighs 2.7–3.6 kilograms. The skin has lost its downy hair, but is still coated with sebum and dead epidermal cells. The scalp is usually covered with hair, the fingers and toes have well-developed nails, and the skull bones are largely ossified. As figure 18.28 shows, the fetus is usually positioned upside down with its head toward the cervix (*vertex position*). Chart 18.1 summarizes the stages of prenatal development.

A number of changes occur in a woman's body as a result of the increased demands of a growing fetus. For example, as the fetus increases in size, the uterus enlarges greatly, and instead of being confined to its normal location in the pelvic cavity, it extends upward and may eventually reach the level of the ribs. At the same time, the abdominal organs are displaced upward and compressed against the diaphragm. Also, as the uterus enlarges, it tends to press on the urinary bladder and cause the woman to feel a need to urinate frequently (figure 18.29).

The size and shape of the uterus may be used as an index of fetal growth. Thus, failure of the uterus to increase in size progressively during pregnancy suggests retarded fetal development, while a sudden increase in growth may indicate the presence of more than one fetus, the formation of excessive amniotic fluid (hydramnios), or an abnormal growth of chorionic tissue (hydatidiform mole).

As the placenta grows and develops, it requires more blood, and as the fetus enlarges, it needs more oxygen and produces greater amounts of wastes that must be excreted. Consequently, the mother's blood volume, cardiac output, breathing rate, and urine production all tend to increase in response to the fetal demands.

The fetal need for increasing amounts of nutrients is reflected in an increased dietary intake by the mother. Her intake must supply adequate nutrients for herself and the fetus. The fetal tissues have a greater capacity to capture available nutrients than do the maternal tissues. Consequently, if the mother's diet is inadequate, her body will usually show symptoms of a deficiency condition before fetal growth is affected.

1. What major changes characterize the fetal stage of development?
2. When can the gender of a fetus be determined?
3. How is a fetus usually positioned within the uterus at the end of the tenth lunar month?

Fetal Circulation

Throughout the fetal stage of development, the maternal blood supplies the fetus with oxygen and nutrients, and carries away its wastes. These substances move between the maternal and fetal blood through the placental membrane, and are carried to and from the fetal body by means of the umbilical blood vessels (figure 18.30). Consequently, the fetal vascular system must be adapted to intrauterine life in special ways.

FIGURE 18.28
A full-term fetus usually becomes positioned
with its head near the cervix.

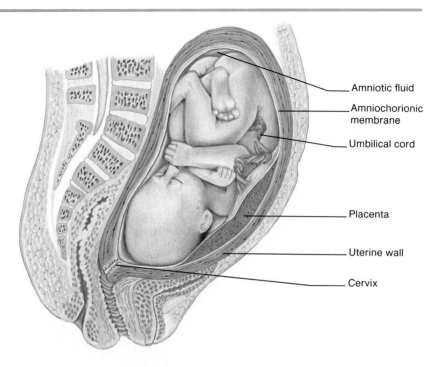

Amniotic fluid

Amniochorionic
membrane

Umbilical cord

Placenta

Uterine wall

Cervix

Chart 18.1 Stages in prenatal development		
Stage	**Time period**	**Major events**
Period of cleavage	First week	Cells undergo mitosis, blastocyst forms; inner cell mass appears; blastocyst becomes implanted in uterine wall.
Embryonic stage	Second through eighth week	Inner cell mass becomes embryonic disk; primary germ layers form; embryo proper becomes cylindrical; main internal organs and external body structures appear; placenta and umbilical cord form; embryo proper is suspended in amniotic fluid.
Fetal stage	Ninth week to birth	Existing structures continue to grow; ossification centers appear in bones; reproductive organs develop; arms and legs achieve final relative proportions; muscles become active; skin is covered with sebum and dead epidermal cells; head becomes positioned toward cervix.

FIGURE 18.29
The uterus enlarges greatly during pregnancy and presses
against the abdominal and pelvic organs.

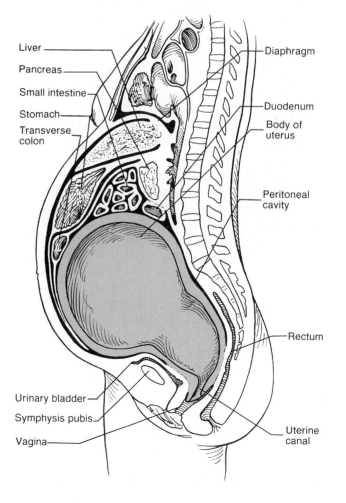

Liver

Pancreas

Small intestine

Stomach

Transverse colon

Diaphragm

Duodenum

Body of uterus

Peritoneal cavity

Rectum

Urinary bladder

Symphysis pubis

Vagina

Uterine canal

In the fetal circulatory system, the *umbilical vein* transports oxygen-rich blood and nutrients from the placenta
to the fetal body. This vein enters the body through the
umbilical ring and travels along the anterior abdominal wall
to the liver. About half the blood it carries passes into
the liver, while the rest enters a vessel called the **ductus
venosus,** which bypasses circulation through the liver
sinusoids.

FIGURE 18.30
Oxygen and nutrients enter the fetal blood from the maternal blood; waste substances enter the maternal blood from the fetal blood.

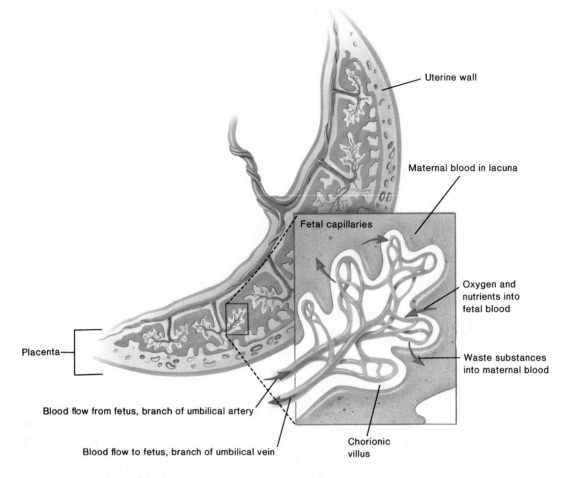

The ductus venosus travels a short distance and joins the inferior vena cava. There the oxygenated blood from the placenta is mixed with deoxygenated blood from the lower parts of the fetal body. This mixture continues through the inferior vena cava to the right atrium.

In an adult heart, blood from the right atrium enters the right ventricle and is pumped through the pulmonary trunk and arteries to the lungs. In the fetus, however, the lungs are nonfunctional, and the blood largely bypasses them. More specifically, as blood from the inferior vena cava enters the fetal right atrium, a large proportion of it is shunted directly into the left atrium through an opening in the atrial septum. This opening is called the **foramen ovale,** and blood passes through it because the blood pressure in the right atrium is somewhat greater than that in the left atrium. Furthermore, a small valve (septum primum) located on the left side of the atrial septum overlies the foramen ovale and helps prevent blood from moving in the reverse direction.

A valve of the inferior vena cava is found at the junction between the inferior vena cava and the right atrium. This valve is large in a fetus and helps direct blood through the foramen ovale.

The rest of the fetal blood entering the right atrium, as well as a large proportion of the deoxygenated blood entering from the superior vena cava, passes into the right ventricle and out through the pulmonary trunk.

Only a small volume of blood enters the pulmonary circuit, because the lungs are collapsed and their blood vessels have a high resistance to the blood flow. However, enough blood reaches the lung tissues to sustain them.

Most of the blood in the pulmonary trunk bypasses the lungs by entering a fetal vessel called the **ductus arteriosus,** which connects the pulmonary trunk to the descending portion of the aortic arch. As a result of this connection, blood with a relatively low oxygen concentration bypasses the lungs as it returns to the heart through the superior vena cava. At the same time, it is prevented from entering the portion of the aorta that provides branches leading to the heart and brain.

FIGURE 18.31

The general pattern of fetal circulation. How does this pattern of circulation differ from that of an adult?

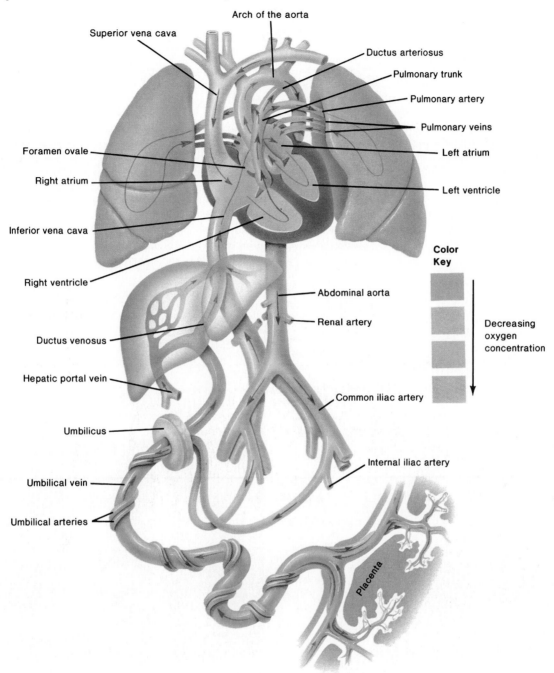

The more highly oxygenated blood that enters the left atrium through the foramen ovale is mixed with a small amount of deoxygenated blood returning from the pulmonary veins. This mixture moves into the left ventricle and is pumped into the aorta. Some of it reaches the myocardium through coronary arteries, while some reaches the brain tissues through the carotid arteries.

The blood carried by the descending aorta is partially oxygenated and partially deoxygenated. Some of it is carried into the branches of the aorta that lead to various parts of the lower regions of the body. The rest passes into the *umbilical arteries,* which branch from the internal iliac arteries and lead to the placenta. There the blood is reoxygenated. (See figure 18.31.)

The umbilical cord usually contains two arteries and one vein. In a small percentage of newborns, however, there is only one umbilical artery. Since this condition is often associated with various cardiovascular disorders, the number of vessels within the severed cord is routinely counted following birth.

Detection of Prenatal Disorders

If prospective parents are concerned about the genetic condition of a developing fetus (prenatal diagnosis), information can sometimes be obtained by testing fetal cells. This procedure, called *amniocentesis*, can be performed in a physician's office. With the aid of sonography (figure 18.32), a small quantity of amniotic fluid is withdrawn from the amniotic cavity by passing a hollow needle through the maternal abdominal and uterine walls (figure 18.33). When this is done between the fourteenth and sixteenth weeks of development, cells of fetal origin (fibroblasts) are usually present in the fluid, and they can be cultured in the laboratory and tested for chromosomal abnormalities. The amniotic fluid obtained by amniocentesis also can be analyzed for the presence of a specific protein

(alpha-fetal protein, or AFP) that is used to detect serious defects in the developing nervous system, such as spina bifida or anencephaly.

Another technique sometimes used to test fetal cells is called *chorionic villi biopsy*. This procedure employs ultrasonography to guide a catheter into a pregnant woman's uterus and uses suction to obtain a sample of the hairlike projections (villi) from the embryonic membrane (chorion) surrounding a young embryo. The cells of the sample can then be analyzed for chromosomal defects. Such a biopsy must be performed between 8 and 10 weeks of pregnancy and has the advantage of providing enough tissue to examine immediately without culturing cells. However, this procedure seems to present a greater risk to the life of the embryo than does amniocentesis.

FIGURE 18.32

A fetus within a uterus as revealed by ultrasonography. (*a*) Frontal view; (*b*) side view.

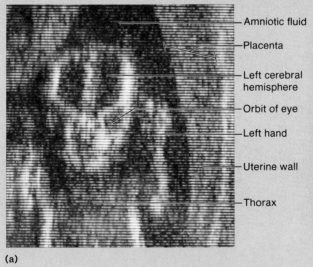

Amniotic fluid
Placenta
Left cerebral hemisphere
Orbit of eye
Left hand
Uterine wall
Thorax

(a)

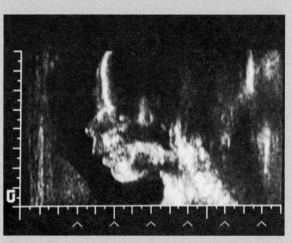

(b)

FIGURE 18.33
Fetal cells can be obtained for examination by means of amniocentesis.

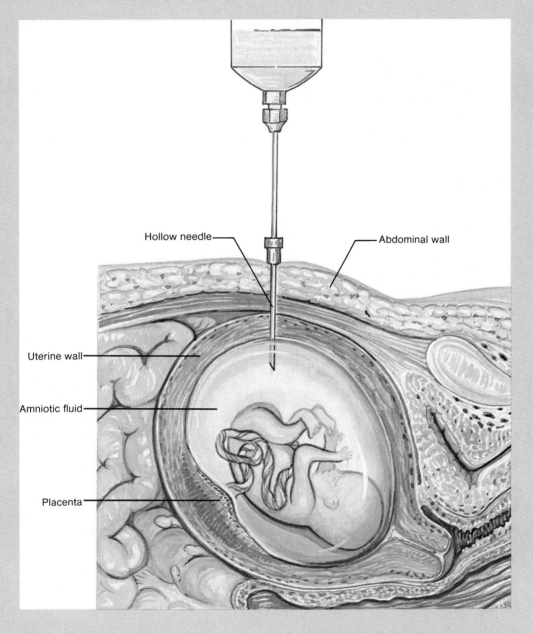

Hollow needle

Abdominal wall

Uterine wall

Amniotic fluid

Placenta

Chart 18.2 summarizes the major features of fetal circulation. At the time of birth, important adjustments must occur in the circulatory system when the placenta ceases to function and the newborn begins to breathe.

1. Which umbilical vessel carries oxygen-rich blood to the fetus?
2. What is the function of the ductus venosus?
3. How does fetal circulation allow blood to bypass the lungs?
4. What characteristic of the fetal lungs tends to shunt blood away from them?

The Birth Process

Pregnancy usually continues for 40 weeks (280 days) or about 9 calendar months (10 lunar months), if it is measured from the beginning of the last menstrual cycle. The pregnancy terminates with the *birth process* (parturition).

Labor is the term for the process in which muscular contractions force the fetus through the birth canal. Once labor starts, rhythmic contractions that begin at the top of the uterus and travel down its length force the contents of the uterus toward the cervix.

Because the fetus is usually positioned with its head downward, labor contractions force the head against the cervix. This action causes the cervix to stretch, which is thought to elicit a reflex that stimulates still stronger labor contractions.

During childbirth, the tissues of the perineum are sometimes torn by the stretching that occurs as the infant passes through the birth canal. For this reason, an incision may be made along the midline of the perineum from the vestibule to within 1.5 centimeters of the anus before the birth is completed. This procedure, called an *episiotomy*, ensures that the perineal tissues are cut cleanly rather than torn.

Chart 18.2 Fetal circulatory adaptations

Adaptation	Function
Umbilical vein	Carries oxygenated blood from placenta to fetus
Ductus venosus	Conducts about half the blood from the umbilical vein directly to the inferior vena cava, thus bypassing the liver
Foramen ovale	Conveys large proportion of blood entering the right atrium from the inferior vena cava, through the atrial septum, and into the left atrium, thus bypassing the lungs
Ductus arteriosus	Conducts some blood from the pulmonary trunk to the aorta, thus bypassing the lungs
Umbilical arteries	Carry blood from the internal iliac arteries to the placenta

As labor continues, abdominal wall muscles are stimulated to contract, and they aid in forcing the fetus through the cervix and vagina to the outside.

Following the birth of the fetus (usually within 10 to 15 minutes), the placenta, which remains inside the uterus, separates from the uterine wall and is expelled by uterine contractions through the birth canal. This expulsion, which is termed the *afterbirth*, is accompanied by bleeding because vascular tissues are damaged in the process. However, the loss of blood usually is minimized by continued contraction of the uterus that compresses the bleeding vessels.

Figure 18.34 illustrates the steps of the birth process.

For several weeks following childbirth, the uterus becomes smaller by a process called *involution*. Also, its endometrium sloughs off and is discharged through the vagina. This is followed by a return of an epithelial lining characteristic of a nonpregnant female.

1. Explain how stretching of the cervix affects labor.
2. How is bleeding controlled naturally after the placenta is expelled?

Neonatal Period

The **neonatal period,** which extends from birth to the end of the first four weeks, begins very abruptly at birth (figure 18.35). At that moment, physiological adjustments must be made quickly, because the newborn (neonate) must suddenly do for itself those things that the mother's body had been doing for it. Thus, the newborn must carry on respiration, obtain nutrients, digest nutrients, excrete wastes, regulate body temperature, and so forth. However, its most immediate need is to obtain oxygen and excrete carbon dioxide, so its first breath is critical.

The first breath must be particularly forceful, because the newborn's lungs are collapsed, and airways are small,

FIGURE 18.34
Stages in the birth process. (*a*) Fetal position before labor begins; (*b*) dilation of the cervix; (*c*) expulsion of the fetus; (*d*) expulsion of the placenta.

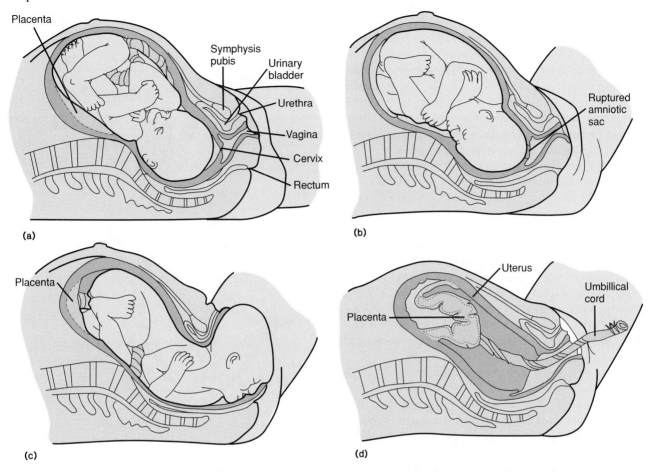

(a)

Placenta
Symphysis pubis
Urinary bladder
Urethra
Vagina
Cervix
Rectum

(b)

Ruptured amniotic sac

(c)

Placenta

(d)

Uterus
Umbillical cord
Placenta

offering considerable resistance to air movement. Also, surface tension holds the moist membranes of the lungs together. However, the lungs of a full-term fetus continuously secrete *surfactant* (see chapter 13), which reduces surface tension. After the first powerful breath begins to expand the lungs, breathing becomes easier.

> Mechanical stimulation of a newborn's lungs, caused by the mother's muscular uterine contractions during natural birth, seems to increase the quantity of surfactant secreted. Related to this is the observation that respiratory distress syndrome occurs more commonly in infants whose births do not include labor.

1. Define the neonatal period of development.
2. Why must the first breath of an infant be particularly forceful?

FIGURE 18.35
The neonatal period extends from birth to the end of the fourth week after birth.

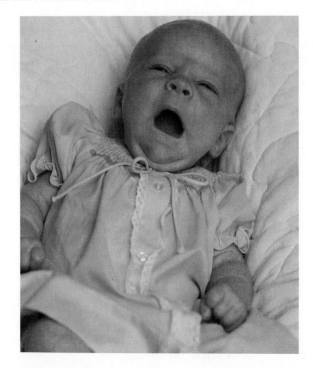

When the placenta ceases to function and breathing begins, changes occur in the circulatory system. For example, following birth, the umbilical vessels constrict. The arteries close first, and if the umbilical cord is not clamped or severed for a minute or so, blood continues to flow from the placenta to the newborn through the umbilical vein, adding to the newborn's blood volume.

The proximal portions of the umbilical arteries persist in the adult as the *superior vesical arteries,* which supply blood to the urinary bladder. The more distal portions become solid cords (lateral umbilical ligaments). The umbilical vein becomes the cordlike *ligamentum teres* that extends from the umbilicus to the liver in an adult.

Similarly, the ductus venosus constricts shortly after birth and is represented in the adult as a fibrous cord (ligamentum venosum), which is superficially embedded in the wall of the liver.

The foramen ovale closes as a result of changes in blood pressure occurring in the right and left atria as fetal vessels constrict. More precisely, as blood ceases to flow from the umbilical vein into the inferior vena cava, the blood pressure in the right atrium drops. Also, as the lungs expand with the first breathing movements, the resistance to blood flow through the pulmonary circuit decreases, more blood enters the left atrium through the pulmonary veins, and the blood pressure in the left atrium increases.

As pressure in the left atrium rises and that in the right atrium falls, a valve on the left side of the atrial septum closes the foramen ovale. In most individuals, this valve gradually fuses with the tissues along the margin of the foramen. In an adult, the site of the previous opening is marked by a depression called the *fossa ovalis.*

The ductus arteriosus, like the other fetal vessels, constricts after birth. After the ductus arteriosus has closed, blood can no longer bypass the lungs by moving from the pulmonary trunk directly into the aorta. In an adult, the ductus arteriosus is represented by a cord called the *ligamentum arteriosum.*

FIGURE 18.36

Major changes that occur in the newborn's circulatory system.

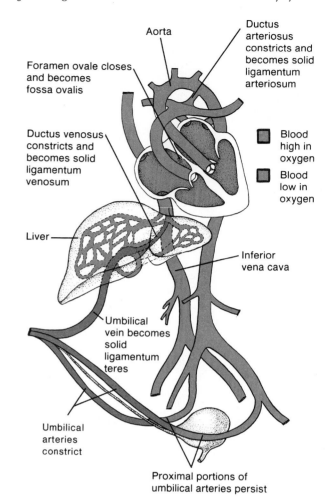

These changes in the newborn's circulatory system do not occur very rapidly. Although the constriction of the ductus arteriosus may be functionally complete within 15 minutes, the permanent closure of the foramen ovale may take up to a year. These circulatory changes are illustrated in figure 18.36 and summarized in chart 18.3.

1. What portions of the umbilical arteries continue to function into adulthood?
2. What is the fate of the foramen ovale? Of the ductus arteriosus?
3. When is the closure of the ductus arteriosus functionally complete?

Chart 18.3 Circulatory adjustments in the newborn

Structure	Adjustment	In the adult
Umbilical vein	Becomes constricted	Becomes ligamentum teres that extends from the umbilicus to the liver
Ductus venosus	Becomes constricted	Becomes ligamentum venosum that is superficially embedded in the wall of the liver
Foramen ovale	Is closed by valvelike septum primum as blood pressure in right atrium decreases and pressure in left atrium increases	Valve fuses along margin of foramen ovale and is marked by a depression called the fossa ovalis
Ductus arteriosus	Constricts	Becomes ligamentum arteriosum that extends from the pulmonary trunk to the aorta
Umbilical arteries	Distal portions become constricted	Distal portions become lateral umbilical ligaments; proximal portions function as superior vesical arteries

Clinical Terms Related to Growth and Development

abortion (ah-bor'shun) the spontaneous or deliberate termination of pregnancy; a spontaneous abortion is commonly termed a miscarriage.

abruptio placentae (ab-rup'she-o plah-cen'ta) a premature separation of the placenta from the uterine wall.

amniocentesis (am"ne-o-sen-te'sis) a technique in which a sample of amniotic fluid is withdrawn from the amniotic cavity by inserting a hollow needle through the mother's abdominal wall.

cesarean section (se-sa're-an sek'shun) the delivery of a fetus through an abdominal incision.

dizygotic twins (di"zi-got'ik twinz) twins resulting from the fertilization of two ova by two sperm cells.

endometritis (en"do-me-tri'tis) inflammation of the uterine lining.

gestation (jes-ta'shun) the entire period of pregnancy.

hydatid mole (hi'dah-tid mol) a type of uterine tumor that originates from placental tissue.

hydramnios (hi-dram'ne-os) the presence of excessive amniotic fluid.

hyperemesis gravidarum (hi"per-e'me-sis grav'i-dar-um) excessive vomiting associated with pregnancy; morning sickness.

intrauterine transfusion (in"trah-u'ter-in trans-fu'zhun) transfusion administered by injecting blood into the fetal peritoneal cavity before birth.

lochia (lo'ke-ah) vaginal discharge following childbirth.

monozygotic twins (mon"o-zi-got'ik twinz) twins resulting from the fertilization of one ovum by one sperm cell.

perinatology (per"i-na-tol'o-je) branch of medicine concerned with the fetus after twenty-five weeks of development and with the newborn for the first four weeks after birth.

postpartum (post-par'tum) occurring after birth.

teratology (ter"ah-tol'o-je) the study of abnormal development and congenital malformations.

trimester (tri-mes'ter) each third of the total period of pregnancy.

ultrasonography (ul"trah-son-og'rah-fe) technique used to visualize the size and position of structures by means of ultrasonic sound waves.

Chapter Summary

Introduction (page 572)
Growth refers to an increase in size; development is the process of changing from one phase of life to another.

Pregnancy (page 572)
1. Transport of sex cells
   a. Movement of the egg cell to the uterine tube is aided by ciliary action.
   b. To move, a sperm cell lashes its tail; its movement within the female body is aided by muscular contractions in the uterus and uterine tube.
2. Fertilization
   a. A sperm cell penetrates an egg cell.
   b. When a sperm cell penetrates an egg cell, the entrance of any other sperm cells is prevented by structural changes that occur in the egg cell membrane.
   c. When the nuclei of a sperm and an egg cell fuse, the process of fertilization is complete.
   d. The product of fertilization is a zygote with 46 chromosomes.

Prenatal Period (page 573)
1. Period of cleavage
   a. Fertilization occurs in a uterine tube and results in a zygote.
   b. The zygote undergoes mitosis.
   c. Each subsequent division produces smaller and smaller cells.
   d. A solid ball of cells (morula) is formed, and it becomes a hollow ball called a blastocyst.
   e. The inner cell mass that gives rise to the embryo proper forms within the blastocyst.
   f. The blastocyst becomes implanted in the uterine wall.
      (1) The endometrium around the blastocyst is digested.
      (2) Fingerlike processes from the blastocyst penetrate into the endometrium.
   g. The period of cleavage lasts through the first week of development.

2. Embryonic stage
   a. The embryonic stage extends from the second through the eighth week.
   b. It is characterized by development of the placenta and the main internal and external body structures.
   c. The cells of the inner cell mass become arranged into primary germ layers.
      (1) Ectoderm gives rise to the nervous system, portions of the skin, lining of the mouth, and lining of the anal canal.
      (2) Mesoderm gives rise to muscles, bones, blood vessels, lymphatic vessels, reproductive organs, kidneys, and linings of body cavities.
      (3) Endoderm gives rise to linings of the digestive tract, respiratory tract, urinary bladder, and urethra.
   d. The embryonic disk becomes cylindrical and is attached to the developing placenta by the connecting stalk.
   e. The embryo develops a head and face, arms, legs, and a mouth, and appears more humanlike.
   f. Chorionic villi develop and are surrounded by spaces (lacunae) filled with maternal blood.
   g. The placental membrane consists of the epithelium of the villi and the epithelium of the capillaries inside the villi.
      (1) Oxygen and nutrients move from the maternal blood through the membrane and into the fetal blood.
      (2) Carbon dioxide and other wastes move from the fetal blood through the membrane and into the maternal blood.
   h. The placenta develops in the disk-shaped area where the chorion remains in contact with the uterine wall.
      (1) The embryonic portion consists of chorion and its villi.
      (2) The maternal portion consists of the uterine wall to which villi are attached.
   i. Fluid-filled amnion develops around the embryo.
   j. The umbilical cord is formed as the amnion envelops the tissues attached to the underside of the embryo.
      (1) The umbilical cord includes two arteries and a vein.
      (2) It suspends the embryo in the amniotic cavity.
   k. The chorion and amnion become fused.
   l. The yolk sac forms on the underside of the embryonic disk.
      (1) It gives rise to blood cells and cells that later form sex cells.
      (2) It helps form the digestive tube.
   m. The allantois extends from the yolk sac into the connecting stalk. It forms blood cells and the umbilical vessels.
   n. By the beginning of the eighth week, the embryo is recognizable as a human.
3. Fetal stage
   a. This stage extends from the end of the eighth week and continues until birth.
   b. Existing structures grow and mature; only a few new parts appear.
   c. The body enlarges, arms and legs achieve final relative proportions, the skin is covered with sebum and dead epidermal cells, the skeleton continues to ossify, the muscles become active, and fat is deposited in subcutaneous tissue.
   d. The fetus is full term at the end of the tenth lunar month and is positioned with its head toward the cervix.
4. Fetal circulation
   a. Blood is carried between the placenta and fetus by umbilical vessels.
   b. Blood enters the fetus through the umbilical vein and partially bypasses the liver by means of the ductus venosus.
   c. Blood enters the right atrium and partially bypasses the lungs by means of the foramen ovale.
   d. Blood entering the pulmonary trunk partially bypasses the lungs by means of the ductus arteriosus.
   e. Blood enters the umbilical arteries from the internal iliac arteries.
5. The birth process
   a. Pregnancy usually lasts 40 weeks.
   b. Uterine muscles are stimulated to contract, and labor begins.
   c. Following the birth of the infant, placental tissues are expelled.

Neonatal Period (page 592)
1. This period extends from birth to the end of the fourth week.
2. The newborn must carry on respiration, obtain nutrients, excrete wastes, and regulate its body temperature.
3. The first breath must be powerful in order to expand the lungs.
4. The circulatory system undergoes changes when placental circulation ceases.
   a. Umbilical vessels constrict.
   b. The ductus venosus constricts.
   c. The foramen ovale is closed by a valve as blood pressure in the right atrium falls and pressure in the left atrium rises.

Clinical Application of Knowledge

1. One of the more common congenital cardiac disorders is a ventricular septum defect in which an opening remains between the right and left ventricles. What problem would such a defect create as blood moves through the heart?
2. What symptoms may occur in a newborn if its ductus arteriosus fails to close?
3. A pregnancy test is always done before a woman has any surgery that uses general anesthesia. (Anesthetic substances circulate in the blood stream.) Explain the reason for this test.
4. Why do you think the procedure of chorionic villi biopsy presents a greater risk to a fetus than does ultrasonography?

Review Activities

1. Define *growth* and *development.*
2. Describe how male and female sex cells are transported within the female reproductive tract.
3. Describe the process of fertilization.
4. Describe the process of cleavage.
5. Distinguish between a blastomere and a blastocyst.
6. Describe the formation of the inner cell mass and explain its significance.
7. Describe the process of implantation.
8. Explain how the primary germ layers form.
9. List the major body parts derived from ectoderm.
10. List the major body parts derived from mesoderm.
11. List the major body parts derived from endoderm.
12. Describe the formation of the placenta and explain its functions.
13. Define *placental membrane.*
14. Distinguish between the chorion and the amnion.
15. Explain the function of amniotic fluid.
16. Describe the formation of the umbilical cord.
17. Explain how the yolk sac and the allantois are related and list the functions of each.
18. Explain why the embryonic period of development is so critical.
19. Define *fetus.*
20. List the major changes that occur during the fetal stage of development.
21. Describe a full-term fetus.
22. Explain how the fetal circulatory system is adapted for intrauterine life.
23. Trace the pathway of blood from the placenta to the fetus and back to the placenta.
24. Discuss the events that occur during the birth process.
25. Describe the circulatory changes that occur in the newborn.

REFERENCE PLATES
Human Development

The following set of figures illustrates the development of the primary germ layers, and some of the organs and systems that develop from them. These diagrams will help you understand some of the changes that occur in the body during development.

PLATE 39

Formation of the primary germ layers. (*a*) An inner cell mass (blue) forms within the blastocyst (green) about the fourth day of development. (*b*) The amniotic cavity appears above the inner cell mass, and the cells of the inner cell mass become organized into a double-layered embryonic disk. The cells of the embryonic disk (blue) give rise to most of the future body cells. (*c*) During the third week of development, a slight depression, called the primitive groove, forms on the surface of the embryonic disk. Many cells of the upper layer of the embryonic disk become detached and migrate into the space below the disk. (*d*) Some of the migrating cells form a middle layer, called mesoderm (red), and others join the lower layer of embryonic disk cells to form the endoderm (yellow). The cells remaining in the upper layer of the embryonic disk are called ectoderm. (*e*) The primitive groove deepens to become the neural groove, and the mesodermal cells become organized into groups. (*f*) The neural groove gives rise to a neural tube, which will develop into the brain and spinal cord. The mesodermal cell masses will give rise to the organs of the skeletal, muscular, cardiovascular, and urinary systems.
(*g*) Outer ectodermal cells give rise to the outer layer of the skin; endodermal cells form the inner lining of the digestive tube and respiratory passages. (*h*) By the end of the fourth week of development, layers of ectodermal and mesodermal cells form the body wall; mesodermal cells give rise to mesentery and the membranes that form the inner linings of the body cavities.

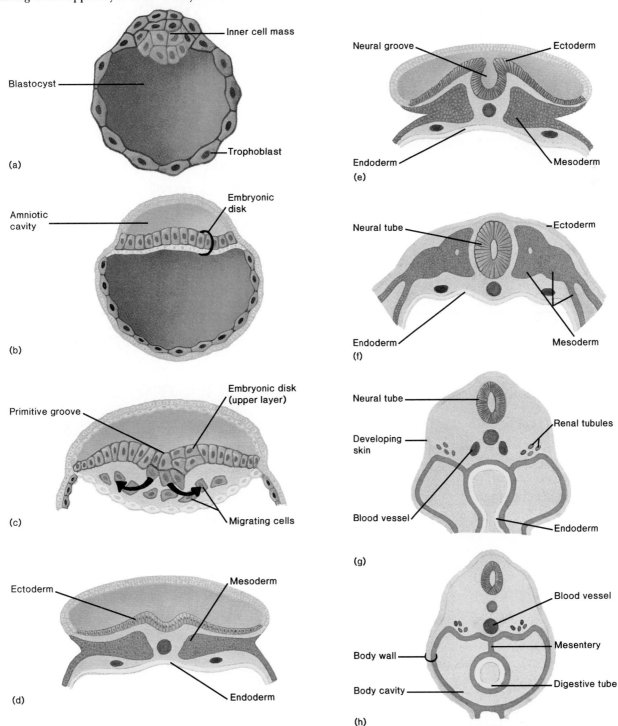

599

PLATE 40

The anterior portion of the neural tube develops into the brain. (*a*) During the fourth week of development, the neural tube (lateral view) forms three major cavities. (*b*) In the fifth week, the anterior cavity divides into two portions, the middle cavity remains undivided, while the posterior cavity divides into two portions. These cavities persist as ventricles and the tubes that connect them within the central nervous system. The wall surrounding these cavities forms the various regions of the brain. (*c*) The wall of the anterior cavity becomes the forebrain; the anterior portion of the forebrain develops into the cerebrum, while the wall of the posterior portion forms the diencephalon. The wall of the middle cavity becomes the midbrain, and the wall of the posterior cavity becomes the hindbrain, which forms the cerebellum, pons, and medulla oblongata. A more rapid growth in some areas of the wall results in a bending of the developing brain. (*d–f*) During the sixth through eleventh weeks, the cerebral hemispheres expand rapidly. As they grow, they cover the diencephalon, the midbrain, and part of the hindbrain.

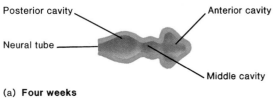

(a) **Four weeks**

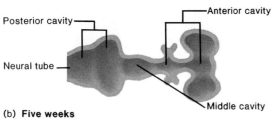
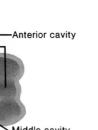

(b) **Five weeks**

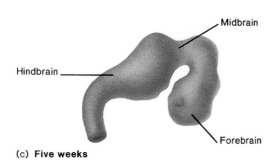

(c) **Five weeks**

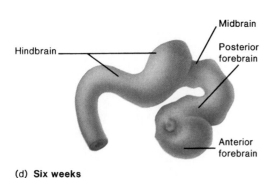

(d) **Six weeks**

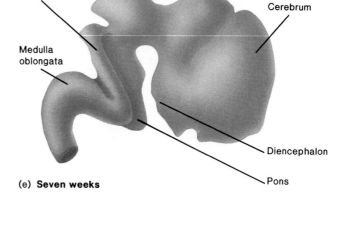

(e) **Seven weeks**

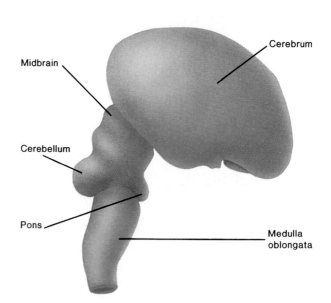

(f) **Eleven weeks**

PLATE 41

(a) During the fourth week of development, an optic stalk bearing an optic vesicle extends outward laterally from each side of the forebrain. (b) The distal portions of these vesicles fold inward to form a double-layered optic cup. (c) At the same time, the surface ectoderm nearest the optic cup also begins to fold inward, first forming a pit, and later developing into a vesicle that will become the lens. (d) The lens vesicle pinches off from the rest of the surface ectoderm during the sixth week. (e) The double-layered optic cup develops into the wall of the eye, the inner layer forming the nerve portion of the retina and the outer layer forming the pigmented portion of the retina. Embryonic connective tissue surrounding the optic cup forms the choroid coat and sclera of the eye. The cornea, which is continuous with the sclera, also develops from the embryonic connective tissue. However, it has an outer covering of epithelium formed from the surface ectoderm. (f) By the tenth week, the major accessory structures of the eye are also formed. (g) The eye of the newborn.

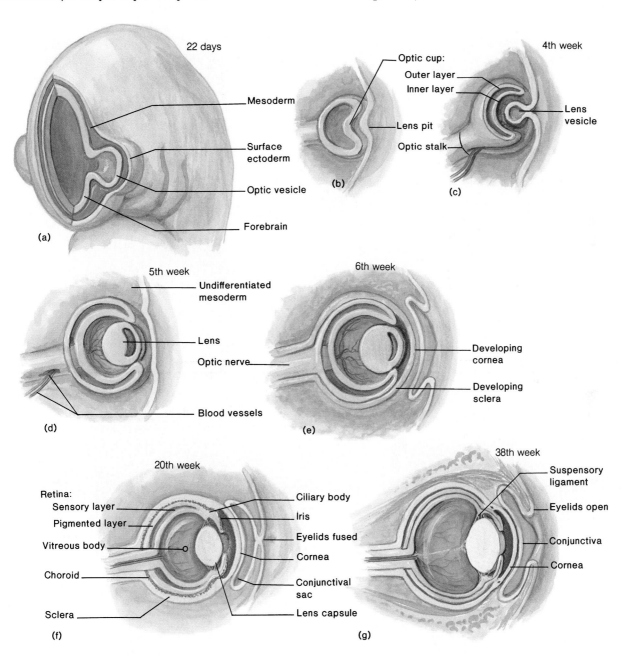

PLATE 42

(Note: Figures *a–d* show anterior views and figures *e–g* show frontal sections.) (*a*) During the fourth week, the heart develops from two tubular parts (heart tubes) that fuse. (*b,c*) The fused heart tubes, shown in anterior view, then bend, forming an S-shaped structure with a single ventricular cavity and a single atrial cavity. The atrium was initially located below the developing ventricle. (*d*) When the heart is bent, the atrium is moved behind the ventricle. At the end of the fourth week, the atrium has moved above the ventricle and formed two bulblike expansions. (*e–g*) From the fifth week to the eighth week, an interatrial septum grows inward from the wall and separates the single atrial cavity into right and left chambers, as shown in these frontal sections. The foramen ovale is the opening that persists between the atrial chambers until birth. During the same time, the interventricular septum grows upward from the wall near the apex of the heart and divides the ventricular cavity into right and left chambers. An interventricular foramen persists until the septum is completely formed during the eighth week (*h*).

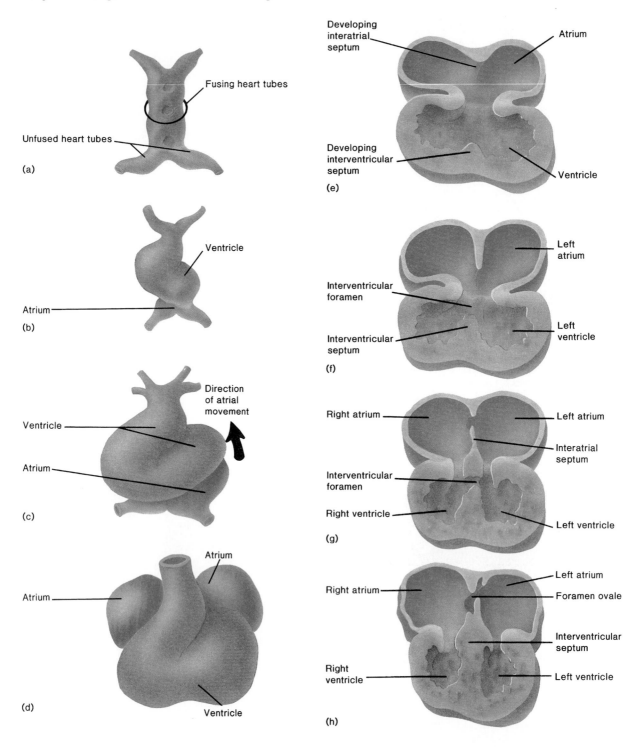

PLATE 43

(a) By the fourth week of development, a sagittal section of the abdominal cavity shows that the digestive system consists of a foregut, midgut, and hindgut. During this time, a portion of the foregut begins to dilate and forms the stomach. The midgut is connected to the yolk sac by a tube called the vitelline duct. Hepatic buds from the midgut begin the formation of the liver and gallbladder. The hindgut leads to a sac called the cloaca. (b) By the fifth week, dorsal and ventral pancreatic buds from the foregut become enlarged. These structures will eventually unite to form a single pancreas. The midgut elongates rapidly, forming a loop. (c,d) In the sixth and seventh weeks, the midgut loop rotates and forms the coils of the small intestine and part of the large intestine. (e) By the tenth week, the large intestine continues its rotation, and the anal canal opens into the amniotic cavity.

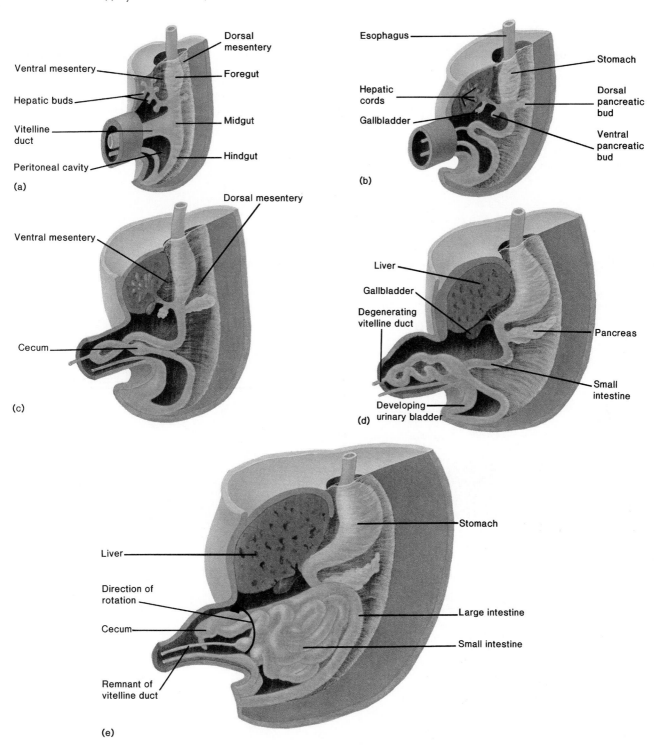

PLATE 44

(Note: Figure *a* shows a lateral view of a midsagittal section and figures *b–g* show anterior views.) The external reproductive organs of both male and female develop from the same embryonic tissues. (*a*) During the fourth week, the genital tubercle forms on the ventral surface between the umbilical cord and the embryonic tail. (*b*) In the sixth week, urogenital folds and labioscrotal folds develop below the tubercle. (*c*) In the seventh and eighth weeks, the genital tubercle lengthens and is called a phallus. The external reproductive organs of male and female remain undifferentiated. During the ninth week, these structures differentiate into male reproductive organs (*d,e*) or female reproductive organs (*f,g*).

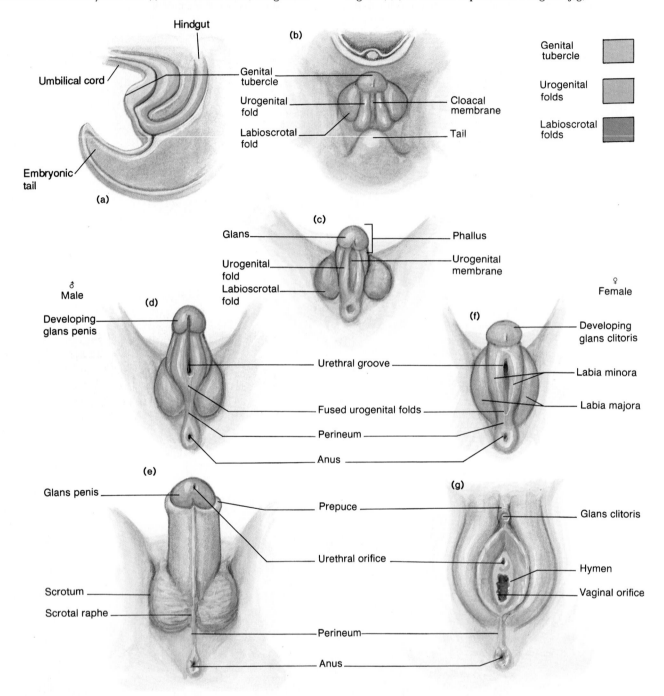

PLATE 45

These lateral views of embryos show some of the developmental changes occurring during the fifth through seventh weeks. (*a–c*) During the fifth week, the head grows rapidly. The maxillary and mandibular processes are visible and will develop into the upper and lower jaws. (*d,e*) During the

sixth week, notches appear in the hand and foot plates. (*f,g*) These notches deepen in the seventh week to further separate the finger and toe rays. Also during this time the tail recedes, the arms and legs lengthen, and the embryo takes on a humanlike appearance.

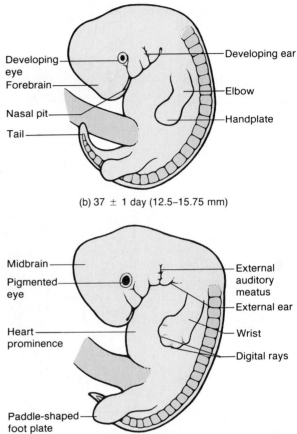

Developing eye
Forebrain
Nasal pit
Tail
Developing ear
Elbow
Handplate

(b) 37 ± 1 day (12.5–15.75 mm)

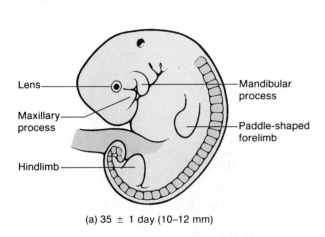

Lens
Maxillary process
Hindlimb
Mandibular process
Paddle-shaped forelimb

(a) 35 ± 1 day (10–12 mm)

Midbrain
Pigmented eye
Heart prominence
Paddle-shaped foot plate
External auditory meatus
External ear
Wrist
Digital rays

(c) 40 ± 1 day (16.0–21.0 mm)

PLATE 45—*Continued*

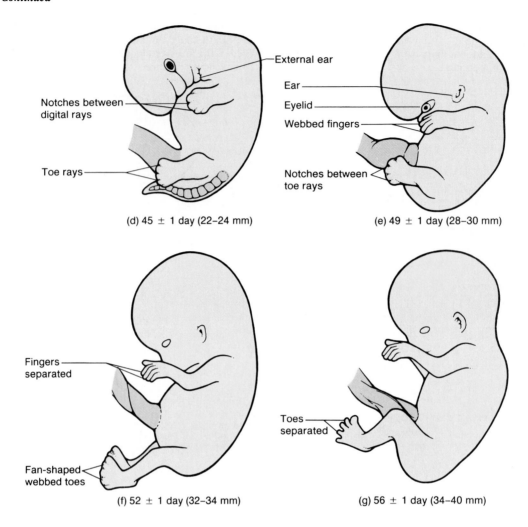

External ear

Notches between
digital rays

Toe rays

(d) 45 ± 1 day (22–24 mm)

Ear

Eyelid

Webbed fingers

Notches between
toe rays

(e) 49 ± 1 day (28–30 mm)

Fingers
separated

Fan-shaped
webbed toes

(f) 52 ± 1 day (32–34 mm)

Toes
separated

(g) 56 ± 1 day (34–40 mm)

REFERENCE PLATES

Human Cadavers

The following set of illustrations includes medial sections, transverse sections, and regional dissections of human cadavers. These photographs will help you visualize the spatial and proportional relationships between the major anatomic structures of actual specimens. The photographs can also serve as the basis for a review of the information you have gained from your study of the human organism.

PLATE 46
Sagittal section of the head and trunk.

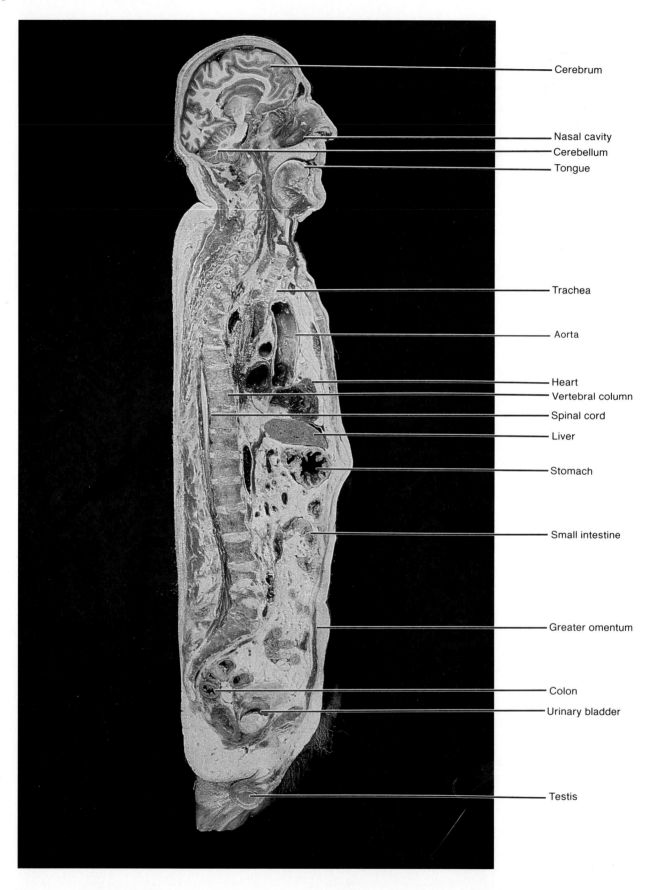

Cerebrum

Nasal cavity
Cerebellum
Tongue

Trachea

Aorta

Heart
Vertebral column
Spinal cord
Liver

Stomach

Small intestine

Greater omentum

Colon
Urinary bladder

Testis

PLATE 47
Sagittal section of the head and neck.

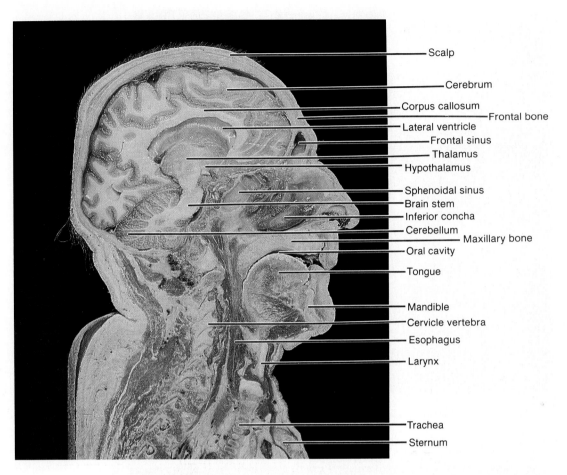

Scalp

Cerebrum

Corpus callosum
Frontal bone

Lateral ventricle

Frontal sinus

Thalamus

Hypothalamus

Sphenoidal sinus

Brain stem

Inferior concha

Cerebellum
Maxillary bone

Oral cavity

Tongue

Mandible

Cervicle vertebra

Esophagus

Larynx

Trachea

Sternum

PLATE 48

Viscera of the thoracic cavity, sagittal section.

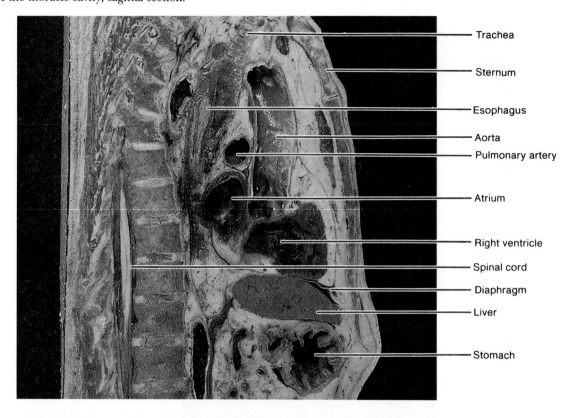

- Trachea
- Sternum
- Esophagus
- Aorta
- Pulmonary artery
- Atrium
- Right ventricle
- Spinal cord
- Diaphragm
- Liver
- Stomach

PLATE 49

Viscera of the abdominal cavity, sagittal section.

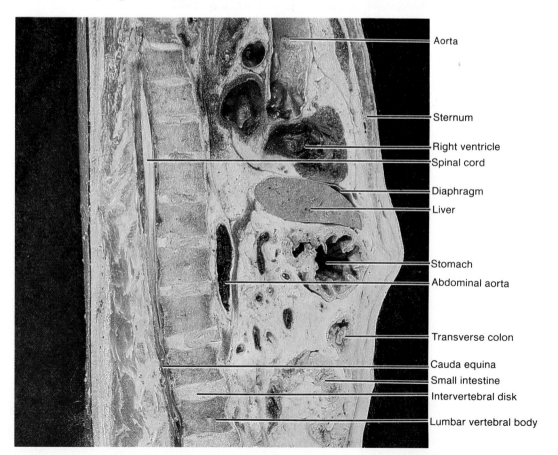

- Aorta
- Sternum
- Right ventricle
- Spinal cord
- Diaphragm
- Liver
- Stomach
- Abdominal aorta
- Transverse colon
- Cauda equina
- Small intestine
- Intervertebral disk
- Lumbar vertebral body

610

PLATE 50
Viscera of the pelvic cavity, sagittal section.

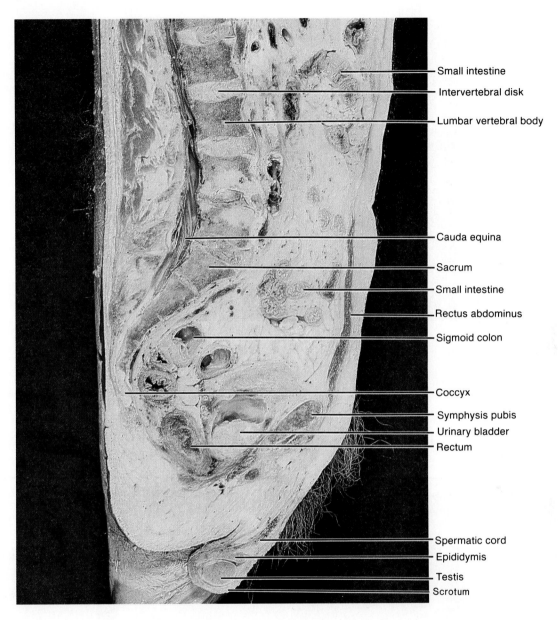

- Small intestine
- Intervertebral disk
- Lumbar vertebral body
- Cauda equina
- Sacrum
- Small intestine
- Rectus abdominus
- Sigmoid colon
- Coccyx
- Symphysis pubis
- Urinary bladder
- Rectum
- Spermatic cord
- Epididymis
- Testis
- Scrotum

PLATE 51

Transverse section of the head above the eyes, superior view.

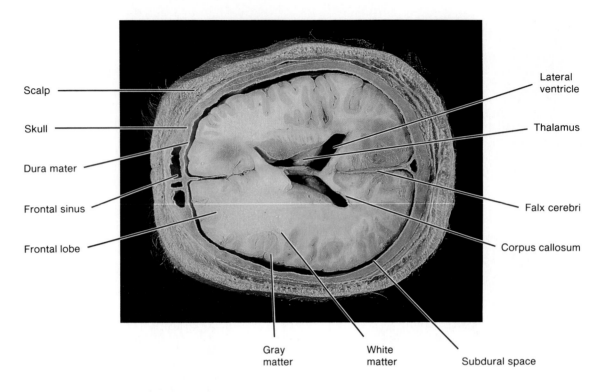

Scalp

Skull

Dura mater

Frontal sinus

Frontal lobe

Lateral ventricle

Thalamus

Falx cerebri

Corpus callosum

Subdural space

Gray matter

White matter

PLATE 52

Transverse section of the head at the level of the eyes, superior view.

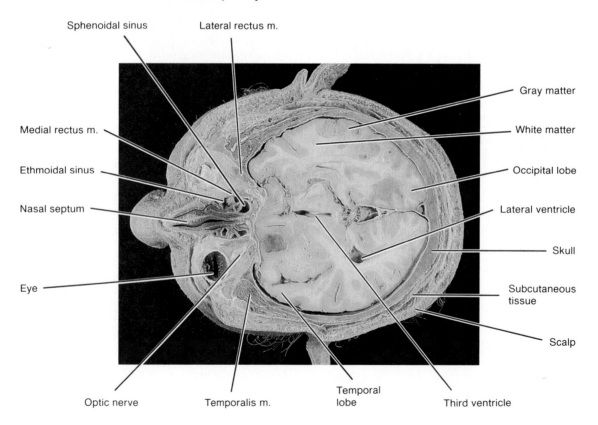

Sphenoidal sinus

Lateral rectus m.

Medial rectus m.

Ethmoidal sinus

Nasal septum

Eye

Gray matter

White matter

Occipital lobe

Lateral ventricle

Skull

Subcutaneous tissue

Scalp

Optic nerve

Temporalis m.

Temporal lobe

Third ventricle

PLATE 53

Transverse section of the neck, inferior view.

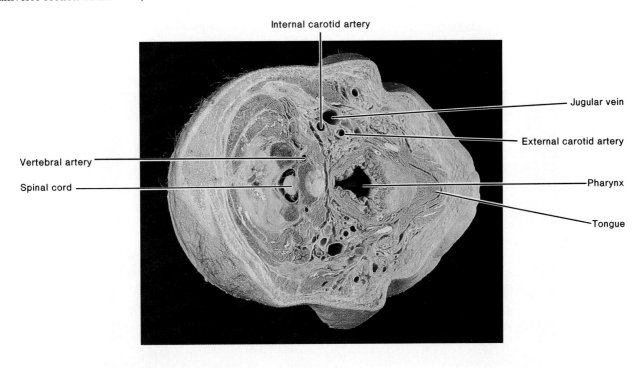

Internal carotid artery

Jugular vein

External carotid artery

Vertebral artery

Spinal cord

Pharynx

Tongue

PLATE 54

Transverse section of the thorax through the base of the heart, inferior view.

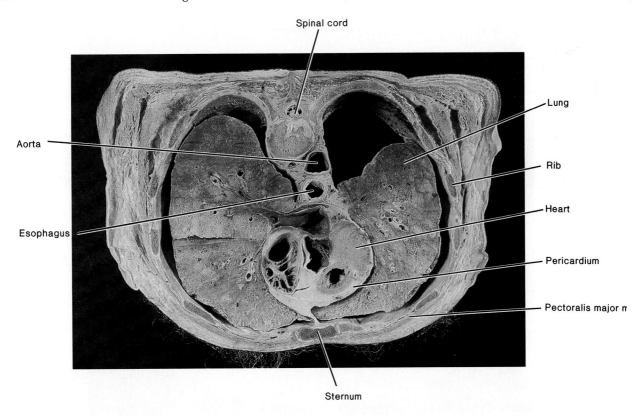

Spinal cord

Lung

Aorta

Rib

Heart

Esophagus

Pericardium

Pectoralis major m

Sternum

PLATE 55

Transverse section of the thorax through the heart, inferior view.

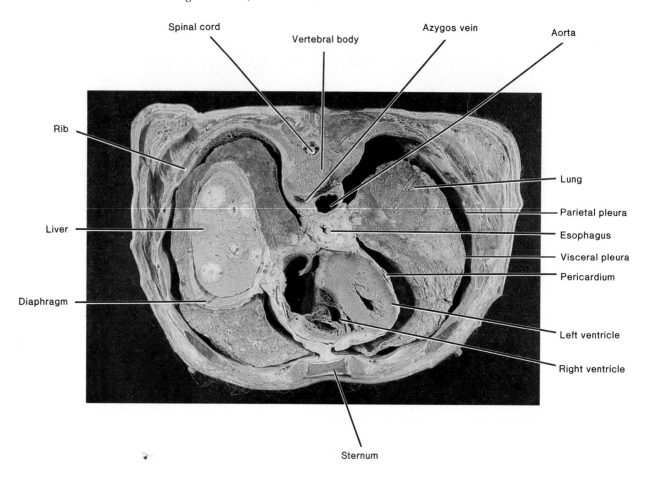

Spinal cord

Vertebral body

Azygos vein

Aorta

Rib

Lung

Parietal pleura

Liver

Esophagus

Visceral pleura

Pericardium

Diaphragm

Left ventricle

Right ventricle

Sternum

PLATE 56

Transverse section of the abdomen through the kidneys, inferior view.

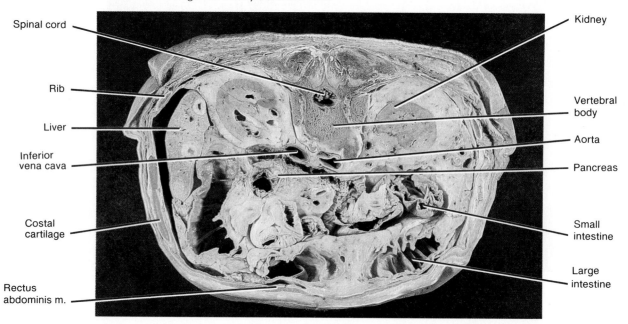

Spinal cord

Kidney

Rib

Vertebral body

Liver

Aorta

Inferior vena cava

Pancreas

Costal cartilage

Small intestine

Rectus abdominis m.

Large intestine

PLATE 57
Transverse section of the abdomen through the pancreas, inferior view.

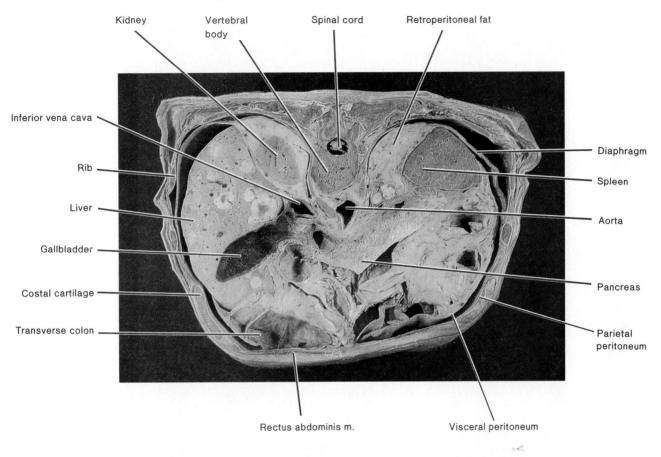

Kidney

Vertebral body

Spinal cord

Retroperitoneal fat

Inferior vena cava

Rib

Liver

Gallbladder

Costal cartilage

Transverse colon

Diaphragm

Spleen

Aorta

Pancreas

Parietal peritoneum

Rectus abdominis m.

Visceral peritoneum

PLATE 58

Transverse section of the male pelvic cavity, superior view.

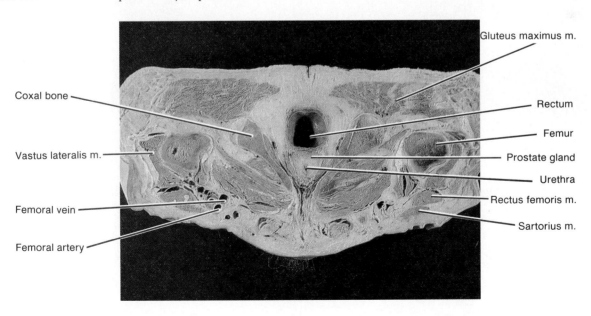

Gluteus maximus m.

Coxal bone

Vastus lateralis m.

Femoral vein

Femoral artery

Rectum

Femur

Prostate gland

Urethra

Rectus femoris m.

Sartorius m.

PLATE 59
Lateral view of the head.

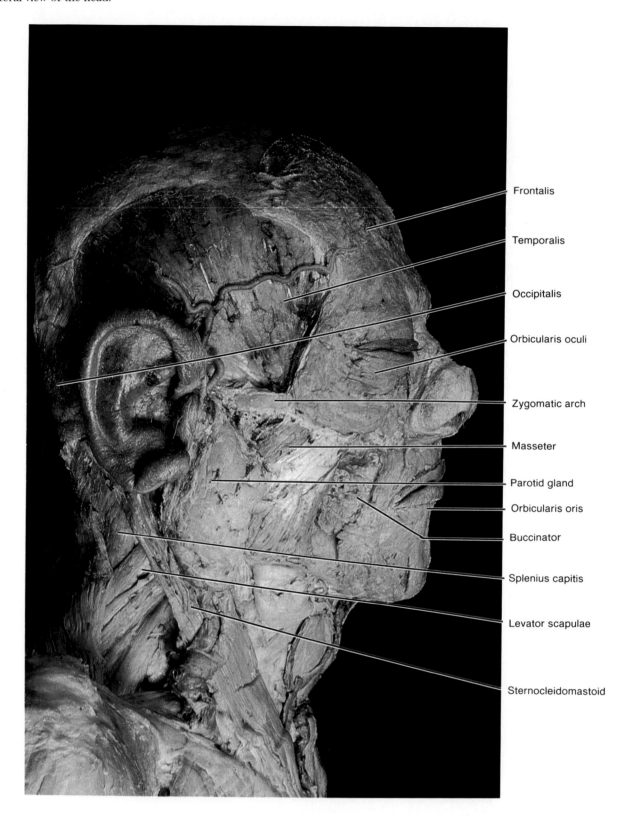

Frontalis

Temporalis

Occipitalis

Orbicularis oculi

Zygomatic arch

Masseter

Parotid gland

Orbicularis oris

Buccinator

Splenius capitis

Levator scapulae

Sternocleidomastoid

PLATE 60
Anterior view of the trunk.

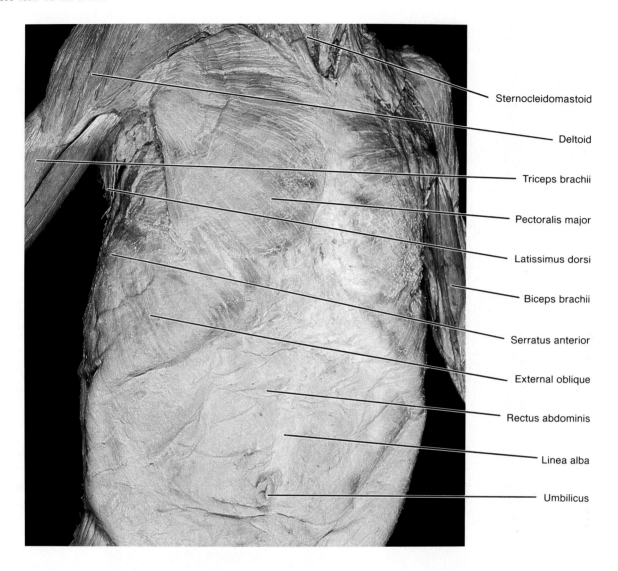

Sternocleidomastoid

Deltoid

Triceps brachii

Pectoralis major

Latissimus dorsi

Biceps brachii

Serratus anterior

External oblique

Rectus abdominis

Linea alba

Umbilicus

PLATE 61
Posterior view of the trunk, with deep thoracic muscles exposed on the left.

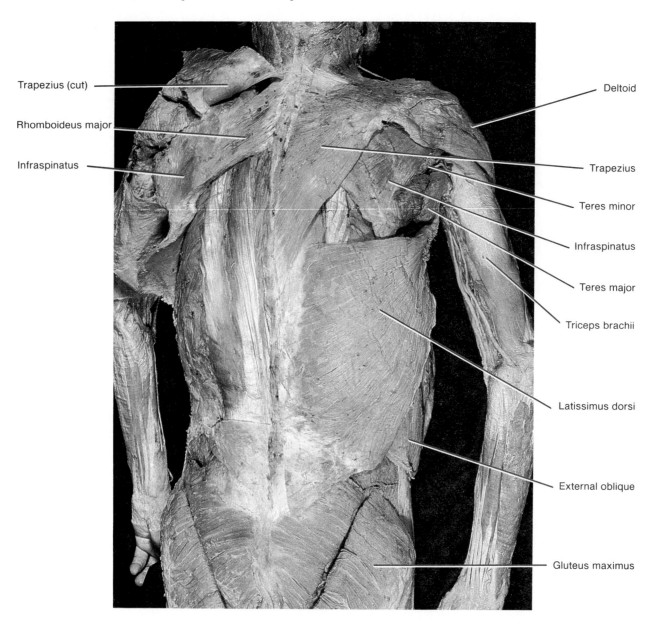

Trapezius (cut)

Rhomboideus major

Infraspinatus

Deltoid

Trapezius

Teres minor

Infraspinatus

Teres major

Triceps brachii

Latissimus dorsi

External oblique

Gluteus maximus

PLATE 62

Posterior view of the right thorax and upper arm.

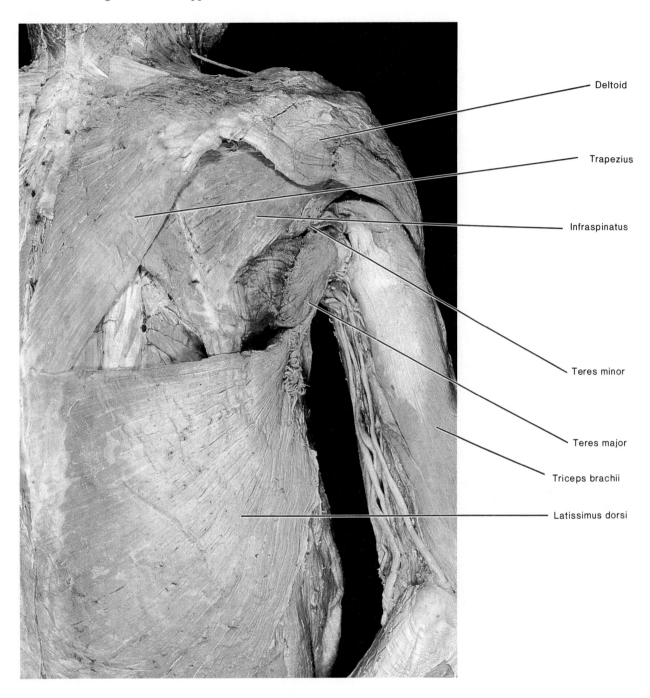

Deltoid

Trapezius

Infraspinatus

Teres minor

Teres major

Triceps brachii

Latissimus dorsi

PLATE 63
Posterior view of the right forearm and hand.

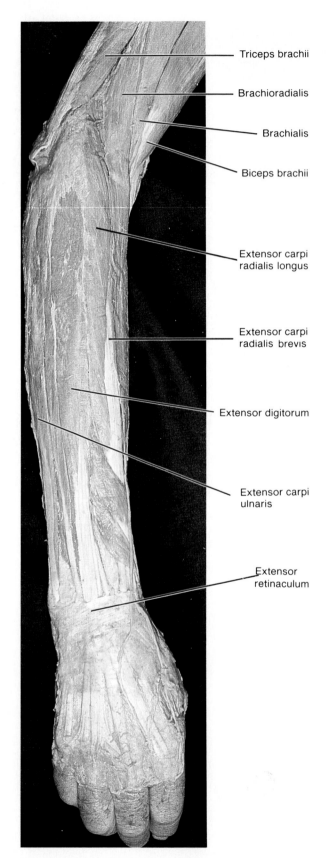

Triceps brachii

Brachioradialis

Brachialis

Biceps brachii

Extensor carpi
radialis longus

Extensor carpi
radialis brevis

Extensor digitorum

Extensor carpi
ulnaris

Extensor
retinaculum

PLATE 64
Anterior view of the right thigh.

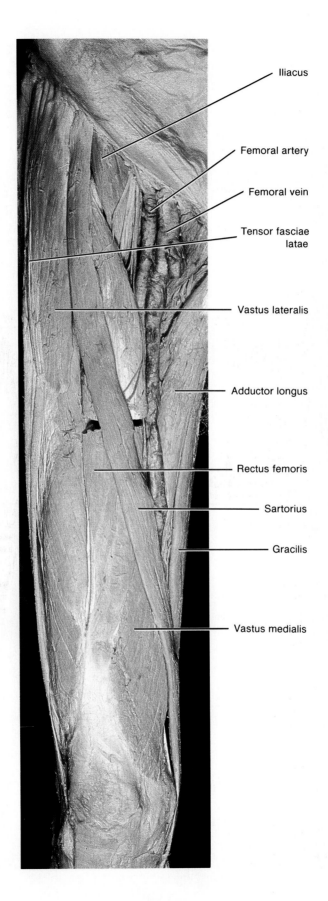

Iliacus

Femoral artery

Femoral vein

Tensor fasciae latae

Vastus lateralis

Adductor longus

Rectus femoris

Sartorius

Gracilis

Vastus medialis

PLATE 65
Posterior view of the right thigh.

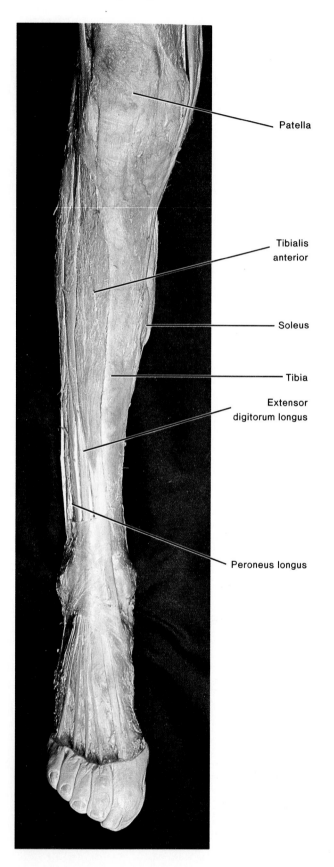

Gluteus medius

Gluteus maximus

Vastus lateralis
(covered by fascia)

Biceps femoris

Semitendinosus

Semimembranosus

PLATE 66
Anterior view of the right leg.

Patella

Tibialis
anterior

Soleus

Tibia

Extensor
digitorum longus

Peroneus longus

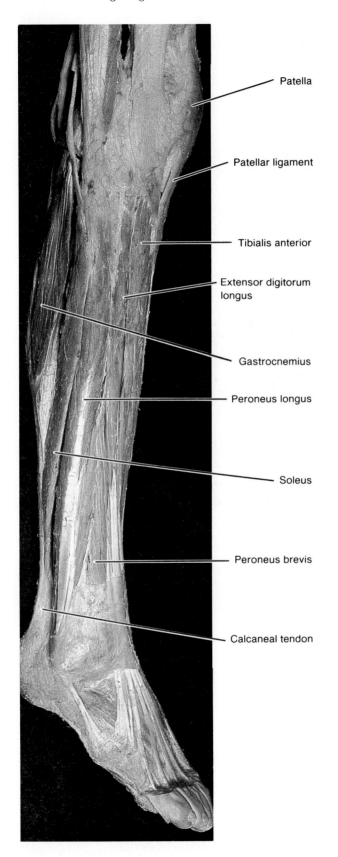

Patella

Patellar ligament

Tibialis anterior

Extensor digitorum longus

Gastrocnemius

Peroneus longus

Soleus

Peroneus brevis

Calcaneal tendon

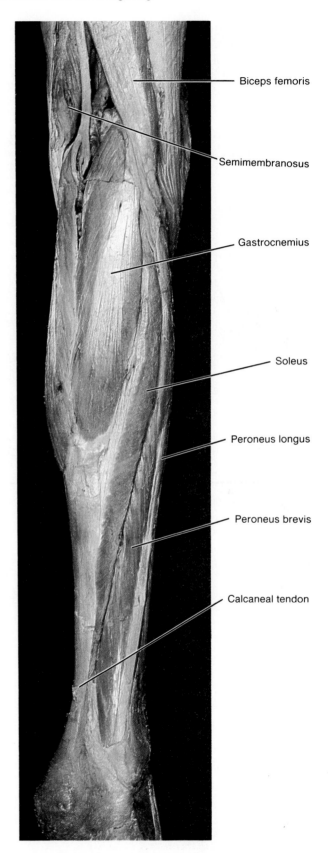

Biceps femoris

Semimembranosus

Gastrocnemius

Soleus

Peroneus longus

Peroneus brevis

Calcaneal tendon

PLATE 69
Thoracic viscera, anterior view. (Brachiocephalic vein has been removed to expose the aorta.)

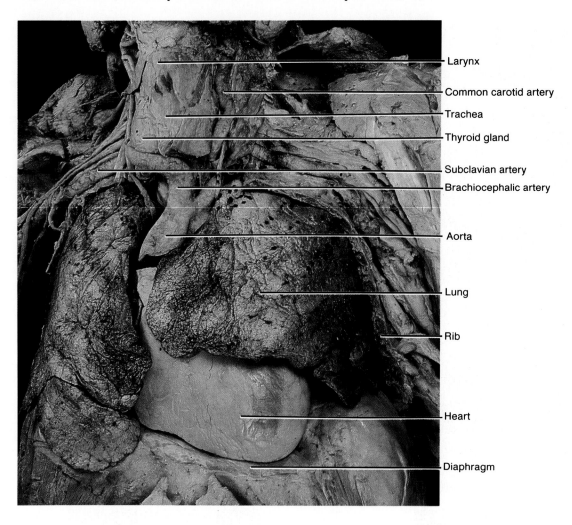

Larynx

Common carotid artery

Trachea

Thyroid gland

Subclavian artery

Brachiocephalic artery

Aorta

Lung

Rib

Heart

Diaphragm

PLATE 70
Thorax with the lungs removed, anterior view.

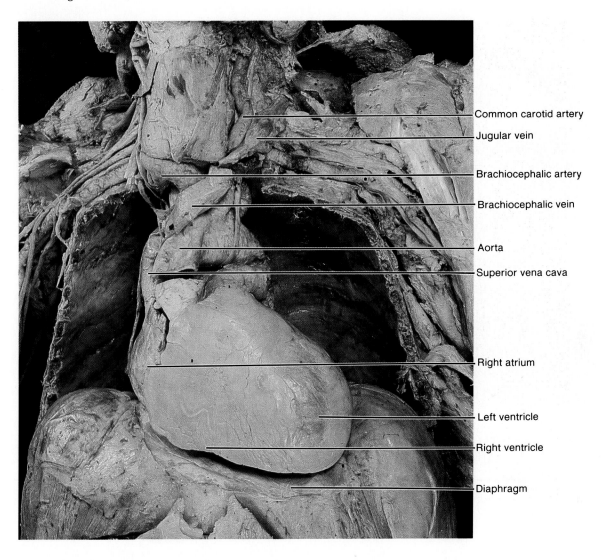

Common carotid artery

Jugular vein

Brachiocephalic artery

Brachiocephalic vein

Aorta

Superior vena cava

Right atrium

Left ventricle

Right ventricle

Diaphragm

PLATE 71
Thorax with the heart and lungs removed, anterior view.

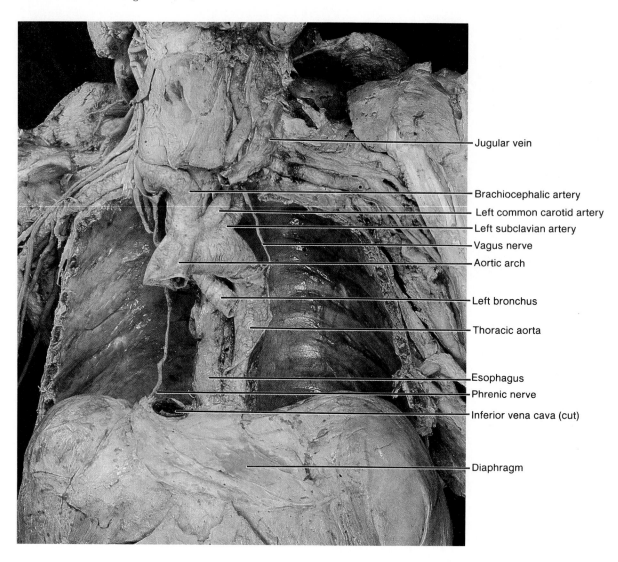

Jugular vein

Brachiocephalic artery

Left common carotid artery

Left subclavian artery

Vagus nerve

Aortic arch

Left bronchus

Thoracic aorta

Esophagus

Phrenic nerve

Inferior vena cava (cut)

Diaphragm

PLATE 72
Abdominal viscera, anterior view.

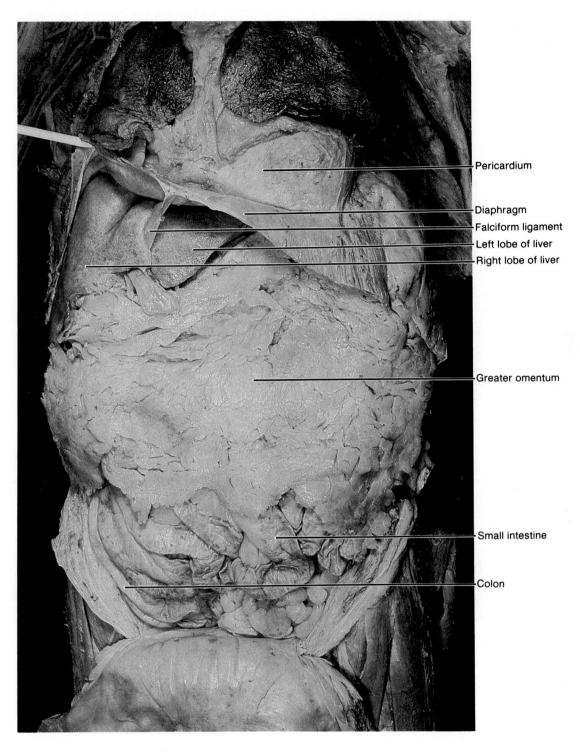

Pericardium

Diaphragm

Falciform ligament

Left lobe of liver

Right lobe of liver

Greater omentum

Small intestine

Colon

PLATE 73
Abdominal viscera with the greater omentum removed. (Small intestine has been displaced to the left.)

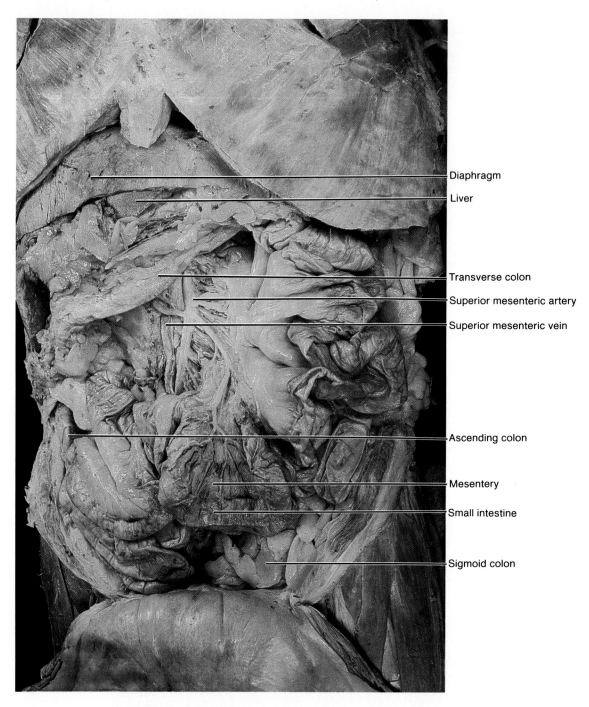

Diaphragm

Liver

Transverse colon

Superior mesenteric artery

Superior mesenteric vein

Ascending colon

Mesentery

Small intestine

Sigmoid colon

APPENDIX A
Units of Measurement and Their Equivalents

Lengths and Their Metric Equivalents

1 yard (yd) =
.9144 meter (m)
91.44 centimeters (cm)
914.4 millimeters (mm)

1 foot (ft) =
.31 meter (m)
30.48 centimeters (cm)
304.8 millimeters (mm)

1 inch (in) =
2.54 centimeters (cm)
25.4 millimeters (mm)

Metric Lengths and Their Equivalents

1 meter (m) =
100. centimeters (cm)
1,000. millimeters (mm)
39.37 inches (in)

1 centimeter (cm) =
.01 meter (m)
10. millimeters (mm)
.39 inches (in)

1 millimeter (mm) =
.1 centimeter (cm)
1,000. micrometer (μm)

1 micrometer (μm) =
.001 millimeter (mm)
1,000. nanometers (nm)

Weights and Their Metric Equivalents

1 ounce (oz) =
0.06 pound (lb)
28.35 grams (g)
28,350. milligrams (mg)

1 pound (lb) =
16. ounces (oz)
453.6 grams (g)
453,600. milligrams (mg)

Volumes and Their Metric Equivalents

1 fluid ounce (fl oz)
0.06 pint (pt)
29.6 milliliters (ml)
29.6 cubic centimeters (cc)

1 pint (pt) =
16. fluid ounces (fl oz)
473. milliliters (ml)
473. cubic centimeters (cc)

Metric Weights and Their Equivalents

1 gram (g) =
0.001 kilogram (kg)
1,000. milligrams (mg)
1,000,000. micrograms (μg)
0.032 ounce (oz)

1 kilogram (kg) =
1,000. grams (g)
1,000,000. milligrams (mg)
1,000,000,000. micrograms (μg)
35.3 ounces (oz)
2.2 pounds (lb)

1 milligram (mg) =
0.000001 kilogram (kg)
0.001 gram (g)
1,000. micrograms (μg)
0.000035 ounce (oz)

Metric Volumes and Their Equivalents

1 liter (l) =
1,000. milliliters (ml)
1,000. cubic centimeters (cc)
2.1 pints (pt)
34. fluid ounces (fl oz)

1 milliliter (ml) =
0.001 liter (l)
1. cubic centimeter (cc)
0.034 fluid ounce (fl oz)

APPENDIX B
Answers to Clinical Application of Knowledge Questions

Chapter 1, page 18

1. Ultrasonography would be preferable since it does not use radiation, but uses very high frequency sound waves.

2. X ray would most likely be used. The pin is made of dense material and therefore would appear very distinct on an X ray. The body organs would appear as shades of gray on the X-ray film, so the location of the pin within an organ could be visualized.

3. To perform an autopsy, a pathologist uses both gross and microscopic anatomy. Organs can be viewed macroscopically for anatomical changes related to disease or injury. Minute pieces of organs may be viewed microscopically for pathological (disease-related) changes.

Chapter 2, page 45

1. The individual with the tumor in the dorsal cavity would probably develop symptoms first. Since the dorsal cavity is smaller, the tumor would exert pressure against the brain or spinal cord, causing symptoms of visual disturbances, headaches, behavioral changes, disequilibrium, disturbances in gait, seizures, uncoordination, or weakness in the extremities.

2. As the uterus increased in size, the pelvic portion of the abdominopelvic cavity would increase in size also. The increase would be in both anterior and superior aspects.

3. Flattening of the diaphragm enlarges the thoracic cavity and compresses the abdominal cavity.

4. The organs in the umbilical region that could be the source of pain include the small intestine (obstruction), pancreas (pancreatitis), abdominal aorta (aneurysm), transverse colon (diverticulitis), or a distended urinary bladder.

Chapter 3, page 71

1. White blood cells normally increase in number during an infection. Exposure to X ray may destroy these cells, along with their ability to engulf and destroy bacteria and produce antibodies against bacteria and viruses.

2. Since the microtubules form spindle fibers, they are important in mitosis. A drug that decreased microtubule formation would therefore slow the rate of mitosis in all cells.

3. Lysosomes engulf and break down excess cellular parts.

4. Electron microscopy would be the most useful technique to observe enlarged mitochondria.

5. Malignant cells have larger nuclei and nucleoli than benign cells. Also, the malignant cells usually are undifferentiated and form disorganized masses.

Chapter 4, page 101

1. Secretions would accumulate in the respiratory passages, impeding the flow of air into and out of the lungs. Microorganisms could also be trapped in the airways, predisposing the individual to respiratory infections.

2. The tissue would become hardened, dry, and tough.

3. Cartilage and (dense) fibrous connective tissue have a limited blood supply, limiting the number of phagocytes, nutrients, and red blood cells (that carry oxygen) reaching the site, thus slowing healing.

4. Connective tissues occur throughout the body and are associated with organs of virtually every body system.

5. Neuroglial cells are capable of carrying out mitosis and are responsible for most tumors in nerve tissue.

Chapter 5, page 117

1. The increased mucus would be likely to block the airways and make breathing more difficult. The decreased serous fluid would make it more difficult for the pleural membranes to slide past each other as breathing occurs, causing pain.

2. The lost functions would include protection from invasion by microorganisms, effects of harmful substances, and excessive water loss. Other lost functions would be the temperature regulation and sensory functions of skin.

3. Ability to regulate body temperature would be decreased and the infant would be susceptible to decreased body temperature.

4. Hair follicles are tubelike structures of epidermis that extend down into the dermis. If the epidermis is lost, hair follicles serve as a source of new, dividing epidermal cells.

5. The major functions lost would be protection (loss of the barrier to infectious agents) and waterproofing.

6. The superficial burn would irritate and thus stimulate nerve endings (pain receptors); the deeper burn would destroy them.

Chapter 6, page 178

1. Children's bones are more flexible and resilient than those of adults, thus they are less susceptible to complete fractures.

2. Difficulties with coordination, balance, and gait.

3. As an individual ages, intervertebral disks lose water and become thinner and more rigid, resulting in compression fractures of the anteriorly located vertebral bodies. These events, in turn, cause the vertebral column to shorten and develop an exaggerated thoracic curvature.

4. The walls of the sinus may press on the eyeball, nasal cavity, or the mouth.

5. When a bone is fractured, a cartilaginous callus is formed between the broken ends. This cartilage is then removed by osteoclasts and bone is formed by osteoblasts.

6. Rate of development—If the posterior fontanel has closed two months after birth, the sphenoid three months after birth, the mastoid twelve months after birth, and the anterior by eighteen months or two years of age, the infant is probably developing on time. Delayed closing of these fontanels may indicate slower than normal development.

Intracranial pressure—Depressed or sunken-in fontanels may indicate decreased intracranial pressure or dehydration. Bulging fontanels may indicate increased intracranial pressure or overhydration.

Chapter 7, page 212

1. Ligaments are composed of dense fibrous connective tissue, which has a poor blood supply. Cartilage is a rigid type of connective tissue that lacks a direct blood supply, resulting in slow healing.

2. The shoulder and hip joints are ball-and-socket joints in which the heads of the humerus and femur, respectively, fit into and are protected by bony sockets. These sockets, in turn, are surrounded by joint capsules, ligaments, and muscles that protect against injuries. The knee joint is of the condyloid and hinge types, has shallow articular surfaces, and is protected only by ligaments, thus making it more susceptible to injuries.

3. The hip joint could be more satisfactorily replaced. The socket of the hip joint is deeper, its ligaments are larger and stronger, and it is surrounded by muscles. It also does not bear as much weight as the knee joint.

4. There would be a loss of matrix from the bones, resulting in bone destruction and brittleness.

5. Keeping the joints mobile prevents stiffness, which leads to immobility. It also prevents contractures, or atrophy and shortening of muscles, which may result in permanent flexion of joints.

6. Ligaments holding the articulating surfaces of the shoulder together are rather weak. Dislocating the shoulder would stretch or strain these ligaments, further weakening them, making future dislocations more likely.

Chapter 8, page 254

1. The levator ani and coccygeus muscles.

2. The gluteus medius muscle covers the superior lateral portion of the ilium. Bone markings that are used to establish the location of this muscle

are the greater trochanter of the femur, the anterior superior iliac spine, posterior iliac spine, and crest of the ilium.

3. Passively moving or electrically stimulating the injured muscle would prevent muscle atrophy and contractures.

4. The quadriceps muscles are the prime movers for extension of the leg at the knee, and the hamstrings muscles are the prime movers for flexion of the leg at the knee. Nonweight-bearing flexion and extension exercises would strengthen the muscles without further injuring the joint.

Chapter 9, page 324

1. (a) Axons of peripheral nerves are able to regenerate due to Schwann cells realigning themselves within the connective tissue endoneurium, which forms a tube in which regenerating axonal sprouts are guided back to their original connections at the neuromuscular junction. Schwann cells also form new myelin around the growing axon. (b) Axons of severed neurons in the central nervous system lack Schwann cells and a connective tissue endoneurium, preventing axonal regeneration.

2. Myelin sheaths in the central nervous system speed impulse conduction along the axons of nerve fibers. Therefore, motor nerve impulses would not be conducted to neuromuscular junctions in individuals with multiple sclerosis due to scarring and degeneration of the myelin sheath.

3. Right occipital lobe—loss of left half of visual field in each eye (left homonymous hemianopsis); right temporal lobe—partial hearing loss in both ears.

4. Olfactory nerves: Identify substances by smell.
Optic nerves: Identify objects by sight.
Oculomotor, trochlear, and abducens nerves: Follow a moving object with the eyes.
Trigeminal nerves: Clench teeth; feel touch and pain on face.
Facial nerves: Raise eyebrows, move lips (smile); taste sweet substance on tip of tongue.

Vestibulocochlear nerves: Hear sounds; maintain balance (with eyes closed).

Glossopharyngeal and vagus nerves: Speak and swallow properly.

Accessory nerves: Elevate scapula and turn head side to side.

Hypoglossal nerves: Speak and move tongue.

5. Descending (motor) anterior, lateral, and corticospinal tracts in the spinal cord would be affected on the same side as the injury, paralysis. Ascending (sensory) lateral spinothalmic tracts for temperature and pain transmission cross over to the opposite side of the spinal cord before ascending, resulting in loss of these sensations below the level of the injury on that side of the body.

6. Neuroglia are more numerous and are capable of mitotic division; mature neurons are incapable of undergoing mitosis.

7. If the biceps and triceps reflexes are present, the injury would be below C7. If the biceps and triceps reflexes are absent, the injury would be above C5. If the biceps reflex is present and the triceps is absent, the injury would be between C5 and C7.

Chapter 10, page 366

1. The bullet would probably cause localized, rather than widespread stimulation of pain receptors, due to acute (A-delta) fibers being stimulated. Crushing of the skin would stimulate more free nerve endings there and in subcutaneous tissues, resulting in stimulation of both acute and chronic (C) pain fibers.

2. Since the cells of the retina would become separated from their supply of oxygen and nutrients, there would be death of retinal cells, progressive loss of vision, and eventual blindness.

3. Shorter, horizontally directed auditory tubes would enable microorganisms to enter the middle ear more easily, since the mucous membrane of the pharynx is continuous with that of the middle ear.

4. Pain nerve fibers from the heart and pain fibers from the skin of the left arm, shoulder, and the base of the neck follow common nerve pathways to the spinal cord and then to the brain.

5. The senses of hearing and equilibrium might be affected.

Chapter 11, page 382

1. The enlarged thyroid gland might press against other nearby organs such as the larynx, trachea, esophagus, or common carotid arteries. This may interfere with their functions.

2. The posterior portions of the thyroid gland should be kept intact because the parathyroid glands are attached. Removal of the entire thyroid would also result in loss of the parathyroid glands.

Chapter 12, page 417

1. Gastric secretions would be greatly reduced. Protein digestion, which normally begins in the stomach, would be decreased or absent. The patient would also be prone to pernicious anemia as a result of the removal of parietal cells of the stomach, which secrete intrinsic factor.

   Removal of 95% of the stomach would also reduce its storage capacity. The patient would need to eat several small meals per day and drink fluids between, rather than with meals.

2. The cystic duct from the gallbladder empties into the common bile duct, which along with the main pancreatic duct, empties into the duodenum at the hepatopancreatic sphincter. Cholecystitis (especially if accompanied by gallstones that block the common bile duct) often causes reflux of bile into the pancreatic duct, which activates pancreatic enzymes, leading to pancreatitis.

3. Since villi greatly increase the surface area in the small intestine, destruction of villi (and microvilli on epithelial cells) would decrease the digestion and absorption of food.

4. If tooth enamel is damaged by any abrasive action, the enamel is not replaced.

Chapter 13, page 446

1. Air entering a tracheostomy would not be warmed, filtered for removal of microorganisms and duct particles, or humidified by the nasal passages or oropharynx. The patient may experience irritation around and inside the tracheostomy opening (due to dryness), coughing, and respiratory infections.

2. Loss of elastic tissue would make both inspiration and expiration more difficult.

3. There would be a decrease or absence of ciliary action and mucus secretion, which would inhibit removal of inhaled dust particles and pathogens through the cough reflex. Inhaled air would not be warmed or humidified before reaching the lungs.

4. The lung, which appears dark in an X-ray film, would be smaller on the affected side.

5. The inferior lobe is separated from the other lobes by connective tissue and is supplied with air by a separate secondary bronchus. Thus, the functioning of one lobe does not depend upon the functioning of others.

Chapter 14, page 497

1. Since the posterior interventricular artery, a branch of the right coronary artery, supplies blood to both ventricles, the ventricular myocardium would receive some blood.

2. The dye failed to stain the brain tissue because of the blood-brain barrier. The dye was unable to move from the brain capillaries to the brain tissue.

3. Blood flow would probably carry the embolus to the pulmonary vessels. Symptoms would include dyspnea, chest pain, rapid heartbeat, cough, spitting up blood (hemoptysis), and restlessness (due to cerebral hypoxia).

4. Femoral artery, external iliac artery, common iliac artery, aorta (abdominal and thoracic), aortic arch, ascending aorta, left coronary artery.

5. Increased capillary pressure could cause varicosities in the thin-walled esophageal veins (known as esophageal varicies), which may rupture, resulting in massive hemorrhage. It could also cause hemorrhoids, caput medusae (dilated cutaneous veins radiating out from the umbilicus), ascities, peripheral edema, and splenomegaly.

6. Brachial vein, axillary vein, subclavian vein, brachiocephalic vein, superior vena cava, heart, aorta, (brachiocephalic artery), common carotid artery, external carotid artery, lingual artery.

Chapter 15, page 517

1. Lymph nodes function to filter out and thus trap microorganisms and cancer cells as they travel between tissues and the blood stream. Lymph node biopsy can therefore be used in diagnosing leukemias, cancers of the lymphatic system, metastatic cancers, and fungal infections (especially of the lungs).

2. The dermis of the skin contains many lymph capillaries.

3. Cancer cells may be transported from one site to another in lymph vessels.

4. Lymph nodes lie along lymphatic pathways. Thus, excising them interrupts the flow of lymph from tissues distal to the excised nodes. The accumulation of tissue fluid (and increased presence of plasma proteins) causes swelling.

5. The infants susceptibility to infections would increase. The thymus gland is the site of T-cell maturation. T-cell deficiency results in the individual having little or no resistance to certain infections.

Chapter 16, page 538

1. Kidney stones are often composed of calcium. Therefore, decreased calcium intake should decrease kidney stone formation.

2. The bladder contacts the anterior wall of the uterus. As the uterus increases in size, it compresses the urinary bladder.

3. Since penicillin is excreted unchanged in the urine, the penicillin will act while the urine is in the urinary bladder. Therefore, the route to the bladder is through the kidneys.

   Absorption into capillaries of the small intestine, venules, superior mesenteric vein, portal vein, liver, hepatic vein, inferior vena cava, heart, aorta, renal arteries, kidneys (glomeruli, glomerular capsule, tubules, collecting ducts, renal pelvis), ureters, urinary bladder.

4. The female urethra is shorter than that of the male. Therefore, microorganisms could ascend into the bladder more readily.

Chapter 17, page 569

1. There would be no significant decrease in secondary sex characteristics following removal of one testis.

   Removal of both testes would result in decreased rate of growth of the beard and body hair due to significant reduction in testosterone production.

   Removal of the prostate gland would have no effect on secondary sex characteristics.

2. Ultrasonography does not use ionizing radiation, which can cause cellular injury to the oocytes within the nearby ovaries.

3. Fluid will still be produced since the seminal vesicles, prostate gland, and bulbourethral glands secrete fluid. However, this fluid will not contain sperm cells.

4. Removing one ovary will have little or no effect on the secondary sexual characteristics. Removal of both ovaries will result in decreased development of mammary glands, decreased deposition of fat in the breasts and buttocks, and decreased vascularization of the skin.

Chapter 18, page 596

1. Problems could include mixing of oxygenated and deoxygenated blood in the right and left ventricles, resulting in cyanosis and hypoxia of body organs. It could also result in increased distension and workload of the right ventricle, which would impede circulation of blood to the lungs and result in already-oxygenated blood being recirculated through the lungs.

2. Blood from the aorta would flow into the pulmonary trunk, causing an increased workload for the right ventricle as well as decreased blood flow to body cells.

3. A general anesthetic that circulates in the mother's blood may be able to cross the placental membrane and enter the blood vessels of an embryo. Consequently, a pregnant woman should not have general anesthesia, since it may affect the developing embryo.

4. Chorionic villi biopsy is an invasive procedure that carries the risk of bleeding and inducing premature labor.

APPENDIX C
Suggestions for Additional Reading

Adams, R. V. 1981. *Principles of neurology.* 2d ed. New York: McGraw-Hill.

Annis, L. F. 1978. *The child before birth.* New York: Cornell Univ. Press.

Avers, C. J. 1988. *Cell biology.* 3d ed. New York: D. Van Nostrand Co.

Balinsky, B. I. 1981. *An introduction to embryology.* 5th ed. Philadelphia: W. B. Saunders.

Basmajian, J. V. 1980. *Grant's method of anatomy.* 10th ed. Baltimore: Williams and Wilkins.

Bellanti, J. A. 1985. *Immunology.* Philadelphia: W. B. Saunders.

Bower, T. G. 1982. *Development in infancy,* 2d ed. San Francisco: W. H. Freeman.

Brooks, F. P., ed. 1978. *Gastrointestinal pathophysiology.* 2d ed. New York: Oxford Univ. Press.

Chewning, E. B. 1979. *Anatomy illustrated.* New York: Simon and Schuster.

Clemente, C. D. 1981. *Anatomy: a regional atlas of the human body.* 2d ed. Philadelphia: Lea and Febiger.

Copenhaver, W. M., et. al. 1978. *Bailey's textbook of histology.* 17th ed. Baltimore, Md.: Williams and Wilkins.

Cummings, G., and Semple, S. 1973. *Disorders of the respiratory system.* Philadelphia: J. B. Lippincott.

DeDuve, C. 1984. *The living cell.* New York: W. H. Freeman and Co.

DiFiore, M. S. 1981. *An atlas of human histology.* 5th ed. Philadelphia: Lea and Febiger.

Durrant, J. D., and Lovrinic, J. H. 1977. *Basis of hearing science.* Baltimore: Williams and Wilkins.

Fawcett, D. W. 1986. *A textbook of histology.* 11th ed. Philadelphia: W. B. Saunders.

Fischer, K., and Lazerson, A. 1984. *Human development: from conception through adolescence.* San Francisco: W. H. Freeman.

Frankel, V. H., and Nordine, M. 1980. *Basic biomechanics of the skeletal system.* Philadelphia: Lea and Febiger.

Freese, A. S. 1977. *The miracle of vision.* New York: Harper and Row.

Grabowski, C. T. 1983. *Human reproduction and development.* Philadelphia: W. B. Saunders.

Helwig, E. B., and Mostofi, F. D., eds. 1980. *The skin.* New York: Krieger.

Higging, J. R. 1977. *Human movement: an integrated approach.* St. Louis: C. V. Mosby.

Hinson, M. M. 1981. *Kinesiology.* 2d ed. Dubuque, Ia.: Wm. C. Brown.

Hurst, J. W., ed. 1979. *The heart.* New York: McGraw-Hill.

Johnson, L. G. 1987. *Biology.* Dubuque, Ia.: Wm. C. Brown.

Kuffler, S. W., et al. 1984. *From neuron to brain: a cellular approach to function of the nervous system.* Sunderland, Mass.: Sinauer Associates.

Last, R. J. 1984. *Anatomy, regional and applied.* 7th ed. Boston: Little, Brown, and Co.

Leeson, T. S., and Leeson, C. R. 1981. *Histology.* 4th ed. Philadelphia: W. B. Saunders.

Lyons, A. S., and Petrucelli, R. J. 1978. *Medicine: an illustrated history.* New York: Harry N. Abrams.

Martin, C. 1985. *Endocrine physiology.* New York: Oxford Univ. Press.

McMinn, R. M. H., and Hutchings, R. T. 1988. *Color atlas of human anatomy.* Chicago: Year Book Medical Publishers.

Moore, K. L. 1982. *The developing human.* 3d ed. Philadelphia: W. B. Saunders.

Nauta, J. H., and Feirtag, M., eds. 1985. *Fundamental neuroanatomy.* San Francisco: W. H. Freeman.

Nilsson, L. 1973. *Behold man.* Boston: Little, Brown.

Pengelley, E. T. 1978. *Sex and human life.* Reading, Mass.: Addison-Wesley.

Platt, W. R. 1979. *Color atlas and textbook of hematology.* 2d ed. Philadelphia: J. B. Lippincott.

Ross, M. H., and Reith, E. J. 1985. *Histology: a text and atlas.* New York: Harper and Row.

Rosse, C., and Clawson, D. K. 1980. *The musculoskeletal system in health and disease.* Philadelphia: Harper and Row.

Shepherd, G. M. 1987. *Neurobiology.* New York: Oxford Univ. Press.

Simon, W. H. 1978. *The human joint in health and disease.* Philadelphia: Univ. of Pennsylvania Press.

Snell, R. S. 1978. *Atlas of clinical anatomy.* Boston: Little, Brown.

Vaughan, J. M. 1981. *The physiology of bone.* 3d ed. New York: Oxford Univ. Press.

Weiss, L., and Greep, R. O. 1983. *Histology.* 5th ed. New York: McGraw-Hill.

Wilson, D. B., and Wilson, J. W. 1983. *Human anatomy.* 2d ed. New York: Oxford Univ. Press.

Wolfe, S. L. 1981. *Biology of the cell.* 2d ed. Belmont, Calif.: Wadsworth.

Woodburne, R. T. 1988. *Essentials of human anatomy.* 8th ed. New York: Oxford Univ. Press.

GLOSSARY

Each word in this glossary is followed by a phonetic guide to pronunciation.

In this guide, any unmarked vowel that ends a syllable or stands alone as a syllable has the long sound. Thus, the word *play* would be spelled *pla*.

Any unmarked vowel that is followed by a consonant has the short sound. The word *tough*, for instance, would be spelled *tuf*.

If a long vowel does appear in the middle of a syllable (followed by a consonant), it is marked with the macron (ˉ), the sign for a long vowel. Thus, the word *plate* would be phonetically spelled plāt.

Similarly, if a vowel stands alone or ends a syllable, but has the short sound, it is marked with a breve (˘).

A

abdomen (ab-do'men) Portion of the body between the diaphragm and the pelvis.

abduction (ab-duk'shun) Movement of a body part away from the midline.

absorption (ab-sorp'shun) The taking in of substances by cells or membranes.

accessory organs (ak-ses'o-re or'ganz) Organs that supplement the functions of other organs; accessory organs of the digestive and reproductive systems.

accommodation (ah-kom''o-da'shun) Adjustment of the lens for close vision.

acetylcholine (as''ĕ-til-ko'lēn) Substance secreted at the axon ends of many neurons that transmits a nerve impulse across a synapse.

adaptation (ad''ap-ta'shun) Adjustment to environmental conditions.

adduction (ah-duk'shun) Movement of a body part toward the midline.

adenoids (ad'ĕ-noids) The pharyngeal tonsils located in the nasopharynx.

adipose tissue (ad'i-pōs tish'u) Fat-storing tissue.

adrenal cortex (ah-dre'nal kor'teks) The outer portion of the adrenal gland.

adrenal glands (ah-dre'nal glandz) Endocrine glands located on the tops of the kidneys.

adrenal medulla (ah-dre'nal me-dul'ah) The inner portion of the adrenal gland.

adrenocorticotropic hormone (ah-dre''no-kor''te-ko-trōp'ik hor'mōn) ACTH; hormone secreted by the anterior lobe of the pituitary gland that stimulates activity in the adrenal cortex.

afferent arteriole (af'er-ent ar-te're-ōl) Vessel that supplies blood to the glomerulus of a nephron within the kidney.

agranulocytes (a-gran'u-lo-sīt) A nongranular leukocyte.

aldosterone (al-dos'ter-ōn) A hormone, secreted by the adrenal cortex.

alimentary canal (al''i-men'tar-e kah-nal') The tubular portion of the digestive tract that leads from the mouth to the anus.

allantois (ah-lan'to-is) A structure that appears during embryonic development and functions in the formation of umbilical blood vessels.

alveolar ducts (al-ve'o-lar dukts') Fine tubes that carry air to the air sacs of the lungs.

alveolar pores (al-ve'o-lar pōrz) Minute openings in the walls of air sacs, which permit air to pass from one alveolus to another.

alveolar process (al-ve'o-lar pros'es) Projection on the border of the jaw in which the bony sockets of the teeth are located.

alveolus (al-ve'o-lus) An air sac of a lung; a saclike structure.

amniocentesis (am''ne-o-sen-te'sis) A procedure in which a sample of amniotic fluid is removed through the abdominal wall of a pregnant woman.

amnion (am'ne-on) An embryonic membrane that encircles a developing fetus and contains amniotic fluid.

amniotic cavity (am''ne-ot'ik kav'i-te) Fluid-filled space enclosed by the amnion.

amniotic fluid (am''ne-ot'ik floo'id) Fluid within the amniotic cavity that surrounds the developing fetus.

anal canal (a'nal kah-nal') The last two or three inches of the large intestine that opens to the outside as the anus.

anaphase (an'ah-fāz) Stage in mitosis during which duplicate chromosomes move to opposite poles of the cell.

anaplasia (an''ah-pla'ze-ah) A change in which mature cells become more primitive; a loss of differentiation.

anastomosis (ah-nas''to-mo'sis) A union of nerve fibers or blood vessels to form an intercommunicating network.

anatomy (ah-nat'o-me) Branch of science dealing with the form and structure of body parts.

androgen (an'dro-jen) A male sex hormone such as testosterone.

aneurysm (an'u-rizm) A saclike expansion of a blood vessel wall.

antagonist (an-tag'o-nist) A muscle that acts in opposition to a prime mover.

antebrachium (an''te-bra'ke-um) The forearm.

antecubital (an''te-ku'bi-tal) The region in front of the elbow joint.

anterior (an-te're-or) Pertaining to the front; the opposite of posterior.

anterior pituitary (an-te're-or pi-tu'i-tār''e) The front lobe of the pituitary gland.

antibody (an'ti-bod''e) A specific substance produced by cells in response to the presence of an antigen; it reacts with the antigen.

antidiuretic hormone (an''tǐ-di''u-ret'ik hor'mōn) Hormone released from the posterior lobe of the pituitary gland; ADH.

antigen (an'tǐ-jen) A substance that stimulates cells to produce antibodies.

anus (a'nus) Inferior outlet of the digestive tube.

aorta (a-or'tah) Major systemic artery that receives blood from the left ventricle.

aortic body (a-or'tik bod'e) A structure associated with the wall of the aorta that contains a group of chemoreceptors.

aortic semilunar valve (a-or'tik sem"ĭ-lu'nar valv) Flaplike structure in the wall of the aorta near its origin that prevents blood from returning to the left ventricle of the heart.

aortic sinus (a-or'tik si'nus) Swelling in the wall of the aorta that contains pressoreceptors.

apneustic area (ap-nu'stik a're-ah) A portion of the respiratory control center located in the pons.

apocrine gland (ap'o-krin gland) A type of sweat gland that responds during periods of emotional stress.

aponeurosis (ap"o-nu-ro'sis) A sheetlike tendon by which certain muscles are attached to other parts.

appendicular (ap"en-dik'u-lar) Pertaining to the arms or legs.

appendix (ah-pen'diks) A small, tubular appendage that extends outward from the cecum of the large intestine.

aqueous humor (a'kwe-us hu'mor) Watery fluid that fills the anterior and posterior chambers of the eye.

arachnoid (ah-rak'noid) Delicate, weblike middle layer of the meninges; arachnoid mater.

arachnoid granulation (ah-rak'noid gran"u-la'shun) Fingerlike structures that project from the subarachnoid space of the meninges into blood-filled dural sinuses and function in the reabsorption of cerebrospinal fluid.

arbor vitae (ar'bor vi'ta) Treelike pattern of white matter seen in a section of cerebellum.

areola (ah-re'o-lah) Pigmented region surrounding the nipple of the mammary gland or breast.

arrector pili muscle (ah-rek'tor pil'i mus'l) Smooth muscle in the skin associated with a hair follicle.

arterial circle (ar-te're-al sir'kl) An arterial ring located on the ventral surface of the brain; circle of Willis.

arterial pathway (ar-te're-al path'wa) Course followed by blood as it travels from the heart to the body cells.

arteriole (ar-te're-ōl) A small branch of an artery that communicates with a capillary network.

arteriosclerosis (ar-te"re-o-sklĕ-ro'sis) Condition in which the walls of arteries thicken and lose their elasticity; hardening of the arteries.

artery (ar'ter-e) A vessel that transports blood away from the heart.

arthritis (ar-thri'tis) Condition characterized by inflammation of joints.

articular cartilage (ar-tik'u-lar kar'tĭ-lij) Hyaline cartilage that covers the ends of bones in synovial joints.

articulation (ar-tik"u-la'shun) The joining together of parts at a joint.

ascending colon (ah-send'ing ko'lon) Portion of the large intestine that passes upward on the right side of the abdomen from the cecum to the lower edge of the liver.

ascending tracts (ah-send'ing trakts) Groups of nerve fibers in the spinal cord that transmit sensory impulses upward to the brain.

association area (ah-so"se-a'shun a're-ah) Region of the cerebral cortex related to memory, reasoning, judgment, and emotional feelings.

astrocyte (as'tro-sīt) A type of neuroglial cell that functions to connect neurons to blood vessels.

atmospheric pressure (at"mos-fer'ik presh'ur) Pressure exerted by the weight of the air; about 760 mm of mercury at sea level.

atom (at'om) Smallest particle of an element that has the properties of that element.

atrioventricular bundle (a"tre-o-ven-trik'u-lar bun'dl) Group of specialized fibers that conduct impulses from the atrioventricular node to the ventricular muscle of the heart; A-V bundle.

atrioventricular node (a"tre-o-ven-trik'u-lar nōd) Specialized mass of muscle fibers located in the interatrial septum of the heart; functions in the transmission of the cardiac impulses from the sinoatrial node to the ventricular walls; A-V node.

atrioventricular orifice (a"tre-o-ven-trik'u-lar or'i-fis) Opening between the atrium and the ventricle on one side of the heart.

atrioventricular sulcus (a"tre-o-ven-trik'u-lar sul'kus) A groove on the surface of the heart that marks the division between an atrium and a ventricle.

atrioventricular valve (a"tre-o-ven-trik'u-lar valv) Cardiac valve located between an atrium and a ventricle.

atrium (a'tre-um) A chamber of the heart that receives blood from veins.

atrophy (at'ro-fe) A wasting away or decrease in size of an organ or tissue.

audiometer (aw"de-om'ĕ-ter) An instrument used to measure the acuity of hearing.

auditory (aw'di-to"re) Pertaining to the ear or to the sense of hearing.

auditory ossicle (aw'di-to"re os'i-kl) A bone of the middle ear.

auditory tube (aw'di-to"re tūb) The tube that connects the middle ear cavity to the pharynx; Eustachian tube.

auricle (aw'ri-kl) An earlike structure; the portion of the heart that forms the wall of an atrium.

autonomic nervous system (aw"to-nom'ik ner'vus sis'tem) Portion of the nervous system that functions to control the actions of the visceral organs and skin.

A-V bundle (bun'dl) A group of fibers that conduct cardiac impulses from the A-V node to the Purkinje fibers; bundle of His.

A-V node (nōd) Atrioventricular node.

axial skeleton (ak'se-al skel'ĕ-ton) Portion of the skeleton that supports and protects the organs of the head, neck, and trunk.

axillary (ak'si-ler"e) Pertaining to the armpit.

axon (ak'son) A nerve fiber that conducts a nerve impulse away from a neuron cell body.

B

basal nuclei (ba'sal nu'kle-i) Mass of gray matter located deep within a cerebral hemisphere of the brain.

basement membrane (bās'ment mem'brān) A layer of nonliving material that anchors epithelial tissue to underlying connective tissue.

basophil (ba'so-fil) White blood cell characterized by the presence of cytoplasmic granules that become stained by basophilic dye.

bicuspid tooth (bi-kus'pid tooth) A premolar that is specialized for grinding hard particles of food.

bicuspid valve (bi-kus'pid valv) Heart valve located between the left atrium and the left ventricle; mitral valve.

bile (bīl) Fluid secreted by the liver and stored in the gallbladder.

bipolar neuron (bi-po'lar nu'ron) A nerve cell whose cell body has only two processes, one serving as an axon and the other as a dendrite.

blastocyst (blas'to-sist) An early stage of embryonic development that consists of a hollow ball of cells.

B-lymphocyte (lim'fo-sīt) Lymphocyte that reacts against foreign substances in the body by producing and secreting antibodies.

brachial (bra'ke-al) Pertaining to the arm.

brain stem (brān stem) Portion of the brain that includes the midbrain, pons, and medulla oblongata.

Broca's area (bro'kahz a're-ah) Region of the frontal lobe that coordinates complex muscular actions of the mouth, tongue, and larynx, making speech possible.

bronchial tree (brong'ke-al trē) The bronchi and their branches that carry air from the trachea to the alveoli of the lungs.

bronchiole (brong'ke-ōl) A small branch of a bronchus within the lung.

bronchus (brong'kus) A branch of the trachea that leads to a lung.

buccal (buk'al) Pertaining to the mouth and the inner lining of the cheeks.

bulbourethral glands (bul"bo-u-re'thral glandz) Glands that secrete a viscous fluid into the male urethra at times of sexual excitement.

bursa (bur'sah) A saclike, fluid-filled structure, lined with synovial membrane, that occurs near a joint.

bursitis (bur-si'tis) Inflammation of a bursa.

C

calcaneal tendon (kal-ka'ne-al ten'don) Tendon in the back of the heel that connects muscles in the posterior lower leg to the calcaneous.

calcification (kal"si-fi-ka'shun) The process by which calcium is deposited within a tissue.

calcitonin (kal"si-to'nin) Hormone secreted by the thyroid gland that helps regulate the level of blood calcium.

canaliculus (kan"ah-lik'u-lus) Microscopic canals that interconnect the lacunae of bone tissue.

cancellous bone (kan'sĕ-lus bōn) Bone tissue with a latticework structure; spongy bone.

capillary (kap'i-ler"e) A small blood vessel that connects an arteriole and a venule.

cardiac conduction system (kar'de-ak kon-duk'shun sis'tem) System of specialized muscle fibers that conducts cardiac impulses from the S-A node into the myocardium.

cardiac cycle (kar'de-ak si'kl) A series of myocardial contractions that constitute a complete heartbeat.

cardiac muscle (kar′de-ak mus′el) Specialized type of muscle tissue found only in the heart.

cardiac output (kar′de-ak owt′poot) A quantity calculated by multiplying the stroke volume by the heart rate in beats per minute.

cardiac veins (kar′de-ak vāns) Blood vessels that return blood from the venules of the myocardium to the coronary sinus.

carina (kah-ri′nah) A cartilaginous ridge located between the openings of the right and left bronchi.

carotid bodies (kah-rot′id bod′ēz) Masses of chemoreceptors located in the wall of the internal carotid artery near the carotid sinus.

carpals (kar′pals) Bones of the wrist.

carpus (kar′pus) The wrist; the wrist bones as a group.

cartilage (kar′ti-lij) Type of connective tissue in which cells are located within lacunae and are separated by a semi-solid matrix.

cataract (kat′ah-rakt) Condition characterized by loss of transparency of the lens of the eye.

cauda equina (kaw ′da ek-wīn′a) A group of spinal nerves that extends below the distal end of the spinal cord.

cecum (se′kum) A pouchlike portion of the large intestine to which the small intestine is attached.

celiac (se′le-ak) Pertaining to the abdomen.

cell (sel) The structural and functional unit of an organism.

cell body (sel bod′e) Portion of a nerve cell that includes a cytoplasmic mass and a nucleus, and from which the nerve fibers extend.

cementum (se-men′tum) Bonelike material that fastens the root of a tooth into its bony socket.

central canal (sen′tral kah-nal′) Tube within the spinal cord that is continuous with the ventricles of the brain and contains cerebrospinal fluid.

central nervous system (sen′tral ner′vus sis′tem) Portion of the nervous system that consists of the brain and spinal cord; CNS.

centriole (sen′tre-ōl) A cellular organelle that functions in the organization of the spindle during mitosis.

centromere (sen′tro-mēr) Portion of a chromosome to which the spindle fiber attaches during mitosis.

centrosome (sen′tro-sōm) Cellular organelle consisting of two centrioles.

cephalic (se-fal′ik) Pertaining to the head.

cerebellar cortex (ser″ĕ-bel′ar kor′teks) The outer layer of the cerebellum.

cerebellum (ser″ĕ-bel′um) Portion of the brain that coordinates skeletal muscle movement.

cerebral aqueduct (ser′ĕ-bral ak′wĕ-dukt″) Tube that connects the third and fourth ventricles of the brain.

cerebral cortex (ser′ĕ-bral kor′teks) Outer layer of the cerebrum.

cerebral hemisphere (ser′ĕ-bral hem′ĭ-sfēr) One of the large, paired structures that together constitute the cerebrum of the brain.

cerebrospinal fluid (ser″ĕ-bro-spi′nal floo′id) Fluid that occupies the ventricles of the brain, the subarachnoid space of the meninges, and the central canal of the spinal cord.

cerebrum (ser′ĕ-brum) Portion of the brain that occupies the upper part of the cranial cavity.

cerumen (sĕ-roo′men) Waxlike substance produced by cells that line the canal of the external ear.

cervical (ser′vi-kal) Pertaining to the neck or to the cervix of the uterus.

cervix (ser′viks) Narrow, inferior end of the uterus that leads into the vagina.

chemoreceptor (ke″mo-re-sep′tor) A receptor that is stimulated by the presence of certain chemical substances.

chief cell (chēf sel) Cell of gastric gland that secretes various digestive enzymes, including pepsinogen.

chondrocyte (kon′dro-sīt) A cartilage cell.

chorion (ko′re-on) Embryonic membrane that forms the outermost covering around a developing fetus and contributes to the formation of the placenta.

chorionic villi (ko″re-on′ik vil′i) Projections that extend from the outer surface of the chorion and help attach an embryo to the uterine wall.

choroid coat (ko′roid kōt) The vascular, pigmented middle layer of the wall of the eye.

choroid plexus (ko′roid plek′sus) Mass of specialized capillaries from which cerebrospinal fluid is secreted into a ventricle of the brain.

chromatid (kro′mah-tid) A member of a duplicate pair of chromosomes.

chromatin (kro′mah-tin) Nuclear material that forms chromosomes during mitosis.

chromosome (kro′mo-sōm) Rodlike structure that appears in the nucleus of a cell during mitosis; contains the genes responsible for heredity.

chyme (kīm) Semifluid mass of food materials that passes from the stomach to the small intestine.

cilia (sil′e-ah) Microscopic, hairlike processes on the exposed surfaces of certain epithelial cells.

ciliary body (sil′e-er″e bod′e) Structure associated with the choroid layer of the eye that secretes aqueous humor and contains the ciliary muscle.

circular muscles (ser′ku-lar mus′lz) Muscles whose fibers are arranged in circular patterns, usually around an opening or in the wall of a tube; sphincter muscles.

circumduction (ser″kum-duk′shun) Movement of a body part, such as a limb, so that the end follows a circular path.

cisternae (sis-ter′ne) Enlarged portions of the sarcoplasmic reticulum near the actin and myosin filaments of a muscle fiber.

cleavage (klēv′ij) The early successive divisions of embryonic cells into smaller and smaller cells.

clitoris (kli′to-ris) Small erectile organ located in the anterior portion of the female vulva; corresponds to the penis of the male.

CNS Central nervous system.

cochlea (kok′le-ah) Portion of the inner ear that contains the receptors of hearing.

collagen (kol′ah-jen) Protein that occurs in the white fibers of connective tissues and in the matrix of bone.

collateral (ko-lat′er-al) A branch of a nerve fiber or blood vessel.

colon (ko′lon) The large intestine.

color blindness (kul′er blīnd′nes) An inability to distinguish colors normally.

colostrum (ko-los′trum) The first secretion of the mammary glands following the birth of an infant.

common bile duct (kom′mon bīl dukt) Tube that transports bile from the cystic duct to the duodenum.

condyle (kon′dīl) A rounded process of a bone, usually at the articular end.

cones (kōns) Color receptors located in the retina of the eye.

congenital (kon-jen′i-tal) Any condition that exists at the time of birth.

conjunctiva (kon″junk-ti′vah) Membranous covering on the anterior surface of the eye.

connective tissue (kŏ-nek′tiv tish′u) One of the basic types of tissue that includes bone, cartilage, and various fibrous tissues.

contraception (kon″trah-sep′shun) The prevention of fertilization of the egg cell or the development of an embryo.

contralateral (kon″trah-lat′er-al) Positioned on the opposite side of something else.

convergence (kon-ver′jens) The coming together of nerve impulses from different parts of the nervous system so that they reach the same neuron.

convolution (kon″vo-lu′shun) An elevation on the surface of a structure caused by an infolding of the structure upon itself.

cornea (kor′ne-ah) Transparent anterior portion of the outer layer of the eye wall.

coronary artery (kor′o-na″re ar′ter-e) An artery that supplies blood to the wall of the heart.

coronary sinus (kor′o-na″re si′nus) A large vessel on the posterior surface of the heart into which the cardiac veins drain.

corpus callosum (kor′pus kah-lo′sum) A mass of white matter within the brain, composed of nerve fibers connecting the right and left cerebral hemispheres.

corpus luteum (kor′pus lu′te-um) Structure that forms from the tissues of a ruptured ovarian follicle and functions to secrete female hormones.

corpus striatum (kor′pus stri-a′tum) Portion of the cerebrum that includes certain basal ganglia.

cortex (kor′teks) Outer layer of an organ such as the adrenal gland, cerebrum, or kidney.

cortical nephron (kor′ti-kl nef′ron) A nephron with its corpuscle located in the renal cortex.

cortisol (kor′ti-sol) A hormone secreted by the adrenal cortex.

costal (kos′tal) Pertaining to the ribs.

cranial (kra′ne-al) Pertaining to the cranium.

cranial nerve (kra′ne-al nerv) Nerve that arises from the brain.

crest (krest) A ridgelike projection of a bone.

cretinism (kre′ti-nizm) A condition resulting from a lack of thyroid secretion in an infant.

cricoid cartilage (kri′koid kar′ti-lij) A ringlike cartilage that forms the lower end of the larynx.

crista ampullaris (kris′tah am-pul′ar-is) Sensory organ located within a semicircular canal that functions in the sense of dynamic equilibrium.

crossing over (kros′ing o′ver) The exchange of genetic material between homologous chromosomes during meiosis.

cubital (ku′bi-tal) Pertaining to the forearm.

cuspid (kus′pid) A canine tooth.

cutaneous (ku-ta′ne-us) Pertaining to the skin.

cystic duct (sis′tik dukt) Tube that connects the gallbladder to the common bile duct.

cytocrine secretion (si′to-krin se-kre′shun) Process by which melanocytes transfer granules of melanin into adjacent epithelial cells.

cytoplasm (si′to-plazm) The contents of a cell surrounding its nucleus.

D

deciduous teeth (de-sid′u-us tēth) Teeth that are shed and replaced by permanent teeth.

dendrite (den′drīt) Nerve fiber that transmits impulses toward a neuron cell body.

dental caries (den′tal kar′ēez) Process by which teeth become decalcified and decayed.

dentin (den′tēn) Bonelike substance that forms the bulk of a tooth.

dermatome (der′mah-tōm) An area of the body supplied by sensory nerve fibers associated with a particular dorsal root of a spinal nerve.

dermis (der′mis) The thick layer of the skin beneath the epidermis.

descending colon (de-send′ing ko′lon) Portion of the large intestine that passes downward along the left side of the abdominal cavity to the brim of the pelvis.

descending tracts (de-send′ing trakts) Groups of nerve fibers that carry nerve impulses downward from the brain through the spinal cord.

desmosome (des′mo-sōm) A specialized junction between cells, which serves as a "spot weld."

detrusor muscle (de-trūz′or mus′l) Muscular wall of the urinary bladder.

diabetes mellitus (di″ah-be′tēz mel-li′tus) Condition characterized by a high blood glucose level and the appearance of glucose in the urine due to a deficiency of insulin.

diaphragm (di′ah-fram) A sheetlike structure composed largely of muscle and connective tissue that separates the thoracic and abdominal cavities; also, a caplike rubber device inserted in the vagina to be used as a contraceptive.

diaphysis (di-af′ĭ-sis) The shaft of a long bone.

diastole (di-as′to-le) Phase of the cardiac cycle during which a heart chamber wall is relaxed.

diencephalon (di″en-sef′ah-lon) Portion of the brain in the region of the third ventricle that includes the thalamus and hypothalamus.

differentiation (dif″er-en″she-a′shun) Process by which cells become structurally and functionally specialized during development.

distal (dis′tal) Farther from the midline or origin; opposite of proximal.

DNA Deoxyribonucleic acid.

dorsal root (dor′sal rōot) The sensory branch of a spinal nerve by which it joins the spinal cord.

dorsal root ganglion (dor′sal rōot gang′gle-on) Mass of sensory neuron cell bodies located in the dorsal root of a spinal nerve.

dorsum (dors′um) Pertaining to the back surface of a body part.

ductus arteriosus (duk′tus ar-te″re-o′sus) Blood vessel that connects the pulmonary artery and the aorta in a fetus.

ductus venosus (duk′tus ven-o′sus) Blood vessel that connects the umbilical vein and the inferior vena cava in a fetus.

duodenum (du″o-de′num) The first portion of the small intestine that leads from the stomach to the jejunum.

dural sinus (du′ral si′nus) Blood-filled channel formed by the splitting of the dura mater into two layers.

dura mater (du′rah ma′ter) Tough outer layer of the meninges.

E

eccrine gland (ek′rin gland) Sweat gland that functions in the maintenance of body temperature.

ectoderm (ek′to-derm) The outermost layer of the primary germ layers, responsible for forming certain embryonic body parts.

effector (ĕ-fek′tor) Organ, such as a muscle or gland, that responds to stimulation.

efferent arteriole (ef′er-ent ar-te′re-ōl) Arteriole that conducts blood away from the glomerulus of a nephron.

elastin (e-las′tin) Protein that comprises the yellow, elastic fibers of connective tissue.

embryo (em′bre-o) An organism in its earliest stages of development.

emission (e-mish′un) The movement of sperm cells from the vas deferens into the ejaculatory duct and urethra.

emphysema (em″fi-se′mah) A condition characterized by abnormal enlargement of the air sacs of the lungs.

enamel (e-nam′el) Hard covering on the exposed surface of a tooth.

endocardium (en″do-kar′de-um) Inner lining of the heart chambers.

endocrine gland (en′do-krin gland) A gland that secretes hormones directly into the blood or body fluids.

endoderm (en′do-derm) The innermost layer of the primary germ layers responsible for forming certain embryonic body parts.

endolymph (en′do-limf) Fluid contained within the membranous labyrinth of the inner ear.

endometrium (en″do-me′tre-um) The inner lining of the uterus.

endomysium (en″do-mis′e-um) The sheath of connective tissue surrounding each skeletal muscle fiber.

endoneurium (en″do-nu′re-um) Layer of loose connective tissue that surrounds individual fibers of a nerve.

endoplasmic reticulum (en-do-plaz′mic rĕ-tik′u-lum) Cytoplasmic organelle composed of a system of interconnected membranous tubules and vesicles.

endothelium (en″do-the′le-um) The layer of epithelial cells that forms the inner lining of blood vessels and heart chambers.

eosinophil (e″o-sin′o-fil) White blood cell characterized by the presence of cytoplasmic granules that become stained by acidic dye.

ependyma (ĕ-pen′di-mah) Membrane, composed of neuroglial cells, that lines the ventricles of the brain.

epicardium (ep″i-kar′de-um) The visceral portion of the pericardium located on the surface of the heart.

epicondyle (ep″i-kon′dīl) A projection of a bone located above a condyle.

epidermis (ep″i-der′mis) Outer epithelial layer of the skin.

epididymis (ep″i-did′i-mis) Highly coiled tubule that leads from the seminiferous tubules of the testis to the vas deferens.

epidural space (ep″i-du′ral spās) The space between the dural sheath of the spinal cord and the bone of the vertebral canal.

epigastric region (ep″i-gas′trik re′jun) The upper middle portion of the abdomen.

epiglottis (ep″i-glot′is) Flaplike cartilaginous structure located at the back of the tongue near the entrance to the trachea.

epimysium (ep″i-mis′e-um) The outer sheath of connective tissue surrounding a skeletal muscle.

epineurium (ep″i-nu′re-um) Outermost layer of connective tissue surrounding a nerve.

epiphyseal disk (ep″i-fiz′e-al disk) Cartilaginous layer within the epiphysis of a long bone that functions as a growing region.

epiphysis (ĕ-pif′i-sis) The end of a long bone.

epithelium (ep″i-the′le-um) The type of tissue that covers all free body surfaces.

erythroblast (ĕ-rith′ro-blast) An immature red blood cell.

erythrocyte (ĕ-rith′ro-sīt) A red blood cell.

erythropoiesis (ĕ-rith″ro-poi-e′sis) Red blood cell formation.

esophageal hiatus (ĕ-sof″ah-je′al hi-a′tus) Opening in the diaphragm through which the esophagus passes.

esophagus (ĕ-sof′ah-gus) Tubular portion of the digestive tract that leads from the pharynx to the stomach.

estrogen (es′tro-jen) Hormone that stimulates the development of female secondary sexual characteristics.

eversion (e-ver′zhun) Movement in which the sole of the foot is turned outward.

excretion (ek-skre′shun) Process by which metabolic wastes are eliminated.

exocrine gland (ek′so-krin gland) A gland that secretes its products into a duct or onto a body surface.

expiration (ek″spi-ra′shun) Process of expelling air from the lungs.

extension (ek-sten′shun) Movement by which the angle between parts at a joint is increased.

extracellular (ek″strah-sel′u-lar) Outside of cells.

extrapyramidal tract (ek″strah-pi-ram′i-dal trakt) Nerve tracts, other than the corticospinal tracts, that transmit impulses from the cerebral cortex into the spinal cord.

extremity (ek-strem′i-te) A limb; an arm or leg.

F

facet (fas′et) A small, flattened surface of a bone.

fascia (fash′e-ah) A sheet of fibrous connective tissue that encloses a muscle.

fasciculus (fah-sik′u-lus) A small bundle of muscle fibers.

feces (fe′sēz) Material expelled from the digestive tract during defecation.

fertilization (fer″ti-li-za′shun) The union of an egg cell and a sperm cell.

fetus (fe′tus) A human embryo after eight weeks of development.

fibril (fi′bril) A tiny fiber or filament.

fibroblast (fi′bro-blast) Cell that functions to produce fibers and other intercellular materials in connective tissues.

fissure (fish′ūr) A narrow cleft separating parts, such as the lobes of the cerebrum.

flagella (flah-jel′ah) Relatively long motile processes that extend out from the surface of a cell.

flexion (flek′shun) Bending at a joint so that the angle between bones is decreased.

follicle (fol′i-kl) A pouchlike depression or cavity.

follicle-stimulating hormone (fol′i-kl stim′u-la″ting hor′mōn) A substance secreted by the anterior pituitary gland. FSH.

follicular cells (fo-lik′u-lar selz) Ovarian cells that surround a developing egg cell and secrete female sex hormones.

fontanel (fon″tah-nel′) Membranous region located between certain cranial bones in the skull of a fetus or infant.

foramen (fo-ra′men) An opening, usually in a bone or membrane (pl. *foramina*).

foramen magnum (fo-ra′men mag′num) Opening in the occipital bone of the skull through which the spinal cord passes.

foramen ovale (fo-ra′men o-val′e) Opening in the interatrial septum of the fetal heart.

forebrain (for′brān) The anteriormost portion of the developing brain that gives rise to the cerebrum and basal nuclei.

fossa (fos′ah) A depression in a bone or other part.

fovea (fo′ve-ah) A tiny pit or depression.

fovea centralis (fo′ve-ah sen-tral′is) Region of the retina, consisting of densely packed cones, which is responsible for the greatest visual acuity.

fracture (frak′chur) A break in a bone.

frenulum (fren′u-lum) A fold of tissue that serves to anchor and limit the movement of a body part.

frontal (frun′tal) Pertaining to the region of the forehead.

G

gallbladder (gawl′blad-er) Saclike organ associated with the liver that stores and concentrates bile.

gamete (gam′ēt) A sex cell; either an egg cell or a sperm cell.

ganglion (gang′gle-on) A mass of neuron cell bodies, usually outside the central nervous system.

gastric gland (gas′trik gland) Gland within the stomach wall that secretes gastric juice.

gastric juice (gas′trik jōōs) Secretion of the gastric glands within the stomach.

germinal epithelium (jer′mi-nal ep″i-the′le-um) Tissue within an ovary that gives rise to sex cells.

germ layers (jerm la′ers) Layers of cells within an embryo that form the body organs during development.

glomerular capsule (glo-mer′u-lar kap′sul) Proximal portion of a renal tubule that encloses the glomerulus of a nephron; Bowman's capsule.

glomerulus (glo-mer′u-lus) A capillary tuft located within the glomerular capsule of a nephron.

glottis (glot′is) Slitlike opening between the true vocal folds or vocal cords.

glucagon (gloo′kah-gon) Hormone secreted by the pancreatic islets of Langerhans.

gluteal (gloo′te-al) Pertaining to the buttocks.

goblet cell (gob′let sel) An epithelial cell that is specialized to secrete mucus.

goiter (goi′ter) A condition characterized by the enlargement of the thyroid gland.

Golgi apparatus (gol′je ap″ah-ra′tus) A cytoplasmic organelle that functions in preparing cellular products for secretion.

Golgi tendon organ (gol″jē ten′dun or′gan) Sensory receptors occurring in tendons close to muscle attachments that are involved in reflexes that help maintain posture.

gomphosis (gom-fo′sis) Type of joint in which a cone-shaped process is fastened in a bony socket.

gonad (go′nad) A sex-cell-producing organ; an ovary or testis.

granulocyte (gran′u-lo-sīt) A leukocyte that contains granules in its cytoplasm.

gray matter (grā mat′er) Region of the central nervous system that generally lacks myelin and thus appears gray.

groin (groin) Region of the body between the abdomen and thighs.

growth (grōth) Process by which a structure enlarges.

growth hormone (grōth hor′mōn) A hormone released by the anterior lobe of the pituitary gland.

H

hair follicle (hār fol′i-kl) Tubelike depression in the skin in which a hair develops.

hematopoiesis (hem″ah-to-poi-e′sis) The production of blood and blood cells; hemopoiesis.

hemocytoblast (he″mo-si′to-blast) A cell that gives rise to blood cells.

hemoglobin (he″mo-glo′bin) Pigment of red blood cells responsible for the transport of oxygen.

hemopoiesis (he″mo-poi-e′sis) The production of blood and blood cells; hematopoiesis.

hepatic (hĕ-pat′ik) Pertaining to the liver.

hepatic lobule (hĕ-pat′ik lob′ūl) A functional unit of the liver.

hepatic macrophage (hĕ-pat′ik mak′ro-fāj) Large, fixed phagocyte in the liver that removes bacterial cells from the blood; Kupffer cell.

hepatic sinusoid (hĕ-pat′ik si′nŭ-soid) Vascular channel within the liver.

heredity (hĕ-red′i-te) The transmission of genetic information from parent to offspring.

hindbrain (hīnd′brān) Posteriormost portion of the developing brain that gives rise to the cerebellum, pons, and medulla oblongata.

histology (his-tol′o-je) The study of the structure and function of tissues.

hormone (hor′mōn) A substance secreted by an endocrine gland that is transmitted in the blood or body fluids.

hydroxyapatite (hi-drok″se-ap′ah-tīt) A type of crystalline calcium phosphate found in bone matrix.

hymen (hi′men) A membranous fold of tissue that partially covers the vaginal opening.

hyperplasia (hi″per-pla′ze-ah) An increased production and growth of new cells.

hyperthyroidism (hi″per-thi′roi-dizm) An excessive secretion of thyroid hormones.

hypertrophy (hi-per′tro-fe) Enlargement of an organ or tissue.

hypochondriac region (hi″po-kon′dre-ak re′jun) The portion of the abdomen on either side of the middle or epigastric region.

hypogastric region (hi″po-gas′trik re′jun) The lower middle portion of the abdomen.

hypoparathyroidism (hi″po-par″ah-thi′roi-dizm) An undersecretion of parathyroid hormone.

hypophysis (hi-pof′i-sis) The pituitary gland.

hypothalamus (hi″po-thal′ah-mus) A portion of the brain located below the thalamus and forming the floor of the third ventricle.

hypothyroidism (hi″po-thi′roi-dizm) A low secretion of thyroid hormones.

I

ileocecal valve (il″e-o-se′kal valv) Sphincter valve located at the distal end of the ileum where it joins the cecum.

ileum (il′e-um) Portion of the small intestine between the jejunum and the cecum.

iliac region (il′e-ak re′jun) Portion of the abdomen on either side of the lower, middle, or hypogastric region.

ilium (il′e-um) One of the bones of a coxal bone or hipbone.

immunity (i-mu′ni-te) Resistance to the effects of specific disease-causing agents.

implantation (im″plan-ta′shun) The embedding of an embryo in the lining of the uterus.

incisor (in-si′zor) One of the front teeth that is adapted for cutting food.

inclusion (in-kloo′zhun) A mass of lifeless chemical substance within the cytoplasm of a cell.

infancy (in′fan-se) Period of life from the end of the first four weeks to one year of age.

inferior (in-fēr′e-or) Situated below something else; pertaining to the lower surface of a part.

inflammation (in″flah-ma′shun) A tissue response to stress that is characterized by dilation of blood vessels and an accumulation of fluid in the affected region.

infundibulum (in″fun-dib′u-lum) The stalk by which the pituitary gland is attached to the base of the brain.

ingestion (in-jes′chun) The taking of food or liquid into the body by way of the mouth.

inguinal (ing′gwi-nal) Pertaining to the groin region.

inguinal canal (ing′gwi-nal kah-nal′) Passage in the lower abdominal wall through which a testis descends into the scrotum.

insertion (in-ser′shun) The end of a muscle that is attached to a movable part.

inspiration (in″spĭ-ra′shun) Act of breathing in; inhalation.

insula (in′su-lah) A cerebral lobe located deep within the lateral sulcus.

insulin (in′su-lin) A hormone secreted by the pancreatic islets of Langerhans.

integumentary (in-teg-u-men′tar-e) Pertaining to the skin and its accessory organs.

intercalated disk (in-ter′kah-lāt′ed disk) Membranous boundary between adjacent cardiac muscle cells.

intercellular (in″ter-sel′u-lar) Between cells.

intercellular fluid (in″ter-sel′u-lar floo′id) Tissue fluid located between cells other than blood cells.

intercellular junction (in″ter-sel′u-lar jungk′shun) A connection between the membranes of adjacent cells.

interneuron (in″ter-nu′ron) A neuron located between a sensory neuron and a motor neuron.

interphase (in′ter-fāz) Period between two cell divisions when a cell is carrying on its normal functions.

interstitial cell (in″ter-stish′al sel) A hormone-secreting cell located between the seminiferous tubules of the testis.

interstitial fluid (in″ter-stish′al floo′id) Same as intercellular fluid.

intervertebral disk (in″ter-ver′tĕ-bral disk) A layer of fibrocartilage located between the bodies of adjacent vertebrae.

intestinal gland (in-tes′tĭ-nal gland) Tubular gland located at the base of a villus within the intestinal wall.

intestinal juice (in-tes′tĭ-nal joos) The secretion of the intestinal glands.

intracellular (in″trah-sel′u-lar) Within cells.

intracellular fluid (in″trah-sel′u-lar floo′id) Fluid within cells.

intramembranous bone (in″trah-mem′brah-nus bōn) Bone that forms from membranelike layers of primitive connective tissue.

inversion (in-ver′zhun) Movement in which the sole of the foot is turned inward.

involuntary (in-vol′un-tār″e) Not consciously controlled; functions automatically.

ipsilateral (ip″sĭ-lat′er-al) Positioned on the same side as something else.

iris (i′ris) Colored muscular portion of the eye that surrounds the pupil and regulates its size.

isometric contraction (i″so-met′rik kon-trak′shun) Muscular contraction in which the muscle fails to shorten.

isotonic contraction (i″so-ton′ik kon-trak′shun) Muscular contraction in which the muscle shortens.

isotope (i′so-tōp) An atom that has the same number of protons as other atoms of an element but has a different number of neutrons in its nucleus.

J

jejunum (je-joo′num) Portion of the small intestine located between the duodenum and the ileum.

joint (joint) The union of two or more bones; an articulation.

juxtaglomerular apparatus (juks″tah-glo-mer′u-lar ap″ah-ra′tus) Structure located in the walls of arterioles near the glomerulus that plays an important role in regulating renal blood flow.

juxtamedullary nephron (juks″tah-med′u-lar-e nef′ron) A nephron with its corpuscle located near the renal medulla.

K

keratin (ker′ah-tin) Protein present in the epidermis, hair, and nails.

keratinization (ker″ah-tin″ĭ-za′shun) The process by which cells form fibrils of keratin and become hardened.

kilogram (kil′o-gram) A unit of weight equivalent to 1,000 grams.

kyphosis (ki-fo′sis) An abnormally increased convex curvature in the thoracic portion of the vertebral column.

L

labor (la′bor) The process of childbirth.

labyrinth (lab′ĭ-rinth) The system of interconnecting tubes within the inner ear, which includes the cochlea, vestibule, and semicircular canals.

lacrimal gland (lak′rĭ-mal gland) Tear-secreting gland.

lactation (lak-ta′shun) The production of milk by the mammary glands.

lacteal (lak′te-al) A lymphatic vessel associated with a villus of the small intestine.

lacuna (lah-ku′nah) A hollow cavity.

lamella (lah-mel′ah) A layer of matrix in bone tissue.

laryngopharynx (lah-ring″go-far′ingks) The lower portion of the pharynx near the opening to the larynx.

larynx (lar′ingks) Structure located between the pharynx and trachea that houses the vocal cords.

lateral (lat′er-al) Pertaining to the side.

leukocyte (lu′ko-sīt) A white blood cell.

lever (lev′er) A simple mechanical device consisting of a rod, fulcrum, weight, and a source of energy that is applied to some point on the rod.

ligament (lig′ah-ment) A cord or sheet of connective tissue by which two or more bones are bound together at a joint.

limbic system (lim′bik sis′tem) A group of interconnected structures within the brain that function to produce various emotional feelings.

linea alba (lin′e-ah al′bah) A narrow band of tendinous connective tissue located in the midline of the anterior abdominal wall.

lingual (ling′gwal) Pertaining to the tongue.

lordosis (lor-do′sis) An abnormally increased concave curvature in the lumbar portion of the vertebral column.

lumbar (lum′bar) Pertaining to the region of the loins.

lumen (lu′men) Space within a tubular structure such as a blood vessel or intestine.

lymph (limf) Fluid transported by the lymphatic vessels.

lymph node (limf nōd) A mass of lymphoid tissue located along the course of a lymphatic vessel.

lymphocyte (lim′fo-sīt) A type of white blood cell that functions to provide immunity.

lysosome (li′so-sōm) Cytoplasmic organelle that contains digestive chemicals.

M

macrophage (mak′ro-fāj) A large phagocytic cell.

macroscopic (mak″ro-skop′ik) Large enough to be seen with the unaided eye.

macula (mak′u-lah) A group of hair cells and supporting cells associated with an organ of static equilibrium.

macula lutea (mak′u-lah lu′te-ah) A yellowish depression in the retina of the eye that is associated with acute vision.

malignant (mah-lig′nant) The power to threaten life; cancerous.

mammary (mam′ar-e) Pertaining to the breast.

marrow (mar′o) Connective tissue that occupies the spaces within bones.

mast cell (mast sel) A cell to which antibodies, formed in response to allergens, become attached.

mastication (mas″ti-ka′shun) Chewing movements.

matrix (ma′triks) The intercellular substance of connective tissue.

matter (mat′er) Anything that has weight and occupies space.

meatus (me-a′tus) A passageway or channel, or the external opening of such a passageway.

mechanoreceptor (mek″ah-no-re-sep′tor) A sensory receptor that is sensitive to mechanical stimulation such as changes in pressure or tension.

medial (me′de-al) Toward or near the midline.

mediastinum (me″de-ah-sti′num) Tissues and organs of the thoracic cavity that form a septum between the lungs.

medulla (mĕ-dul′ah) The inner portion of an organ.

medulla oblongata (mĕ-dul′ah ob″long-gah′tah) Portion of the brain stem located between the pons and the spinal cord.

medullary cavity (med′u-lār″e kav′i-te) Cavity within the diaphysis of a long bone occupied by marrow.

megakaryocyte (meg″ah-kar′e-o-sīt) A large bone marrow cell that functions to produce blood platelets.

meiosis (mi-o′sis) Process of cell division by which egg and sperm cells are formed.

melanin (mel′ah-nin) Dark pigment normally found in skin and hair.

melanocyte (mel′ah-no-sīt″) Melanin-producing cell.

melatonin (mel″ah-to′nin) A hormone thought to be secreted by the pineal gland.

meninges (mĕ-nin′jēz) A group of three membranes that covers the brain and spinal cord (sing. *meninx*).

menisci (men-is′si) Pieces of fibrocartilage that separate the articulating surfaces of bones in the knee.

menstrual cycle (men′stroo-al si′kl) The female reproductive cycle that is characterized by regularly reoccurring changes in the uterine lining.

mesentery (mes′en-ter″e) A fold of peritoneal membrane that attaches an abdominal organ to the abdominal wall.

mesoderm (mez′o-derm) The middle layer of the primary germ layers, responsible for forming certain embryonic body parts.

metacarpals (met″ah-kar′pals) Bones of the hand between the wrist and finger bones.

metaphase (met′ah-fāz) Stage in mitosis when chromosomes become aligned in the middle of the spindle.

metastasis (mĕ-tas′tah-sis) The spread of disease from one body region to another; a characteristic of cancer.

metatarsals (met″ah-tar′sals) Bones of the foot between the ankle and toe bones.

microfilament (mi″kro-fil′ah-ment) Tiny rod of protein that occurs in cytoplasm and functions in causing various cellular movements.

microglia (mi-krog′le-ah) A type of neuroglial cell that helps support neurons and acts to carry on phagocytosis.

microscopic (mi″kro-skop′ik) Too small to be seen with the unaided eye.

microtubule (mi″kro-tu′būl) A minute, hollow rod found in the cytoplasm of cells.

microvilli (mi″kro-vil′i) Tiny, cylindrical processes that extend outward from some epithelial cell membranes and increase the membrane surface area.

micturition (mik″tu-rish′un) Urination.

midbrain (mid′brān) A small region of the brain stem located between the diencephalon and the pons.

mitochondrion (mi″to-kon′dre-on) Cytoplasmic organelle that contains enzymes responsible for aerobic respiration (pl., *mitochondria*).

mitosis (mi-to′sis) Process by which body cells divide to form two identical daughter cells.

mitral valve (mi′tral valv) Heart valve located between the left atrium and the left ventricle; bicuspid valve.

mixed nerve (mikst nerv) Nerve that includes both sensory and motor nerve fibers.

molar (mo′lar) A rear tooth with a somewhat flattened surface adapted for grinding food.

molecule (mol′ĕ-kūl) A particle composed of two or more atoms bound together.

monocyte (mon′o-sīt) A type of white blood cell that functions as a phagocyte.

morula (mor′u-lah) An early stage in embryonic development; a solid ball of cells.

motor area (mo′tor a′re-ah) A region of the brain from which impulses to muscles or glands originate.

motor end plate (mo′tor end plāt) Specialized portion of a muscle fiber membrane at a neuromuscular junction.

motor nerve (mo′tor nerv) A nerve that consists of motor nerve fibers.

motor neuron (mo′tor nu′ron) A neuron that transmits impulses from the central nervous system to an effector.

motor unit (mo′tor unit) A motor neuron and the muscle fibers associated with it.

mucosa (mu-ko′sah) The membrane that lines tubes and body cavities that open to the outside of the body; mucous membrane.

mucous cell (mu′kus sel) Glandular cell that secretes mucus.

mucous membrane (mu′kus mem′brān) Mucosa.

mucus (mu′kus) Fluid secretion of the mucous cells.

multipolar neuron (mul″ti-po′lar nu′ron) Nerve cell that has many processes arising from its cell body.

muscle spindle (mus′el spin′dul) Modified skeletal muscle fiber that can respond to changes in muscle length.

myelin (mi′ĕ-lin) Fatty material that forms a sheathlike covering around some nerve fibers.

myocardium (mi″o-kar′de-um) Muscle tissue of the heart.

myofibril (mi″o-fi′bril) Contractile fibers found within muscle cells.

myometrium (mi″o-me′tre-um) The layer of smooth muscle tissue within the uterine wall.

myoneural junction (mi″o-nu′ral jungk′shun) Site of union between a motor neuron axon and a muscle fiber.

myxedema (mik″sĕ-de′mah) Condition resulting from a deficiency of thyroid hormones in an adult.

N

nasal cavity (na′zal kav′i-te) Space within the nose.

nasal concha (na′zal kong′kah) Shell-like bone extending outward from the wall of the nasal cavity; a turbinate bone.

nasal septum (na′zal sep′tum) A wall of bone and cartilage that separates the nasal cavity into two portions.

nasopharynx (na″zo-far′ingks) Portion of the pharynx associated with the nasal cavity.

neonatal (ne″o-na′tal) Pertaining to the period of life from birth to the end of four weeks.

nephron (nef′ron) The functional unit of a kidney, consisting of a renal corpuscle and a renal tubule.

nerve (nerv) A bundle of nerve fibers.

neurilemma (nu″ri-lem′ah) Sheath on the outside of some nerve fibers due to the presence of Schwann cells.

neurofibrils (nu″ro-fi′brils) Fine, cytoplasmic threads that extend from the cell body into the processes of neurons.

neuroglia (nu-rog′le-ah) The supporting tissue within the brain and spinal cord, composed of neuroglial cells.

neuromuscular junction (nu″ro-mus′ku-lar jungk′shun) Myoneural junction.

neuron (nu′ron) A nerve cell that consists of a cell body and its processes.

neurotransmitter (nu″ro-trans-mit′er) Chemical substance secreted by the terminal end of an axon that stimulates a muscle fiber contraction or an impulse in another neuron.

neutrophil (nu′tro-fil) A type of phagocytic leukocyte.

Nissl bodies (nis′l bod′ēz) Membranous sacs that occur within the cytoplasm of nerve cells and have ribosomes attached to their surfaces.

nucleic acid (nu-kle′ik as′id) A substance composed of nucleotides bound together; RNA or DNA.

nucleolus (nu-kle′o-lus) A small structure that occurs within the nucleus of a cell and contains RNA.

nucleoplasm (nu′kle-o-plazm″) The contents of the nucleus of a cell.

nucleus (nu′kle-us) A body that occurs within a cell and contains relatively large quantities of DNA; the dense core of an atom that is composed of protons and neutrons.

nutrient (nu′tre-ent) A chemical substance that must be supplied to the body from its environment.

O

occipital (ok-sip′i-tal) Pertaining to the lower, back portion of the head.

olfactory (ol-fak′to-re) Pertaining to the sense of smell.

olfactory nerves (ol-fak′to-re nervz) The first pair of cranial nerves, which conduct impulses associated with the sense of smell.

oligodendrocyte (ol″i-go-den′dro-sīt) A type of neuroglial cell that functions to connect neurons to blood vessels and to form myelin.

oocyte (o′o-sīt) An immature egg cell.

oogenesis (o″o-jen′ĕ-sis) The process by which an egg cell forms from an oocyte.

ophthalmic (of-thal′mik) Pertaining to the eye.

optic (op′tik) Pertaining to the eye.

optic chiasma (op′tik ki-az′mah) X-shaped structure on the underside of the brain created by a partial crossing over of fibers in the optic nerves.

optic disk (op′tik disk) Region in the retina of the eye where nerve fibers leave to become part of the optic nerve.

oral (o′ral) Pertaining to the mouth.

organ (or′gan) A structure consisting of a group of tissues that performs a specialized function.

organelle (or″gah-nel′) A living part of a cell that performs a specialized function.

organism (or′gah-nizm) An individual living thing.

orifice (or′i-fis) An opening.

origin (or′i-jin) End of a muscle that is attached to a relatively immovable part.

oropharynx (o″ro-far′ingks) Portion of the pharynx in the posterior part of the oral cavity.

osseous tissue (os′e-us tish′u) Bone tissue.

ossification (os″i-fi-ka′shun) The formation of bone tissue.

osteoblast (os′te-o-blast″) A bone-forming cell.

osteoclast (os'te-o-klast") A cell that causes the erosion of bone.

osteocyte (os'te-o-sīt) A mature bone cell.

osteon (os'te-on) A cylinder-shaped unit containing bone cells that surround an osteonic canal; Haversian system.

osteonic canal (os'te-o-nik kah-nal') A tiny channel in bone tissue that contains a blood vessel; Haversian canal.

otolith (o'to-lith) A small particle of calcium carbonate associated with the receptors of equilibrium.

otosclerosis (o"to-sklĕ-ro'sis) Abnormal formation of spongy bone within the ear that may interfere with the transmission of sound vibrations to hearing receptors.

oval window (o'val win'do) Opening between the stapes and the inner ear.

ovarian (o-va're-an) Pertaining to the ovary.

ovary (o'var-e) The primary reproductive organ of a female; an egg-cell-producing organ.

oviduct (o'vĭ-dukt) A tube that leads from the ovary to the uterus; uterine tube or fallopian tube.

ovulation (o"vu-la'shun) The release of an egg cell from a mature ovarian follicle.

ovum (o'vum) A mature egg cell.

oxytocin (ok"sĭ-to'sin) Hormone released by the posterior lobe of the pituitary gland.

P

pacemaker (pās'māk-er) Mass of specialized muscle tissue that controls the rhythm of the heartbeat; the sinoatrial node.

pain receptor (pān re"sep'tor) Sensory nerve ending associated with the feeling of pain.

palate (pal'at) The roof of the mouth.

palatine (pal'ah-tīn) Pertaining to the palate.

palmar (pahl'mar) Pertaining to the palm of the hand.

pancreas (pan'kre-as) Glandular organ in the abdominal cavity that secretes hormones and digestive enzymes.

pancreatic (pan"kre-at'ik) Pertaining to the pancreas.

papilla (pah-pil'ah) Tiny nipplelike projection.

papillary muscle (pap'ĭ-ler"e mus'el) Muscle that extends inward from the ventricular walls of the heart and to which the chordae tendineae are attached.

paralysis (pah-ral'ĭ-sis) Loss of ability to control voluntary muscular movements, usually due to a disorder of the nervous system.

parasympathetic division (par"ah-sim"pah-thet'ik di-vizh'un) Portion of the autonomic nervous system that arises from the brain and sacral region of the spinal cord.

parathyroid glands (par"ah-thi'roid glandz) Small endocrine glands that are embedded in the posterior portion of the thyroid gland.

paravertebral ganglia (par"ah-ver'tĕ-bral gang'gle-ah) Sympathetic ganglia that form chains along the sides of the vertebral column.

parietal (pah-ri'ĕ-tal) Pertaining to the wall of an organ or cavity.

parietal cell (pah-ri'ĕ-tal sel) Cell of a gastric gland that secretes hydrochloric acid and intrinsic factor.

parietal pleura (pah-ri'ĕ-tal ploo'rah) Membrane that lines the inner wall of the thoracic cavity.

parotid glands (pah-rot'id glandz) Large salivary glands located on the sides of the face just in front and below the ears.

parturition (par"tu-rish'un) The process of childbirth.

pathogen (path'o-jen) Any disease-causing agent.

pathology (pah-thol'o-je) The study of disease.

pectoral (pek'tor-al) Pertaining to the chest.

pectoral girdle (pek'tor-al ger'dl) Portion of the skeleton that provides support and attachment for the arms.

pelvic (pel'vik) Pertaining to the pelvis.

pelvic girdle (pel'vik ger'dl) Portion of the skeleton to which the legs are attached.

pelvis (pel'vis) Bony ring formed by the sacrum and coxal bones.

penis (pe'nis) External reproductive organ of the male through which the urethra passes.

pericardial (per"ĭ-kar'de-al) Pertaining to the pericardium.

pericardium (per"ĭ-kar'de-um) Serous membrane that surrounds the heart.

perichondrium (per"ĭ-kon'dre-um) Layer of fibrous connective tissue that encloses cartilaginous structures.

perilymph (per'ĭ-limf) Fluid contained in the space between the membranous and osseous labyrinths of the inner ear.

perimetrium (per-ĭ-me'tre-um) The outer serosal layer of the uterine wall.

perimysium (per"ĭ-mis'e-um) Sheath of connective tissue that encloses a bundle of striated muscle fibers.

perineal (per"ĭ-ne'al) Pertaining to the perineum.

perineum (per"ĭ-ne'um) Body region between the scrotum or urethral opening and the anus.

perineurium (per"ĭ-nu're-um) Layer of connective tissue that encloses a bundle of nerve fibers within a nerve.

periodontal ligament (per"e-o-don'tal lig'ah-ment) Fibrous membrane that surrounds a tooth and attaches it to the bone of the jaw.

periosteum (per"e-os'te-um) Covering of fibrous connective tissue on the surface of a bone.

peripheral (pĕ-rif'er-al) Pertaining to parts located near the surface or toward the outside.

peripheral nervous system (pĕ-rif'er-al ner'vus sis'tem) The portions of the nervous system outside the central nervous system.

peristalsis (per"ĭ-stal'sis) Rhythmic waves of muscular contraction that occur in the walls of various tubular organs.

peritoneal (per"ĭ-to-ne'al) Pertaining to the peritoneum.

peritoneal cavity (per"ĭ-to-ne'al kav'ĭ-te) The potential space between the parietal and visceral peritoneal membranes.

peritoneum (per"ĭ-to-ne'um) A serous membrane that lines the abdominal cavity and encloses the abdominal viscera.

peritubular capillary (per"ĭ-tu'bu-lar kap'ĭ-ler"e) Capillary that surrounds a renal tubule and functions in reabsorption and secretion during urine formation.

permeable (per'me-ah-bl) Open to passage or penetration.

peroxisome (pĕ-roks'ĭ-sōm) Membranous cytoplasmic vesicle that contains enzymes responsible for the production and decomposition of hydrogen peroxide.

phalanx (fa'langks) A bone of a finger or toe (plural, *phalanges*).

pharynx (far'ingks) Portion of the digestive tube between the mouth and the esophagus.

photoreceptor (fo"to-re-sep'tor) A nerve ending that is sensitive to light energy.

physiology (fiz"e-ol'o-je) The branch of science dealing with the study of body functions.

pia mater (pi'ah ma'ter) Inner layer of meninges that encloses the brain and spinal cord.

pineal gland (pin'e-al gland) A small structure located in the central part of the brain.

pituitary gland (pĭ-tu'ĭ-tār"e gland) Endocrine gland that is attached to the base of the brain and consists of anterior and posterior lobes; the hypophysis.

placenta (plah-sen'tah) Structure by which an unborn child is attached to its mother's uterine wall and through which it is nourished.

plantar (plan'tar) Pertaining to the sole of the foot.

plasma (plaz'mah) Fluid portion of circulating blood.

platelet (plāt'let) Cytoplasmic fragment formed in the bone marrow that functions in blood coagulation.

pleural (ploo'ral) Pertaining to the pleura or membranes investing the lungs.

pleural cavity (ploo'ral kav'ĭ-te) Potential space between the pleural membranes.

pleural membranes (ploo'ral mem'brānz) Serous membranes that enclose the lungs.

plexus (plek'sus) A network of interlaced nerves or blood vessels.

pneumotaxic area (nu"mo-tax'ik a're-ah) A portion of the respiratory control center located in the pons of the brain.

polar body (po'lar bod'e) Small, nonfunctional cell produced as a result of meiosis during egg cell formation.

polymorphonuclear leukocyte (pol"e-mor"fo-nu'kle-ar lu'ko-sīt) A leukocyte or white blood cell with an irregularly lobed nucleus.

pons (ponz) A portion of the brain stem above the medulla oblongata and below the midbrain.

popliteal (pop"lĭ-te'al) Pertaining to the region behind the knee.

posterior (pos-tēr'e-or) Toward the back; opposite of anterior.

postganglionic fiber (pōst"gang-gle-on'ik fi'ber) Autonomic nerve fiber located on the distal side of a ganglion.

postnatal (pōst-na'tal) After birth.

preganglionic fiber (pre"gang-gle-on'ik fi'ber) Autonomic nerve fiber located on the proximal side of a ganglion.

pregnancy (preg'nan-se) The condition in which a female has a developing offspring in her uterus.

prenatal (pre-na'tal) Before birth.

presbycusis (pres"bĭ-ku'sis) Loss of hearing that accompanies old age.

presbyopia (pres″be-o′pe-ah) Condition in which the eye loses its ability to accommodate due to loss of elasticity in the lens; farsightedness of age.

pressoreceptor (pres″o-re-sep′tor) A receptor that is sensitive to changes in pressure.

primary reproductive organs (pri′ma-re re″pro-duk′tiv or′ganz) Sex-cell-producing parts; testes in males and ovaries in females.

prime mover (prīm mōōv′er) Muscle that is mainly responsible for a particular body movement.

projection (pro-jek′shun) Process by which the brain causes a sensation to seem to come from the region of the body being stimulated.

prolactin (pro-lak′tin) Hormone secreted by the anterior pituitary gland.

pronation (pro-na′shun) Movement in which the palm of the hand is moved downward or backward.

prophase (pro′fāz) Stage of mitosis during which chromosomes become visible.

proprioceptor (pro″pre-o-sep′tor) A sensory nerve ending that is sensitive to changes in tension of a muscle or tendon.

prostate gland (pros′tāt gland) Gland located around the male urethra below the urinary bladder that adds its secretion to seminal fluid during ejaculation.

protraction (pro-trak′shun) A forward movement of a body part.

proximal (prok′si-mal) Closer to the midline or origin; opposite of distal.

puberty (pu′ber-te) Stage of development in which the reproductive organs become functional.

pulmonary (pul′mo-ner″e) Pertaining to the lungs.

pulmonary circuit (pul′mo-ner″e ser′kit) System of blood vessels that carries blood between the heart and the lungs.

pulse (puls) The surge of blood felt through the walls of arteries due to the contraction of the ventricles of the heart.

pupil (pu′pil) Opening in the iris through which light enters the eye.

Purkinje fibers (pur-kin′je fi′berz) Specialized muscle fibers that conduct the cardiac impulse from the A-V bundle into the ventricular walls.

pyloric sphincter muscle (pi-lor′ik sfingk′ter mus′l) Sphincter muscle located between the stomach and the duodenum; pylorus.

pyramidal cell (pi-ram′i-dal sel) A large, pyramid-shaped neuron found within the cerebral cortex.

R

radiation (ra″de-a′shun) A form of energy that includes visible light, ultraviolet light, and X rays.

rectum (rek′tum) The terminal end of the digestive tube between the sigmoid colon and the anus.

red marrow (red mar′o) Blood-cell-forming tissue located in spaces within bones.

referred pain (re-ferd′ pān) Pain that feels as if it is originating from a part other than the site being stimulated.

reflex (re′fleks) A rapid, automatic response to a stimulus.

reflex arc (re′fleks ark) A nerve pathway, consisting of a sensory neuron, interneuron, and motor neuron, that forms the structural and functional bases for a reflex.

releasing hormone (re-le′sing hor′mōn) A substance secreted by the hypothalamus whose target cells are in the anterior pituitary gland.

renal (re′nal) Pertaining to the kidney.

renal corpuscle (re′nal kor′pusl) Part of a nephron that consists of a glomerulus and a Bowman's capsule; Malpighian corpuscle.

renal cortex (re′nal kor′teks) The outer portion of a kidney.

renal medulla (re′nal mě-dul′ah) The inner portion of a kidney.

renal pelvis (re′nal pel′vis) The hollow cavity within a kidney.

renal tubule (re′nal tu′būl) Portion of a nephron that extends from the renal corpuscle to the collecting duct.

reproduction (re″pro-duk′shun) The process by which an offspring is formed.

resorption (re-sorp′shun) The process by which something is lost as a result of physiological activity.

respiratory center (re-spi′rah-to″re sen′ter) Portion of the brain stem that controls the depth and rate of breathing.

respiratory membrane (re-spi′rah-to″re mem′brān) Membrane composed of a capillary and an alveolar wall through which gases are exchanged between the blood and the air.

reticulocyte (rě-tik′u-lo-sīt) A young red blood cell that has a network of fibrils in its cytoplasm.

reticuloendothelial tissue (rě-tik″u-lo-en″do-the′le-al tish′u) Tissue composed of widely scattered phagocytic cells.

retina (ret′i-nah) Inner layer of the eye wall that contains the visual receptors.

retraction (rě-trak′shun) Movement of a part toward the back.

retroperitoneal (ret″ro-per″i-to-ne′al) Located behind the peritoneum.

rhythmicity area (rith-mis′i-te a′re-ah) A portion of the respiratory control center located in the medulla.

ribosome (ri′bo-sōm) Cytoplasmic organelle that consists largely of RNA and functions in the synthesis of proteins.

rod (rod) A type of light receptor that is responsible for colorless vision.

rotation (ro-ta′shun) Movement by which a body part is turned on its longitudinal axis.

round window (rownd win′do) A membrane-covered opening between the inner ear and the middle ear.

S

saccule (sak′ūl) A saclike cavity that makes up part of the membranous labyrinth of the inner ear.

sagittal (saj′i-tal) A plane or section that divides a structure into right and left portions.

salivary gland (sal′i-ver-e gland) A gland, associated with the mouth, that secretes saliva.

S-A node (nōd) Sinoatrial node.

sarcolemma (sar″ko-lem′ah) The cell membrane of a muscle fiber.

sarcomere (sar′ko-mēr) The structural and functional unit of a myofibril.

sarcoplasm (sar′ko-plazm) The cytoplasm within a muscle fiber.

sarcoplasmic reticulum (sar″ko-plaz′mik rě-tik′u-lum) Membranous network of channels and tubules within a muscle fiber, corresponding to the endoplasmic reticulum of other cells.

Schwann cell (shwahn sel) Cell that surrounds a fiber of a peripheral nerve and forms the neurilemmal sheath and myelin.

sclera (skle′rah) White fibrous outer layer of the eyeball.

scoliosis (sko″le-o′sis) Abnormal lateral curvature of the vertebral column.

scrotum (skro′tum) A pouch of skin that encloses the testes.

sebaceous gland (sě-ba′shus gland) Gland of the skin that secretes sebum.

sebum (se′bum) Oily secretion of the sebaceous glands.

semen (se′men) Fluid discharged from the male reproductive tract at ejaculation that contains sperm cells and the secretions of various glands.

semicircular canal (sem″i-ser′ku-lar kah-nal′) Tubular structure within the inner ear that contains the receptors responsible for the sense of dynamic equilibrium.

seminiferous tubule (sem″i-nif′er-us tu′būl) Tubule within the testes in which sperm cells are formed.

sensation (sen-sa′shun) A feeling resulting from the interpretation of sensory nerve impulses by the brain.

sensory area (sen′so-re a′re-ah) A portion of the cerebral cortex that receives and interprets sensory nerve impulses.

sensory nerve (sen′so-re nerv) A nerve composed of sensory nerve fibers.

sensory neuron (sen′so-re nu′ron) A neuron that transmits an impulse from a receptor to the central nervous system.

serous cell (se′rus sel) A glandular cell that secretes a watery fluid with a high enzyme content.

serous fluid (se′rus floo′id) The secretion of a serous membrane.

serous membrane (ser′us mem′brān) Membrane that lines a cavity without an opening to the outside of the body.

sesamoid bone (ses′ah-moid bōn) A round bone that may occur in tendons adjacent to joints.

sigmoid colon (sig′moid ko′lon) S-shaped portion of the large intestine between the descending colon and the rectum.

sinoatrial node (si″no-a′tre-al nōd) Group of specialized tissue in the wall of the right atrium that initiates cardiac cycles; the pacemaker; S-A node.

sinus (si′nus) A cavity or hollow space in a bone or other body part.

skeletal muscle (skel′ě-tal mus′l) Type of muscle tissue found in muscles attached to skeletal parts.

smooth muscle (smōōth mus′el) Type of muscle tissue found in the walls of hollow visceral organs; visceral muscle.

somatic cell (so-mat′ik sel) Any cell of the body other than the sex cells.

special sense (spesh'al sens) Sense that involves receptors associated with specialized sensory organs, such as the eyes and ears.

spermatid (sper'mah-tid) An intermediate stage in the formation of sperm cells.

spermatocyte (sper-mat'o-sīt) An early stage in the formation of sperm cells.

spermatogenesis (sper''mah-to-jen'ĕ-sis) The production of sperm cells.

spermatogonium (sper''mah-to-go'ne-um) Undifferentiated spermatogenic cell found in the germinal epithelium of a seminiferous tubule.

spermatozoa (sper''mah-to-zo'ah) Male reproductive cells; sperm cells.

sphincter (sfingk'ter) A circular muscle that functions to close an opening or the lumen of a tubular structure.

spinal (spi'nal) Pertaining to the spinal cord or to the vertebral canal.

spinal cord (spi'nal kord) Portion of the central nervous system extending downward from the brain stem through the vertebral canal.

spinal nerve (spi'nal nerv) Nerve that arises from the spinal cord.

spleen (splēn) A large, glandular organ located in the upper left region of the abdomen.

spongy bone (spunj'e bōn) Bone that consists of bars and plates separated by irregular spaces; cancellous bone.

squamous (skwa'mus) Flat or platelike.

sterility (stĕ-ril'ĭ-te) An inability to produce offspring.

stimulus (stim'u-lus) A change in the environmental conditions that is followed by a response by an organism or cell.

stomach (stum'ak) Digestive organ located between the esophagus and the small intestine.

strabismus (strah-biz'mus) A condition characterized by lack of visual coordination; crossed eyes.

stratified (strat'ĭ-fid) Arranged in layers.

stratum basale (stra'tum ba-sale) The deepest layer of the epidermis in which the cells undergo mitosis.

stratum corneum (stra'tum kor'ne-um) Outer horny layer of the epidermis.

subarachnoid space (sub''ah-rak'noid spās) The space within the meninges between the arachnoid mater and the pia mater.

subcutaneous (sub''ku-ta'ne-us) Beneath the skin.

sublingual (sub-ling'gwal) Beneath the tongue.

submaxillary (sub-mak'sĭ-ler''e) Below the maxilla.

submucosa (sub''mu-ko'sah) Layer of connective tissue that underlies a mucous membrane.

sulcus (sul'kus) A shallow groove, such as that between adjacent convolutions on the surface of the brain.

superficial (soo''per-fish'al) Near the surface.

superior (su-pe're-or) Pertaining to a structure that is higher than another structure.

supination (soo''pĭ-na'shun) Rotation of the forearm so that the palm faces upward when the arm is outstretched.

surface tension (ser'fas ten'shun) Force that tends to hold moist membranes together due to an attraction that water molecules have for one another.

surfactant (ser-fak'tant) Substance produced by the lungs that reduces the surface tension within the alveoli.

suture (soo'cher) An immovable joint, such as that between adjacent flat bones of the skull.

sympathetic nervous system (sim''pah-thet'ik ner'vus sis'tem) Portion of the autonomic nervous system that arises from the thoracic and lumbar regions of the spinal cord.

symphysis (sim'fĭ-sis) A slightly movable joint between bones separated by a pad of fibrocartilage.

synapse (sin'aps) The junction between the axon end of one neuron and the dendrite or cell body of another neuron.

synaptic knob (sĭ-nap'tik nob) Tiny enlargement at the end of an axon that secretes a neurotransmitter substance.

synchondrosis (sin''kon-dro'sis) Type of joint in which bones are united by bands of hyaline cartilage.

syncytium (sin-sish'e-um) A mass of merging cells.

syndesmosis (sin''des-mo'sis) Type of joint in which the bones are united by relatively long fibers of connective tissue.

syndrome (sin'drōm) A group of symptoms that together characterize a disease condition.

synergist (sin'er-jist) A muscle that assists the action of a prime mover.

synovial fluid (sĭ-no've-al floo'id) Fluid secreted by the synovial membrane.

synovial joint (sĭ-no've-al joint) A freely movable joint.

synovial membrane (sĭ-no've-al mem'brān) Membrane that forms the inner lining of the capsule of a freely movable joint.

synthesis (sin'thĕ-sis) The process by which substances are united to form more complex substances.

system (sis'tem) A group of organs that act together to carry on a specialized function.

systemic circuit (sis-tem'ik ser'kit) The vessels that conduct blood between the heart and all body tissues except the lungs.

systole (sis'to-le) Phase of the cardiac cycle during which a heart chamber wall is contracted.

T

target tissue (tar'get tish'u) Specific tissue on which a hormone acts.

tarsus (tar'sus) The bones that form the ankle.

taste bud (tāst bud) Organ containing the receptors associated with the sense of taste.

telophase (tel'o-fāz) Stage in mitosis during which daughter cells become separate structures.

tendon (ten'don) A cordlike or bandlike mass of white fibrous connective tissue that connects a muscle to a bone.

testis (tes'tis) Primary reproductive organ of a male; a sperm-cell-producing organ.

testosterone (tes-tos'tĕ-rōn) Male sex hormone secreted by the interstitial cells of the testes.

thalamus (thal'ah-mus) A mass of gray matter located at the base of the cerebrum in the wall of the third ventricle.

thermoreceptor (ther''mo-re-sep'tor) A sensory receptor that is sensitive to changes in temperature; a heat receptor.

thoracic (tho-ras'ik) Pertaining to the chest.

thrombocyte (throm'bo-sīt) A blood platelet.

thymosin (thi'mo-sin) A hormone secreted by the thymus gland that affects the production of certain types of white blood cells.

thymus (thi'mus) A two-lobed glandular organ located in the mediastinum behind the sternum and between the lungs.

thyroid gland (thi'roid gland) Endocrine gland located just below the larynx and in front of the trachea that secretes thyroid hormones.

thyroxine (thi-rok'sin) A hormone secreted by the thyroid gland.

tissue (tish'u) A group of similar cells that performs a specialized function.

T-lymphocyte (lim'fo-sīt) Lymphocytes that interact directly with antigen-bearing particles and are responsible for cell-mediated immunity.

trabecula (trah-bek'u-lah) Branching bony plate that separates irregular spaces within spongy bone.

trachea (tra'ke-ah) Tubular organ that leads from the larynx to the bronchi.

transverse colon (trans-vers' ko'lon) Portion of the large intestine that extends across the abdomen from right to left below the stomach.

transverse tubule (trans-vers' tu'būl) Membranous channel that extends inward from a muscle fiber membrane and passes through the fiber.

tricuspid valve (tri-kus'pid valv) Heart valve located between the right atrium and the right ventricle.

trochanter (tro-kan'ter) A broad process on a bone.

trochlea (trok'le-ah) A pulley-shaped structure.

trophoblast (trof'o-blast) The outer cells of a blastocyst that help form the placenta and other embryonic membranes.

tubercle (tu'ber-kl) A small, rounded process on a bone.

tuberosity (tu''bĕ-ros'ĭ-te) An elevation or protuberance on a bone.

tympanic membrane (tim-pan'ik mem'brān) A thin membrane that covers the auditory canal and separates the external ear from the middle ear; the eardrum.

U

umbilical cord (um-bil'ĭ-kal kord) Cordlike structure that connects the fetus to the placenta.

umbilical region (um-bil'ĭ-kal re'jun) The central portion of the abdomen.

umbilicus (um-bil'ĭ-kus) Region to which the umbilical cord was attached; the navel.

unipolar neuron (u''ni-po'lar nu'ron) A neuron that has a single nerve fiber extending from its cell body.

ureter (u-re′ter) A muscular tube that carries urine from the kidney to the urinary bladder.

urethra (u-re′thrah) Tube leading from the urinary bladder to the outside of the body.

uterine (u′ter-in) Pertaining to the uterus.

uterine tube (u′ter-in tūb) Tube that extends from the uterus on each side toward an ovary and functions to transport sex cells; fallopian tube or oviduct.

uterus (u′ter-us) Hollow muscular organ located within the female pelvis in which a fetus develops.

utricle (u′trĭ-kl) An enlarged portion of the membranous labyrinth of the inner ear.

uvula (u′vu-lah) A fleshy portion of the soft palate that hangs down above the root of the tongue.

V

vacuole (vak′u-ōl) A space or cavity within the cytoplasm of a cell.

vagina (vah-ji′nah) Tubular organ that leads from the uterus to the vestibule of the female reproductive tract.

varicose veins (var′ĭ-kōs vānz) Abnormally swollen and enlarged veins, especially in the legs.

vasa recta (va′sah rek′tah) A branch of the peritubular capillary that receives blood from the efferent arterioles of juxtamedullary nephrons.

vascular (vas′ku-lar) Pertaining to blood vessels.

vas deferens (vas def′er-ens) Tube that leads from the epididymis to the urethra of the male reproductive tract (pl., *vasa deferentia*).

vasoconstriction (vas″o-kon-strik′shun) A decrease in the diameter of a blood vessel.

vasodilation (vas″o-di-la′shun) An increase in the diameter of a blood vessel.

vein (vān) A vessel that carries blood toward the heart.

vena cava (vēn′ah kāv′ah) One of two large veins that convey deoxygenated blood to the right atrium of the heart.

ventral root (ven′tral rōot) Motor branch of a spinal nerve by which it is attached to the spinal cord.

ventricle (ven′trĭ-kl) A cavity, such as that in the brain that is filled with cerebrospinal fluid, or that of the heart that contains blood.

venule (ven′ūl) A vessel that carries blood from capillaries to a vein.

vermiform appendix (ver′mĭ-form ah-pen′diks) Appendix.

vesicle (ves′ĭ-kal) Membranous cytoplasmic sac formed by an action of the cell membrane.

villus (vil′us) Tiny, fingerlike projection that extends outward from the inner lining of the small intestine.

visceral (vis′er-al) Pertaining to the contents of a body cavity.

visceral peritoneum (vis′er-al per″ĭ-to-ne′um) Membrane that covers the surfaces of organs within the abdominal cavity.

visceral pleura (vis′er-al ploo′rah) Membrane that covers the surfaces of the lungs.

vitreous humor (vit′re-us hu′mor) The substance that occupies the space between the lens and the retina of the eye.

vocal cords (vo′kal kordz) Folds of tissue within the larynx that create vocal sounds when they vibrate.

voluntary (vol′un-tār″e) Capable of being consciously controlled.

vulva (vul′vah) The external reproductive parts of the female that surround the opening of the vagina.

Y

yellow marrow (yel′o mar′o) Fat storage tissue found in the cavities within certain bones.

Z

zygote (zi′gōt) Cell produced by the fusion of an egg and sperm; a fertilized egg cell.

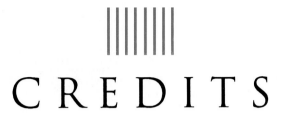

CREDITS

ILLUSTRATORS

Laurel Antler: 3.13b, 3.27, 18.13.

Ernest Beck: 18.25a, 18.33.

Todd Buck: Plates 1, 5, 6, and 7; figures 6.1, 6.2, 6.4a, 6.7, 6.11, 6.12, 6.16a, 6.23, 6.24, 6.25, 6.28, 6.29, 6.32, 6.35, 6.36, 6.37, 6.39, 6.40, 6.43, 6.45, 6.46, 6.48, 6.49, 6.51, 6.52, 6.53, 6.55, 6.56, 6.58a,b, 6.59, 6.61, 6.62, 6.63, 6.64, 7.5, 10.24, 13.3, 16.23a,b, 16.24a, 18.30, 18.31.

Barbara Cousins: 1.4, 1.21, 2.18.

Chris Creek: 9.52, 9.54.

Fineline Illustrations, Inc.: 2.1, 2.14.

Peg Gerrity: Plates 2, 3, and 4; figures 2.2, 2.7, 2.8, 2.9, 2.10, 2.11, 4.1a, 4.2a, 4.3a, 4.5a, 4.6a, 4.14a, 4.15a, 4.16a, 4.19a, 4.20a, 4.21a, 4.22a, 4.23a, 4.32a, 4.36a, 4.37a, 4.38a, 9.6, 9.33, 10.1, 10.13, 12.13, 12.20, 12.30, 13.33, 14.3, 14.11, 14.13, 14.19, 14.38, 14.41a, 15.8a, 17.24a, 17.35.

Rob Gordon: 9.27.

Rob Gordon/Tom Waldrop: 10.15.

Susan Hakola: Plates 39, 40, 42, and 43; figures 3.10, 7.4, 7.9b, 7.15, 7.22a, 8.11, 8.13, 8.15b, 9.19a,b, 9.22, 9.39, 9.42, 9.44, 9.45, 9.47, 10.7, 12.24a, 13.9, 13.12, 13.14a, 14.2, 14.14, 14.17, 14.54, 15.4, 15.10, 17.5, 17.6, 17.7.

Keith Kasnot: 9.59, 9.60, 10.23, 10.28, 10.29a, 10.31.

Keith Kasnot/Todd Buck: 10.21.

Ruth Krabach: 1.23, 6.6a, 7.6, 7.7, 7.13, 7.14a, 7.16, 7.17a, 7.18, 7.20a, 7.21, 7.23, 9.30, 9.35, 9.36, 17.18, 18.28.

Rictor Lew: 10.18.

Bill Loechel: 5.6a, 9.14, 11.15, 12.2, 12.3, 12.15, 12.16, 12.18, 12.22, 12.23, 12.26, 12.28, 12.31, 12.32, 12.35, 12.36, 12.37, 12.38, 13.4, 13.26, 13.32, 16.3, 16.4, 16.5, 16.7, 16.10, 16.12a, 16.14, 16.19, 16.20, 17.3.

Patrick Lynch: 2.17, 12.8, 14.44, 14.47a, 14.49, 14.51, 14.55, 14.56.

Robert Margulies: 14.29, 14.34, 18.14, 18.15, 18.24.

Robert Margulies/Tom Waldrop: 8.1, 8.8, 8.9, 14.43.

Nancy Marshburn: 3.2, 3.5a, 3.6b, 3.7b, 3.8b, 4.26a, 9.3, 9.20, 9.25, 9.41, 10.34, 10.39, 12.4, 14.1, 14.6a, 14.6b.

Steve Moon: 1.5a,b, 1.18c, 3.3, 5.2a, 5.10, 5.13, 6.18, 9.1, 9.8, 9.9, 9.10, 9.13, 9.15, 9.16, 9.57, 10.9, 10.14, 10.25, 10.27, 11.9, 11.13, 12.5, 12.6, 12.10, 12.12, 13.7, 13.8, 13.10a,b, 13.11, 13.22, 13.34, 13.35, 14.16, 14.26a, 14.40, 15.6, 15.7, 15.11, 15.12, 15.13, 15.14, 15.15, 16.1, 17.32.

Diane Nelson & Associates: 2.12, 6.19, 6.20, 6.21, 6.22, 6.26, 6.27, 6.30, 6.31, 6.34, 7.2A, 8.27, 10.4, 10.17, 10.38a,b, 11.1, 11.4, 13.19, 14.10, 14.21, 14.23, 14.42a, 14.45, 14.46, 14.50, 14.52, 14.53, 15.1, 15.2, 17.9, 17.31, 18.16, 18.22.

Diane Nelson & Associates/Bill Loechel: 12.21a,b.

John Nyquist: 3.4b, 14.7b, 14.8, 14.9b, 14.12, 14.27, 14.30a.

Ron McLean: 17.2.

Felecia Paras: 9.56, 9.58.

June Pedigo: 10.40, 13.28, 14.33, 14.37.

Mildred Rinehart: 5.9.

Rolin Graphics: 3.14b, 3.15b, 6.13.

Nancy Sally: 10.16.

Mike Schenk: 1.8, 2.15, 2.16, 3.1, 3.19a, 3.21a, 3.26a, 4.8, 4.9, 6.17, 7.1, 7.8a–c, 7.8d–f, 9.21a, 9.26, 9.34, 9.38, 9.43, 9.46, 9.49, 9.50, 9.53, 9.55, 11.2, 11.18, 12.1, 12.9, 13.1, 13.2, 13.6, 16.6, 17.8b, 18.1, 18.4, 18.19, 18.34.

Tom Sims: 10.5, 10.33, 10.37, 14.20, 16.15a, 16.18, 16.24b.

Tom Sims/Mike Schenk: 2.3, 2.13b, 9.29, 10.32, 13.24, 16.13b.

Catherine Twomey: 3.18, 3.20a, 3.22a, 3.23a, 3.24a, 18.5, 18.8, 18.9.

Tom Waldrop: Plates 41 and 44; figures 2.4, 2.5, 2.6a, 2.6b, 4.33, 4.34a, 4.35, 5.4b, 8.2, 8.4a, 8.5, 8.6, 8.7, 8.10, 8.12, 8.14, 8.15a, 8.16, 8.17, 8.18, 8.19a,b, 8.19c–c, 8.20, 8.21, 8.22, 8.23, 8.24a,b, 8.24c–g, 8.25, 8.26, 8.28, 8.29, 8.30a,b, 8.30c–c, 8.31, 9.18, 9.28, 9.31, 10.6, 11.3, 11.5, 13.17, 13.23, 16.22, 17.1a, 17.1b, 17.16, 17.17, 17.25, 17.29, 18.2.

John Walters & Associates: 10.20.

Marcia Williams: 1.22, 4.25, 5.1, 7.9a, 7.10, 7.11, 9.4a, 9.4b, 9.17, 13.29, 13.30, 14.4a, 14.18, 15.17, 18.21.

Charles Wood: 7.3, 9.23, 9.24, 10.26, 14.39.

LINE ART

Fig. 1.3a: Reprinted with the permission of Macmillan Publishing Company from *Antony Van Leeuwenhoek and His "Little Animals"* by Clifford E. Dobell. Copyright © Russell & Russell, Inc.

Fig. 1.5a: From Kent M. Van De Graaff and Stuart Ira Fox, *Concepts of Human Anatomy and Physiology*, 3d ed. Copyright © 1992 Wm. C. Brown Communications, Inc., Dubuque, Iowa. All Rights Reserved. Reprinted by permission.

Fig. 2.3: From Kent M. Van De Graaff and Stuart Ira Fox, *Concepts of Human Anatomy and Physiology*, 3d ed. Copyright © 1992 Wm. C. Brown Communications, Inc., Dubuque, Iowa. All Rights Reserved. Reprinted by permission.

Fig. 2.13 (bottom right): From Kent M. Van De Graaff and Stuart Ira Fox, *Concepts of Human Anatomy and Physiology*, 1st ed. Copyright © 1986 Wm. C. Brown Communications, Inc., Dubuque, Iowa. All Rights Reserved. Reprinted by permission.

Figs. 2.15 and 2.16: From Kent M. Van De Graaff, *Human Anatomy*, 3d ed. Copyright © 1992 Wm. C. Brown Communications, Inc., Dubuque, Iowa. All Rights Reserved. Reprinted by permission.

Fig. 3.19a: From Leland G. Johnson, *Biology*, 2d ed. Copyright © 1987 Wm. C. Brown Communications, Inc., Dubuque, Iowa. All Rights Reserved. Reprinted by permission.

Fig. 4.8: From Kent M. Van De Graaff, *Human Anatomy*, 3d ed. Copyright © 1992 Wm. C. Brown Communications, Inc., Dubuque, Iowa. All Rights Reserved. Reprinted by permission.

Fig. 4.9: From Kent M. Van De Graaff, *Human Anatomy*, 2d ed. Copyright © 1989 Wm. C. Brown Communications, Inc., Dubuque, Iowa. All Rights Reserved. Reprinted by permission.

Fig. 6.17: From Kent M. Van De Graaff, *Human Anatomy*, 3d ed. Copyright © 1992 Wm. C. Brown Communications, Inc., Dubuque, Iowa. All Rights Reserved. Reprinted by permission.

Figs. 6.19, 6.21, 6.22, 6.27, 6.30, 7.8a,c–f: From Kent M. Van De Graaff, *Human Anatomy*, 3d ed. Copyright © 1992 Wm. C. Brown Communications, Inc., Dubuque, Iowa. All Rights Reserved. Reprinted by permission.

Figs. 8.1 and 8.8: From Kent M. Van De Graaff and Stuart Ira Fox, *Concepts of Human Anatomy and Physiology*, 3d ed. Copyright © 1992 Wm. C. Brown Communications, Inc., Dubuque, Iowa. All Rights Reserved. Reprinted by permission.

Fig. 8.4a: From Stuart Ira Fox, *Human Physiology*, 4th ed. Copyright © 1993 Wm. C. Brown Communications, Inc., Dubuque, Iowa. All Rights Reserved. Reprinted by permission.

Fig. 8.9: From Kent M. Van De Graaff and Stuart Ira Fox, *Concepts of Human Anatomy and Physiology*, 3d ed. Copyright © 1992 Wm. C. Brown Communications, Inc., Dubuque, Iowa. All Rights Reserved. Reprinted by permission.

Fig. 8.27: From Kent M. Van De Graaff and Stuart Ira Fox, *Concepts of Human Anatomy and Physiology*, 2d ed. Copyright © 1989 Wm. C. Brown Communications, Inc., Dubuque, Iowa. All Rights Reserved. Reprinted by permission.

Fig. 9.1: From Kent M. Van De Graaff and Stuart Ira Fox, *Concepts of Human Anatomy and Physiology*, 3d ed. Copyright © 1992 Wm. C. Brown Communications, Inc., Dubuque, Iowa. All Rights Reserved. Reprinted by permission.

Fig. 9.4b: From Stuart Ira Fox, *Human Physiology*, 4th ed. Copyright © 1993 Wm. C. Brown Communications, Inc., Dubuque, Iowa. All Rights Reserved. Reprinted by permission.

Fig. 9.12: From Kent M. Van De Graaff and Stuart Ira Fox, *Concepts of Human Anatomy and Physiology*, 3d ed. Copyright © 1992 Wm. C. Brown Communications, Inc., Dubuque, Iowa. All Rights Reserved. Reprinted by permission.

Fig. 9.16: From Stuart Ira Fox, *Human Physiology*, 3d ed. Copyright © 1990 Wm. C. Brown Communications, Inc., Dubuque, Iowa. All Rights Reserved. Reprinted by permission.

Fig. 9.21a: From Kent M. Van De Graaff, *Human Anatomy*, 3d ed. Copyright © 1992 Wm. C. Brown Communications, Inc., Dubuque, Iowa. All Rights Reserved. Reprinted by permission.

Fig. 9.26a,b: From Kent M. Van De Graaff, *Human Anatomy*, 2d ed. Copyright © 1989 Wm. C. Brown Communications, Inc., Dubuque, Iowa. All Rights Reserved. Reprinted by permission.

Fig. 9.27: From Kent M. Van De Graaff, *Human Anatomy*, 3d ed. Copyright © 1992 Wm. C. Brown Communications, Inc., Dubuque, Iowa. All Rights Reserved. Reprinted by permission.

Fig. 9.29: From Kent M. Van De Graaff and Stuart Ira Fox, *Concepts of Human Anatomy and Physiology*, 2d ed. Copyright © 1989 Wm. C. Brown Communications, Inc., Dubuque, Iowa. All Rights Reserved. Reprinted by permission.

Figs. 9.38, 9.43: From Kent M. Van De Graaff, *Human Anatomy,* 3d ed. Copyright © 1992 Wm. C. Brown Communications, Inc., Dubuque, Iowa. All Rights Reserved. Reprinted by permission.

Fig. 9.46: From Kent M. Van De Graaff, *Human Anatomy,* 2d ed. Copyright © 1989 Wm. C. Brown Communications, Inc., Dubuque, Iowa. All Rights Reserved. Reprinted by permission.

Figs. 9.49a,b, 9.50, 9.52, 9.54: From Kent M. Van De Graaff, *Human Anatomy,* 3d ed. Copyright © 1992 Wm. C. Brown Communications, Inc., Dubuque, Iowa. All Rights Reserved. Reprinted by permission.

Figs. 9.56, 9.58: From Kent M. Van De Graaff and Stuart Ira Fox, *Concepts of Human Anatomy and Physiology,* 3d ed. Copyright © 1992 Wm. C. Brown Communications, Inc., Dubuque, Iowa. All Rights Reserved. Reprinted by permission.

Fig. 10.5: From Kent M. Van De Graaff and Stuart Ira Fox, *Concepts of Human Anatomy and Physiology,* 2d ed. Copyright © 1989 Wm. C. Brown Communications, Inc., Dubuque, Iowa. All Rights Reserved. Reprinted by permission.

Fig. 10.15: From Kent M. Van De Graaff and Stuart Ira Fox, *Concepts of Human Anatomy and Physiology,* 3d ed. Copyright © 1992 Wm. C. Brown Communications, Inc., Dubuque, Iowa. All Rights Reserved. Reprinted by permission.

Fig. 10.18: From Stuart Ira Fox, *Human Physiology,* 3d ed. Copyright © 1990 Wm. C. Brown Communications, Inc., Dubuque, Iowa. All Rights Reserved. Reprinted by permission.

Fig. 10.20: From Stuart Ira Fox, *Human Physiology,* 4th ed. Copyright © 1993 Wm. C. Brown Communications, Inc., Dubuque, Iowa. All Rights Reserved. Reprinted by permission.

Figs. 10.32, 10.37, 11.5: From Kent M. Van De Graaff and Stuart Ira Fox, *Concepts of Human Anatomy and Physiology,* 3d ed. Copyright © 1992 Wm. C. Brown Communications, Inc., Dubuque, Iowa. All Rights Reserved. Reprinted by permission.

Fig. 11.18: From Kent M. Van De Graaff and Stuart Ira Fox, *Concepts of Human Anatomy and Physiology,* 2d ed. Copyright © 1989 Wm. C. Brown Communications, Inc., Dubuque, Iowa. All Rights Reserved. Reprinted by permission.

Fig. 12.1: From Kent M. Van De Graaff, *Human Anatomy,* 3d ed. Copyright © 1992 Wm. C. Brown Communications, Inc., Dubuque, Iowa. All Rights Reserved. Reprinted by permission.

Fig. 12.3: From Kent M. Van De Graaff and Stuart Ira Fox, *Concepts of Human Anatomy and Physiology,* 3d ed. Copyright © 1992 Wm. C. Brown Communications, Inc., Dubuque, Iowa. All Rights Reserved. Reprinted by permission.

Fig. 12.9: From Kent M. Van De Graaff, *Human Anatomy,* 3d ed. Copyright © 1992 Wm. C. Brown Communications, Inc., Dubuque, Iowa. All Rights Reserved. Reprinted by permission.

Fig. 12.21a: From Kent M. Van De Graaff, *Human Anatomy,* 3d ed. Copyright © 1992 Wm. C. Brown Communications, Inc., Dubuque, Iowa. All Rights Reserved. Reprinted by permission.

Fig. 12.21b: From Kent M. Van De Graaff and Stuart Ira Fox, *Concepts of Human Anatomy and Physiology,* 2d ed. Copyright © 1989 Wm. C. Brown Communications, Inc., Dubuque, Iowa. All Rights Reserved. Reprinted by permission.

Figs. 12.37, 12.38: From Kent M. Van De Graaff and Stuart Ira Fox, *Concepts of Human Anatomy and Physiology,* 3d ed. Copyright © 1992 Wm. C. Brown Communications, Inc., Dubuque, Iowa. All Rights Reserved. Reprinted by permission.

Figs. 13.1, 13.2, 13.5, 13.24: From Kent M. Van De Graaff, *Human Anatomy,* 3d ed. Copyright © 1992 Wm. C. Brown Communications, Inc., Dubuque, Iowa. All Rights Reserved. Reprinted by permission.

Fig. 13.32: From E. Peter Volpe, *Biology and Human Concerns,* 3d ed. Copyright © 1983 Wm. C. Brown Communications, Inc., Dubuque, Iowa. All Rights Reserved. Reprinted by permission.

Fig. 13.34: From Kent M. Van De Graaff, *Human Anatomy,* 3d ed. Copyright © 1992 Wm. C. Brown Communications, Inc., Dubuque, Iowa. All Rights Reserved. Reprinted by permission.

Fig. 14.20: From Kent M. Van De Graaff and Stuart Ira Fox, *Concepts of Human Anatomy and Physiology,* 3d ed. Copyright © 1992 Wm. C. Brown Communications, Inc., Dubuque, Iowa. All Rights Reserved. Reprinted by permission.

Fig. 14.21: From Kent M. Van De Graaff, *Human Anatomy,* 3d ed. Copyright © 1992 Wm. C. Brown Communications, Inc., Dubuque, Iowa. All Rights Reserved. Reprinted by permission.

Figs. 14.26a, 14.43: From Kent M. Van De Graaff and Stuart Ira Fox, *Concepts of Human Anatomy and Physiology,* 3d ed. Copyright © 1992 Wm. C. Brown Communications, Inc., Dubuque, Iowa. All Rights Reserved. Reprinted by permission.

Fig. 14.46: From Kent M. Van De Graaff and Stuart Ira Fox, *Concepts of Human Anatomy and Physiology,* 1st ed. Copyright © 1986 Wm. C. Brown Communications, Inc., Dubuque, Iowa. All Rights Reserved. Reprinted by permission.

Figs. 14.48, 15.2: From Kent M. Van De Graaff, *Human Anatomy,* 3d ed. Copyright © 1992 Wm. C. Brown Communications, Inc., Dubuque, Iowa. All Rights Reserved. Reprinted by permission.

Fig. 16.6: From Kent M. Van De Graaff, *Human Anatomy,* 2d ed. Copyright © 1988 Wm. C. Brown Communications, Inc., Dubuque, Iowa. All Rights Reserved. Reprinted by permission.

Fig. 16.13b: From Kent M. Van De Graaff and Stuart Ira Fox, *Concepts of Human Anatomy and Physiology,* 2d ed. Copyright © 1989 Wm. C. Brown Communications, Inc., Dubuque, Iowa. All Rights Reserved. Reprinted by permission.

Figs. 16.15a, 16.18: From Kent M. Van De Graaff and Stuart Ira Fox, *Concepts of Human Anatomy and Physiology,* 3d ed. Copyright © 1992 Wm. C. Brown Communications, Inc., Dubuque, Iowa. All Rights Reserved. Reprinted by permission.

Fig. 16.24: From Kent M. Van De Graaff, *Human Anatomy,* 3d ed. Copyright © 1992 Wm. C. Brown Communications, Inc., Dubuque, Iowa. All Rights Reserved. Reprinted by permission.

Fig. 17.3: From Kent M. Van De Graaff, *Human Anatomy,* 2d ed. Copyright © 1989 Wm. C. Brown Communications, Inc., Dubuque, Iowa. All Rights Reserved. Reprinted by permission.

Figs. 17.8b, 17.16: From Kent M. Van De Graaff and Stuart Ira Fox, *Concepts of Human Anatomy and Physiology,* 3d ed. Copyright © 1992 Wm. C. Brown Communications, Inc., Dubuque, Iowa. All Rights Reserved. Reprinted by permission.

Fig. 17.21b: From Stuart Ira Fox, *Human Physiology,* 3d ed. Copyright © 1990 Wm. C. Brown Communications, Inc., Dubuque, Iowa. All Rights Reserved. Reprinted by permission.

Figs. 17.25, 17.32, 18.2: From Kent M. Van De Graaff and Stuart Ira Fox, *Concepts of Human Anatomy and Physiology,* 3d ed. Copyright © 1992 Wm. C. Brown Communications, Inc., Dubuque, Iowa. All Rights Reserved. Reprinted by permission.

Fig. 18.4: From Kent M. Van De Graaff, *Human Anatomy,* 3d ed. Copyright © 1992 Wm. C. Brown Communications, Inc., Dubuque, Iowa. All Rights Reserved. Reprinted by permission.

Fig. 18.25a: From Stuart Ira Fox, *Human Physiology,* 4th ed. Copyright © 1993 Wm. C. Brown Communications, Inc., Dubuque, Iowa. All Rights Reserved. Reprinted by permission.

Fig. 18.26: From Scammon, R. E., and Calkins, L. A. *The Development and Growth of External Dimensions of the Human Body in the Fetal Period.* Minneapolis: University of Minnesota Press, 1929. Reprinted by permission.

Fig. 18.34: From Kent M. Van De Graaff and Stuart Ira Fox, *Concepts of Human Anatomy and Physiology,* 3d ed. Copyright © 1992 Wm. C. Brown Communications, Inc., Dubuque, Iowa. All Rights Reserved. Reprinted by permission.

Fig. 18.36: From Stuart Ira Fox, *Human Physiology,* 4th ed. Copyright © 1993 Wm. C. Brown Communications, Inc., Dubuque, Iowa. All Rights Reserved. Reprinted by permission.

Plates 41, 44, 45: From Kent M. Van De Graaff, *Human Anatomy,* 3d ed. Copyright © 1992 Wm. C. Brown Communications, Inc., Dubuque, Iowa. All Rights Reserved. Reprinted by permission.

PHOTOS

Plates 8–20: © Jack Hole; 21–31: © Dr. Sheril D. Burton; 32, 33, 35, 36, 37: © Leestma/Custom Medical Stock Photo; 34, 38: General Electric Medical Systems; 46–73: © Wm. C. Brown Communications/Karl Rubin Photographer; p. 256: © John C. Mese.

Chapter 1

Fig. 1.1: From the works of Andreas Vesalius of Brussels by J. B. de C. D. Saunders and Charles P. O'Malley, Dover Publications, Inc., N.Y., 1973; 1.2: Studio Fotofast; 1.3b: Southern Illinois University/Photo Researchers, Inc.; 1.5c: © Will McIntyre/Photo Researchers, Inc.; 1.6a: © Z. Binor/Custom Medical Stock Photo; 1.6b: © Michael English, M.D./Custom Medical Stock Photo; 1.7: © Manfred Kage/Peter Arnold, Inc.; 1.9a: © Larry Mulvehill/Science Source/Photo Researchers, Inc.; 1.9b: © Malcolm S. Kirk/Peter Arnold, Inc.; 1.10: © Rod W. Orme/Visuals Unlimited; 1.11a, 1.13: © Martin M. Rotker; 1.11b: © Dr. Keith Porter; 1.11c: © Dr. Anderjs Liepins/Science Photo Library/Photo Researchers, Inc.; 1.12: © Larry Mulvehill/Photo Researchers, Inc.; 1.14: © James Shaffer; 1.15a,b: Science Photo Library/Photo Researchers, Inc.; 1.15c: © CNRI/Science Photo Library/Photo Researchers, Inc.; 1.16: Omikron/Photo Researchers, Inc.; 1.17a: © Tsiaras/Photo Researchers, Inc.; 1.17b: © Kent Van De Graaff; 1.18a: © Bob Coyle; 1.18b: © Southern Illinois University/Peter Arnold, Inc.; 1.19: Photo by Monte S. Buchsbaum, M.D.; 1.20a: © Lester Bergman and Associates, Inc.; 1.20b: Alliance Imaging, Inc./Mobile MRI Provider, Finley Hospital.

Chapter 2

Fig. 2.13a: © A. Glauberman/Photo Researchers, Inc.; 2.13b: © Patrick J. Lynch/Photo Researchers, Inc.; 2.13c: © Biophoto Associates/Photo Researchers, Inc.

Chapter 3

Figs. 3.4a, 3.7a, 3.13a: © Gordon Leedale/Biophoto Associates; 3.5b–d: © J. Gennero, Jr./Photo Researchers, Inc.; 3.6a: © David Zielenirc; 3.6d, 3.11, 3.14c: © Dr. Keith Porter; 3.8a: © Dr. Keith Porter/Photo Researchers, Inc.; 3.9: © Don W. Fawcett/Photo Researchers, Inc.; 3.14a: American Lung Association; 3.15a: © Martin M. Rotker; 3.16: © Stephen L. Wolfe; 3.19b: © E. J. Duprew; 3.19c: Grant Heilman Photography, Inc.; 3.20b, 3.21b, 3.22b, 3.23b, 3.26b: © Edwin Reschke; 3.25a–c: Springer-Verlag Heidelberg; 3.28a,b: Science Photo Library/Photo Researchers, Inc.

Chapter 4

Figs. 4.1b, 4.1c, 4.2b, 4.5b, 4.7a, 4.14b, 4.15b, 4.16b, 4.19b, 4.20b, 4.23b, 4.24, 4.30, 4.31, 4.32b, 4.36b, 4.39: © Edwin Reschke; 4.3b, 4.37b, 4.38b: © Manfred Kage/Peter Arnold, Inc.; 4.4: © Fawcett/Hirokawa/Heuser/Photo Researchers, Inc.; 4.6b: © Fred Hossler/Visuals Unlimited; 4.10: © Keith R. Porter/Photo Researchers, Inc.; 4.11: © Jean-Paul Revel; 4.12: © Veronica Burmeister/Visuals Unlimited; 4.13: © Dr. Jerome Gross/Lovett Group Developmental Biology; 4.17, 4.18, 4.29: © Martin M. Rotker; 4.21b: © John Cunningham/Visuals Unlimited; 4.22b: © Victor B. Eichler, Ph.D.; 4.22c: © BioPhoto Associates/Photo Researchers, Inc.; 4.26b: © Bill Longcore/Photo Researchers, Inc.; 4.27: © Warren Rosenberg/BPS; 4.28: © Edwin Reschke/Peter Arnold, Inc.; 4.34b: © Lester V. Bergman & Associates, Inc.; 4.37c: Courtesy Paul Heidger/University of Iowa.

Chapter 5

Fig. 5.2b: © Edwin Reschke; 5.3, 5.6b: © Victor B. Eichler, Ph.D.; 5.4a: © M. Schlwia/Visuals Unlimited; 5.5: © Science Photo Library/Photo Researchers, Inc.; 5.7: © CNRI/Photo Researchers, Inc.; 5.8: © Frank M. Hanna, Ph.D./Visuals Unlimited; 5.11: © John D. Cunningham/Visuals Unlimited; 5.12: © Nancy Hamilton/Photo Researchers, Inc.

Chapter 6

Fig. 6.3a: © Lester V. Bergman & Associates, Inc.; 6.3b, 6.3c, 6.10, 6.16b, 6.58c,d, 6.61c: © Jack Hole; 6.4b: Courtesy of Professors Richard G. Kessel and Randy H. Kardon, University of Iowa; 6.5: © Biophoto Associates/Photo Researchers, Inc.; 6.6b, 6.44: © Victor B. Eichler, Ph.D.; 6.8: © James Shaffer; 6.9: R. G. Kessel and R. H. Kardon. *Tissues and Organs: A Text Atlas of Scanning Electron Microscopy,* 1979, W. H. Freeman Company; 6.15a,b: *New England Journal of Medicine;* 6.33a,b: © Jan Halaska/Photo Researchers, Inc.; 6.38, 6.41, 6.42: © Courtesy of Kent Van De Graaff, Ph.D.; 6.47: © Courtesy of Eastman Kodak; 6.50, 6.54, 6.57, 6.60, 6.65a: © Martin M. Rotker; 6.65b: © Ted Conde; 6.66: © Larry Mulvehill/Science Source/Photo Researchers, Inc.

Chapter 7

Figs. 7.2c, 7.12, 7.19a,b: Jack Hole; 7.14b, 7.17b, 7.20b, 7.22b: © Paul Reimann; 7.24: NMSB/Custom Medical Stock Photo; 7.25: English/Custom Medical Stock Photo.

Chapter 8

Fig. 8.3: Courtesy of Professors Richard G. Kessel and Randy H. Kardon, University of Iowa; 8.4b: © Victor B. Eichler, Ph.D.

Chapter 9

Fig. 9.2: © Ed Reschke; 9.5a: © H. Webster and John Hubbard *The Vertebrate Peripheral Nervous System* (1974) Plenum Press, 1974; 9.5b: © Biophoto Associates/Photo Researchers, Inc.; 9.7, 9.40: Courtesy of Professors Richard G. Kessel and Randy H. Kardon, University of Iowa; 9.11: © Don Fawcett/Photo Researchers, Inc.; 9.21b: © Per H. Kieldsen; 9.32: Kent Van De Graaff; 9.37: © Courtesy of Igatu Shoin, LTD.

Chapter 10

Figs. 10.2, 10.3: © Ed Reschke; 10.8: © Bruce Iverson, Photomicrography; 10.10: © Omikron/Photo Researchers, Inc.; 10.11: © Victor B. Eichler, Ph.D.; 10.12: Kessel & Kardon, *Tissues and Organs: A Text Atlas of Scanning Electron Micrography;* fig. 2, p. 132, 1979, W. H. Freeman Company; 10.19a: © John D. Cunningham/Visuals Unlimited; 10.19b: © Fred Hossler/Visuals Unlimited; 10.22: © Dean E. Hellman; 10.29b: © 1991 Martin M. Rotker; 10.30: © Science Photo Library/Photo Researchers, Inc.; 10.35: © Per H. Kjeldson, University of Michigan at Ann Arbor; 10.36: © Carroll W. Weiss/Camera M. D. Studios; 10.38c: © Frank S. Werblin.

Chapter 11

Figs. 11.6, 11.16: © John D. Cunningham/Visuals Unlimited; 11.7: Library of Congress Collection; 11.8a–d: © Department of Illustrations, Washington University School of Medicine and American Journal of Medicine 20 (Jan. '56), p. 133; 11.10: © Fred Hossler/Visuals Unlimited; 11.11: © Courtesy of F. A. Davis Co., Philadelphia, and Dr. R. H. Kampmeier; 11.12: © Lester V. Bergman and Associates; 11.14: © BioPhoto Associates/Photo Researchers, Inc.; 11.17: © R. C. Calentine/Visuals Unlimited; 11.19: © Ed Reschke.

Chapter 12

Fig. 12.7: © Jack Hole; 12.11a, 12.11c: © Bruce Iverson; 12.11b: © BioPhoto Associates/Science Source/Photo Researchers, Inc.; 12.14, 12.19, 12.21c, 12.33a,b, 12.40, 12.41: © Edwin Reschke; 12.17: Kent Van De Graaff; 12.24b, 12.39: Kessel and Kardon, *Tissues and Organs: A Text Atlas of Scanning Electron Microscopy,* 1979, W. H. Freeman Company; 12.25: © Victor B. Eichler, Ph.D.; 12.27: © Carroll H. Weiss/Camera M.D. Studios; 12.29: © Armed Forces Institute of Pathology; 12.34: © K. R. Porter.

Chapter 13

Fig. 13.5: © Courtesy of Eastman Kodak; 13.13a,b: © Edwin Reschke; 13.13c, 13.18, 13.25: American Lung Association; 13.14b: Biophoto Associates/Photo Researchers, Inc.; 13.15: © John Watney/Photo Library; 13.16: © J. Croyle/Custom Medical Stock Photo; 13.20: © Dwight Kuhn Photography; 13.21: Courtesy of Professors Richard G. Kessel and Randy H. Kardon, University of Iowa; 13.27: © Murray, John F., *The Normal Lungs,* 2/e, W. B. Saunders Co., 1986; 13.31a,b: © Victor B. Eichler, Ph.D.

Chapter 14

Fig. 14.4b: D. W. Fawcett; 14.5a,b: © 1991/Martin M. Rotker; 14.7a, 14.9a: © Courtesy of Igaku Shoin, LTD; 14.15a: © Carroll Weiss/Camera M.D. Studios; 14.15b: © Donald S. Baim, from Hurst et al., *The Heart,* 5/e, McGraw-Hill Book Company, 1982; 14.22b: Dwight R. Kuhn Photography; 14.24a, 14.31c: Kessel and Kardon, *Tissues and Organs: A Text Atlas of Scanning Electron Microscopy.* © 1979, W. H. Freeman Company; 14.24b, 14.47b: © BioPhoto Associates/Photo Researchers, Inc.; 14.25: *American Journal of Anatomy,* Patricia Phelps and J. Luft, Electron Study of Relaxation and Constriction in Frog Arterioles, Vol. 125, p. 409, figs. 2 and 3, 1969; 14.26b: © T. Kuwabara from Bloom, W., and D. W. Fawcett, *A Textbook of Histology,* 10/e, 1975, W. B. Saunders; 14.28: © D. W. Fawcett; 14.30b, 14.31a, 14.32: © Edwin Reschke; 14.31b: © Victor B. Eichler, Ph.D.; 14.36: © American Heart Association, Dallas, TX; 14.41b: © Courtesy Utah Valley Hospital; 14.42b: © From *Practische OntleedKundi,* J. Dankmeyer, H. G. Lambers, and J. M. F. Landsmees, Bohn, Scheltema & Holkema.

Chapter 15

Fig. 15.3: © Ed Reschke; 15.5: © Courtesy of Eastman Kodak; 15.8b: © John Watney/Photo Researchers, Inc.; 15.9, 15.18: © Igaku Shoin, LTD; 15.16: © John D. Cunningham/Visuals Unlimited; 15.19: © Biophoto Associates/Photo Researchers, Inc.; 15.21: © Courtesy of Memorial Sloan-Kettering Cancer Center.

Chapter 16

Fig. 16.2: © CNRI/SPL/Photo Researchers, Inc.; 16.8: © Lester V. Bergman & Associates; 16.9: Courtesy of Professors Richard G. Kessel and Randy H. Kardon, University of Iowa; 16.11: © R. B. Wilson; 16.12b: David M. Phillips/Visuals Unlimited; 16.13a: © D. Friend; 16.15b: © Dwight Kuhn Photography; 16.16, 16.25: © Edwin Reschke; 16.17a: BioPhoto Associates/Photo Researchers, Inc.; 16.17b: Manfred Kage/Peter Arnold, Inc.; 16.21: © Per H. Kjeldson, University of Michigan at Ann Arbor; 16.23c: © John D. Cunningham/Visuals Unlimited.

Chapter 17

Figs. 17.4, 17.12: Courtesy of Professors Richard G. Kessel and Randy H. Kardon, University of Iowa; 17.8a: BioPhoto Associates/Photo Researchers, Inc.; 17.10: © David M. Phillips/The Population Council/Taurus Photos, Inc.; 17.11, 17.13, 17.21a, 17.22a, 17.27, 17.30: © Edwin Reschke; 17.12: Courtesy of Professors Richard G. Kessel and Randy H. Kardon, University of Iowa; 17.14, 17.15: © Manfred Kage/Peter Arnold, Inc.; 17.20: Bloom & Fawcett. *A Textbook of Histology,* W. B. Saunders Company © D. W. Fawcett; 17.22b: Hole, 4/c, fig. 22.26, p. 831; 17.23: © Dr. Landrum Shettles, M.D.; 17.24b: © Bloom/Fawcett, *Histology,* 10/e, W. B. Saunders Co.; 17.26: © Don Fawcett/Photo Researchers, Inc.; 17.28: © Michael Peres; 17.33a,b: © SIU School of Medicine; 17.34: © BioPhoto Associates/Photo Researchers, Inc.

Chapter 18

Fig. 18.3: © Mia Tegner, J. J., and Epel, D., *Science* 179 (2–16–73), 685–88, AAAS; 18.6a: © Alexander Tsiaras/Science Source/Photo Researchers, Inc.; 18.6b: © Omikron/Photo Researchers, Inc.; 18.7: © R. G. Edwards; 18.10: © Roman O'Rahilly/Carnegie Labs of Embryology, University of California; 18.11: © Carnegie Institute of Washington, Department of Embryology, Davis Division; 18.12: © Donald Yaeger/Camera M.D. Studios; 18.17a,b: © Dr. Landrum B. Shettles, M.D.; 18.17c: © Petite Format/Nestle/Science Source/Photo Researchers, Inc.; 18.18a: © Donald Yaeger/Camera M.D. Studios; 18.18b: © Dr. Landrum Shettles, M.D.; 18.20: © Petit Format/Nestle/Photo Researchers, Inc.; 18.25b: © Martin M. Rotker, 1993; 18.27a: © Petit Format/Nestle/Photo Researchers, Inc.; 18.27b: © Donald Yeager/Camera M.D. Studios; 18.32a,b: © Gregory Dellore, M.D. and Steven L. Clark, M.D.; 18.35: © Donna Jernigan.

INDEX

AIDS TO UNDERSTANDING ANATOMICAL TERMINOLOGY

a-, without: amorphous
abduc-, to separate: abduction
adduc-, to bring toward: adduction
adip-, fat: adipose tissue
af-, toward: afferent arteriole
alb-, white: albino
aliment-, food: alimentary canal
allant-, sausage-shaped: allantois
alveol-, small cavity: alveolus
angio-, vessel: angiogram
annul-, ring: annular ligament
ante-, before: antebrachium
append-, to hand something:
  appendicular
-ar, pertaining to: lobar bronchus
arbor-, like a tree: arbor vitae
arc-, like a bow: arciform artery
areol-, space: areola
aris-, pertaining to: orbicularis oris
arth-, joint: arthrology
astr-, starlike: astrocyte
ather-, porridge: atherosclerosis
atri-, entrance: atrium
aud-, to hear: auditory canal
aur-, ear: auricle
ax-, axis: axial skeleton
axill-, armpit: axillary artery
bas-, base: basilar artery
bi-, two: bicuspid valve
bio-, life: biology
-blast, budding or developing:
  osteoblast
blephar-, eyelid: blepharitis
brachi-, arm: brachial region
bronch-, windpipe: bronchus
burs-, pouch: bursa
calat-, something inserted: intercalated
  disk
calcan-, heel: calcaneus
calyc-, small cup: major calyx
canal-, channel: canaliculus
carcin-, spreading sore: carcinoma
cari-, decay: dental caries
carin-, keel-like: carina
cardi-, heart: pericardium
carp-, wrist: carpals
caud-, tail: cauda equina
cavernos-, hollow: corpora cavernosa

cec-, blindness: cecum
centr-, point: centromere
cephal-, head: cephalic region
-ceps, head: biceps brachii
cerbr-, brain: cerebrum
cervic-, neck: cervical vertebrae
chiasm-, cross: optic chiasma
chondr-, cartilage: chondrocyte
chorio-, skin: chorion
choroid-, skinlike: choroid coat
chrom-, color: chromatin
-clast, broken: osteoclast
clav-, bar: clavicle
cleav-, to divide: cleavage
cochlea-, snail: cochlea
col-, large intestine: colon
condyl-, knob: condyle
corac-, beaklike: coracoid process
corn-, horn: cornea
corp-, body: corpus callosum
cran-, helmet: cranial
cribr-, sievelike: cribriform plate
cric-, ring: cricoid cartilage
-crin, to secrete: endocrine
crist-, ridge: crista galli
crur-, lower part: crura
cusp-, projection: tricuspid valve
cut-, skin: subcutaneous
cyst-, bladder: cystitis
cyt-, cell: cytoplasm
dart-, like skin: dartos muscle
deglut-, to swallow: deglutination
dendr-, tree: dendrite
derm-, skin: dermis
detrus-, to force away: detrusor muscle
di-, two: diencephalon
diastol-, dilation: diastole
digit-, finger: digital artery
dors-, back: dorsal
ect-, outside: ectoderm
ejacul-, to shoot forth: ejaculation
encephal-, head: encephalitis
endo-, within: endoplasmic reticulum
ependym-, tunic: ependyma
epi-, upon: epithelial tissue
erg-, work: synergist
erythr-, red: erythrocyte
ethm-, like a sieve: ethmoid bone

exo-, outside: exocrine gland
falx-, sickle-shaped: falx cerebelli
fasc-, bundle: fasciculus
femur-, thigh: femur
fimb-, fringe: fimbriae
flagell-, whip: flagellum
follic-, small bag: hair follicle
fore-, before: forebrain
foss-, ditch: fossa ovalis
fov-, pit: fovea capitis
frenul-, restraint: frenulum
funi-, small cord or fiber: funiculus
gangli-, swelling: ganglion
gastr-, stomach: gastric gland
gladi-, sword: gladiolus
glen-, joint socket: glenoid cavity
-glia, glue: neuroglia
glom-, little ball: glomerulus
glut-, buttocks: gluteus maximus
gracil-, slender: gracilis
gubern-, to guide: gubernaculum
gust-, to taste: gustatory receptor
gyn-, woman: gynecology
hem-, blood: hemoglobin
hemi-, half: hemiplegia
hepat-, liver: hepatic duct
hiat-, opening: esophageal hiatus
hist-, fabric: histology
hol-, entire: holocrine gland
hormon-, to excite: hormone
hy-, U-shaped: hyoid bone
hyal-, glass: hyaline cartilage
im- (or *in-*), not: imbalance
immun-, free: immunity
inflamm-, setting on fire: inflammation
infra-, below: infraorbital nerve
inhal-, to breathe in: inhalation
insul-, island: insula
inter-, between: interphase
intra-, within: intracellular
iris, rainbow: iris
jugul-, throat: jugular vein
junct-, uniting: junctional fiber
juxta-, near to: juxtaglomerular
  nephron
kerat-, horn: keratin
kyph-, crooked: kyphosis
labr-, lip: glenoidal labrum